ROUTLEDGE HANDBOOK OF PHYSICAL ACTIVITY POLICY AND PRACTICE

Physical activity, inactivity and their relationship to health are serious concerns for governments around the world. This is the first book to critically examine the policy and practice of physical activity from a multi-disciplinary, social-scientific perspective. Moving beyond the usual biophysical and epidemiological approaches, it defines and explores the key themes that are shaping the global physical activity debate.

Unrivalled in its scale and scope, it presents the latest data on physical activity from around the world, including case studies from Europe, North and South America, Africa and Asia. Drawing on social, economic and behavioural sciences, it covers contexts from the global to the local and introduces the dominant ideas which inform the study of physical activity. Its 41 chapters examine the use of different forms of evidence in policymaking, the role of organisations in advocating physical activity, and the practical realities of public health interventions.

The *Routledge Handbook of Physical Activity Policy and Practice* is a landmark publication for all students, academics, policymakers and practitioners interested in the social-scientific study of sport, exercise, physical activity and public health.

Joe Piggin is a Senior Lecturer in Sport Policy and Management in the School of Sport, Exercise and Health Sciences at Loughborough University, UK. Joe's research covers two main areas, namely sport policy translation into marketing and programmes, and physical activity policy. He has published articles on physical activity policy in New Zealand, the UK and in a global context. Joe holds a PhD from the University of Otago, New Zealand.

Louise Mansfield is research lead for welfare, health and wellbeing (Institute for Environment, Health and Societies) and Senior Lecturer in Sport, Health and Social Sciences at Brunel University London, UK. Her research focusses on the relationship between sport, physical activity and public health. She is interested in partnership and community approaches to physical activity engagement and issues of health, wellbeing, inequality and diversity. She has led research projects for the Department of Health, Youth Sport Trust, Sport Scotland, ESRC, Medical Research Council, Macmillan Cancer Support, Public Health England and Sport England. She sits on the editorial boards for *Leisure Studies*, *Qualitative Research in Sport, Exercise and Health* and the *International Review for the Sociology of Sport*.

Mike Weed is Pro Vice-Chancellor (Research and Enterprise) and Professor of Applied Policy Sciences at Canterbury Christ Church University, UK. Drawing on a wide range of social science disciplines, including social psychology, sociology, economics, geography and policy science, his work has focussed on informing, improving and interrogating policy in the applied domains of public health, physical activity, physical education, sport, tourism, transport, urban development and major events. Professor Weed is Strategic Director of the Centre for Sport, Physical Education and Activity Research (SPEAR), editor-in-chief of the *Journal of Sport and Tourism*, and sits on the editorial boards of *Qualitative Research in Sport, Exercise and Health* and *Psychology of Sport and Exercise*.

ROUTLEDGE HANDBOOK OF PHYSICAL ACTIVITY POLICY AND PRACTICE

Edited by
Joe Piggin, Louise Mansfield
and Mike Weed

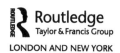

LONDON AND NEW YORK

First published 2018
by Routledge
2 Park Square, Milton Park, Abingdon, Oxon OX14 4RN

and by Routledge
711 Third Avenue, New York, NY 10017

Routledge is an imprint of the Taylor & Francis Group, an informa business

British Library Cataloguing-in-Publication Data
A catalogue record for this book is available from the British Library

Library of Congress Cataloging-in-Publication Data
A catalog record for this book has been requested

ISBN: 978-1-138-94308-7 (hbk)
ISBN: 978-1-315-67277-9 (ebk)

Typeset in Bembo
by Keystroke, Neville Lodge, Tettenhall, Wolverhampton

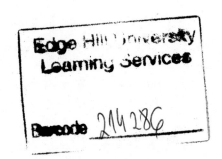
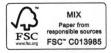

MIX
Paper from
responsible sources
FSC™ C013985
www.fsc.org

Printed in the United Kingdom
by Henry Ling Limited

CONTENTS

Contents

CONTRIBUTORS

Anna Aggestål is a PhD student at the Department of Education, Umeå University, Sweden. In her PhD project, she investigates the use of voluntary sport organisations in implementation of physical activity policy. More specifically, she studies the Swedish Sports Confederation (and affiliated organisations) and its role in public health promotion.

Stephanie Alexander, PhD, is a post-doctoral fellow at the Collège d'études mondiales, in the research chair of anthropology & global health in Paris, France. Her doctoral research examined how children's play is being transformed within physical activity interventions and her post-doctoral research ethnographically investigates global physical activity partnerships (i.e., Canada-Kenya) and examines how global ideas about children's play, health and physical activity are taken up, transformed and promoted locally.

Marco Antonio Bettine de Almeida is with the School of Arts, Sciences and Humanities, University of São Paulo, in Brazil.

Mahfoud Amara is assistant professor in sport management and policy at the College of Arts and Sciences (Sport Science Program). Before joining Qatar University he worked at the School of Sport and Health Sciences at Loughborough University. Dr Amara has a specific interest in sport business, culture, and politics in Arab and Muslim contexts. He has numerous publications on sport in colonial and post-colonial contexts, sport and the business of media broadcasting, the sport and modernisation debate; sport development and development through sport. His other research interest is sport, multiculturalism and intercultural dialogue, including the provision of sport for ethnic minorities/ sport and social inclusion/sport and integration. He has published a new book on *Sport Politics and Society in the Arab World*, and more recently an edited book of Alberto Testa on *Sport in Islam and in Muslim Communities*.

Nana Kwame Anokye, PhD is a senior health economist at Brunel University in the UK. Having won the Walduck Prize for Research Impact, Nana's work further secured prestigious UK Department of Health funding to conduct the first ever English general population survey on the economics of physical activity. His interests in public health are wide-ranging. How primary care can improve health outcomes; whether financial incentives improve maternal and child health; and what the link between shopping vouchers and breastfeeding may be, are some of the public health questions Nana is keen to answer.

Alan Bairner is professor of sport and social theory at Loughborough University. He studied politics at the University of Edinburgh, gained a PGCE from Moray House College of Education and was awarded his PhD at the University of Hull for a thesis on the social and political theory of Antonio Gramsci. He is co-editor of the *Routledge Handbook of Sport and Politics* published in 2016. He is also the editor-in-chief of the *Asia Pacific Journal of Sport and Social Science*. His current research focuses on the relationships between sport and national identity and between sport, leisure and urban spaces.

Hugh Barton is Emeritus Professor of planning, health and sustainability at WHO Collaborating Centre for Healthy Urban Environments, UWE, Bristol. Hugh has written a series of innovative books and guides on the planning of healthy, sustainable settlements, including most recently *City of Well-being: A Radical Guide to Planning* (Routledge 2017). Some of his conceptual models and practical tools have been widely adopted by public health and planning professionals. He is now retired but still working!

Fay Beck completed a PhD in tobacco control policy, to explore whether NHS stop smoking services were effectively meeting women's needs. She has since gained extensive experience working for the NHS delivering behaviour change interventions and evaluating services, and for two years worked as a knowledge transfer fellow in a local council-university partnership project to evaluate and improve an exercise referral scheme. She currently works for NHS England as a senior analytical lead.

Paul Bretherton was awarded a PhD in sport and leisure policy from Loughborough University in 2014. His research focuses mainly on the Olympic Games and sport mega events, sport sponsorship and corporate social responsibility in sport.

Sean Bulger, EdD is an associate professor in the College of Physical Activity and Sport Sciences at West Virginia University, United States. His teaching and research interests include the use of multi-component approaches to promoting children's physical activity. He has over 25 years of experience working with individuals across a developmental perspective in a variety of physical activity intervention contexts including school, community and family-based programming.

Richard J. Buning, PhD, a lifelong cyclist, is a lecturer in event management in the tourism cluster at The University of Queensland Business School. His research focuses on cycling, sport tourism, event management and sport development.

Pippa Chapman, PhD is a teaching fellow at Durham University, UK. She had a broad research interest in sport policy and management with specific interests in elite sport systems, youth sport and leadership in sport. She holds a PhD in elite sport policy from Loughborough University. She has previously taught at Brunel University and Loughborough University on subjects including sport policy, international development and coaching. She has also worked in the sport sector with England Netball, UK Sport and Women in Sport.

Danielle Keylla Alencar Cruz works with the Brazilian Ministry of Health.

John Day is a doctoral candidate and university instructor in sociology of sport and sport and leisure policies and a PhD candidate at Canterbury Christ Church University. His research explores the physical activity of family members and the implications for wellbeing using a life histories approach. He is also a member of Canterbury's sport and body cultures research group.

Aman Dhall completed his Master's degree at Loughborough University's School of Sport, Exercise and Health Sciences. Aman lives in India and is an entrepreneur and a marketing communications specialist. He carries more than 15 years of combined experience as an athlete, journalist and management professional. He is a founder of two sport development ventures A national-level table tennis player and a county player in the UK, he has observed the Indian sports system as an athlete, scrutinised it as a journalist, and is now seeking to bring positive changes in the system as a consultant.

Angela Dobele is the deputy head of research and innovation, in the School of Economics, Finance and Marketing, RMIT University. Dr. Dobele's research considers engagement through social enterprise, both online, including viral marketing, and traditional referrals. She also researches academic workload and performance, considering both academic staff and students.

Paul Downward is professor of economics in the School of Sport, Exercise and Health Sciences at Loughborough University. He has long standing research interests in sport, leisure and tourism as interconnected aspects of the consumption of time, as well as the economics of sport more generally. He also has long-standing research interests in research philosophy, methodology and ethics. He is currently exploring the economic, social, health, crime and well-being impacts of participation. He has worked with major stakeholders in sport and leisure, including the Department for Digital, Culture, Media and Sport, UK Sport, Sport England, Sustrans, Streetgames and UEFA.

Markus Duncan is a PhD candidate in the School of Kinesiology at the University of British Columbia. He received his MSc in Exercise Sciences from the University of Toronto in 2014 with a thesis examining affective responses to physical activity among individuals with schizophrenia. His current research is focused on measuring physical activity in clinical populations and the impact of physical activity on mental health.

Eloise Elliott, PhD serves as the Ware Distinguished Professor in the College of Physical Activity and Sport Sciences at West Virginia University, United States. Her work primarily focuses on children's health, specifically physical activity, nutrition and obesity prevention, and on pedagogy and curriculum development. In West Virginia, Elliott is the co-director of the WV CARDIAC Project in the WVU School of Medicine (state-wide children's health surveillance and intervention initiative).

Dale Esliger is a senior lecturer in physical activity measurement at the National Centre for Sport and Exercise Medicine at Loughborough University. His research focuses on enhancing accelerometry-based measurements of physical activity and sedentary behaviour. Dale's research recently incorporated continuous physiological sensing in an effort to advance our understanding of the interplay between physical activity, sedentary behaviour, and health. Dale has published over 60 manuscripts and has attracted research and enterprise funding exceeding £2.5 million.

Josef Fahlén is an associate professor in education at Umeå University, Sweden, and Visiting Professor at the Norwegian School of Sport Sciences. His research is concerned with the governance, organisation and management of voluntary, non-profit and membership-based club sport. Fahlén's publications cover sport policymaking and implementation in general and more specifically the use of sport clubs as vehicles for social change.

Guy Faulkner is a professor in the School of Kinesiology at the University of British Columbia, and is a Canadian Institutes of Health Research-Public Health Agency of Canada (CIHR-PHAC) Chair in Applied Public Health. Broadly, his research has focused on two interrelated themes: the development and evaluation of physical activity interventions, and physical activity and mental health. He is a founding editor of the Elsevier journal *Mental Health and Physical Activity*.

Abby Foad is research director for the Centre for Sport, Physical Education and Activity Research (spear) at Canterbury Christ Church University. Abby is responsible for directing spear's programme of contract research, including the Change4Life Sports Club programme for the Department of Health and Youth Sport Trust. The Centre's research is funded by a range of national and international funders and delivers world-leading impact by informing investment, policy, provision and practice, particularly around the physical activity and sport participation of young people, hard to reach and less active populations.

Michael Gard is an associate professor at the School of Human Movement and Nutrition Sciences at the University of Queensland. He has a Master's degree in exercise science, PhD in the sociology and history of dance, has published four books on topics including obesity, science and public health policy. His current research is on schools and public health and the history of sport.

Heather J. Gibson is a professor and faculty member in the Department of Tourism, Recreation and Sport Management at the University of Florida. She researches in the area of leisure, sport and tourism behaviour with a focus on gender and lifespan.

Fiona Gillison is a senior lecturer and chartered health psychologist at the University of Bath. After working in the NHS in public engagement, smoking cessation and weight management, she undertook a PhD exploring motivation and health behaviour change and now conducts research into the prevention and reduction of obesity. Fiona's current focus is on applying psychological theories to explore support for how we can promote health behaviour change at the individual, community or policy level.

Billy Graeff is a Brazillian scholar interested in physical education and sociology of pports. He is completing his PhD at Loughborough University in the UK. His research includes teacher training, sports teaching, social trajectory of skateboarders and sport mega events.

Ken Green is professor of sociology of physical education and youth sport and head of sport and exercise sciences at the University of Chester, UK, as well as a visiting professor at Inland Norway University of Applied Sciences. He is editor-in-chief of the *European Physical Education Review* and his publications include *The Routledge Handbook of Youth Sport* (2016; Routledge), co-edited with Andy Smith, and *Key Themes in Youth Sport* (2010; Routledge).

Margaret Heffernan is an academic in the School of Management, RMIT University. Dr Heffernan's research examines cross-cultural communications within a socio-ecological framework, and particularly the phenomenon of transubstantive error within public health promotion. Her work has resulted in several awards for cross-cultural collaborations and resource developments across Australia and internationally.

Michael Horswell is a senior lecturer at the University of the West of England. His work involves a number of multidisciplinary teams – providing the specialist knowledge and skills to integrate a 'spatial view' into projects. He has participated in research ranging from environmental management to urban planning to health.

Barbara Humberstone is professor of sociology of sport and outdoor education at Bucks New University. Her research interests include nature-based sport and the senses, wellbeing and outdoor pedagogies; physical activity and ageing healthily. Her concern is the interconnections in embodiment and social and environmental action/justice. She is co-editor of *Routledge International Handbook of Outdoor Studies* (2016), *Seascapes: Shaped by the Sea* (2015), *Urban Nature: Inclusive Learning Through Youth Work and School Work* (2014) and editor-in-chief of the *Journal of Adventure Education and Outdoor Learning*. She is a keen windsurfer, yogini and swimmer.

Emily Jones, PhD, is with the School of Kinesiology and Recreation, at Illinois State University. Her research interests include school and community-based physical activity program and initiatives and the training of teachers to integrate instructional technology in physical education. She has also taught PE at the elementary and middle school levels.

Tess Kay is professor of sport and social sciences at Brunel University London and leads the Brunel Sport, Health and Wellbeing (B-SHaW) research group. She has more than 25 years' experience of research into sport, inclusion, diversity and development in the UK and internationally including in-depth studies with unemployed young people, disaffected youth, members of minority ethnic groups, 'non-sporty' girls and young people with disabilities. She is a fellow of the Academy of Social Sciences.

Andrew Kingsnorth graduated from the University of Birmingham with a BSc in sport and exercise sciences before undertaking a MSc in physical activity and public health at Loughborough University. Furthering his studies at Loughborough, Andrew has recently completed his PhD (Spring 2017), which focused on the objective measurement and novel processing of sedentary and physical activity data, to establish links with chronic disease and acute physiology, including interstitial glucose levels.

Tracy L. Kolbe-Alexander is with the Centre for Research on Exercise, Physical Activity and Health, School of Human Movement and Nutrition Sciences, University of Queensland, Brisbane, Australia, as well as the Research Unit for Exercise Science and Sports Medicine, Department of Human Biology, Faculty of Health Sciences, University of Cape Town, South Africa.

Emily Knox completed her PhD at Loughborough University and is now a research fellow with the Division of Nursing in the School of Health Sciences at the University of Nottingham, UK.

Estelle V. Lambert is a professor at the Research Unit for Exercise Science and Sports Medicine, Department of Human Biology, Faculty of Health Sciences, University of Cape Town, South Africa.

Jessica Lee, PhD is a senior lecturer in health promotion in Griffith University's School of Medicine. Jessica's main focus in research is in critical perspectives in health and physical activity promotion, obesity and public health. Key research projects to date are the Life Activity Project, contradictions and tensions in the UK's Change4Life and the assembling of Healthier.Happier, a Queensland Government preventive health campaign.

David Lubans received his PhD from the University of Oxford and is currently a professor and the theme leader for school-based research within the University of Newcastle's Priority Research Centre for Physical Activity and Nutrition. In addition, Professor Lubans is an Australian Research Council Future Fellow. His research interest is focused on the design, implementation and evaluation of school-based physical activity interventions.

Rodney Lyn received his PhD from Georgia State University in 2008 and is currently an associate professor and the associate dean for academic affairs in the School of Public Health at Georgia State University. Dr Lyn's research specialisations include childhood obesity, physical activity, school and community health and health policy.

Dominic Malcolm is reader in the sociology of sport at Loughborough University, UK. He has published widely in the sociology of sport including *Sport and Sociology* (2012) and *Globalizing Cricket* (2013). His research on sport, health and medicine explores the embodied experiences of injury, practices harmful to athletes' health and the problems of practicing medicine within sport. He has published *The Social Organization of Sports Medicine* (2012, co-edited with Parissa Safai) and, most recently, *Sport, Medicine and Health: The Medicalization of Sport?*

Lois Mansfield, PhD is a principal lecturer in the Department of Science, Natural Resources and Outdoor Studies at the University of Cumbria and the research lead for the ecosystem services strand of the Centre for National Parks and Protected Areas. A geographer, her main areas of research interest revolve around the multifunctional management of upland resources through a transdisciplinary approach, around which her forthcoming textbook focuses (*Managing Upland Resources: New Rural Approaches*).

Louise Mansfield, PhD is senior lecturer in sport, health and social sciences at Brunel University London, UK. Her research focuses on the relationship between sport, physical activity and public health. She is interested in partnership and community approaches to physical activity engagement and issues of health, wellbeing, inequality and diversity. She has led research projects for the Department of Health, Youth Sport Trust, Sport Scotland, ESRC, Medical Research Council, Macmillan Cancer Support, Public Health England and Sport England. She sits on the editorial boards for *Leisure Studies, Qualitative Research in Sport, Exercise and Health* and the *International Review for the Sociology of Sport*.

Carolynne Mason, PhD is a lecturer in sport management within the School of Sport Exercise and Health Sciences at Loughborough University. She has conducted research with children and young people for many years, particularly those living in disadvantaged communities within the UK, with a focus on participation, citizenship, health and wellbeing.

Jim McKenna is professor of physical activity and health and the 12-year head of the Centre for Active Lifestyles at Leeds Beckett University, following almost 20 years' service at the University of Bristol. He has accumulated an extensive portfolio of PhD completions, grants and peer-reviewed papers. Beyond being an award-winning academic, Jim works with underserved groups, like hard-to-reach men, that others get their daily PA running away from! He is currently learning about the neuroscientific basis of learning and behaviour and is leading the evaluation of the BattleBack Centre programme for service personnel, funded by The Royal British Legion.

David McGillivray is professor in event and digital cultures at the University of the West of Scotland. David's research interests focus on the socio-cultural analysis of a variety of sport, physical activity and event-related themes. His PhD focused on a Foucauldian analysis of organisational wellness, and he has continued to consider the value of ideas of self-discipline, body politics and technologies of the self as they increase in importance within a neo-liberalised health and fitness narrative. He has taken this work into the fields of sport, health and fitness and the workplace.

Jenny McMahon is a senior lecturer in health and physical education at the University of Tasmania. Jenny is a former elite swimmer, having represented Australia on numerous occasions. She has conducted qualitative research on athlete wellbeing in sport; sporting cultures; coaching practices; coach education; body pedagogies and creative analytical practices. She currently teaches health and physical education; sports coaching and physical pursuits.

Paul Millar was a contributing author on the chapter entitled 'Neighbourhood Accessibility and Active Travel', along with Hugh Barton and Michael Horswell.

Nanette Mutrie has been chair of physical activity for health at the University of Edinburgh since July 2012. She directs the Physical Activity for Health Research Centre (PAHRC) in the Institute for Sport, Physical Education and Health Sciences. Nanette is a chartered psychologist with the British Psychological Society and a fellow of the British Association of Sport and Exercise Sciences. She has been involved with policy making, including 'Let's make Scotland more active' and the National Institute of Health and Clinical Excellence (NICE) programmes on physical activity and the environment and the promotion of walking and cycling. She is currently a member of the National Strategic Oversight Group for Physical Activity in Scotland. In 2015 Nanette was awarded an MBE for services to physical activity for health in Scotland.

Mark Norman received his PhD from University of Toronto in 2015, where his dissertation research focused on sport and physical culture in Canadian prisons. He is currently a sessional lecturer at University of Toronto and Ryerson University, and a project manager at the Centre for Sport Policy Studies at the University of Toronto.

Cassandra Phoenix, PhD is a reader (associate professor) in the Department for Health at the University of Bath. Her research currently spans three complementary themes: the embodiment of ageing and physical activity; everyday experiences of chronic illness and impairment; and the use of outdoor spaces to manage and promote wellbeing. Edited collections include: *Sport and Physical Activity in Later Life: Critical Perspectives* and *The World of Physical Culture in Sport and Exercise: Visual Methods for Qualitative Research*.

Joe Piggin is a senior lecturer in sport policy and management at the School of Sport, Exercise and Health Sciences at Loughborough University. Joe's research covers two main areas, namely sport policy translation into marketing and programmes, and physical activity policy. He has published articles on physical activity policy in New Zealand, the UK and in a global context. Joe holds a PhD from the University of Otago (New Zealand).

Darren Powell, PhD is now a lecturer at the University of Auckland in health and physical education. His research interrogates the role of corporations – mostly food companies – and charities in schools. This includes a critical analysis of the various healthy lifestyles education resources and programmes that are provided free to primary schools and the ways in which certain notions of health are reproduced in ways that align with the private sectors' best interests, but not necessarily the children's.

Heather Prince, PhD is associate professor of outdoor and environmental education and principal lecturer in collaborative and experiential learning at the University of Cumbria, UK. She designs, develops and teaches on undergraduate and postgraduate courses in outdoor studies, and is interested in pedagogic practice of outdoor learning in schools and higher education. She is convenor of the *Journal of Adventure Education and Outdoor Learning,* co-editor of the *Routledge International Handbook of Outdoor Studies* and a principal fellow of the Higher Education Academy, UK. She loves physical activity through adventure in wild places, and attempting to live life sustainably.

Andy Pringle, PhD is reader in physical activity and public health and research lead for physical activity and health in the Centre for Active Lifestyles at Leeds Beckett University. He is a fellow of the Royal Society of Public Health and a Topic Expert on the Public Health Advisory Committee for the National Institute for Health and Care Excellence. Andy conducts research into the effectiveness of physical activity interventions. He led the National Evaluation of the Local Exercise Action Pilots, the Premier League Men's Health programme and mapping of health improvement services in the 72 Football League Clubs.

Emma Pullen is a post-doctoral researcher at Bournemouth University. Her research focus is on the sociology of the body, cutting across fields of health, medicine and physical activity policy and practices.

Thiago Hérick de Sá is an urban health researcher at the World Health Organization working with urban, transport and land use planning issues. He has previously worked at the Centre for Epidemiological Research in Nutrition and Health, School of Public Health, University of São Paulo.

Bernadette Sebar is a senior lecturer in Griffith University's School of Medicine. Her research takes a postmodern perspective and focuses on the impact of discourse and power on understandings of health and health behaviour. In particular, she is interested in how gendered discourses influence men's and women's access to health.

Michelle Secker is research manager for the Centre for Sport, Physical Education and Activity Research (spear) at Canterbury Christ Church University. Michelle's project manages spear's contract research, overseeing the Centre's programme of research. Prior to her work with spear, Michelle worked in policy development and review for a London Borough. In recent years, Michelle has contributed to research design, methodology, delivery and analysis on multiple spear projects, including the Change4Life Sports Club evaluation for the Department of Health and Youth Sport Trust.

Lauren Sherar is a senior lecturer in physical activity and public health at the National Centre for Sport and Exercise Medicine at Loughborough University. Her research aims to develop, implement and evaluate interventions to positively impact the health and wellbeing of young people and clinical populations through an increase in physical activity and a decrease in sedentary behaviours. Lauren currently has over 65 papers published and a number of funded projects in this area.

Aaron Smith is a professor in the Graduate School of Business and Law at RMIT University, Australia. His research and extensive publications encompass the management of psychological, organisational and policy change in business, sport, health, religion and society. He has consulted globally with multi-national corporations, professional and national sporting entities, media companies and government.

Andy Smith is professor of sport and physical activity in the Department of Sport and Physical Activity at Edge Hill University, UK. His publications include *The Routledge Handbook of Youth Sport, Doing Real World Research in Sports Studies* and *Sport Policy and Development.* He is also former co-editor of the *International Journal of Sport Policy and Politics*.

Brett Smith is professor in physical activity and health and a leading expert on disability, health and physical activity. He is also internationally recognised as a methodologist in qualitative research. He is founding editor-in-chief of the international journal *Qualitative Research in Sport, Exercise and Health* and Associate Editor of *Psychology of Sport and Exercise*. Brett is co-author of *Qualitative Research Methods in Sport, Exercise and Health: From Process to Product.* He is also co-editor of two handbooks, *The Routledge International Handbook of Sport Psychology*, and *The Routledge International Handbook of Qualitative Methods in Sport and Exercise*.

Jordan Smith received his PhD in 2015 and is currently a lecturer in physical education at the University of Newcastle. Dr Smith's PhD thesis evaluated the effects of a school-based obesity prevention program for disadvantaged adolescent boys. His current research involves physical activity promotion within school and community settings, with a focus on the promoting resistance training for health.

Constantino Stavros is an associate professor in Marketing at RMIT University in Australia. Associate Professor Stavros is the editor of *Sport, Business and Management: An International Journal* and has published in a variety of areas within sport, including marketing, economics, sociology and communications. His research interests include social media, athlete and fan behavior and marketing strategy.

Miranda Thurston is professor of public health at Inland Norway University of Applied Sciences. She is author of *Key Themes in Public Health* (2014, Routledge).

Emmanuelle Tulle, PhD is a reader (associate professor) in sociology in the Department of Social Sciences, Media and Journalism at Glasgow Caledonian University. She has written widely on age, embodiment and anti-ageing science, focusing more specifically on master sport, physical activity and sedentary behaviour. She is currently undertaking research on contemporary women mountaineers. Edited collections include *Old Age and Agency, Sport and Physical Activity in Later Life: Critical Perspectives* and is the author of *Ageing, the Body and Social Change: Running in Later Life*.

Philippa Velija, PhD is head of subject for sport education and development at Southampton Solent University. Her research applies sociological theories to understanding gender relations in sport. She has previously published peer-reviewed articles on women's cricket, national identity and women's cricket, governance and gender in sport, women and the martial arts and female jockeys.

Mike Weed is pro vice-chancellor (research and enterprise) and professor of applied policy sciences at Canterbury Christ Church University. Drawing on a wide range of social science disciplines, including social psychology, sociology, economics, geography and policy science, his work has focussed on informing, improving and interrogating policy in the applied domains of public health, physical activity, physical education, sport, tourism, transport, urban development and major events. Professor Weed is strategic director of the Centre for Sport, Physical Education and Activity Research (spear), editor-in-chief of the *Journal of Sport and Tourism* and sits on the editorial boards of *Qualitative Research in Sport, Exercise and Health* and *Psychology of Sport and Exercise*.

Kate Westberg is an associate professor in marketing at RMIT University in Australia. She has published in a variety of sport-related areas including sponsorship, sport management and fan engagement. Associate Professor Westberg also has an interest in social marketing and has undertaken research in areas pertaining to obesity, gambling and alcohol.

Benjamin Williams, PhD is a lecturer in health and physical education in Griffith University's School of Education and Professional Studies. His research focuses on pedagogies of movement and how knowledge is produced, expertise is recognised and research is translated in this field.

Toni Williams, PhD is a senior lecturer in sport and exercise psychology. Her research broadly explores disability, health and physical activity, and has been published in leading international journals including *Health Psychology Review* and *International Journal of Qualitative Studies on Health and Well-being*. Toni's research interests also include narrative inquiry, disability studies, psychology of injury and rehabilitation and qualitative meta-synthesis. She has also published book chapters on the use of qualitative methods to conceptually advance the field of sport and exercise science.

Mads de Wolff completed his PhD at Loughborough University in 2016. His dissertation focused on post-Lisbon EU sport policy and, in particular, the role of the so-called 'trio Presidency'.

Catherine Woods, PhD works in physical activity psychology and public health in Dublin City University's School of Health and Human Performance. In Ireland, Catherine is part of SAGO, a Special Action Group on Obesity who advises the Minister of Health on the prevention and management of obesity in Ireland. Catherine is a member of the WHO network on health enhancing physical activity, where she is chair of the working group on children and young people.

Stephen Zwolinsky is a research officer within the Centre for Active Lifestyles at Leeds Beckett University. He has extensive experience of undertaking applied research and consultancy projects for a range of organisations including the NHS, local government departments and commercial enterprises. He has published extensively within the field of physical activity and health in a range of different formats including project reports, blogs, books, letters and journal articles. He is currently funded by Leeds City Council to determine the prevalence and clustering of the proximal lifestyle risk factors that underpin non-communicable disease and their links to long-term conditions.

INTRODUCTION

In 2012, 32 international scholars, writing in *The Lancet* as *The Lancet* Physical Activity Series Working Group warned us that the 'pandemic of physical inactivity' is now the fourth leading cause of death worldwide (Kohl et al, 2012: 294). Four years later, members of this group provided a 'progress report' that not much had changed, but added that almost 300,000 new cases of dementia could be avoided globally each year if all people were active (Sallis et al, 2016: 1329), and that the costs of physical inactivity to the global economy were $67.5 billion (£51.2bn) (Ding et al, 2016: 1317). The editors of *The Lancet* concluded that it is now time for policy makers to take physical activity seriously, and for people to take physical activity regularly (Das & Horton, 2016: 1255).

Not surprisingly, the apparent international scientific consensus that this work appeared to represent added further weight to calls that something must be done, and governments and agencies re-doubled their efforts following the warnings of The Lancet Group. Public Health England now wants 'everybody active every day' (PHE, 2014), the Centers for Disease Control and Prevention says 'physical activity builds a healthy and strong America' (CDC, 2016), whilst the Australian Department of Health wants you to 'make your move – be active for life!' (Department of Health, 2014). Globally, the World Health Organization has called for a 10 per cent reduction in physical inactivity by 2025, and has more recently produced a new global action plan for physical activity (WHO, 2017). Following the apparent scientific consensus an international policy consensus also seems to have emerged.

However, the emergence of these common consensuses is characterised by a distinct lack of debate. It is difficult to identify a diversity of voices and perspectives that might challenge and test some of the assumptions and approaches that have shaped the scientific consensus, or the common policy response. A lack of diversity and debate suggests that there may be limits to the common consensuses that have emerged, boundaries beyond which ideas and opportunities have not been explored.

It is this lack of debate and diverse voices that has motivated us to produce this *Routledge Handbook of Physical Activity Policy and Practice*. We want to stimulate debate about the politics of physical activity, and we do this by selecting chapters written by scholars from a range of disciplinary perspectives which critically examine the policy and practice of physical activity around the world. Seventy-five authors have contributed to the 41 chapters in the Handbook which are organised into three parts and a series of identified themes.

Part 1 focuses on Policy Issues in Physical Activity. Theme A identifies and addresses Policy Concepts and Contexts that inform and frame physical activity policy. The chapters examine how policy for physical activity has been shaped, has come to be understood and the key disciplines and discourses with which it intersects and overlaps. Theme B considers Evidence and Policy, exploring diverse evidence bases and their influence on policy agendas and goals. Theme C addresses debates about Policy Communities and Physical Activity; the sets of actors who coalesce around, and shape, policymaking. Chapters here develop understanding about who makes decisions about physical activity, how they do so and in whose interests those decisions are made.

Part 2 focuses on Practices. Theme D includes chapters on People, Places and Physical Activity. Discussions variously focus on the ways that difference and diversity are both reinforced and challenged in policymaking and practice in the physical activity sector. Furthermore, the spatialised aspects of contextual diversity are highlighted as central to peoples' physical activity experiences. Theme E turns attention to critical discussions about Understanding and Evaluating Practices and Programmes. Chapters explore issues and challenges in implementing and evaluating physical activity interventions in different contexts and for different population groups.

Part 3 considers International Perspectives on Physical Activity Policy and Practice. Theme F focuses on Physical Activity Policy and Practice Around the World. This final theme presents a series of regional and country-specific case studies. The chapters explore historic and current policy initiatives, the pertinent political, economic and cultural priorities of the area which inform policy and a description of the dominant forms of physical activity in the area's occupations, leisure and education systems.

In a handbook of this scale and scope, and given the complexity of emerging debates, we have not been able to include every possible issue in physical activity policy and practices. We look forward to seeing further discussions and writing about the connection between the mass media, social media and physical activity for example. Likewise, there is space for addressing physical activity policy and practice issues for a range of specific demographic and social groups. Further, there is certainly more to learn about physical activity policy and practice from a range of other countries and regions around the world. We do not intend this to be the final word in debates about physical activity policy and practice. Instead we imagine the Handbook as providing a starting point for further discussion amongst academics, policymakers and practice experts.

References

Centers for Disease Control and Prevention. (2016). Physical activity builds a healthy and strong America. www.cdc.gov/physicalactivity/downloads/healthy-strong-america.pdf. Accessed 29 August 2017.

Das, P., Horton, R. (2016). Physical activity – Time to take it seriously and regularly. *The Lancet*, 388:1254–5.

Department of Health. (2014). Australia's physical activity and sedentary behaviour guidelines. www.health.gov.au/internet/main/publishing.nsf/content/health-pubhlth-strateg-phys-act-guidelines. Accessed 29 August 2017.

Ding, D., Lawson, K. D., Kolbe-Alexander, T. L., Finkelstein, E. A., Katzmarzyk, P. T., van Mechelen, W., Pratt, M., for *The Lancet* Physical Activity Series 2. (2016). The economic burden of physical inactivity: A global analysis of major non-communicable diseases. *The Lancet*, Sept. 24; 388(10051): 1311–24. doi: 10.1016/S0140-6736(16)30383-X.

Kohl, H. W., Craig, C. L., Lambert, E. V., Inoue, S., Alkandari, J. R., Leetongin, G., et al, for *The Lancet* Physical Activity Series Working Group. (2012). The pandemic of physical inactivity: Global action for public health. *The Lancet*, 380:294–305. doi: 10.1016/S0140-6736(12)60898-8.

Public Health England. (2014). *Everybody active, every day: An evidence-based approach to physical activity.* London, UK: Public Health England.

Sallis, J. F., Bull, F., Guthold, R., et al, for *The Lancet* Physical Activity Series 2 Working Group. (2016). Progress in physical activity over the Olympic quadrennium. *The Lancet.* http://dx.doi.org/10.1016/S0140-6736(16)30581-5.

WHO. (2017). Governance: Development of a draft global action plan to promote physical activity. www.who.int/ncds/governance/physical_activity_plan/en/. Accessed 29 August 2017.

PART I

Policy issues in physical activity

THEME A INTRODUCTION
Policy concepts and contexts

The Handbook's first theme focuses on the concepts and contexts that inform and frame physical activity policy. It contains four original contributions and two reprinted discussions and collectively addresses how policy for physical activity has been shaped, has come to be understood and the key disciplines and discourses with which it intersects and overlaps. Discussions focus on the influence and responsibility of individuals and structures or systems in relation to physical activity, claims about the extent to which physical activity is, or should be, the norm and the positioning of physical activity policy within discourses of medicine, wellbeing and public health.

In the first chapter, Joe Piggin sets out some of the core concepts and theories that have come to be dominant in the construction of physical activity policy. Starting out with a foundational discussion of structure and agency, the chapter then explores the extent to which systems theories have been presented as a response, or even a solution, to the structure and agency interaction. However, Piggin subsequently focuses on the logic of interventions and shows that, despite longstanding debate and discussion about what shapes behaviours, interventions to change behaviour have remained relatively simple and relatively blunt, focusing on the individual and attempting to either regulate or incentivise behaviours. Various frameworks, conceptualised by their proponents as a ladder, a wheel and a pyramid are set out, and their usefulness, or not, in shaping and informing physical activity policy are critiqued.

The next two chapters, both reprints, have been selected because of the different perspectives and, more fundamentally, the different discourses they present on the global development of physical activity policy. Catherine Woods and Nanette Mutrie, writing in 2012, argue that physical activity has more to offer than purely health benefits, but also contextualise their discussions of how global and national policy should be developed with reference to World Health Organization guidelines for health-enhancing physical activity and the Toronto Charter for Physical Activity. Contextualising their perspectives within an ecological model, Woods and Mutrie set out what they see as the characteristics of a successful physical activity policy, and outline what they suggest countries or states should do to promote physical activity, discussing the potential of such policies to support the physical, social and mental wellbeing of populations.

Joe Piggin and Alan Bairner, writing in 2014, offer in contrast a critique of some of the normative ideas about physical activity policy, exploring the rhetorical construction of the 'global inactivity pandemic'. They suggest that idealistic recommendations and problematic claims of what is and what is not normal and abnormal should be considered more rigorously and extensively. In exploring claims about physical activity programmes and, by implication, policies, they argue that effects are more contentious than they are sometimes presented to be, and that the increasingly popular systems or ecological models deployed to address physical (in)activity contain inherent contradictions.

The next two chapters explore physical activity in relation to medicine and wellbeing. In the first of these, Dominic Malcolm and Emma Pullen present a sociological perspective on the Exercise Is Medicine movement, questioning the extent to which it is legitimate to conceptualise physical activity in the same way as a pharmaceutical. Implicit in Malcolm and Pullen's argument is that the trademarked Exercise Is Medicine concept may be more about professional prominence and legitimacy than what is or is not beneficial to populations. They also argue that there are ethical problems in reconceptualising what it means to be healthy or unwell, and that this is disempowering for citizens.

Drawing on concepts from economics relating to choice and the potential for health and wellbeing to be competing outcomes, Paul Downward explores whether the most prominent benefits of physical activity in the form of sport participation are those set out in health guidelines. Downward presents data to demonstrate that, in relation to sport at least, it is wider wellbeing outcomes associated with social interaction that appear to be valued and reflected in people's participation choices, rather than the physical health guidelines that policymakers more prominently pursue.

Finally in this theme, Louise Mansfield explores physical activity in relation to the field of public health, setting out the historical development of modern approaches to public health. Mansfield shows that, despite the explicit conceptualisation of public health as being about the health of populations, dominant public health discourses that emphasise health lifestyle behaviours and choices place the responsibility for health within the realm of the individual. She therefore argues that there is a need for greater collaboration, cross-sector knowledge exchange and an emphasis on community-based approaches if the public health goals for the physical activity of populations are to be achieved.

1

CONCEPTS AND THEORIES IN PHYSICAL ACTIVITY POLICY

Joe Piggin

Introduction – What is physical activity policy?

Policy can be thought of in different ways. First, it may be defined as an *ideal, aspiration, or a call to action*. For instance, the catchphrase "More People! More Active! More Often" can be seen in physical activity documents in England, Australia, the European Union, Ireland, New Zealand and Italy. Such phrasing suggests idealised communities of ever-increasingly active citizens and residents. Second, policy can be conceived of as *resource allocation*, whereby an organisation commits recourses, such as staff, money, time or materials to achieving a particular outcome. Therefore, policy influences (and sometime can dictate) what citizens have access to, spend their time thinking about and doing and what they spend their money on. Third, policy can be thought of as a *process*. Thinking of policy as a process means considering the way in which major decisions are made, implemented and evaluated.

This chapter focuses on the **main concepts and theories** which currently inform how physical activity policy is conceived of and operationalised. This includes

- ideas about human nature,
- ideas about influential structures in society,
- ideas about how to intervene to promote physical activity.

Agency and structure

It is necessary to start with a discussion of two concepts which inform all policy researchers and policy makers in some way: agency and structure. When constructing physical activity policy, both researchers and policy writers make assumptions about human nature. As such, all policies bring with them assumptions about agency and structure – the extent to which individuals are in control of their own life situations. Health promoters who emphasise *agency* believe that people have an ability to make choices, take action and be an active "agent" in their lives. Ideas about "free will" feature prominently for these advocates. Popular sports brands embrace this logic, with messages such as "Just do it" and "Impossible is nothing", insinuating that if only individuals commit to living physically active lives, they can accomplish this goal. People are supposed to be "personally responsible" for their own health. This logic includes the belief that individuals should "know" what is good for them, and therefore a failure to be active (and healthy) is predominantly the fault of the individual.

This viewpoint can be contrasted with researchers and policy makers who focus on *structure* – the factors that shape and constrain a person's ability to act in the world. Policy makers who focus on structure would argue that people are born into already constituted societies, with limits imposed on them. While policy makers would not usually argue that people's lives are *totally* predetermined, they do often emphasise the significant effects of social structures. For example, family upbringing is well recognised as a major, dominant factor in a person's wellbeing. Extending the influence of structure further, research suggests that many disease processes may begin before birth, in the mother's womb (McGill et al., 2010). Further, consider how the World Health Organization (WHO) (2002) takes into account a wide array of factors when calculating health risks around the world:

> The need to view such risks in their local context is obvious when analysing percep-tions of risk in [developing] countries, especially when risk factors are considered alongside life-threatening diseases such as tuberculosis, malaria and HIV/AIDS. There are also other daily threats, such as poverty, food insecurity and lack of income. In addi-tion, families may face many other important 'external' risks, such as political instability, violence, natural disasters and wars.

Therefore, policy makers emphasising structure tend to focus on factors and barriers (such as economics, education and physical environment) that potentially influence health. Because of the increasing attention on structural factors that influence the physical activity levels of a population (and the corresponding recognition that people are not simply either intrinsically motivated or extrinsically "inspired" to be active), researchers and policy makers alike have recently devoted more attention to "systems" which influence physical activity rates.

Systems and ecological approaches

Systems models are one way of thinking about a social problem by taking into account a wide variety of interrelated actors and components. The apparent benefit of systems thinking is that a view of the "whole" might lead to better solutions. So, in order to understand the "system" of physical activity, a policy maker would need to account for a wide range of factors, from the built environment and the weather, to the education system and the economic environment.

Forester (1993) notes that systems-based paradigms have been advocated as the only way in which governments can solve *complex, profound and interdependent social problems*. However, in epidemiology, systems thinking is relatively new. As recently as 2010, Galea et al. argued that isolating "causes" has emerged as one of the central foci in policy decades, and so "epidemiological thinking needs to broaden its conception of causes, and that such thinking may well be served by the adoption of complex systems dynamic models" (p. 102). King (2015) also notes that many complex models await empirical application and support, though acknowledges this is difficult when complex systems tend to be nonlinear, unpredictable and dynamic.

An important component of systems thinking is the starting point of the policy maker/intervener. Stewart and Ayres (2001) write that those engaged in systems approaches believe that trying to discover a single cause of a problem is futile. They write that in a systems approach:

> the "problem" is itself a manifestation of a set of inter-related elements, at least some of which reflect the effects of past policy choices. In other words, there is a problem situ-ation, rather than an identifiable causal factor. Consequently, there will be many causes, rather than one, of the identified difficulty.

Strengths of this approach include the ability to account for factors that may otherwise have been ignored. The approach allows policy makers to see "the big picture". Also, systems thinking allows policy makers to consider solutions which may not have been obvious. Policy makers can become more aware, and therefore make more informed decisions than a policy maker focused only on traditional conceptions of a problem and traditional ways of addressing it. Therefore systems thinking might be particularly suited to physical activity promotion, since the problem is commonly considered to be complex.

One of the most well known cases of systems thinking is the "Full Obesity Systems Map" published by the UK Government Office for Science in 2007. The map featured over 100 different macro, meso and micro level components and included sections on food production, food consumption, physiology, individual psychology, social psychology, individual physical activity and the physical activity environment. Despite this apparent comprehensive delineation, some of the map could still be described as overly simplistic. For example, the influence attributed to "education" was relatively minor compared to the influence attributed to "media consumption". The hope to see *everything* affecting a problem is particularly short-sighted, as all models are by definition simplifications. As Boulding (1956) noted, "we always pay for generality by sacrificing content, and all we can say about practically everything is almost nothing" (p. 197). Policy makers must be aware that any model of a system will need to balance a general knowledge with specific knowledge.

Two versions of the systems framework featured prominently in recent physical activity literature. In a 2012 special issue of *The Lancet* on Physical Activity, the physical inactivity pandemic was framed as complex. Kohl et al. (2012) acknowledged the complexity of social life, suggesting even a well designed intervention might result in a "net zero gain" due to unintended consequences. Bauman et al. (2012) described an adapted ecological model of the determinants of physical activity. It offers individual, interpersonal, environmental, policy and global factors, along with the added dimension of "life-course". While this model does

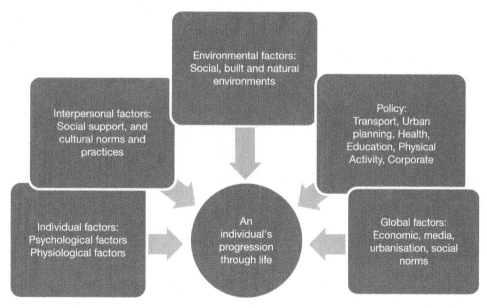

Figure 1.1 Typical physical activity ecological model

Source: Adapted from Bauman et al., 2012

not have the particularities of the UK Government's (2007) "full obesity system map", the addition of the life-course aspect does add to the complexity of the model.

In the final chapter in the 2012 *The Lancet* series, Kohl et al. offered a systems model, and compared this with a "traditional behavioural or environmental intervention strategy". At the centre of their systems model are a variety of elements and factors which inform the process on the outer region of the model. For example, the built environment, unintended consequences and competing actions are all offered as potential barriers to the successful implementation of behaviour change. The authors write that:

> there is an acknowledgment of issues, such as delay functions, adaptation, unintended consequences, competing interests, and feedback that could negatively affect an approach to increase physical activity. Various characteristics might also accelerate or inhibit the speed of the effectiveness of the strategies.
>
> *p. 72*

Indeed this model demonstrates that significant change might not be possible, despite the best intentions from health promoters. With this in mind, it is important to consider the limitations of systems.

While there are many benefits of adopting a systems approach, operationalising systems thinking can be fraught with tension and potential contradictions. Take the example of the sport of football as a site to increase population physical activity. Football, and the Football World Cup in particular, are often praised for inspiring participation in football around the world. However, numerous examples can be listed to show why we should be sceptical of the Football World Cup to contribute to physical activity. In 2015 the governing body, the Fédération Internationale de Football Association (FIFA), became embroiled in allegations of corruption. FIFA has also been accused of holding the Football World Cup in countries which have been criticised for major human rights violations. Further, FIFA's corporate sponsors have faced allegations of worker abuses and the promotion of unhealthy food. A systems approach would need to account for these ambiguous, contradictory and paradoxical aspects of "the system". When opportunities arise for physical activity promoters to work with FIFA (and to use their wide reach and branding), a systems approach gives little advice on navigating such ethically problematic issues. A health promoter using a systems approach would by definition be obliged to consider the repercussions of problematic aspects of a system.

There is also a necessity at some point to place a boundary on a systems analysis. With systems thinking, all boundaries are artificially constructed by the creator of the model. As such the articulation of a system is inherently political. How much weight is given to one factor over another? Which factors are ignored due to time constraints? Rich and Ashby (2013) take this thinking one step further to consider that "health" (as measured by longevity and socially acceptable behaviour) is often not the greatest desire or motivation for people. They argue there are other things that people value, beside "health". For example, despite clear road rules, many drivers often drive at unlawful speeds, thereby increasing risk of injury or death to oneself and others. "Health", in this case, takes a back seat.

Overall, it appears that systems thinking is becoming the model par excellence in the physical activity promotion and policy scholarship, despite being a relatively recent way of conceiving of a social problem, and despite being difficult to operationalise in interventions. Certainly, systems thinking is useful in provoking academics and policy makers to consider what change is possible in various sectors of the environment. At the same time, we should not forget that the reductive nature of systems mapping can make a relationship between two aspects appear as simple as a unidirectional arrow. Such simplification is highly problematic, and would likely lead the most optimistic policy maker or practitioner into difficulty when attempting to implement an intervention.

Interventions

It is easy to defer to the ***state*** when thinking about the main levers for interventions. After all, health knowledge about physical activity is often produced by state funded universities, and disseminated through state-funded schools and health care systems. The models presented in this chapter often refer to "populations", implying nations or geographic areas. However, it is important to acknowledge that in many countries there is an enormous diversity of non-governmental organisations, companies and civil society groups involved in promoting physical activity. Indeed, grassroots civil movements, from self-organised hiking clubs to charity cycle fundraising events, operate predominantly outside of state control. For the purposes of this chapter however, the focus is mainly on state policy.

Interventions are informed by how a problem is framed, what evidence is available and what resources policy makers have at their disposal. First, how the problem is framed will be shaped by the existing political ideology. Arguably, most Western, neo-liberal democracies emphasise autonomy when it comes to the physical activities that citizens engage in. Therefore interventions (particularly with adults) tend to focus on encouraging and incentivising people to become more active. Second, the evidence currently available is also influential. The relative amount and strength of evidence accrued for the efficacy and effectiveness of a policy intervention will contribute to various options being considered. Third, the resources at the disposal of policy makers will determine which of an array of interventions will be deployed.

The adverse consequences of inactivity in terms of physical health, quality of life and wellbeing are well documented. To offer one of many examples, a major study in 2015 of European adults suggested that "physical inactivity is responsible for more than twice as many deaths as general obesity" (Ekelund et al., 2015). Further, physical activity is an important way in which people "exercise" their rights, create meaning and accomplish goals throughout their lifetimes. As such, physical activity policy has the potential to not only alleviate poor health, but also can enable and liberate people to live more fulfilled, satisfied lives. Therefore, justifying physical activity policies is unlike many other health and social policies. For example, while anti-smoking policies are predominantly informed by ideas about individual wellbeing and public health budgets, physical activity policies are of interest for professionals working in other fields. There is a growing body of literature detailing the benefits that accrue from regular participation in physical activity. Along with "physical health", there is growing evidence about mental health (Mason & Holt, 2012), social inclusion (Forde et al., 2015), economic benefits (Pereira et al., 2015), educational improvements (Singh et al., 2012), crime prevention (Roman et al., 2013), sustainability (Gerike et al., 2016), et cetera. By being associated with these social goods, physical activity has become a utility; something which is used to accomplish *other* goals.

A consequence of the expansion of costs and benefits associated with physical activity has been that PA policies increasingly emphasise "*everyone*" and *all* places – work, home, school, leisure and transport. This means that physical activity becomes a multi-dimensional issue, potentially affecting people in all countries, of all ages, in all settings.

Policy interventions imply a claim or warrant about what can be expected to happen if a particular action is taken (Dunn, 1981). However, making good physical activity policy is difficult, because the notion of "intervening" is problematic. There are various reasons why policies fail, as noted by Hogwood and Gunn (1993). Table 1.1 provides examples of why physical activity policies might fail.

Table 1.1 Hogwood and Gunn's (1997) reasons for policy failure, with physical activity examples

Reason for policy failure	Physical activity example
External circumstances impose constraints.	A lack of time, people or expertise and financial restrictions all severely affect PA interventions.
Required resources are not available.	There is a perception that physical activity has been undervalued in terms of its importance and therefore under-resourced. One aim from the London Olympics Games was to "inspire a generation". However, this was perceived by some to be unachievable because not enough funding was dedicated to the goal.
Policy makers do not take into account all causes and effects.	This is a common issue for policy makers who "simplify" a problem such as physical inactivity rates to a matter of individual motivation. The dynamic nature of the policy environment can also influence success.
Dependency relationships have an influence.	Physical activity promoters are often reliant on a range of stakeholders. Funding bodies which provide critical resources may decide to halt funding, or a law may change which inhibits a PA policy from being sustainably organised.
There is confusion about objectives.	This issue is relevant for the people involved in implementing physical activity policies. PA policies have various aims, such as increasing awareness or knowledge or inspiring people to take action. Specific aims may be misinterpreted or misunderstood by promoters and practitioners involved in the policy.
A lack of knowledge about objectives.	Following the previous point, promoters and practitioners may simply not be informed about the specific goals. Further, they may not have the required expertise and skills to undertake the actions required.
Tasks are completed out of order.	The dynamic nature of the practical world may prohibit a "perfect" sequencing of policy tasks. For example, a mass media physical activity campaign encouraging people to get off the couch and into sport would not be effective if there is not an existing sports structure which welcomes beginners.
Communication and coordination is lacking.	This is one of the most common difficulties faced in physical activity policy. Many objectives relate specifically to behaviour change, which in turn requires interpersonal communication. Crafting effective messages for targeted groups is very difficult.
Perfect compliance cannot be obtained.	The success of a PA policy relies on an inactive group to become active. While policy makers often acknowledge that not "everyone" will obey the suggestions offered, there are often ongoing issues regarding people who relapse into inactive lifestyles.

Aside from the practical difficulties involved in intervening, there are also ethical issues involved. Interventions can suggest an imposition by some outside force upon a person, organisation or community (and can conflict with dominant liberal attitudes toward personal freedom in many societies). While policy interventions are often undertaken with the most benevolent of intentions, there are always tensions between private rights and the public good, and between the individual and the community. In recent years, public policy attention has increasingly focused upon the importance of physical activity in contributing to healthy, productive and wealthy societies. Some research has already examined how different types of intervention seek to nudge (Vallgårda, 2012), police (Piggin, Jackson, & Lewis, 2007), empower (Bercovitz, 1998), inspire (Evans, 2013), exhort (Garvin & Eyles, 1997) and educate (Gard & Wright, 2011). Here we discuss the two policy instruments most commonly used to intervene with regard to physical activity: rules and inducements.

Inducements and rules

Inducements and rules are the two main instruments utilised by health promoters, and both are fraught with difficulty in their implementation. *Inducements* aim to bring individual goals in line with community goals. Deborah Stone (2002) writes that employing inducements assumes people are rational, adaptable, unitary and oriented towards the future. One example of inducements can be seen in the UK's Change4Life (healthy eating and physical activity) marketing strategy. The strategy discussed how there was a need to convince the public that change was "imperative", but yet proceeded to promote changes as something that the population "should" do. This approach has been described as "nudging", and is a popular way in which a population is then encouraged to change their physical activity behaviour (Vallgårda, 2012). This strategy presupposes that individuals should be free to choose how to live their lives with respect to diet and physical activity, and, therefore, should not be forced to change their behaviour, but rather encouraged, or nudged, to adopt healthy forms of behaviour. Stone argues, however, that it is very difficult for policy makers to decide on appropriate inducements. For example, while it may seem a good idea to offer subsidised cycles to incentivise active transport, commuters who already walk to work may feel unfairly treated, since they receive no immediate extra benefit for their existing healthy behaviour.

Rules, or commands to make people behave a certain way, are a contentious policy tool with respect to physical activity in neo-liberal societies. The idea of "enforcing" physical activity upon people is viewed as unacceptable. Even in schools, where physical education is often a compulsory element of the curriculum, there are usually many other regulations which over-ride or disrupt a rule instructing students to be physically active. For example, teachers have discretion in making and enforcing rules, and students can look for ways to avoid punishment for breaking a rule. Some potential rules in health policy are to a large extent "unthinkable". Seldom do health promotion scholars recommend compulsory intervention in people's lives. For example, an entire community partaking in communal physical activity are usually framed as the epitome of authoritarian, totalitarian regimes.

Types of public health interventions: The Ladder, Wheel and Pyramid

Health agencies and academics use various models to explain the type and purpose of various policies. One template that has gained in popularity in recent years is the idea of an "Intervention Ladder" (see Figure 1.2, adapted from Nuffield Council on BioEthics, 2007). At one end is individual freedom and at the other is imposition of state-mandated policies. This model considers actions by taking into account both the benefits to individuals and society, and the potential for erosion of individual freedom. This point is particularly pertinent in the realm of physical activity. While it is widely accepted that school-aged children can "be told" to participate in school physical education lessons, free adults do not tend to be faced with compulsory physical activity of any sort. Along with this tension, the economic costs and benefits are weighed against the potential health and societal benefits.

The creators of the Ladder note that the model is not intended as a formulaic device, but rather a way of appreciating the different levels of intrusiveness and likely acceptability of various interventions. Of course, as with any interventions, there are choices to be made

Table 1.2 A physical activity intervention ladder

Intervention type	Explanation and physical activity examples
Eliminate choice	Regulate in such a way as to entirely eliminate choice. For example, making able children complete a one mile run every morning at school.
Restrict choice	Regulation is imposed so that options available to people are restricted. For example, limiting the number of car parks at a workplace might contribute to people choosing other ways of commuting.
Guide choice through disincentives	Disincentives such as monetary penalties can be put in place to influence people not to pursue certain activities. For example through charging more money for car use and car parking.
Guide choices through incentives	Regulations which induce socially desired behaviour. For example, offering fiscal incentives such as discounts for employee cycle use.
Guide choices through changing the default policy	An organisation alters their focus and policy to contribute to behaviour change. For example, instead of a school providing cricket as a standard physical education class, students might be offered breakdancing or triathlon, where participants are more active session.
Enable choice	Enable individuals to change their behaviours. For example, a city council might construct a range of new free leisure opportunities, such as outdoor gyms, skate parks and walking tracks.
Provide information	Offer useful information to people outlining the benefits of certain behaviours. For example, emphasising the various benefits of taking part in health enhancing physical activity.
Do nothing	Continue with the status quo.

Source: Adapted from Nuffield, 2007

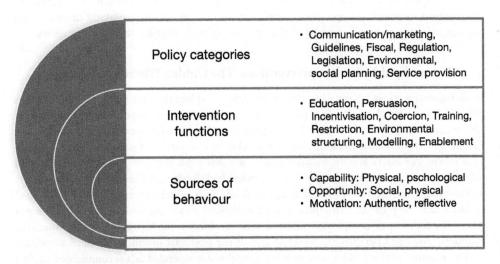

Figure 1.2 A Behaviour Change Wheel

Source: Adapted from Michie et al., 2011

about what level of intervention is acceptable in the pursuit of particular outcomes. These choices will be informed by a number of factors, including the policy maker's personal politics, their budget and their time constraints. Every step in the ladder has the potential for significant ethical and practical problems to arise. For example, "providing information" about physical activity might be a relatively innocuous intervention for many people, but culturally conservative groups might question what is appropriate physical activity, where and for whom? Further, as we move up the ladder towards restricting and eliminating choice, there is potential for protest about the curtailing of previously acceptable civil liberties. Also policy makers should not assume that restricting or eliminating choice will lead to a particular result. There are often unintended consequences of restrictive policies, whereby the target population resists or finds ways around the desired behaviour.

Another popular way to separate interventions is to examine them based on where their focus lies, such as with individuals, populations or systems. The **traditional intervention wheel** was first proposed in 1998 by the Minnesota Department of Health to address these different levels. The wheel showcases a wide variety of interventions, from marketing to counselling to advocacy and surveillance. It extends the broad logic of the Intervention Ladder to consider more specific tools that physical activity policy makers can draw upon.

Table 1.3 Interventions and policies involved in the Behaviour Change Wheel

Interventions	Definition and example
Education	Physical education is an important element, though education can extend throughout the life course.
Persuasion	Inducing positive or negative feelings or stimulate action. The threat of years lost from being physically active may be less persuasive than promoting the social benefits and joy derived from activity.
Incentivisation	Creating expectation of reward. Weight loss is a popular incentive to promote physical activity.
Coercion	Creating expectation of punishment or cost. For physical activity, costs are often explained in terms of the possibility of future ill health.
Training	Imparting skills. Many discretionary leisure activities involve an element of training to develop competence of an activity. Often training is the largest component of formal sports.
Restriction	Using rules to increase the opportunity to engage in the target behaviour. Restricting sitting by installing standing desks at work is a subtle form of restriction.
Environmental structuring	Changing the physical or social context. Local councils might make incremental changes such as installing trial cycle lanes, or more radical changes by prohibiting vehicle use in community centres.
Modelling	Providing an example for people to aspire to or imitate. Promoters of physical activity often utilise elite sportspeople to promote messages about healthy eating and physical activity to children.
Enablement	Increasing means/reducing barriers to increase capability or opportunity. Offering free use of public facilities to low income earners is one idea of increasing inclusive physical activity.

(continued)

Table 1.3 Interventions and policies involved in the Behaviour Change Wheel *(continued)*

Interventions	Definition and example
Policy categories	
Communication/ marketing	Using various media forms. Mass media campaigns are popular, and while awareness is often high in the target population, these are not usually sufficient by themselves to change behaviour significantly.
Guidelines	Creating documents that recommend or mandate practice and service provision. In recent years there has been much lobbying for formal, national level physical activity policy.
Fiscal	Using the tax system to reduce or increase the financial cost. Physical activity advocates claim that increasing population-wide physical activity will result in significant tax expenditure on health care.
Regulation	Establishing rules or principles of behaviour or practice. Organisations might limit working hours in order to promote balanced lifestyles.
Legislation	Making or changing laws. Making physical education compulsory in schools is influential legislation, though there are many other spaces to change laws, such as changing road laws to prioritise cyclists' rights.
Environmental, social planning	Designing and/or controlling the physical or social environment. By prioritising public health, town planners can develop urban areas in order to encourage incidental and planned physical activity.
Service provision	Delivering a service. Many professional football clubs now offer physical activity schemes for older adult fans, including training at the stadium.

Source: Adapted from Michie et al., 2011

All of these tools have various strengths and weaknesses for targeting different aspects of a complex issue. It is broadly agreed, however, that for a policy issue as complex as physical activity, interventions would need to be multi-sectorial, multi-level and sustainable. This is perhaps the reason why recent World Health Organization policy around physical activity has escalated in tone in recent years and has increasingly identified many different sectors as needing to be involved in the solution. Another "wheel" is the "Behaviour Change Wheel".

The various elements which contribute to the wheel are described in more detail below. The logic of the wheel is that a "behaviour system" is made up of three essential conditions (capability, opportunity and motivation) which influence and are influenced by the surrounding intervention functions and policy categories. By considering these factors in relation to one another and how they might influence behaviour change, researchers and practitioners can decide where and how to focus their attention. The examples offered here are illustrative only; in the wide variety of countries, cultures and settings around the world, there will be an enormous array of possibilities for intervention and policy.

The creators of the Behaviour Change Wheel acknowledge various limitations. For example, some of the terms used can overlap with each other, such as with "education" and "training". Also they note that any given intervention could possibly perform more than one behaviour change function, and that there are near infinite ways of classifying interventions and intervention functions. However, the purported strength is that the Wheel incorporates the previously under-theorised and under-investigated context of interventions. If indeed context is essential to good policy making, then it should feature in modelling.

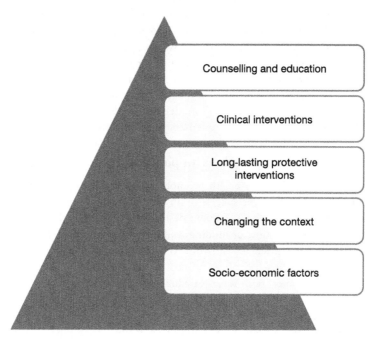

Figure 1.3   The Health Impact Pyramid

Source: Adapted from Frieden, 2010

Another way of thinking about the types of interventions available is the **Health Impact Pyramid**, which demonstrates the varying effects interventions have on a population. The model suggests that while some interventions rely on a significant amount of public input, they might often yield limited results, whereas major structural changes in socio-economic status have the greatest effect. Frieden (2010) notes that interventions focusing on lower levels of the pyramid tend to be more effective because they have a wider reach and require less individual effort. However, concurrent interventions at each of the levels can achieve the greatest sustained public health benefit.

By considering the relative weight of these impacts, it becomes apparent that while mass media campaigns imploring people to "move more" might be the most visible manifestations of health promotion, there are many other *structural factors* that are potentially more effective in promoting physical activity, despite being less publicly visible. Like the Behaviour Change Wheel model, the Pyramid encourages us to critically consider the context in which interventions take place. Further, the model takes into account the size of the impact of various interventions. Of course, since socio-economic factors are incredibly difficult to change through targeted public policy (because of budget and political will constraints), the interventions with less potential impact are the more popular choices for public health interventions.

By perusing these various intervention models, policy makers and action researchers might wonder if there is one best model to conceptualise intervening and to increase the likelihood of an intervention succeeding. The answer, until proven otherwise, is no. Whether or not an intervention succeeds is dependent on a wide array of circumstances. Different models simply provide a frame on which to hang policy ideas, and help those involved to include, exclude and organise various programmes and practices.

Each policy setting will be unique and will require those involved to address a range of questions. How many factors should be taken into account? Is the policy short term or long term? Is the policy small or large scale? How great is the imposition of the policy? Do inducements contribute to favourable outcomes or do rules need to be enforced? What resources are available to make structural change? And, of course, how is success measured? Policy makers, practitioners and researchers alike should compare and contrast the variety of models available to them, adapt existing models where they see fit and even construct new ways of understanding how to best implement physical activity programmes.

Implications for policy and practice

Researchers, policy makers and health promoters alike are faced with limited budgets and time constraints which affect the success of physical activity policy. Couple this with policy makers who, aside from having a genuine desire to improve population health, might also possess limited experience, time or funding, and it becomes apparent that modifying physical activity levels becomes particularly difficult. And this is of course to say nothing of the target population, who are themselves often defined as "hard to reach", living in poverty, time-pressed, with low incomes, poor levels of education, living isolated lives or in an otherwise marginalised group. Given the complexity of the lived experiences of many who are deemed to be "physically inactive" and therefore worthy of scrutiny, policy makers would be well placed to consider both agency and structure as contributors to physical activity rates. It is envisaged here that if policy makers consider both agency and structure as influential in physical activity rates at a population level, more sympathetic and appropriate interventions will be produced.

This chapter also aimed to offer a sense of the various models which are used in physical activity policy. Ideally, these concepts and theories *inform* how policy makers think and speak about physical activity. Are these models always transferred into practice by policy makers? Probably not. It is clear there is often a disconnection between theory and practice. Rather, it is more likely that at different times, aspects of these models are foregrounded, backgrounded and omitted as different practical realities are dealt with. As Hogwood and Gunn show, there is seldom such a thing as the perfect implementation of a policy. However, having an understanding of the variety of ideas which can and do inform policy production will put the reader in good stead to consider alternatives to existing or failing policy.

References

Bauman, A. E., Reis, R. S., Sallis, J. F., Wells, J. C., Loos, R. J. F., & Martin, B. W., for *The Lancet* Physical Activity Series Working Group (2012). Correlates of physical activity: Why are some people physically active and others not? *The Lancet, 380*(9838), 258–271. doi:10.1016/S0140-6736(12)60735-1.

Bercovitz, K. (1998) Canada's Active Living policy: A critical analysis. *Health Promotion International, 13*(4), 319–328.

Boulding, K. E. (1956) General systems theory – The skeleton of science. *Management Science, 2*(3), 197–208.

Dunn, W. (1981) *Public policy analysis: An introduction.* Beverly Hills: SAGE.

Ekelund, U. et al., (2015) Physical activity and all-cause mortality across levels of overall and abdominal adiposity in European men and women: The European prospective investigation into cancer and nutrition study. *American Journal of Clinical Nutrition.* 10.3945/ajcn.114.100065.

Evans, J. (2013) Physical education as porn! *Physical Education and Sport Pedagogy, 18*(1), 75–89. doi:10.1080/17408989.2011.631002.

Forde, S. D., Lee, D. S., Mills, C., & Frisby, W. (2015) Moving towards social inclusion: Manager and staff perspectives on an award winning community sport and recreation program for immigrants. *Sport Management Review, 18*, 126–138.

Forester, J. (1993) *Critical theory, public policy and planning practice: Towards a critical pragmatism.* Albany: State University of New York Press.

Frieden, T. R. (2010) A framework for public health action: The health impact pyramid. *American Journal of Public Health, 100*(4), 590–595.

Galea, S., Riddle, M., & Kaplan, G. A. (2010) Causal thinking and complex system approaches in epidemiology. *International Journal of Epidemiology,* 39, 97–106.

Gard, M. and Wright, J. (2001) Managing uncertainty: Obesity discourses and physical education in a risk society. *Studies in Philosophy and Education, 20*:6, 535–549.

Garvin, T. & Eyles, J. (1997) The sun safety metanarrative: Translating science into public health discourse. *Policy Sciences, 30*(2), 47–70. doi:10.1023/A:1004256124700.

Gerike, R., et al. (2016) Physical activity through sustainable transport approaches (PASTA): A study protocol for a multicentre project. *BMJ Open.* doi:10.1136/bmjopen-2015-009924.

Hogwood, B. & Gunn, L. (1993) Why "perfect" implementation is unattainable, in: M. Hill (Ed.) *The policy process,* London: Harvester Wheatsheaf.

King, A. C. (2015) Theory's role in shaping behavioral health research for population health. *International Journal of Behavioral Nutrition and Physical Activity,* 12, 146. doi:10.1186/s12966-015-0307-0.

Kohl, H. W., et al. for *The Lancet* Physical Activity Series Working Group. (2012) The pandemic of physical inactivity: Global action for public health. *The Lancet,* 380, 294–305. doi:10.1016/S0140-6736(12)60898-8.

Mason, O. J., & Holt, R. (2012) Mental health and physical activity interventions: A review of the qualitative literature. *Journal of Mental Health, 21*(3), 274–284.

McGill, H. C. Jr,, McMahan C. A., & Gidding S. S. (2010) Childhood obesity, atherogenesis, and adult cardiovascular disease. *Pediatric Obesity.* New York: Springer, 265–78.

Michie, S. M., van Stralen, M., & West, R. (2011) The Behaviour Change Wheel: A new method for characterising and designing behaviour change interventions. *Implementation Science,* 6, 42.

Nuffield Council on BioEthics (2007) *Public Health: Ethical Issues.* London: Nuffield.

Pereira, M. J., Coombes, B. K., Comans, T. A., & Johnston, V. (2015) The impact of onsite workplace health-enhancing physical activity interventions on worker productivity: A systematic review. *Occup Environ Med, 72*(6), 401–412.

Piggin, J., Jackson, S., & Lewis, M. (2007). Classify, divide and conquer: Shaping physical activity discourse through National Public Policy. *New Zealand Sociology,* 22, 274–293.

Rich, L. E. & Ashby, M. A. (2013) From personal misfortune to public liability: The ethics, limits, and politics of public health saving ourselves from ourselves. *Journal of Bioethical Inquiry, 10*(1), 1–5.

Roman, C. G., Stodolska, M., Yahner, J. & Shinew, K. (2013) Pathways to outdoor recreation, physical activity, and delinquency among urban Latino adolescents. *Annals of Behavioral Medicine, 45*(1), 151–161.

Singh, A., Uijtdewilligen, L., Twisk, J. W., van Mechelen, W., & Chinapaw, M. J. (2012) Physical activity and performance at school: A systematic review of the literature including a methodological quality assessment. *The Archives of Pediatrics & Adolescent Medicine, 166*(1), 49–55.

Stewart, J. & Ayres, R. (2001) Systems theory and policy practice: An exploration. *Policy Science, 34*(1), 79–94.

Stone, D. A. (2002) *Policy paradox: The art of political decision making.* New York: W.W. Norton.

UK Government. (2007) *Government office for science. Foresight. Tackling obesities: Future choices.* London: UK Office for Science.

Vallgårda, S. (2012) Nudge: A new and better way to improve health? *Health Policy, 104*(2), 200–203. doi: 10.1016/j.healthpol.2011.10.013.

World Health Organization. (2002) *Reducing risks, promoting healthy life, the World Health Report.* www.who.int/.

2

PUTTING PHYSICAL ACTIVITY ON THE POLICY AGENDA

Catherine Woods and Nanette Mutrie

Physical inactivity involves little or no movement and has recently been identified as the fourth leading risk factor for mortality in the world (http://www.globalpa.or.uk). Physical activity involves any bodily movement that is produced by the contraction of the skeletal muscles and that substantially increases energy expenditure (Caspersen, Powell, & Christenson, 1985). Regular participation in health-enhancing physical activity (activity that is sufficiently above baseline activity to produce health gain) has numerous health benefits, including a reduction in coronary heart disease and stroke, diabetes, hypertension, colon cancer, breast cancer, and depression (World Health Organization, 2003; Mathers, Stevens, & Mascarenhas, 2009). The majority of most populations do not engage in sufficient physical activity to gain these health benefits. The high risk and high prevalence of inactivity in most countries around the world make the promotion of physical activity a major public health concern. In addition, physical inactivity contributes substantially to direct and indirect healthcare costs. Such an important health behaviour should be central to education programs and activities.

Yet physical activity has more to offer than purely individual or societal health benefits. Physical education, the systematic introduction to, and education in, sport, exercise, and physical activity as part of the school curriculum, provides children with opportunities to not only learn about movement skills, but also to learn through these activities about other aspects of knowledge (Hardman, 2008). Physical activity can also help promote sustainable development; urban design principles or transport policies that promote pedestrian and bicycle travel give people the chance to opt to walk or cycle as a form of transport, thus potentially reducing greenhouse gas emissions, congestion, and air pollution (Heath et al., 2006).

The global recommendations on physical activity for health published by the World Health Organization (WHO) in 2010 aim to provide scientifically informed guidance on how much physical activity (in terms of frequency, intensity, time, and type) different population subgroups should do in order to accrue health benefits (World Health Organization, 2010a). According to these recommendations, all children and young people (aged 5–17 years) should accumulate at least 60 minutes of moderate to vigorous-intensity physical activity daily. While most of this activity will be aerobic in nature, the importance of incorporating activities that strengthen muscle and bone at least three times per week was also suggested. For this age group opportunities to be active should be facilitated through the family, the school, and the community where the child lives, and include activities like play, games, sports, transportation, recreation, physical education, or planned exercise. Clearly education has a major role to play both in educating children about the level of activity they should be doing to gain health benefits, but also in giving children the skills and attitudes which will help them lead a physically active life. A main contributor to this education will be the physical education opportunities available to children. For adults (aged 18–64 years), the WHO recommends participation in at least 150 minutes of moderate-intensity aerobic activity per week, or at least 75 minutes of vigorous-intensity aerobic activity weekly, or an equivalent combination of moderate- and vigorous-intensity activity (with activity performed in bouts of at least 10-minute duration). Additional benefits can be accrued relative to increasing the duration of the activity at each intensity level. Similar aerobic physical activity recommendations exist for older adults (65 years plus), with the addition of advice for those with poor mobility, or other health conditions that might limit their ability to engage in physical activity. Additionally, engaging in muscle-strengthening activities which involve the major muscle groups on at least two days per week is encouraged for all adults.

These guidelines have been adopted by numerous countries worldwide (Department of Health and Children, 2009; OECD, 2010; U.S. Department of Health and Human Services, 2008; UK Department of Health, 2004; Chief Medical Officers, 2011). Physical activity guidelines are important because they clarify for individuals, physical activity professionals, physical education teachers, and other key stakeholders in physical activity promotion how much physical activity is required to benefit current and future health. This is important advocacy information as it can be used to inform physical activity policy formation, by, for example, providing starting points from which to set targets for physical activity promotion at population level or to justify the need for curriculum time for physical education and extra-curricular activities. Guidelines also inform surveillance of population levels of physical activity, allowing for monitoring over time and inter-country comparisons to be determined and can also be used by those in charge of quality control in education to determine if schools are achieving goals in relation to physical education and related activity.

However, levels of physical activity in most populations are low, with levels of physical inactivity rising in many countries. In Europe, approximately one in five children meet the physical activity guidelines for developing their current and future health (Currie et al., 2008; OECD, 2010). In 2001, 45.4 per cent of U.S. adults self-reported achieving the US physical activity recommendations (Centers for Disease Control and Prevention, 2003). More than half of the total adult population across the European Union (EU) and across the US are now overweight or obese, and the rate of obesity has more than doubled over the past 20 years in most EU countries (OECD, 2010; Flegal, Carrol, Ogden, & Curtin, 2010). Physical inactivity is a public health issue.

From this background it is clear that intervention is needed to promote population levels of physical activity. Traditional physical activity programs that focus on the individual have had limited success in promoting long-term adherence to physical activity (Mutrie & Woods, 2003). Obstacles can prevent even the most motivated individual from being active. These obstacles include car- as opposed to pedestrian-orientated transportation systems, sedentary jobs, poor physical education provision leading to a lack of skill, competence, or understanding, lack of or poorly maintained parks and other green spaces, and community designs that require driving (King & Sallis, 2009). An ecological approach to the promotion of physical activity is recognized as having potential to meet this grand challenge. Ecological models recognize the importance of individual influences (intra-individual) on health behaviour, but they also identify the contribution of social and environmental factors (extra-individual) (Sallis, Owen, & Fisher, 2008). They also adhere to the Ottawa Charter for Health Promotion (World

Health Organization, 1986). Figure 2.1 gives an example of how an ecological model works; it posits that behaviour is influenced by intra-individual (e.g. attitudes, knowledge, skill), and extra-individual (at (1) interpersonal, for example, teacher-child relationship; (2) organizational, for example, provision of physical education within a school setting; (3) community, for example, relationships between schools in how they address the needs of children and youth in after-school sport; and (4) public policy, for example, educational policy on frequency and duration of physical education classes within the school timetable) factors.

At the public policy level, the initiation, co-ordination, and implementation of policies that promote physical activity, enhance opportunities for whole populations to be active, and develop environments that promote active choices are necessary (Bull, Bellew, Schoppe, & Bauman, 2004). This policy-based approach is endorsed by the World Health Assembly (in 2004, and again in 2008) in Resolution WHA57.17: Global Strategy on Diet, Physical Activity and Health, and Resolution WHA61.14: Prevention and Control of Non-communicable Diseases (NCD), and most recently in the High-level Meeting of the United Nations General Assembly on the prevention and control of NCD (World Health Organization, 2004; World Health Organization, 2008; United Nations General Assembly, 2011). The resolutions urged member states and governments to develop national physical activity action plans and policies, with the ultimate aim of increasing physical activity levels in their populations. Prior to these resolutions, the Center for Disease Prevention and Health Promotion (CDC) and the World Health Organization (WHO) set up the CDC WHO Collaborating Center for Physical Activity and Health Promotion. This centre is located within the Division of Nutrition and Physical Activity at the CDC, and over the past decade it has helped focus global health policy on physical activity promotion by (1) building an evidence base for interventions, (2) developing tools for surveillance of population levels of physical activity, (3) evaluation, and (4) building capacity of those working in physical

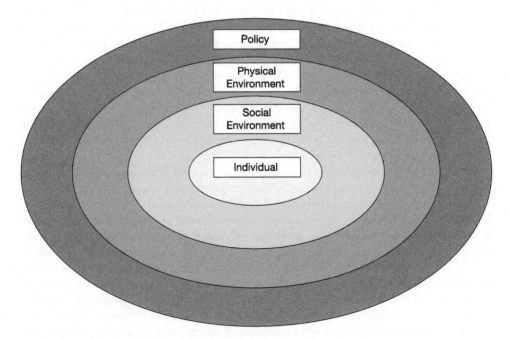

Figure 2.1 Graphic representation of the social-ecological model

activity and health promotion (Pratt, Epping, & Dietz, 2009). Pratt and colleagues indicated that today physical activity is central to good public health practice globally and nationally; however, they identified a future challenge as the development of this practice at state and local level. The development of physical activity policy is central to this change in practice, as a co-ordinated approach where global, national, regional, state, and local level policies that promote, enhance, and develop opportunities for individuals, groups, and whole populations to be physically active are supported (irrespective of their origin—health, education, sport and recreation, transport, and so on). The remainder of this manuscript will discuss what a physical activity policy is, guidelines on how to write one, and examples of good practice that include practice in physical education. Although reference is drawn throughout to a "national" physical activity policy, this information equally applies to physical activity policy written for state, regional, or local areas.

What is physical activity policy?

A policy is a statement of intent. Policy may be conceptualized as "formal written codes, regulations or decisions bearing legal authority . . . as written standards that guide choices or . . . as unwritten social norms that influence or guide behaviour" (Schmid, Pratt, & Witmer, 2006, p. S22). Health-related public policy is when public policy impacts directly or indirectly on health, by for example, at a national level through legislation creating supportive environments for individuals to engage in health-promoting behaviour. This can occur at a national level (for example, a law preventing individuals from smoking in workplaces) or at a local level (for example, a school or a school district adopting a physical activity policy that facilitates active school transport). A physical activity policy is an example of a public health policy. It is a document that defines physical activity as a priority area; that identifies specific population goals and targets; and that provides a framework for action, or an action plan to achieve these goals (Bellew et al., 2008). Ideally, a physical activity policy should also define of roles and responsibilities of involved partners, allocation of resources, and clearly identify accountability for implementation of specific components of the policy aligned to a realistic and achievable timeframe (Bull et al., 2004).

Why is PA policy important?

A successful national physical activity policy has the potential to influence the health and wellbeing of an entire population. Successful state or local policies have the potential to influence all of the individuals within their geographical area, or specific setting, for example, a school or workplace. Policy can give support, coherence, and visibility at the political level, while also making it possible for the organizations involved at national, regional, and local levels—for example, national government sectors, regional or local authorities, stakeholders, and the private sector—to be logical and consistent in their actions to achieve a shared goal (World Health Organization, 2010b). It can give all relevant organizations a mandate to adopt shared strategies based on identified roles and responsibilities.

This policy approach to the promotion of physical activity requires collaboration and interaction among policy makers from several different sectors, each tackling the physical activity goal for different reasons but with the same agenda to get the population or population subgroup more active. A number of different government sectors can play a role in achieving national physical activity goals. Although the main policy focus of these different sectors is probably not "to increase levels of population physical activity," if the policy makers within each sector can be convinced that physical inactivity is a problem that needs to be addressed, then they can change their public policy or allocate their public funds in ways designed to address this problem (Leyden, Reger-Nash, Bauman, & Bias, 2008). Additionally, advocacy in partnership for adequate resources and accountability for use of these resources as well as acknowledgment of contribution could potentially lead to a better policy. However, this leveraging of existing sector assets requires active engagement and cooperation across a number of sectors (Mowen & Baker, 2009). WHO recently outlined the potential role of different government sectors, identifying the specific roles that can be played by public health, transport, environment, sport, and education sectors in the promotion of physical activity. For example, in Ireland, the Smarter Travel Policy (Department of Transport, 2009) states that there is a need to "minimize the negative impacts of transport on the local and global environment through reducing localized air pollutants and greenhouse gas emissions" (p. 27), and one strategy it proposes to do this is

> of all travel modes, cycling and walking have the lowest environmental impact. If we are to successfully promote cycling and walking as realistic alternatives to the private car we need to ensure that they are, as far as possible, a safe and pleasant experience.
>
> *p. 42*

The focus here is not on health, but on sustainability and environmental impact, yet with close collaboration, both the health and the sustainability goals can be achieved. Similarly, the promotion of mixed land use or urban planning strategies that facilitate physical activity would come under the remit of the environment sector, creating school environments (not just curricula) that promote and encourage active lifestyles would be the remit of education, and so on.

The Toronto Charter for Physical Activity was launched in May 2010 by the Global Advocacy Council for Physical Activity (see www.globalpa.org.uk). This document is a call for action and an advocacy tool; its aim is to create sustainable opportunities for physically active lifestyles for everyone. Within the Toronto Charter there are nine guiding principles listed for a population-based approach to physical activity. These guiding principles identify the importance of evidence-based approaches, of embracing equity by reducing social and health inequalities or removing disparities in access to physical activity. Importantly, the principles acknowledge the need to move beyond the individual to include environmental and social determinants of physical inactivity. Other principles identify sustainability, a life-course approach to promoting activity, and the need to garner political support and resource commitment at the highest level. Four key action areas are identified; each area makes a unique contribution but also builds and is shaped by the other areas. Each area requires action in partnership, and the actors are listed as government, civil society, academic institutions, professional associations, the private sector, and other organizations as well as the communities themselves.

Area one: Implement a national policy and action plan

The Toronto Charter outlines how the presence of such a policy or plan will unify the many different sectors in working together to achieve a common goal. It also states how it would help clarify political and financial commitment to the promotion of physical activity. Key components of such a policy or plan include: engaging relevant stakeholders, identifying clear leadership, knowing roles and actions of all stakeholders, having an implementation plan that identifies timelines, funding, and accountability. Ensuring that evidence-based guidelines on physical activity and health are adopted and having a repertoire of different strategies that are evidence-informed and inclusive of different social, cultural, and economic backgrounds is also recommended. Even though the Toronto Charter stresses the importance of this area as a key population-based approach, it suggests that the absence of such a policy or plan should not prevent, nor delay, regional, state, or local efforts to increase physical activity or to develop relevant policy at their levels (www.globalpa.org.uk).

Area two: Introduce policies that support physical activity

This area highlights supportive policy and the regulatory environment in which this is placed. It cites examples such as urban planning and design to support sustainable transport options, fiscal policies to subsidize physical activity participation, or educational policies to ensure quality opportunities are provided to all children both within and outside the curriculum timetable at the school setting.

Area three: Reorient services and funding to prioritize physical activity

This area explains how different government sectors can still deliver their core business, but change their priorities to focus on health-enhancing physical activity goals. This would allow for multiple benefits to be achieved, but these would need to be recognized as important and given adequate priority. For example in sport, parks, and recreation, changing the focus away from elite or competitive sport participation to include a mass participation, an inactive or a disabilities focus, and consequently provide staff training to build capacity in these areas. In health this would involve giving greater priority to primary prevention and health promotion, as opposed to secondary or tertiary prevention.

Area four: Develop partnerships for action

Programs that focus on changing health behaviour of individuals within one sector can be labour-, time-, and money-intensive. Rather partnership that links programs across sectors, for example, education, transport, sports, parks, and recreation and other sectors, could create efficiencies, enhance use of community-based physical activity programmes, and increase physical activity (Mowen & Baker, 2009). Examples of different partnerships and collaborations across national, regional, and local levels are given within the Toronto Charter (see www.globalpa.org.uk).

Characteristics of successful physical activity policy

Based on a review of literature and on consensus meetings representing experiences of writing physical activity policies from around the world, a set of characteristics for generating successful physical activity policy were published (Bellew et al., 2008). These criteria, described by the acronym HARDWIRED, are explained in Table 2.1 and reflect the "characteristics absolutely essential for national physical activity policy development" (p. 2). The authors go on to suggest that these need to be embedded for the long term in order to deliver successful outcomes.

Table 2.1 HARDWIRED: Criteria for writing a national physical activity policy

Highly consultative in development (from grassroots to strategic policy makers).

Active through multi-strategic, multi-level partnerships (across government sectors, non-government agencies, and private sector).

Resourced adequately (with stable and suitable financial and human resources).

Developed in stand-alone and synergistic policy modes.

Widely communicated.

Independently evaluated (including process, impact, and outcome indicators of success).

Role-clarified and performance-delineated.

Evidence-informed and evidence-generating.

Defined national guidelines for health-enhancing physical activity.

Source: Adapted from Bellew et al., 2008.

What should countries or states do to promote physical activity?

Global Advocacy for Physical Activity and leading academics and practitioners from around the world reviewed evidence for interventions that were effective in increasing physical activity levels. This review led to the production of a companion document to the Toronto charter titled "Seven investments that work" (www.globalpa.org.uk/investments). These seven approaches are:

1   Whole of school programs in which schoolchildren are encouraged to be active on the journey to and from school, during school break times, and after school and via quality physical education programs at all ages.
2   Transport policies and systems that prioritize walking, cycling, and public transport.
3   Urban design regulations and infrastructure that provide for equitable and safe access for recreational physical activity, and recreational and transport-related walking and cycling across the life course.
4   Physical activity and non-communicable disease prevention integrated into primary healthcare systems.
5   Public education, including mass media, to raise awareness and change social norms on physical activity.
6   Community-wide programs involving multiple settings and sectors and that mobilize and integrate community engagement and resources.
7   Sports systems and programs that promote "sport for all" and encourage participation across the life span.

This document allows educators to argue for resources in their countries to enable the whole of school approach which has evidence of being an effective way of improving health (see www.globalpa.org.uk/investments for supporting references).

Examples of PA policies in action

Bornstein and colleagues published a review of six countries' national physical activity policies. A national physical activity plan was defined as a "comprehensive document that provided overall goals of the country's physical activity plan, details for how the plan was created, policy and/or practice recommendations, and epidemiological evidence to support their recommendations" (Bornstein, Pate, & Pratt, 2009, p. S246). Initial searches yielded 252 documents from 52 countries or regions, but following an inclusion criteria, for example, excluding documents that did not represent one country, a total of six documents from six countries emerged and were included in the review. The countries represented were Australia, United Kingdom, Scotland, Sweden, Northern Ireland, and Norway (Health Promotion Agency for Northern Ireland, 1997; The Strategic Inter-Governmental Forum on Physical Activity and Health, 2005; National Food Administration & National Institute of Public Health, 2005; Scottish National Physical Activity Task Force, 2003; Ministry of Health and Care Services, 2005; UK Department of Health, 2009). In common, all plans included key elements like consultation with key stakeholders; development of coalitions across government, non-government and private sectors; use of individual and environmental strategies for intervention. Most plans were found to be remiss in including details on funding for implementation or evaluation of the plan, two of the key compulsory elements highlighted by Bellew and colleagues (Bellew et al., 2008). Evaluation and review of the plan were conducted by only two countries, Northern Ireland and Scotland respectively.

Bornstein and colleagues (Bornstein et al., 2009) provide an overview of the process that different countries went through in order to develop their physical activity plans. This process gives details on the consultation methodology and/or the relevant national documents that were published prior to the publication of the physical activity plan, but were important in paving the way for the national plan to be adopted. Their paper outlines the subpopulations targeted, for example, people aged 50+ (N. Ireland), children (Australia), and adults (Scotland, Norway), and it provides details on the overall vision and the strategic objectives of each country's plan. The vision statements for each country are different, but include reference to increasing levels of health-related physical activity, to decreasing sedentary or inactive behaviour, to increasing population health and wellbeing through physical activity and to populations enjoying the benefits of physical activity as part of their everyday life. From the vision statements, numerous strategic objectives are highlighted. These objectives are presented under different sector headings including business/industry, education, healthcare, mass media, parks/recreation/fitness/sport, public health, transportation/urban design/ community planning, volunteer and non-profit, and an "other" category. This supports the importance of following the HARDWIRED criteria in order to ensure that all potential partners are engaged in a strategic manner in order to tackle the challenge of inactivity.

Similar findings are reported by the World Health Organization in their recent policy content analysis, "Promoting sport and enhancing health in European Union (EU) countries" (World Health Organization, 2011). Twenty-five national documents from 15 EU member states were identified from a total of 130 documents (27 EU member states) as meeting the inclusion criteria. These were analysed, and it was found that they were issued mainly by government ministries (for example, education, culture and sport, health, welfare, or local government), had a specified timeframe (this varied from two to 20 years) and gave some information on the policy development process (although the quality of this information was mixed, ranging from alluding to a consultation process through to a detailed account of all stakeholders and the approach taken to engage these key groups). They also had defined participation targets that covered the continuum from elite sport to sport for all and to health-enhancing physical activity. Target groups, settings, and implementation strategies were presented, for example, children were targeted in all strategies, mainly in the school setting and through physical education (p. 32). WHO highlighted the Dutch strategy "Time for Sport" as an example of good practice for budget allocation. Under its focus "Participation through

Sport" it allocated a specific budget for each target set, for example, "Education through sport and school," one of six areas under this focus was allocated a budget of C1.5 million per year for a total of five years to achieve its objectives (World Health Organization, 2011, p. 36). One critique by WHO was that although most of the documents analyzed mentioned evaluation, the specific evaluation information provided along with measurable outcome indicators was varied and quite often absent. Adhering to a "HARDWIRED" criteria would stress the importance of evaluation, and ideally the independent quality of this evaluation.

Will these policies help educators?

We have already pointed out that the existence of global or national policies can help educators argue for resources, provide evidence for approaches that are effective, and provide a framework for monitoring progress. However, the efficacy of such an intervention strategy is yet to be determined (Hoehner et al., 2008; Mowen & Baker, 2009). Evaluating whether or not policy has been effective in this regard is not straightforward, and change can be attributed to many causes. We will use examples from our own countries—Scotland and Ireland—to show how different approaches, one based on policy, the other lack of policy, have potential impact for provision of physical education within the school setting.

In Scotland, a national policy was agreed by all political parties in 2003. The policy was entitled "let's make Scotland more active." The policy had a broad aim of increasing the proportion of people in Scotland leading physically active lives. In particular, the policy set a target for 2022 of 50 per cent of adults and 80 per cent of children meeting the minimum levels of physical activity for health gain. Several priorities emerged, including children and young people. One part of the policy suggested that all schools (from nursery to senior) should provide a minimum of two hours of quality physical education in curriculum time each week and adopt a "whole of school" approach to helping children achieve a minimum of 60 minutes of activity each day. In 2005, it was reported that less than 5 per cent of schools achieved the minimum of two hours of physical education. However, in 2010 the percentage of schools providing the two hours of physical education had risen to 50 per cent. While it is difficult to say that the policy caused this change in time spent in physical education, it is also difficult to see alternative explanations for the observed increase. The national policy for physical activity in Scotland preceded a review of the whole school curriculum (including all subjects, not just physical education or health education) and in forming our new approach "the curriculum for excellence" a health and well-being strand was informed by the need for physical activity in general and also for quality physical education in primary and secondary schools. Education Scotland has in turn supplied in-service courses and on line resources to help head teachers, class room teachers, and physical education teachers deliver this health and wellbeing strand of the new curriculum. In this way, education policy was influenced by global and national policy and appears to have had a positive effect on the percentage of schools providing the minimum requirement of two hours of physical education. To achieve this, more specialist physical education teachers have been trained and more curriculum resources have been provided. The policy was reviewed in 2009 by a panel of independent experts. The conclusions from the review were that the policy was still relevant and the 2022 targets could be met if efforts were sustained and refined. Refinements included more attention to segments of the population seen from National Health Survey data to be making slow progress towards the 2022 targets. Two particular target groups were noted: older adults and adolescent girls. This re-statement of the policy and refinement of target groups may help deliver the increased physical activity goals for Scotland and may also influence how schools tackle the low levels of activity for adolescent girls in particular. As a result of the review a summit was organized involving educators, local service providers, practitioners, and academics to make suggestions on how to improve activity levels for adolescent girls within and beyond school (www.paha.org.uk/Resource/teenage-girls-physical-activity-summit). This is another example of how educators can benefit from physical activity policy.

In Ireland, no national physical activity policy exists. Consequently, a national vision for physical activity with clear goals, a strategic plan of action, an identification of resources, partners, nor evaluation mechanisms exist. There are many policy documents within different government sectors that identify physical activity promotion as part of their agenda. The "Ready, Steady, Play! A national play policy" (National Children's Office, 2004) outlines the need "to plan for an increase in public play facilities and thereby improve quality of life of children living in Ireland, providing them with more quality play opportunities" (p. 8). The Department of Transport's policy for Ireland 2009–2020 encourages schools to adopt "active travel plans," advocates for "a strong cycling culture in the cities, towns, villages, and rural areas of Ireland" (Department of Transport, 2009, p. 42) and "Teenspace: A national recreation policy—12–18 year olds" has, as its second objective, the "need to develop increased opportunities for dance and physical activity, and tackle gender issues around provision in sport" (Office for the Minister of Children and Youth Affairs, 2007). However, without a "clear stand along/single issue physical activity policy statement" (Bellew et al., 2008, p. 2) these related strands of physical activity policy embedded within other agendas may be less effective. Without the backing of a national physical activity policy, within which there is a defined role for education (particularly physical education), then it is more difficult to convince decision makers of its contribution, need, and importance. In 2010, a working group was set up by the Health Services Executive (HSE), and its purpose was to provide the Department of Health and Children with an initial draft national physical activity plan. Membership of this group included representatives from the sectors of health, transport, education, environment, sport, local authorities, non-governmental organizations, and academics. It was chaired by the HSE. The academics on the working group were invited from three different third-level institutions in the Republic of Ireland and one from the North of Ireland to provide a whole-island approach to the promotion of physical activity. The academics represented the areas of sport and exercise science, physical activity, and public health and physical education teacher education. Their role was to provide scientific information and to lead on the writing of the draft plan. This important advocacy opportunity, although outside the academic remit of research or teaching, provided a unique chance to ensure that current scientific information was available to a key group of policy decision makers from a number of different government sectors in Ireland. Information provided included the evidence base for why physical activity is an important public health issue, statistics on the prevalence of physical activity and inactivity in Ireland (and compared to other countries), advice on the recommended minimum amounts of physical activity necessary for health benefit and perspective on current capacity in physical education, sport, and physical activity and on the need for evidence-based intervention in different areas was highlighted. The role of quality physical education was clearly documented and is included in the draft plan, along with the need to provide children and young people with a broad range of opportunities to engage in physical activity outside of school, recommendations relevant to other sectors are also present. The first draft of the national physical activity plan is with the HSE, and it is hoped that it will influence the writing of the current national public health policy by strengthening the inclusion of physical activity as a determinant of health. The challenge will be to ensure that it is circulated widely to all key stakeholders, for example physical education teachers, coaches, parents, architects, engineers, planners, urban designers, and so on, for consideration and feedback prior to finalization, consistent with the HARDWIRED criteria. Upon completion of the consultation, an implementation plan will then need to be drawn up.

Conclusion

In conclusion, this paper has provided an overview of what a physical activity policy is, why it is important, and key criteria that can influence the success of such a document. Recent physical activity policy documents have been referenced, and two case studies discussed. The policy space that any country devotes to the physical activity needs of its citizens is varied; good policy does not guarantee better resources, but it has the potential to influence practice through formal written codes, regulations, or standards to guide choices. Consequently, policy has the potential to increase the likelihood that quality physical education is offered to all children and young people, that opportunities to be active are enhanced through urban design, planning, and transport policies that facilitate active modes of travel, that national targets are set, monitored, and evaluated ensuring accountability is determined. Ultimately, a national or state physical activity policy has the potential to increase the likelihood that the physical, social, and mental wellbeing that can be achieved through regular health-enhancing physical activity for all the population is achieved. The role of the academic in this development is clear; they need to be able to produce good scientific evidence—found in physical education, physiology, psychology, public health, planning, and transport, etc.—into meaningful advice and recommendations for the key policy makers in the various government sectors in order to ensure that the potential of physical activity in the promotion of health (in its broadest sense) is realized.

This chapter has been adapted from: Woods, C. B. & Mutrie, N. (2012). Putting physical activity on the policy agenda. *Quest, 64*(2), 92–104, DOI: 10.1080/00336297.2012.669318.

References

Bellew, B., Schoppe, S., Bull, F. C., & Bauman, A. (2008). The rise and fall of Australian physical activity policy 1996–2006: A national review framed in an international context. *Australia and New Zealand Health Policy, 5*(18), 1–10.

Bornstein, D. B., Pate, R. R., & Pratt, M. (2009). A review of the national physical activity plans of six countries. *Journal of Physical Activity and Health, 6*(S2), S245–S264.

Bull, F., Bellew, B., Schoppe, S., & Bauman, A. (2004). Developments in national physical activity policy: An international review and recommendations towards better practice. *Journal of Science and Medicine in Sport, 7*(1), S93–S104.

Caspersen, C., Powell, K. E., & Christenson, G. (1985). Physical activity, exercise and physical fitness: Definitions and distinctions for health-related research. *Public Health Reports, 100*(2), 126–131.

Centers for Disease Control and Prevention (2003). Prevalence of physical activity, including lifestyle activities among adults—United States, 2000–2001. *MMWR, 5*(32), 764–769.

Chief Medical Officers (2011). *Start active, stay active: A report on the physical activity for health from the four home countries.* London: UK Department of Health.

Currie, C. E., NiGabhainn, S., Godeau, E., Roberts, C., Smith, R., & Currie, D. (2008). *Inequalities in young people's health: HBSC international report from 2005–2006 survey.* Edinburgh: HBSC International Coordinating Centre, World Health Organization.

Department of Health and Children (2009). *The national physical activity guidelines for Ireland.* Dublin: The Stationary Office.

Department of Transport (2009). *Smarter travel: A sustainable transport future. A new transport policy for Ireland 2009–2020.* Dublin: Department of Transport.

Flegal, K., Carrol, M., Ogden, C., & Curtin, L. (2010). Prevalence and trends in obesity among US adults, 1999–2008. *Journal of the American Medical Association, 303*(3), 235–241.

Hardman, K. (2008). Physical education in schools: A global perspective. *Kinesiology, 40*(1), 5–28.

Health Promotion Agency for Northern Ireland (1997). *Physical activity: An investment in public health. The Northern Ireland Physical Activity Strategy Action Plan 1998–2002*. Belfast: HPANI.

Heath, G. W., Brownson, R. C., Kruger, J., Miles, R., Powell, K. E., Ramsey, L. T., et al. (2006). The effectiveness of urban design and land use and transport policies and practices to increase physical activity: A systematic review. *Journal of Physical Activity and Health, 3*(S1), S55–S76.

Hoehner, C. M., Soares, S., Perez, D., Riberio, I. C., Joshu, C. E., & Pratt, M. (2008). Physical activity interventions in Latin America: A systematic review. *American Journal of Preventive Medicine, 34*(3), 224–233.

King, A. C., & Sallis, J. F. (2009). Why and how to improve physical activity promotion: Lessons from behavioral science and related fields. *Preventive Medicine, 49*(4), 286–288.

Leyden, K. M., Reger-Nash, B., Bauman, A., & Bias, T. (2008). Changing the hearts and minds of policy makers: An exploratory study associated with the West Virginia Walks Campaign. *American Journal of Health Promotion, 22*(3), 204–207.

Mathers, C., Stevens, G., & Mascarenhas, M. (2009). *Mortality and burden of disease attributable to selected major risks*. Geneva: World Health Organization.

Ministry of Health and Care Services (2005). *The action plan on physical activity 2005–2009. Working together for physical activity*. Norway: Ministry of Health and Care Services.

Mowen, A. J., & Baker, B. L. (2009). Park, recreation, fitness and sport sector recommendations for a more physically active America: A white paper for the United States National Physical Activity Plan. *Journal of Physical Activity and Health, 6*(S2), S236–S244.

Mutrie, N., & Woods, C. B. (2003). How can we get people to become more active? A problem waiting to be solved. In J. McKenna & C. Riddoch (Eds.), *Perspectives on health and exercise* (1st ed., p. 129–152). Basingstoke, UK: Palgrave Macmillan.

National Children's Office (2004). *Ready, steady, play! A national play policy*. Dublin: National Children's Office.

National Food Administration & National Institute of Public Health (2005). *Background material to the action plan for healthy dietary habits and increased physical activity*. Uppsala, Sweden: National Food Administration.

OECD (2010). *Health at a glance: Europe 2010*. OECD Publishing. Retrieved from www.oecd.org/

Office for the Minister of Children and Youth Affairs (2007). *Teenspace: A national recreation policy for young people*. Dublin: Minister for Children and Youth Affairs.

Pratt, M., Epping, J. N., & Dietz, W. H. (2009). Putting physical activity into public health: A historical perspective from the CDC. *Preventive Medicine, 49*(4), 301–302.

Sallis, J., Owen, N., & Fisher, E. B. (2008). Ecological models of health behavior. In K. Glanz, B. K. Rimer, & K. Viswanath (Eds.), *Health behavior and health education. Theory, research and practice* (4th ed.). San Francisco, CA: Jossey-Bass.

Schmid, T., Pratt, M., & Witmer, L. (2006). A framework for physical activity policy research. *Journal of Physical Activity and Health, 3*(1), S20–S29.

Scottish National Physical Activity Task Force (2003). *Let's make Scotland more active: A strategy for physical activity*. Edinburgh: Scottish Executive.

The Strategic Inter-Governmental Forum on Physical Activity and Health (2005). *National public health partnership, Be Active Australia: A framework for health sector action for physical activity 2005–2010*. Melbourne, Australia: National Public Health Partnership.

UK Department of Health (2004). *At least five a week: Evidence on the impact of physical activity and its relationship to health. A report from the Chief Medical Officer*. London: Department of Health.

UK Department of Health (2009). *Be active, be healthy: A plan for getting the nation moving*. London: Department of Health.

United Nations General Assembly (2011). Political declaration of the high-level meeting of the general assembly on the prevention and control of non-communicable diseases, p. 1–12. Retrieved from www.globalpa.org.uk/.

U.S. Department of Health and Human Services (2008). *Physical activity guidelines for Americans*. Retrieved from www.health.gov/paguidelines/.

World Health Organization (1986). *The Ottawa charter for health promotion*. Retrieved from www.euro.who.int/pubrequest/.

World Health Organization (2003). *Health and development through physical activity and sport*. Geneva: World Health Organization. Retrieved from www.euro.who.int/pubrequest/.

World Health Organization (2004). *Resolution WHA57.17. Global strategy on diet, physical activity, and health. In: Fifty-seventy World Health Assembly, Geneva, 17–22 May 2004. Resolutions and decisions, annexes*. Geneva: World Health Organization. Retrieved from www.euro.who.int/pubrequest/.

World Health Organization (2008). *2008–2013 Action plan for the global strategy for the prevention and control of noncommunicable diseases*. Geneva: World Health Organization. Retrieved from www.euro.who.int/pubrequest/.

World Health Organization (2010a). *Global recommendations on physical activity for health*. Geneva: World Health Organization. Retrieved from www.euro.who.int/pubrequest/.

World Health Organization (2010b). *Review of physical activity promotion policy development and legislation in European Union Member States* (Rep. No. 10). Copenhagen: World Health Organization. Retrieved from www.euro.who.int/pubrequest/.

World Health Organization (2011). *Promoting sport and enhancing health in European Union countries: A policy content analysis to support action*. Copenhagen: World Health Organization Regional Office for Europe. Retrieved from www.euro.who.int/pubrequest/.

3

THE GLOBAL PHYSICAL INACTIVITY PANDEMIC

An analysis of knowledge production

Joe Piggin and Alan Bairner

Introduction

The promotion of health is inherently political, and it is well established that the causes of and solutions to all social problems are contested through rhetoric, discourse and narrative (Petersen and Lupton, 1996; Stone, 2002). Roe (1994) describes the importance of 'meta-narratives' in constructing a hegemonic approach to a specific policy issue. A metanarrative is a dominant story that is developed over time by one or more parties involved in the social problem. These stories are used to establish and stabilise the assumptions for policymaking in response to the issue's uncertainty, complexity or polarisation (Roe, 1994).

One recent metanarrative is the *global physical inactivity pandemic*, an important contribution to which is *The Lancet* Physical Activity Series (*The Lancet*, 2012). This both defines and actively constructs how 'we' (the scientific and academic communities at least and the human population at most) should think about physical activity. Understanding more about the production dynamics of physical activity knowledge is important for various reasons. How any pandemic is framed will have important consequences for proposed health outcomes and the distribution of various resources. Any such problem requires that action is taken, whether this is in the form of government funding to address the problem, new laws to decrease the prevalence of the problem or the modification of a population's behaviour to minimise the problem (Parsons, 1995). As a lobbying tool, the pandemic is potentially very powerful, since a significant amount of resources might be directed towards measuring, scrutinising and encouraging people to behave in particular ways and for particular reasons. The ideas espoused might also govern how a range of organisations use physical activity, and influence how agents and causes are (re)framed. Further, ideas about physical activity can impact on how individuals think about the activities in which they partake and also about their own and others' bodies.

This research builds on the growing attention given to the various narratives and discourses through which physical activity policies and programmes are used to nudge (Vallgårda, 2011), police (Piggin, Jackson and Lewis, 2007), empower (Bercovitz, 1998), inspire (Evans, 2013), exhort (Garvin and Eyles, 1997), intervene (Mansfield and Rich, 2013) and educate (Gard and Wright, 2001). It is also situated at a specific moment with regard to the obesity epidemic. Gard (2011: 4) contends that the obesity epidemic is essentially over: 'by 2010 a new phase in the obesity epidemic had been reached, marking the end of a period of consciousness raising or hyperbole . . . and a transitioning to something else'. That 'something else', we argue, is the physical inactivity pandemic. This new problem shifts the focus from what we are, to how we act.

Some focus has also been directed towards the ways in which ideas about public health pandemics are produced and framed (Abeysinghe and White, 2010; 2011). In research on a recent flu pandemic policy, Holmes (2010: iii) concluded that 'despite a history of critical research on constructions of disease, social sciences literature on pandemics is primarily practical'. Holmes's research concluded that a variety of discursive elements, including active language and statistics, recalling the past as key to the future, reference to expert knowledge and conferring moral responsibility on the public to feel at risk constructed a pandemic flu as inevitable, significant and manageable. Regarding the framing of health debates, recent research has focused on contests between public health organisations and corporations, for example in relation to obesity (Kwan, 2009; Jenkin, Signal and Thomson, 2011; Kim and Willis, 2007). Some research exists regarding the messages of physical activity policies. In the Australian policy context Fullagar (2002) examined health promotion campaigns with regard to the rationalities and ethics through which individuals are encouraged to govern their own healthy lifestyle practices in the name of freedom. In particular she examined the ways in which individuals may come to govern their own subjectivity through 'healthy' lifestyles and leisure practices. This current research builds on Fullagar's work in two ways. First, we extend the analysis to investigate ideas which inform physical activity promotion at a global level. Second, we incorporate the increasingly diverse interest groups beyond state governments which seek to change the behaviour of populations. The lobbying potential of physical activity scholars is considered explicitly.

In order to understand more about the physical activity narratives involved and the rhetoric that sustains them, this research focuses its attention on a specific case study which has produced a declaration of a global physical inactivity pandemic. We explore how knowledge is created about physical activity in the prestigious and influential medical journal, *The Lancet*. We examine the knowledge produced about physical activity with the following questions in mind. What ideas about physical activity are foregrounded? Are these ideas coherent? Are these ideas always appropriate? The way in which facts are disseminated is also important to consider. Petersen and Lupton (1996: 33) note that 'like other scientific facts, epidemiological facts gain their credence from being published in scholarly journals, in which process the historical and sociocultural dimensions of their construction . . . are effectively hidden'. In the case of the *Lancet* series on physical activity, the journal's reputation as a renowned health publication bestows a sense of legitimacy upon the claims made. It is these hidden and possibly unaccounted-for dynamics of construction that we attempt to illuminate here. It is not our goal to construct a perfect, coherent story about the history and meaning of physical activity. Rather, by exposing misrepresentations and contradictions by world leading experts involved in *The Lancet*, we might first encourage scepticism about grand proclamations and, second, open space to develop a critical and ethical approach to physical activity promotion.

Research approach

Given the purported multidimensional nature of the physical inactivity pandemic, the current study merges a variety of methodological perspectives. Our theoretical framework is broadly informed by writings on governmentality (Foucault 1994; Rose, 1990; Rose and Miller,

1992; Markula and Pringle, 2006). Foucault (1994) uses governmentality to describe the regulation of individuals' lives, which involves procedures, analyses, calculations and tactics that allow for the exercise of power through the governing of others. Rose (1990: xxii) goes on to note that it is through these interlocking apparatuses for the programming of various dimensions of life that we are 'urged, incited, encouraged, exhorted and motivated to act'. Rose and Miller (1992: 174) assert that these various forms of power are used by governments to ensure citizens believe in 'a kind of regulated freedom'. By understanding more about these dynamics (with particular regard to physical activity), one can begin to either support or question the impact of such espoused meanings and interventions in the lives of citizens. Propositions such as those put forward in *The Lancet* about physical activity provide a significant moment to examine 'a whole complex of knowledges' (Foucault, 1994: 220). In examining the text of various *Lancet* articles, we are also guided by critical health psychology (Hepworth, 2006) and an adapted policy-as-discourse perspective (Bacchi, 2000), both of which interrogate the construction processes and outcomes in the realm of public policy. While *The Lancet* is not official public policy, we consider its global reputation sufficient to warrant its 'official' pronouncements of pandemics as authoritative.

A specific set of documents is analysed, and is limited to *The Lancet* Physical Activity Series published in July 2012. The *Series* consists of five 'comments', one 'article' and five further articles under the heading 'Series'. The selection of these articles for analysis is considered and deliberate, since it captures the moment of the announcement of the physical activity pandemic, the description of the 'landscape' in which to address the pandemic, the proposed actions that are needed and the important actors and institutions.

The data analysis involved a number of stages. An initial, cursory reading of the Physical Activity Series revealed numerous tensions and inconsistencies. This was the catalyst for a formal study, whereby the researchers systematically and critically read the *Lancet* articles. The 'critical' lens came from the researchers comparing and contrasting claims made in *The Lancet* against one another. As well as this, the researchers juxtaposed various claims with other ways of thinking about population health, which might disrupt the ostensibly unproblematic, positive claims about physical activity and health. That is, the researchers examined the continuity, coherence and appropriateness of ideas that emanate from *The Lancet* about physical activity. Following this, in line with the governmentality theme, the issues were then shortlisted and examined in detail with regard to how they might impact on health promoters' and citizens' understandings of physical activity.

Ultimately, the aim of undertaking this analysis is to disrupt the taken-for-granted assumptions and 'facts' which 'govern' the ideas presented in *The Lancet* before any major policy initiatives are rolled out in order to combat physical inactivity. Not only may these result in the inefficient distribution of scarce resources, but potentially harm citizens' understandings about physical activity. To paraphrase Pringle and Pringle (2012), in this study we critique the validity of the truth claims surrounding physical activity while also drawing on the notion of 'health' as justification for rejecting some of the ideas proposed.

Context: *The Lancet* and the global physical inactivity pandemic

According to its own website, *The Lancet* journal is an authoritative voice in global medicine. With an 'impact factor' of 38.28 at the time of writing, which is amongst the highest of all academic journals, it is clearly influential in the medical community. In July 2012, *The Lancet* published a *Series* of physical activity commentaries and articles about the physical inactivity pandemic and called for a 'social revolution . . . towards an active physical and mental life'

(Das and Horton, 2012: 189–190).[1] The global significance of physical inactivity was highlighted on numerous occasions. The pandemic is said to be affecting all nations in the world (Das and Horton, 2012). According to the *Series*, 'physical inactivity is the fourth leading cause of death worldwide' (Kohl et al., 2012: 294) and is said to be responsible for '6–10% of all deaths from the major NCDs. . . . [and] more than 5.3% of the 57 million deaths that occurred worldwide in 2008' (Lee at al., 2012: 219).

While the *Lancet Series* contains much large-scale quantitative data about the benefits of physical activity, it also includes a significant amount of rhetoric and argumentation to shape the physical inactivity pandemic. Claiming that physical inactivity is 'pandemic' is an important moment in health promotion discourse. It suggests a rhetorical and policy shift in attention away from physical inactivity being a component of the 'obesity epidemic', thereby requiring alterations in how population health is perceived and addressed by a range of stakeholders.

The call to action that culminates in *The Lancet* requires a wide array of organisations in every nation to change their practices, including transnational organisations such as the UN and WHO, national governments, companies, voluntary organisations and academics and individuals. By considering the growing field of physical activity scholarship as a potent policy domain, this current research examines how the problem of the pandemic is rhetorically constructed and how solutions are proposed.

Analysis: The disunity of what is known about physical activity

First we examine what is claimed to be known about physical activity by the various authors of the *Series* and by so doing we uncover what is contested. In the first commentary, Das and Horton (2012: 189) state that the goal of the Series (and the 'first step' in this social revolution towards active physical lives) had been 'to assemble the best experts in the field and the *best evidence* to understand what we know about the relationship between human health and physical activity' (italics added). However, with regard to establishing what we know about human health and physical activity, it is demonstrably apparent in the *Series* that, in fact, there is much confusion about what 'we' (the scientific community) know.

On the first page of the *Series*, Das and Horton (2012: 189) claim that 'unlike other NCD risk factors . . . *the importance of physical activity has been slow to be recognised*' (italics added). However, this is difficult to reconcile with a statement on the second page, where Hallal et al. (2012:190) claim that '*[f]or millennia, exercise has been recommended by physicians and scholars*' (italics added). Other disparate claims are made. Wen and Wu (2012: 192) assert that *'[exercise] receives little respect from doctors or society'* (italics added), whereas Heath et al. (2012: 272) state that '*[i]nterventions to increase physical activity in whole populations are now prominent* with community-based informational, behavioural, social, policy, and environmental approaches' (italics added). For this range of oscillating statements regarding societal knowledge and action about physical activity and exercise to be made within the first few pages of one of the world's leading medical journals is particularly problematic. Specifically, this poses a problem for establishing a starting point for addressing the pandemic. If much is known about physical activity and many interventions are in place, then any policy action would surely differ vastly from a situation where physical activity has little respect and where interventions are lacking.

To be clear, we do not believe that these statements are intended to be contrary. At no point do the authors argue against one another over these claims. The remarks appear independently throughout the *Series* as common-sense claims which then lead to suggestions for policy and practice changes. However, when compared, rather than articulating *what is known* about physical activity, these equivocal statements would leave readers wondering about the importance of physical activity, the extent to which exercise is respected by society/ies and about the prominence of interventions.

The multifarious claims, while usually presented as common sense and even banal, set the tone for the ambition to rid the world of the pandemic. If we are to regard *The Lancet*'s reputation sufficient to proclaim the emergence of a physical inactivity pandemic, it appears problematic that such contrary statements would be published. To be clear, both authors of this article suggest that physically active lifestyles are worthy of promotion to populations around the world and appreciate that disagreement is often the way that scientific understanding moves forward. However, the contradictory claims inherent within *The Lancet* should be attended to with rigor consistent with that of the accompanying statistical analyses which are intended to provide evidence to justify the pandemic. If a history of physical activity and exercise is to be offered in *The Lancet*, more rigorous research about the claims that are made should be undertaken.

Perhaps even more problematic than the aforementioned ambiguity is the claim by Kohl et al. (2012: 302) that a '*complete understanding* of all stakeholders, their interactions, and how their interactions make up the whole is crucial to understanding of the systems that impede progress on physical activity' (italics added). While we believe the goal of attaining 'complete understanding' is ultimately futile, it is disturbing that this would be a goal at all. We ask, what does 'complete' mean in the physical activity domain? What knowledge about individuals is 'fair game' for physical activity researchers pursuing this goal? What surveillance techniques might be utilised to attain this 'complete understanding'? Where do individual rights fit in with such a plan? We argue these questions must be given attention by physical activity scholars, particularly since ideas about surveillance also feature prominently in the *Series*.

The attempted rewriting of the history of physical activity

Numerous statements in the *Series* use both recent and 'ancient' history as important reference points to justify focusing on physical activity. However, many of these claims fail to contain sufficient rigor in their production. In an article that provides much statistical evidence for a physical activity revolution, Lee et al. (2012: 219, italics added) write:

> Ancient physicians – including those from China in 2600 BC and Hippocrates around 400 BC – believed in the value of physical activity for health. By the 20th century, however, a diametrically opposite view – that exercise was dangerous – *prevailed instead*.

This claim uses various rhetorical devices to create a powerful narrative about physical activity. It invokes the wisdom of the 'Ancients' from Greece and China and suggests that their espousal of health practices had somehow been usurped and subjugated by forces not identified in the text. This is a powerful story of decline whereby 'in the beginning, things were pretty good. But they got worse. In fact, they are nearly intolerable. Something must be done' (Stone, 2002: 138). However, we argue this narrative is both inaccurate and is itself also used by other authors in the *Series* to propagate further misrepresentations.

First, it is unreasonable to use the 20th century as the time during which scepticism about exercise prevailed. Further it is inaccurate to claim that an opposing view 'prevailed *instead*'. Tracing the literature that Lee et al. use to support their own claim illuminates this. The evidence offered for the 'prevailing' view that 'exercise was dangerous' originated from a *British Medical Journal* article by Rook (1954) which reported on an investigation into 'the longevity of Cambridge sportsmen'. The article by Rook claimed that '*[m]any observers, both in ancient and in more modern times*, have pointed out the alleged dangers of such activities' (p. 774, italics added). In turn, Rook cites Hartley and Llewellyn (1939) who wrote that concerns have existed about strenuous exercise since 'the earliest times' (p. 657). These historical debates, both ancient and recent, about the concerns about exercise are omitted by Lee et al. in favour of a more dramatic, though inaccurate, narrative.

The transformation of the narrative continues, when Wen and Wu use the claims by Lee et al. as a reference in the assertion that '[s]ocially, being inactive is perceived as normal, and in fact doctors order patients to remain on bed rest far more often than they encourage exercise' (p. 192). This is inaccurate in two respects. First, Lee et al. do not claim that 'being inactive is perceived as normal'. Second, Lee et al. *actually* write that '[d]uring the early 20th century, complete bed rest was prescribed for patients with acute myocardial infarction' (p. 219) which is totally incongruent with Wen and Wu's assertion. We argue that it is important that the narrative regarding physical activity promotion does not include dramatic statements such as 'in fact doctors order patients to remain on bed rest far more often than they encourage exercise' without supporting evidence. The problematic climax to this series of inaccuracies is the claim by Wen and Wu that '[t]his passive attitude towards inactivity, where exercise is viewed as a personal choice, is anachronistic, and is reminiscent of the battles still being fought over smoking' (p. 192). This view is derived from a series of misrepresentations by various authors within *The Lancet*, and therefore should be treated with scepticism. These narratives are powerful to the extent that they attempt to justify the research that follows. The simplifications and misrepresentations suggest a need for a more critical approach by physical activity scholars to understanding what societies *do* think about physical activity. We argue that these grand proclamations require more rigorous consideration by the various researchers in the first instance and more scrutiny by editors and reviewers of *The Lancet* in the second.

The rhetorical technique of nostalgically referencing a bygone age is also apparent in another aspect of *The Lancet*. The cover page of the *Lancet Series* is adorned with an image (which is repeated on the first page) of a painting of what appears to be children playing. Indeed the painting is called *Children's Games (Kinderspiele)* from 1560, by Pieter Bruegel. The image portrays a town square full of young people playing both outside and in the surrounding buildings. We suggest the intention of including the image (twice) is to imply that populations have indeed neglected or forgotten the goodness of games.

A cursory analysis of *Children's Games*, however, reveals various activities which would surely be deemed detrimental to physical or mental health today. They include a child poking and stirring what appears to be excrement with a stick, someone urinating only a few metres from where others are playing, a group of children kicking the legs of others, another group seemingly manhandling an uncooperative person and a child being bullied by having their hair pulled by a group of others.[2] We suggest it is unlikely this image would have been purposefully selected had this range of health-diminishing activities been recognised. Regarding the interpretation of these images, we are not arguing against the wide variety of benefits that come from different types of physical activity. We are drawing attention to the various, often contradictory ideas about what 'physical activity' involves. That is, it is clear that both hundreds of years ago and currently, the realm of physical activity involves more than 'brisk walking'.

Also on the first page is a quote from the 'ancient' Plato which reads '[l]ack of activity destroys the good condition of every human being while movement and methodical physical exercise save it and preserve it'. Both the quote and a general view of the painting promote a naïvely nostalgic view of what life used to be like and advocate a return to particular traditional ideas and practices of yesteryear. It is interesting to note that the origins of nostalgia are to be found in medicine itself. As Boym (2007: 7) points out:

> It would not occur to us to demand a prescription for nostalgia. Yet in the seventeenth century nostalgia was considered to be a curable disease, akin to a severe common cold. Swiss doctors believed that opium, leeches, and a journey to the Swiss Alps would take care of nostalgic symptoms.

Whilst we would not promote such remedies, we do agree with Boym's (2007: 9–10) claim that '[t]he danger of nostalgia is that it tends to confuse the actual home with the imaginary one', in this case the past, in which premature death was a fact of life, and the imagined past in which children were physically active and, as a result, healthy.

In many cases generalisations about yesteryear and 'the Ancients' are relied upon to contextualise the issue under discussion. However, we argue that such grand summations simplify the debated and contested history of thought about physical activity. Of course, these arguments are not the main focus of the *Lancet* articles. Historical anecdotes are mostly offered as introductions to the research and policy suggestions that follow. However, this 'scene setting' is important when considering the range of claims that are made about what is, or is not appropriate physical activity. Despite these contrary statements mentioned above, as rhetorical devices, all of the claims contribute to a narrative that something must be done. In the course of doing so, the claims rule in and rule out certain types of action and certain types of knowledges which can be used to regulate the behaviour of a population. This is explored in the next section.

Abnormal, design and failure: The politics of regulating populations

In both subtle and explicit ways, particular types of physical activity are promoted and marginalised in *The Lancet*. Foucault referred to these as dividing practices; 'the judges of normality are present everywhere. We're in the society of the teacher-judge, the doctor-judge ... It is on them that the universal reign of the normative is based' (Foucault, 1979: 304). Here we consider which ideas are promoted as acceptable (or 'normal') in the *Series*.

In the final call to action, Kohl et al. claim that '[t]he freedom and opportunity for individuals to participate in physical activity should be viewed as a basic human right' (p. 300). 'Freedom' is a wholly worthwhile principle, and in one significant way, it is addressed in a *Series* article by Rimmer and Marques entitled 'Physical activity for people with disabilities' (2012: 193). Rimmer and Marques propose that more is done to promote physical activity for the more than one billion people worldwide who have disabilities. However, while ideas about 'freedom' and 'rights' do feature, there are also other ideas which work against these ideas. For example, there are instances where 'normality' is referred to in a way which deviates from other, more inclusive discourse. We focus our attention in particular on Wen and Wu's (2012, p. 193, italics added) suggestion that

> In addition to doctors' traditional advocacy of the health benefits of exercise, stressing the harms of inactivity could strengthen our battle against inactivity. *We need to view the inactive population as abnormal* and consider them at high risk of disease.[3]

We argue that describing people as 'abnormal' when considering physical activity promotion is wholly inappropriate. This idea is particularly worrying. The plethora of literature which exists around problematic aspects of the obesity epidemic alone should alert us to the possibility of stigma associated with being labelled as inactive (see Gard and Wright, 2005; Puhl, 2011; Puhl and King, 2013). In their *Lancet* text, Wen and Wu (2012, p. 192, italics added) also state:

> To individuals, *the failure* to spend 15–30 min a day in brisk walking increases the risk of cancer, heart disease, stroke, and diabetes by 20–30%, and shortens lifespan by 3–5 years.

In a similarly normative manner, Das and Horton (2012, p. 189) state that the *Series* is concerned with

> using the body that we have in the way it was designed, which is to walk often, run sometimes, and move in ways where we physically exert ourselves regularly whether that is at work, at home, in transport to and from places, or during leisure time in our daily lives.

These quotes are concerning for two reasons. First, using '15–30 min a day in brisk walking' is overly normative, and does not reflect the range of disabilities which people around the world face. Any promotion of physical activity should extend to people who, for a wide variety of reasons, can neither walk nor run. Second, the idea that individuals 'fail' at this task is in total opposition to a systems approach advocated by many of the authors in the *Series* who focus more on structural factors.[4] In light of the significant attention given to promoting surveillance within the *Series*, we urge reflection with regard to people who, no matter how they were 'designed', do not obey these normative descriptions and prescriptions. There is surely space for physical activity scholars to produce more inclusive definitions of what physical activity can be. These definitions should take into account ideas about diversity of movement as well as the diverse meanings attached to physical activity. Scholars in physical education and pedagogy have demonstrated time and again that they are willing to be self-critical and to examine new ways in which physical activity amongst young people can be increased and improved (see Quennerstedt, 2008). As Stidder (2013: 19) notes, 'critical self-reflection and pedagogy through the use of reflexivity in physical education can contextualise and illustrate various topics of educational debate as well as inform research and provide the impetus for innovation and change'. There is little evidence to date of such self-analysis amongst the overwhelming majority of physical activity scholars who might consider the evidence base for some of their espoused truths.

Foucault writes that there are powerful effects of claims about normality: 'each individual, wherever he (sic) may find himself, subjects to [normative ideas] his body, his gestures, his behavior, his aptitudes, his achievements' (Foucault, 1979: 304). While regular physical activity might indeed contribute to healthy, able bodies, physical activity scholars would benefit from integrating the diversity of human life more fully into their proclamations. There is space in the domain of physical activity policy 'for further consideration with respect to how to talk about the fit body' (Neville, 2013: 490).

Olympic legacy claims: Denial, lamentation or praiseworthy?

While many organisations are integrated into *The Lancet*'s call to action, there is a significant amount of attention given to the International Olympic Committee and the Olympic Games.

Throughout the *Series* however, it is clear that there is much contention about the value of the Olympic Games in promoting physical activity. This case study of rhetoric about the Olympic Games demonstrates that even though various *Lancet* authors promote a systems approach, the complexity of any issue can become so great as to stifle any positive action. Hallal et al. (2012, p. 190, italics added) unequivocally claim that

> The popularity of the Olympic Games and elite sports such as professional soccer *has not been, and will not be, translated into mass participation in exercise and physical activity* that will improve the health of the world's population.

Refuting the claim that worldwide physical activity from the Olympic Games will occur is a powerful rhetorical device. It adds to the problem, since it alerts the reader to the possibility that some aims are not being achieved (despite the fact that no person or organisation is cited as having made the claim in the first place). This denial differs from the *Lancet* editorial for the *Series*, which suggests that the Olympic Games are actually *detrimental* to health. The editorial criticises the involvement of sponsors such as Coca Cola, Cadbury's and McDonald's and laments 'the long-term effect of Games-associated junk food advertising on people's hearts and waistlines – definitely one Olympic legacy the world can do without' (p. 188).

This 'villain' narrative is certainly popular, although a critical ecological approach might consider two problematic aspects of this view. First, the tone of these claims about the 'Olympic effect' differs significantly from that of another commentary in the *Series* in which Malta and Silva write (2012: 196) about efforts in Brazil to promote physical activity using the Olympic Games. They write that 'the Brazilian government launched a strategic plan to tackle NCDs in 2011'. Part of this strategic plan is to use the 2016 Olympic Games to promote physical activity:

> Furthermore, educational measures that foster healthy habits and the practice of daily physical activity are underway as part of the legacy of two major sporting events that will be held in Brazil: the 2014 World Cup and the Olympic Games in 2016.
>
> *p. 196*

Adding to the contention about the value of the Olympic Games, in the final call to action this Brazilian strategic plan is *praised*

> Ideally, national policies and action plans are designed not for implementation solely by governments, but rather for mobilisation of both governmental and non-governmental collaboration towards advancement of physical activity and reduction of physical inactivity. The recent Brazilian experience is one from which many such lessons can be learned. Similar action is needed worldwide.
>
> *Kohl et al., 2012: 296*

What all of this highlights, amongst other things, is a failure to engage with research conducted by social scientists into legacy issues associated with the Olympic Games and other mega events. Long before the London Olympics of 2012 took place, it was being pointed out that, if large-scale changes in sports participation were to occur, these would be the consequence of interaction between numerous factors, including improved infrastructure for grass-roots activities (Coalter, 2004). Any suggestion that simply by hosting a mega event such interaction will inevitably follow is idealistic in the extreme. Post-2012, there is little evidence that youth sport participation has increased since the Games. As Judy Murray, mother of British tennis gold-medal winner Andy, has pointed out, there is a dearth of new talent in her sport not least because several schemes to improve free-to-use public courts in deprived urban areas have failed to materialise (Parkhouse, 2013). Inspiring a generation, which was the aim of London 2012, is one thing, but if there are insufficient facilities and coaches to meet demand, the inspired generation will become quickly disillusioned. In addition, figures show that 'there are now fewer adults playing sport regularly than before the London 2012 Olympics' (Gibson, 2013). Indeed, as Bell (2013: 175) concludes, 'despite the excitement and interest London 2012 generated, delivering an inspirational and successful Olympics/Paralympics was not sufficient on its own to get more people taking part in sport – as many had already predicted'. None of this is to suggest that participation levels will never increase after the staging of a mega event, such as the Olympic Games. The point is, however, that apparently unbeknown to some *Lancet* authors, there has long been a significant and well-informed debate on such matters which they ignore to their detriment.[5]

The *Lancet* statements illuminate not only the stark contradictions that characterise the debate about the 'Olympic effect' but also reveal that some of these contradictions come from authors in the same *Lancet* Physical Activity Series Working Group. To extrapolate this point, the sentiments of denial and lamentation above cannot be reconciled with the advice in the climactic 'call to action' article which encourages the private sector to:

> Orient marketing, advertising, and promotional messages to encourage physical activity and discourage physical inactivity and sedentary behaviours [and] Collaborate with government and non-governmental organisations in the creation and promotion of opportunities to promote and engage in physical activity.
>
> *Kohl et al., 2012: 302*

That is, the call to action specifically *encourages* private companies to promote physical activity. This case demonstrates the non-linear and multifaceted nature of appeals to 'health'. It also illustrates the governmental forces at work, whereby there are interlocking (but not necessarily synergistic) apparatuses which contribute to lived environments. These apparatuses 'form a force field through which we are urged, incited, encouraged, exhorted and motivated to act' (Rose, 1990: xxii). One might argue that the *Lancet* Series does promote acknowledging these multifaceted understandings through a systems approach. In their call to action, Kohl et al. argue that a variety of 'different areas are needed to tackle the global pandemic of physical inactivity because multidisciplinary work is essential' (p. 294). However, a more concerted systems approach would acknowledge this paradox of the Olympics as at once hindering and assisting health in order to establish a more nuanced appreciation of the complexities associated with corporate sponsorship of sport events. Certainly, these paradoxes demonstrate the need for urgent review focused on existing policies and practices. We suggest that by acknowledging the multiplicity of these corporate and non-governmental arrangements, a more 'ecological' context can be presented.

Conclusion

While the Physical Activity Series is well intended, there remain concerns regarding the continuity, coherence and appropriateness of various ideas that emanate from it. We applaud the idea of encouraging people to partake in more physical activity. However, the complexities inherent within the global pandemic metanarrative disrupt the possibility of rigorous argument. The concerns expressed here are not intended to derail momentum being generated in relation to physically active lifestyles. Instead, by giving more rigorous attention to defining and discussing the context and meanings of physical activity, fairer, more respectful and more effective promotion can result. The institutionalised, population-wide study of physical activity is relatively new, and, as Bull and Bauman note, physical inactivity might be described as the 'Cinderella' of NCD risk factors, with a 'poverty of policy attention and resourcing proportionate to its importance' (2011: 13). There is clearly space, then, for physical activity scholars to reflect on what stories are being (and should be) told about physical activity, in order to develop a more nuanced approach to engaging with it.

The *Lancet Series* frames the physical inactivity pandemic as complex. Claiming a social problem is complex allows for it to be conceived, explained and measured in particular ways, in this case requiring a 'systems approach' (Kohl et al., 2012: 294) or an 'ecological' model (Bauman et al., 2012: 258). According to Kohl et al. (2012: 300):

> a systems approach acknowledges the complex non-linearity of health behaviours, including the many interactions, delays in adoption, adaptations, competing actions, and unintended consequences that can occur within a system. A systems approach acknowledges such complexities and allows for planning to counteract the unintended consequences.

We argue that a systems approach would also need to account for and attempt to mitigate the complexities, competing ideas and unintended consequences inherent within its own propositions. It is apparent that various authors in *The Lancet* make bold, definitive and binary claims about physical activity and sport. These claims are of significant import given their possible influence in public health policy formulation and subsequent resource allocation. However, not only are these claims at times contradictory, but they are difficult to reconcile with a proposed systems approach which purportedly aims to consider unintended effects. Various claims acknowledge the complexity of social life (such as Kohl et al.'s suggestion that even a well designed intervention might result in a 'net zero gain' due to unintended consequences). At other times however, complexity is dismissed in favour of grand generalisations and definitions.

The ways in which the Physical Activity Series is transformed into policy and practice are yet to be seen. Given that physical activity is indeed a complex arena, we caution physical activity researchers to avoid elevating any physical health justifications for engaging in physical activity above other meanings that motivate people to be active. Using walking as one example, Bairner (2012: 373) argued the physical health benefits accrued from walking 'may well be of secondary importance to the lessons that can be learned from the pedagogies of the street'. Therefore, at the very least, we encourage physical activity promoters not to lose sight of the benefits and meanings of certain activities simply because they lack physical exertion. To reiterate Fullagar's (2002: 73) remarks: 'What is at stake here is the way that health policy discourses do or do not engage with other logics and modes of embodiment when promoting active leisure as something more than a risk-reducing physical activity.' We suggest here that more consideration of the implications of adopting a systems approach is needed before advancing the call to action further. We endorse Mansfield and Rich's (2013: 356) suggestion of institutional 'border crossings' by physical activity scholars so that 'counter perspectives and critical voices offering alternative health paradigms' will not be systematically marginalised or silenced.

This analysis provides an opportunity to acknowledge the dangers of what is at times a totalising response, particularly regarding surveillance. What is required is a weighing up of competing values (such as 'complete understanding' versus privacy) and competing stories (such as the various histories of health). Although *The Lancet* is undoubtedly a world leading medical journal, it is not the only, or even the dominant, producer of truth about physical activity. Academic journals are situated within a wider milieu of diverse truth claims, institutions, cultures and histories. There is a vast array of issues, a myriad of organisations and a complex nexus of research, policies, treatments and behaviours involved in managing population health around the world. The *Series*'s ideas will only be influential to the extent populations can be mobilised by a willing 'activity-force'. We do not reject the *Series*'s call to action. Rather, we encourage that it is reformed.

This chapter has been adapted from: Piggin, J. and Bairner, A. (2014), The global physical inactivity pandemic: An analysis of knowledge production. *Sport, Education and Society, 21*:2, 131–147.

Notes

1 Eight years earlier in 2004, Manson et al. also announced escalating global pandemics of sedentary lifestyles and inactivity and also wrote a 'call to action' for clinicians (Manson et al., 2004).
2 Lupton (1995) notes that 'from medieval times well into the closing years of the Victorian era, European towns and cities were characterised by filthy streets littered with human and animal excrement and rotting garbage' (p. 26).
3 The term 'normal' also appears in other places as common sense. Wen and Wu claim that 'being inactive is perceived as *normal*' (p. 192, italics added). Lee et al. also imagine 'if all obese people in the USA were to attain *normal* weight' (p. 228, italics added).
4 The idea of 'failure' features in a profile interview in another *Series* in *The Lancet*, where one author makes a specific claim about physical education: 'The truth is that physical educators have failed . . . Physical education itself hasn't delivered physical activity benefits to children in schools' (Khan, in Holmes, 2012: 20). This type of accusation in a world leading medical journal that physical educators have failed has been responded to by physical education scholars as being the pursuit of not only illusory but also dangerous ideals (see Evans, Rich and Davies, 2004).
5 Also, a systems approach would cast a critical eye over the alleged altruism of the IOC, an organisation which has been subject to a range of critiques focussed on corruption which would surely undermine its capacity to promote physical activity around the world (Jennings, 2011; Lenskyj, 2008).

References

Abeysinghe, S. and White, K. (2010), Framing disease: The avian influenza pandemic in Australia. *Health Sociology Review, 19*:3, 369–381.
Abeysinghe, S. and White, K. (2011), The avian influenza pandemic: Discourses of risk, contagion and preparation in Australia, Health, *Risk & Society, 13*:4, 311–326.
Bacchi, C. (2000), Policy as discourse: What does it mean? Where does it get us? *Discourse: Studies in the Cultural Politics of Education, 21*:1, 45–57.
Bairner, A. (2012), Urban walking and the pedagogies of the street, *Sport, Education and Society, 16*:3, 371–384.
Bauman, A.E., Reis, R.S., Sallis, J.F., Wells, J.C., Loos, R.J.F. and Martin, B.W., for *The Lancet* Physical Activity Series Working Group. (2012), Correlates of physical activity: Why are some people physically active and others not? *The Lancet, 380*:9838, 258–271.
Bell, B. (2013), 'From podium to park' in Mark Perryman (ed.), *London 2012: How was it for us?* (164–176). London: Lawrence and Wishart.
Bercovitz, K. (1998), Canada's Active Living policy: A critical analysis. *Health Promotion International, 13*:4, 319–328.
Boym, S. (2007), Nostalgia and its discontents. *The Hedgehog Review*, Summer, 7–18.

Bruegel, P. (1560), *Kinderspiele (Children's Games)* (oil on panel), Kunsthistorisches Museum, Vienna, Austria/The Bridgeman Art Library.

Bull, F.C. and Bauman, A.E. (2011), Physical inactivity: The 'Cinderella' risk factor for noncommunicable disease prevention. *Journal of Health Communication: International Perspectives, 16*:sup2, 13–26.

Coalter, F. (2004), 'Stuck in the Blocks? A sustainable sporting legacy', in Anthony Vigor, Melissa Mean and Charlie Tims (eds.), *After the Goldrush: A sustainable Olympics for London* (93–108). London: IPPR and Demos.

Das, P. and Horton, R. (2012), Rethinking our approach to physical activity. *The Lancet, 380*:9838, 189–190.

Evans, J. (2013), Physical education as porn! *Physical Education and Sport Pedagogy, 18*:1, 75–89.

Evans, J., Rich, E. and Davies, B. (2004), The emperor's new clothes: Fat, thin, and overweight: The social fabrication of risk and ill health. *Journal of Teaching in Physical Education, 23*:4, 372–391.

Foucault, M. (1979), *Discipline and punish: The birth of the prison.* Harmondsworth: Penguin Books.

Foucault, M. (1994), 'Governmentality', in James Faubion (ed.), *Michel Foucault: Power: Essential works of Foucault 1954–1984*, Vol. 3 (p. 201–222). London: Penguin.

Fullagar, S. (2002), Governing the healthy body: Discourses of leisure and lifestyle within Australian health policy. *Health, 6*:1, 69–84.

Gard, M. (2011), *The end of the obesity epidemic.* London: Routledge.

Gard, M. and Wright, J. (2001), Managing uncertainty: Obesity discourses and physical education in a risk society. *Studies in Philosophy and Education, 20*:6, 535–549.

Gard, M. and Wright, J. (eds.) (2005), *The obesity epidemic: Science and ideology.* London: Routledge.

Garvin, T. and Eyles, J. (1997), The sun safety metanarrative: Translating science into public health discourse. *Policy Sciences, 30*:2, 47–70.

Gibson, O. (2013), 'Fewer adults playing sport since London Olympics', *Guardian*, 14 June (http://aggregga.com/kennethp80/post/632080/fewer-adults-playing-sport-since-london-olympics). Retrieved 6 July, 2013.

Hallal, P.C., Bauman, A.E., Heath, G.W., Kohl, H.W., Lee, I. and Pratt, M. (2012), Physical activity: More of the same is not enough. *The Lancet, 380*:9838, 190–191.

Hartley, P.H-S. and Llewellyn, G.F. (1939), The longevity of oarsmen: A study of those who rowed in the Oxford and Cambridge boat race from 1829–1928. *British Medical Journal, 1*: 657–662.

Heath, G.W., Parra, D.C., Sarmiento, O.L., Andersen, L.B., Owen, N., Goenka, S., Montes, F. and Brownson, R.C., for *The Lancet* Physical Activity Series Working Group. (2012), Evidence-based intervention in physical activity: Lessons from around the world. *The Lancet, 380*:9838, 272–281.

Hepworth, J. (2006), The emergence of critical health psychology: Can it contribute to promoting public health? *Journal of Health Psychology, 11*:3, 331–41.

Holmes, B. (2010), *Constructing the coming plague: A discourse analysis of the British Columbia Pandemic Influenza Preparedness Plan*, doctoral thesis, Simon Fraser University. http://summit.sfu.ca/item/11398.

Holmes, D. (2012), Profile: Karim Khan: Good sport. *The Lancet, 380*:9836, 20.

Jenkin, G., Signal, L. and Thomson, G. (2011), Framing obesity: The framing contest between industry and public health at the New Zealand inquiry into obesity. *Obesity Reviews, 12*:12, 1022–30.

Jennings, A. (2011), Investigating corruption in corporate sport: The IOC and FIFA. *International Review for the Sociology of Sport, 46*:4, 387–398.

Kim, S. and Willis, L. (2007), Talking about obesity: News framing of who is responsible for causing and fixing the problem. *Journal of Health Communication, 12*:4, 359–76.

Kohl, H.W., Craig, C.L., Lambert, E.V., Inoue, S., Alkandari, J.R., Leetongin, G. and Kahlmeier, S., for *The Lancet* Physical Activity Series Working Group. (2012), The pandemic of physical inactivity: Global action for public health. *The Lancet, 380*:9838, 294–305.

Kwan, S. (2009), Framing the fat body: Contested meanings between government, activists, and industry. *Social Inq, 79*:1, 25–50.

Lancet. (2012), Chariots of fries. *The Lancet, 380*:9838, 188.

Lee, I.M., Shiroma, E.J., Lobelo, F., Puska, P., Blair, S.N. and Katzmarzyk, P.T, for *The Lancet* Physical Activity Series Working Group. (2012), Effect of physical inactivity on major non-communicable diseases worldwide: An analysis of burden of disease and life expectancy. *The Lancet, 380*:9838, 219–229.

Lenskyj, H.J. (2008), *Olympic industry resistance: Challenging Olympic power and propaganda.* U.S.A.: State University of New York Press.

Lupton, D. (1995), *The imperative of health: Public health and the regulated body*. Australia: Sage Publication Ltd.

Malta, D.C. and Silva, J.B. (2012), Policies to promote physical activity in Brazil. *The Lancet*, *380*:9838, 195–196.

Mansfield, L. and Rich, E. (2013), Public health pedagogy, border crossings and physical activity at every size. *Critical Public Health*, *23*:3, 356–370.

Manson, J.E., Skerrett, P.J., Greenland, P. and VanItallie, T.B. (2004), The escalating pandemics of obesity and sedentary lifestyle: A call to action for clinicians. *Archives of Internal Medicine*, *164*:3, 249–258.

Markula, P. and Pringle, R. (2006), *Foucault, sport and exercise: Power, knowledge and transforming the self*. USA: Routledge.

Neville, R.D. (2013), Considering a complemental model of health and fitness. *Sociology of Health & Illness*, *35*:3, 479–492.

Parkhouse, S. (2013) 'Judy Murray: Lack of free courts is keeping tennis elitist', *Observer*, 23 June (www.guardian.co.uk/sport/2013/jun/23/judy-murray-elitist-tennis). Retrieved 24 June, 2013.

Parsons, W. (1995), *Public policy*. Aldershot: Edward Elgar.

Petersen, A.R. and Lupton, D. (1996), *The new public health: Discourses, knowledges, strategies*. Australia: Allen and Unwin.

Piggin, J., Jackson, S. and Lewis, M. (2007), Classify, divide and conquer: Shaping physical activity discourse through national public policy. *New Zealand Sociology*, *22*:2, 274–293.

Pringle, R. and Pringle, D. (2012), Competing obesity discourses and critical challenges for health and physical educators. *Sport, Education and Society*, *17*:2, 143–161.

Puhl, R.M. (2011), Weight stigmatization toward youth: A significant problem in need of societal solutions. *Childhood Obesity*, *7*:5, 359–363.

Puhl, R.M. and King, K.M. (2013), Weight discrimination and bullying. *Best Practice & Research Clinical Endocrinology & Metabolism*, http://dx.doi.org/10.1016/j.beem.2012.12.002.

Quennerstedt, M. (2008), Exploring the relation between physical activity and health – A salutogenic approach to physical education. *Sport, Education and Society*, *13*:3, 267–283.

Rimmer, J.H. and Marques, A.C. (2012), Physical activity for people with disabilities. *The Lancet*, *380*:9838, 193–195.

Roe, E. (1994), *Narrative policy analysis: Theory and practice*. Durham: Duke University Press.

Rook, A. (1954, Apr 3), An investigation into the longevity of Cambridge sportsmen. *British Medical Journal*, *1*:4865, 773–777.

Rose, N. (1990), *Governing the soul: The shaping of the private self*. London: Routledge.

Rose, N. and Miller, P. (1992), Political power beyond the state: Problematics of government. *British Journal of Sociology*, *43*:2, 173–205.

Stone, D. (2002), *Policy paradox: The art of political decision making*. New York: W.W. Norton.

Stidder, G. (2013), 'The value of reflexivity for inclusive practice in physical education', in Gary Stidder and Sid Hayes (eds.), *Equity and inclusion in physical education and sport, second edition* (17–33). London: Routledge.

Vallgårda, S. (2011), Nudge – A new and better way to improve health? *Health Policy*, *104*:2, 200–203.

Wen, C.P. and Wu, X. (2012), Stressing harms of physical inactivity to promote exercise. *The Lancet*, *380*:9838, 192–193.

4

IS EXERCISE MEDICINE?

A critical sociological examination

Dominic Malcolm and Emma Pullen

Exercise is Medicine (EiM) was launched in November 2007 as a collaborative initiative of the American College of Sports Medicine (ACSM) and the American Medical Association (AMA) (Sallis 2009a). Its introduction was justified alongside the citation of a range of 'costs' associated with physical inactivity (e.g. 3.3 million deaths per year globally, $102 billion direct cost to the US healthcare system), and a range of benefits (i.e. the lower incidence of conditions such as diabetes, heart disease, arthritis, osteoporosis and various cancers) that are believed to stem from 150 minutes per week of 'moderate intensity' physical activity which induces slight breathlessness. Its explicit aims are two-fold:

> To make physical activity and exercise a standard part of a disease prevention and treatment medical paradigm in the United States;
>
> For physical activity to be considered by all healthcare providers as a vital sign in every patient visit, and that patients are effectively counselled and referred as to their physical activity and health needs, thus leading to overall improvement in the public's health and longer term reduction in healthcare cost.
>
> *Jonas and Phillips 2009:p.ix*

EiM seeks to build coalitions with three primary constituencies: healthcare professionals; the public; and those working in the fitness industries. It seeks to strengthen the scientific evidence base, influence policy makers and stage patient-oriented marketing campaigns. It also seeks to disseminate best practice, tools and techniques via various on-line resources. A central aspect of this educational work has been the publication of a book called *ACSM's Exercise is Medicine: A clinician's guide to exercise prescription* (Jonas and Phillips 2009), which in many ways is an instruction manual for those charged with implementing EiM.

EiM belongs to the vast and seemingly ever-growing number of physical activity health promotion (PAHP) policies. For instance, a review of national documents published in the 27 EU member states between 2000 and 2009 identified 112 which 'mentioned health-enhancing physical activity and contained overall goals on participation in sport and physical activity and/or on health promotion' (WHO 2011:p.42). However, because EiM was first established in perhaps the major loci of global cultural diffusion, it has developed from being a national programme to having international ambitions and reach, with branches established in 43 countries and across six continents. EiM hosted its inaugural 'World Congress' in 2010, attended by delegates from over 60 countries (Neville 2013). But alongside its typicality and global relevance EiM has a third feature that gives it wider resonance and makes it particularly sociologically interesting. For while there is a long history of exercise being advocated for its health-promoting properties (Berryman 2010) this movement uniquely contains the claim (or aspiration) that exercise and medicine have (or should) become synonymous in some respects.

What are the implications of the assertion that exercise is medicine? Of course, the statement could be metaphorical. Indeed at times this is exactly what is claimed (Phillips and Capell 2009a:p.33; Phillips et al. 2009a:p.89). But, the enthusiasm with which this and similar policies are pursued, the hyperbole within which they are couched and the degree to which EiM has globally diffused suggest that a more literal meaning is intended. Indeed, for Neville (2013:p.615) Exercise is Medicine 'is now something of a platitude'. In a literal sense the word 'medicine' can have two main meanings. It can be used as a noun referring to the treatment of illness, or a drug/pharmaceutical for such treatment. But it can also be used in a wider sense to refer to a practice – the art and science of healing – which has, since the mid-1800s, been monopolized by a specific discipline/profession and which has subsequently become an increasingly influential social institution (Freidson 1970). Contained within the EiM initiative are references to 'medicine' in both senses. Both, we go on to demonstrate, are problematic.

This chapter seeks to provide a critical sociological examination (Malcolm 2017) of the claim that exercise is medicine, both in relation to the specifics of the EiM initiative, but also the broader cultural phenomenon of PAHP. It begins with a deconstruction of the EiM claim considering the multiple meanings implied and locating these in the context of key processes underlying the development of contemporary medicine. It then outlines existing sociological critiques of public health campaigns in general and illustrates their relevance for EiM in particular. It concludes that rather than being unequivocally celebrated as some kind of 'miracle cure' (AMRC 2015) the repositioning of exercise as a form of medicine represents a fundamental social change which has major and potentially negative implications for the citizens of contemporary societies. In so doing it presents ethical issues for the medical profession.

Exercise as a medicine

Within the EiM documentation, exercise is at various times referred to as a form of 'medication' (Jonas 2009a:p.3), a pill, and 'the much needed vaccine to prevent chronic disease and premature death' (Sallis 2009a:p.3). The documentation describes the act of getting a patient to take up exercise as the equivalent of interventions for medications or medical procedures. Moreover, the 'exercise pill' is claimed to have miraculous effects: 'If we had a pill that conferred all the confirmed health benefits of exercise would we not do everything humanly possible to see to it that everyone had access to this wonder drug?' (Sallis 2009a:p.3).

There is, however, a lack of reflexivity in this usage. Here, medicine is assumed to be fundamentally benign, if not essentially beneficial. However, as English idioms embracing medicine indicate – 'to take one's medicine', 'to have a taste of one's own medicine' – medicine is frequently seen to be unpalatable or unpleasant. Medicines are not always unequivocally positive for patients, and researchers have been critical of the process of pharmaceuticalization which has led to a social dependence on such substances (Williams et al. 2011). As the historical use of thalidomide and contemporary debates about the use of statins demonstrate, it would be naive to assume that the use of pharmaceutical substances can only enhance the human condition.

Indeed it is for this reason that substances categorized as medicines are normally subject to regulation in modern societies. For instance, what distinguishes a medicine from water is not that the former helps maintain or enhance good health but that, in most countries, it is licensed by the state. The pathway to license depends on testing procedures, the 'gold standard' of which are 'double blind control trials' and, once licensed, the medicine is (or should be) accompanied by guidance on appropriate dosage and potential side effects. In addition to this, the dosage of any particular medicine is normally reduced or stopped (as are the risk of side effects) as the person becomes healthier. In these three interconnected respects (dosage, side effects, prognosis), exercise seems to diverge from medicine as conventionally understood.

First, recommended exercise dosages are highly generalized rather than carefully controlled. For instance, the UK Government Chief Medical Officer's guidelines on physical activity recommend that under-5s (who can walk unsupported) are active for 180 minutes per day, that 5–18 year olds should engage in moderate to vigorous activity for 60 minutes per day and that adults undertake 150 minutes of moderate or 75 minutes of vigorous activity per week (PHE 2014). Second, the evidence base for exercise as medicine is relatively weak in the sense that a placebo control group is impossible. Indeed, despite the recent concentration of research in this area, the recommended dosage has not fundamentally changed for 20 years. This could either imply that exercise is an unusual medicine in that knowledge of its efficacy cannot be improved, or be indicative of the underlying social construction of physical activity related medical knowledge. The advocacy of 'five a day' in relation to fresh fruit and vegetables has been shown to be influenced by conceptions of what degree of behavioural change is achievable, and the sceptical might draw parallels with the advocacy in EiM of 30 minutes of moderate activity five or more times a week (Sallis 2009b:p.viii; see also DoH 2004). Indeed, the highly unusual practice of offering 'patients' a choice of dosages supports the contention that its prescription is as much socially as medically defined. Third, the extent to which the appropriate dosage of exercise is achieved is somewhat imprecise (i.e. slight breathlessness, enabling one to talk but not sing) and, rather than professionally controlled, largely dependent on a layperson's relatively subjective assessment. This may, for instance, account for the discordance between self-report measures of activity (which show a slow increase over time) and accelerometry data (Scarborough et al. 2011). Fourth, the more regularly or longer a person exercises, the greater the intensity required to achieve 'moderate' levels of activity. Thus by definition, if exercise is (a) medicine, the appropriate dosage will not only 'increase' over time, but will do so especially when its application is successful and an individual gets 'healthier' through increased fitness. If exercise is medicine, the healthier you are the more medication you need. EiM conforms with PAHP policies more generally in this regard (e.g. DoH 2004). Sallis (2009a:p.4; emphasis added), for instance, exhorts clinicians to 'collectively urge *all* patients to become *more* active and stay active throughout their lives'. While it is conceded that 'either too much or too little [exercise] can be harmful' (Phillips et al. 2009b:p.149), the overriding message is that 'the more intense the activity, that is the more aerobic it is, the more benefit there is to be gained from it' (Jonas 2009a:p.11). Exercise cannot be a *miracle* cure because it isn't actually a cure.

The position that *everybody* would benefit from increased levels of activity is only sustainable in light of a final but key anomaly: the reluctance to embrace the possibility that exercise might have negative side effects which it would be socially beneficial to control. While exercise is clearly different to pharmaceuticals, and this is perhaps one reason why

PAHP in general has met with relatively little critique or resistance, it would be false to assume that it cannot negatively impact on health. There is not space to challenge this assumption in detail. Indeed the assessment of sport-related injury (SRI) is notoriously difficult and hotly debated. For instance, while most SRI research prioritizes acute injuries because they are both more routinely presented to medical practitioners and more easily linked to a particular aetiology (e.g. sports participation), there is evidence to suggest that particular sporting populations experience relatively high levels of conditions as diverse as asthma (Elers et al. 2011) and osteoarthritis (Kuijta et al. 2012). The longer-term impact of sport-related head injuries is an emerging and controversial field. But regardless of these significant grey areas, there is a consensus amongst epidemiologists that participation in exercise (and particularly sport) can have negative health impacts (i.e. sports injuries), that certain activities entail particularly high rates of injury and that the dangers increase as the intensity of activity (the 'dosage') increases.

Despite this, EiM documentation recommends that people pursue higher risk activities, suggesting that more competitive settings and taking part in sports rather than exercise will facilitate continued participation (Jonas 2009b). Moreover it portrays injury as the product of individual actions caused, e.g., by 'trying to go too far, too fast, too frequently' (Jonas 2009a:p.11). Thus injury is deemed largely avoidable, and the recommendation for avoiding 'intrinsic injuries' (to muscles, tendons, etc.) 'is simply not to overdo it' while injuries caused by external events can be avoided by being 'aware of your surroundings' (Phillips et al. 2009a:p.96).[1] It gives no indication that SRI can be chronic as well as acute (see Nicholl et al. 1995 below). It is fundamentally problematic, therefore, that EiM ignores the research which shows that both acute and chronic injury is inherent to the structure of exercise and sport in particular.

In contrast to EiM's portrayal of the risks, epidemiology continually shows that sports injuries are a relatively frequent occurrence. Again the field is hotly debated, hampered by highly diverse findings and the absence of a standardized way to contextualize data (Pollock 2014). For example, studies have found that the proportion of the population to have suffered from SRI in the previous year varies between 3.1 per cent in Germany (Schneider et al. 2006), 5.9 per cent in Australia (Egger 1991), 7.4 per cent in Ontario (McClaren 1996), 10.1 per cent in Canada (McCutcheon et al. 1997), 16.6 per cent in Queensland (Mummery et al. 2002) and 18 per cent in the Netherlands (van der Sluis et al. 1998). A study of the adult population in England and Wales reported that 8.1 per cent incurred a SRI in the four weeks prior to survey which equated to 18 per cent of the sports-active population (Nicholl et al. 1995). On this basis Nicholl et al. estimate that there are 19.3 million new sports injuries a year in England and Wales, plus 10.4 million recurrent injuries, making a total of 29.7 million SRIs per year in England and Wales. The Association of British Insurers similarly recorded 20 million SRIs during 1994 (cited in White 2004). The relatively consistent pattern of injuries shows them to be a structural feature of exercise (and especially sport) which is neither peripheral nor insignificant.

Unfortunately, no data exist on which we could make holistic comparisons of cost-benefit, and indeed a critical sociological investigation would fundamentally reject the use of measures such as Quality Adjusted Life Years for the underlying premise that it is meaningful to quantify essentially qualitative experiences (most qualitative health researchers would favour the analysis of biographical disruption; for instance, see Malcolm 2017). But if we restrict ourselves to narrower and therefore more like-for-like comparisons we can see that the evidence for the cost savings of promoting physical activity are far from straightforward. For instance, 20 years ago the estimated direct cost of treating sports injuries in England and

Wales was £420 million per year (Nicholl et al. 1995), or approximately 45 per cent of the *current* estimated cost of physical inactivity (Scarborough et al. 2011). Implicitly evoking reference to EiM, a prominent campaigner for the greater recognition of the injury risks of sport, Allyson Pollock (2014:p.11), has argued that 'if rugby were a new medical drug it would be withheld until its efficacy and safety had been proven'.

Thus if exercise is *a* medicine, it is a particularly unusual kind of medicine. It is prescribed for entire populations regardless of symptoms, in general rather than specific dosages and with a subtext that there is no limit to how much is good for you. Most particularly, if exercise *is* medicine, it is prescribed with a disregard for what clearly can be significant potential side effects. But what of the synonym of exercise and medicine in the second sense identified; that exercise and the medical profession are increasingly merging. It is to this that we now turn.

Exercise and the medical profession

A central implication of the second reading of EiM is that (parts of) the medical discipline/profession have become consumed within the sport and exercise industry and/or vice versa. As we will see, this meaning is similarly conspicuous in the broader EiM literature. However, due to the greater complexity of the social consequences of this conflation, we need to undertake a more detailed consideration of the developmental trajectory of medicine. While medicine 'originated as a response to human suffering' and the 'pursuit . . . of the relief of suffering' 'remains one of the central, defining goals of medicine' (Edwards and McNamee 2006:p.104), over time medicine has become increasingly involved in prevention rather than cure (Nettleton 2006). In addition to this medicine has also become prominent as an arbitrator of social problems and a moralistic voice on the conduct of individuals and groups and the organization of society (Conrad 1992). Key concepts in this respect are surveillance, medicalization and the New Public Health (NPH). If exercise is medicine, what kind of medicine is it, and how will social relations be altered by this new configuration?

Exercise is Medicine and medicalization

Fundamental to the development of medicine during the twentieth century has been the changing locations in which it is performed – from domestic bedsides, to hospitals, to the wider society – and the impact of this on medical practice (Armstrong 1995). Whereas bedside medicine occurred in the patient's home, the development of what Armstrong has termed 'surveillance medicine' entails a shift in the social space of practice into the community at large. Whereas bedside medicine was characterized by patient-initiated diagnosis, surveillance medicine entails profession-initiated interventions. The increasing focus on prevention also shifts medicine's focus to the environmental and social context and to prescriptions about the structure of societies and the agency of lifestyle choice. Interventions such as population screening constitute fundamentally *different kinds* of experiment which alter understanding of the human condition and so shift our understanding of the distinction between health and illness (Armstrong 1995). The experience of disease and risk of disease converge as more detailed understanding leads to the identification of disease precursors on a 'continuum of abnormalities' (Aronowitz 2009:p.425). 'Diagnosis creep' entails identifying and treating predisease states (Kreiner and Hunt 2013). The experience of being at risk of developing a disease becomes indistinguishable from the illness experience of symptomatic patients for whom medical intervention has become characterized by disease management rather than treatment.

The EiM movement epitomizes these processes. EiM represents community rather than clinical intervention. EiM focuses primarily on lifestyle choices, on 'change and how to make it, choices to be made and how to make them' (Jonas 2009a:p.1). In advocating the 'prescription' of 'medicine' to entire populations, EiM contributes to the blurring of the health-illness distinction by converging the lived experience of being either well or unwell. Uniquely though, EiM extends/refracts surveillance back on to the medical profession itself, not only encouraging 'physicians and other healthcare providers to be physically active themselves' (Jonas and Phillips 2009:p.ix), but presenting this as a moral obligation: 'we heartily recommend that, if you are not presently a regular exerciser yourself, you seriously consider becoming one, both for your own benefit *and that of your patients*' (Jonas 2009a:p.7. Emphasis added).

In the terms of a critical sociology of medicine, therefore, EiM represents an extension of the medicalization of social life (Davis 2006). Medicalization was initially a term used to refer to the expansion of medical authority through the definition of certain deviant practices as medically classifiable, and medicine's subsequent jurisdictional monopoly over their treatment (Zola 1972). Medicalization was latterly identified as the embrace of a range of natural aspects of the life-course (e.g. childbirth and ageing) into the domain of medical practice. Initially, critical analyses of medicalization were largely based on concerns about the legitimacy of the medical profession's expansion, but Illich (1975) further argued that medicalization meant that the profession not only cured illness and relieved suffering, but created iatrogenesis, or medically generated/exacerbated illness or social problems. Finally, medicalization has come to refer to instances where medical language or a medical framework structures our understanding of a particular aspect of social life (Conrad 1992).

In conflating exercise and medicine in their manifestations as disciplines, practices and professions, EiM represents medicalization in most of the multiple senses that sociologists have used the term. For instance, EiM represents an attempt to redefine a previously mundane aspect of social life as medically essential. It threatens to subsume previously important motivational drives for sports participation – e.g. risk taking, emotional stimulation, the quest for excitement (Elias and Dunning 1986) – under the goals of health, and encourages the evaluation of health outcomes through the use of technology such as heart rate monitors (Neville 2013). Despite couching this development within an emphasis on social and lifestyle factors, stressing the multidimensional nature of problems and the necessity of multiagency solutions, the EiM initiative effectively expands the social role, and consolidates the social influence, of (sports) medicine. Indeed EiM explicitly identifies this as a process of paradigmatic change, and in reaching out to its three primary constituencies – healthcare professions, the public and those working in the fitness industries – EiM evokes questions of jurisdictional legitimacy. Sallis (2009a:p.4) for instance urges that 'we must begin to merge the fitness industry with the healthcare industry if we are going to improve the world'; 'I believe that sports medicine physicians around the world are the best advocates for Exercise is Medicine'. EiM can therefore be read as an explicit attempt on the part of (sports) medicine to colonize a sphere of social life that was previously beyond its ambit. Finally, in its reluctance to fully acknowledge the risks of activity-induced injury, EiM may either cause or exacerbate human suffering and thus lead to iatrogenesis as Illich (1975) identified.

Exercise is Medicine and the New Public Health

The notions of surveillance and medicalization underpin aspects of the sociological critique of health promotion, and the NPH in particular. Nettleton (2006) argues that a new health promotion agenda – the New Public Health (NPH) – emerged in the late 1970s/early 1980s stimulated by four key developments: the diminishing returns of investments in technology; the changing disease burden from infection to chronic non-communicable diseases; the ageing population; and financial pressures on health services. The explicit principles of the NPH are informed patient choice, partnership and personalization, but while NPH focuses on the social causes of disease and the facilitation of healthy lifestyles, it also exploits strategies such as persuasion, personal counselling and legislation. Critical sociological commentaries on the NPH largely focus on three inter-related issues: structure, surveillance and consumption (Burrows et al. 1995).

EiM resonates with the critiques of NPH in a variety of senses. First, as evidenced by the range of health benefits exercise is said to engender (cited in the introduction to this chapter), it stems from the significance of chronic conditions with the overall health 'burden'. Second, it is justified directly in relation to existing costs endured by the healthcare system. However, in exemplifying the three overarching critiques of NPH identified above – *structure, surveillance* and *consumption* – EiM is indicative of how PAHP is contoured by the broader trajectory of public health within the development of medicine. The parallels with each of these critiques merit elaboration.

Structurally health promotion has been criticized for failing to recognize the importance of material (dis-)advantage in mediating lifestyle and disregarding the role of poverty and living conditions in contouring the choices that people can make. Consequently, health promotion campaigns frequently perpetuate and reinforce inequalities and, in advocating individual freedom and responsibility for health, can lead to victim-blaming and stigmatization.

EiM similarly obscures the structural conditions which impact upon sport and exercise participation seeking essentially to position such pursuits as lifestyle choices. For example, rather than addressing the highly gendered pattern of sport participation or the variegated influences of socio-economic class, ethnicity and (dis)ability, there is a fundamental bias towards the psychologization of behaviour (Horrocks and Johnson 2014). Specifically physical inactivity is explicitly described as a behavioural rather than a structural factor, described as 'the one major factor affecting our health and longevity that is almost entirely under our control' (Sallis 2009a:p.3). While no specific cost to the individual who exercises is identified, EiM alludes to the kind of cost-benefit analysis to decision-making common in health promotion policies (Horrocks and Johnson 2014), citing an estimated 'cost' of physical inactivity to the US healthcare system of $330 per person per year (ACSM 2014). (It is somewhat ironic therefore that *A Clinician's Guide* advocates the benefits of joining a gym – access to personnel trained to assist and monitor exercise, variety of equipment, etc. – and estimates that the average cost of membership is about $500 per year). The (in)decision to be physically active is projected as an essentially personal and individual (ir)responsibility. Clinicians are advised that their 'patient . . . knows that he "should" be more active' (Phillips et al. 2009a:p.91).

Second, health promotion has been criticized for monitoring and regulating populations through *surveillance*, in a compatible but extended sense to Armstrong's use of the term. This critique argues that under the NPH the population becomes 'profiled' into distinct social groups. Because healthy living becomes not something one merely does, but part of a broader personal philosophy of continuous self-improvement, new social identities are constructed. In perhaps the most renowned and extensive critique of NPH, Deborah Lupton (1995) argues that we have seen the development of *The Imperative of Health*, through which citizens come to continuously yet 'voluntarily' compel themselves to live healthy lives. Health promotion constructs and normalizes a subject who is 'autonomous, directed at self-improvement, self-regulated, desirous of self-knowledge, a subject who is seeking happiness and healthiness' (Lupton, 1995:p.11). But this increased emphasis on self-management has been described as 'insidious population governance' because its consequence is to 'provide opportunities for self-fulfilment for some responsible and independent citizens and abandonment for others' (Moore et al. 2015:p.4). Health promotion takes medical surveillance above and beyond the intrusion into the populations' everyday life into something which consulting doctors alone could never achieve.

Surveillance is writ large in the EiM initiative. An explicit goal of EiM is that physical activity should become a 'vital sign' which physicians check at every patient consultation, regardless of a patient's reasons for medical consultation, self-report of symptoms or any other contextual factor. This represents not just a considerable outreach into citizens' lives – a shift from patient autonomy to professional direction - but blurs the health-illness distinction by redefining physical inactivity as a pre-disease state (Aronowitz 2009). Moreover, the secondary goal - that the counselling of patients 'become consistently effective' (Jonas and Phillips 2009:p.ix) - suggests that the emphasis of EiM is *not* about providing advice for individuals to make informed decisions, but ensuring compliance with recommendations for behavioural change. As Jonas (2009a:p.1) argues, *A Clinician's Guide* is 'about how you can assist them [patients] in . . . making those changes and choices'. Third, there are expressed desires to create a 'broad awareness' of the desirability of exercise (Jonas and Phillips 2009:p.ix), and to ensure that this awareness becomes *normalized* through the construction of patient expectations (i.e. if you visit a physician you should expect to be asked about your physical activity). Fourth, the generalized and imprecise prescription in EiM creates open-ended physical activity targets and so fosters a context in which citizens internalize the goals of continuous self-improvement and thus strict self-management. As Jonas (2009a:p.7) notes, 'being a regular exerciser is like being on a never-ending journey . . . no final destination is ever reached'. Fifth, and crucially, EiM concludes with aspirations to develop self-regulation through identifying the individual as culpable for non-compliance. Specifically, within a statement about advising patients of the benefits of regular physical activity is the clause; 'Regular exercise can be fun, *if you let it be fun!*' (Jonas 2009a:p.6; emphasis added). The implication here is that the individual who does not recognize the inherent pleasure of exercising is personally at fault for failing to do so.

Finally it has been argued that the blurring of health and consumer culture in NPH leads to the creation of distinct lifestyles which consolidate the stratification of society. Health becomes not simply a state of being, nor a state to be pursued, but something which we can purchase. Jennifer Smith-Maguire (2008) uses the phrase 'fit for consumption, fit to be consumed', to illustrate in a Bourdieuian sense the deeply interconnected nature of physical and economic capital. Specifically, the wealthier (and therefore those with longer, and higher quality, life expectancy) are better able to join gyms etc. and so become increasingly healthy. This contributes to greater physical capital which in turn helps generate greater wealth.

EiM mirrors this trend, for while the initiative is located in evidence of health benefits, advocacy is consistently also couched in terms of lifestyle benefits. For example, in advising clinicians how to respond to patients who ask why they should exercise, the rationales of risk reduction and/or illness management are presented alongside advice such as: 'It makes you feel better'; 'It makes you look better'; and 'It makes you feel better about yourself' (Jonas 2009a:p.5). Similarly, included amongst the seven major benefits of taking regular exercise, are that it 'can help you feel younger and act that way too'; it 'can help spark your sex life' (Jonas 2009a:p.6). In addition to this the claim that exercise 'is the only way to "get in shape"' illustrates that fitness is here evoked as both a medical and corporeal concept. Prominent in what is advocated, therefore, is that citizens 'buy into' a lifestyle. The fundamental flaw with this thinking is that if, as Bourdieu's (1978) sociological analysis tells us, lifestyles are fundamental to the accrual of social status, exercise cannot be a panacea for all but simply an additional mechanism by which populations are stratified.

While in this respect EiM has developed in parallel with other forms of health promotion, a further but distinct aspect of this initiative and indeed PAHP in general, is the coalition of public and private interests. Whereas the other primary targets of public health campaigns – alcohol, tobacco and diet – have large and proactive commercial lobbies which provide a counter-weight to promotional materials, EiM encounters no such resistance. For example the 'global partners' of EiM include *Anytime Fitness* (gym franchise), *Technogym* (manufacturers of gym equipment), *United Health Foundation* (a not-for-profit arm of the United Health Group involved, for instance, in the sale of health insurance), *Optum* (suppliers of information and technology-enabled healthcare services) and *Coca-Cola*. Why is this important? The concern must be that all of these partners, with the exception of *Coca-Cola* (whose interest may be to divert criticism of the high sugar content of its drinks through an association with health promoting activities), stand to directly and financially benefit from higher physical activity levels which either reduce health costs overall or shift the expenditure burden onto the individual consumer (and thus boost profits). Specifically EiM recommends gym membership (which will potentially benefit *Anytime Fitness* and *Technogym*) and the use of cardiac monitoring equipment (benefiting *Optum*).

It is fairly well established that big businesses 'invest directly in research and lobbying . . . [to support] policies that do not threaten their interests' (Baum and Fisher 2014:p.219). The public health community is acutely aware of the role of tobacco companies in this respect (Pollock 2014) but the relationship between the fitness industry and PAHP needs to be similarly critiqued. In this respect EiM is not unique in incorporating this convergence of interests. One of the most prominent examples of this wider trend is the Nike commissioned report, *Designed to Move* (Nike et al. 2012). This report has become highly influential, cited for example in four UK PAHP documents published in 2014 (Malcolm 2017). But as Piggin (2015) has noted, despite presenting evidence which identified the workplace as the major locus for the reduction in physical activity in recent years, *Designed to Move* targets leisure as the solution. In so doing, it clearly promotes behavioural change which closely aligns with its own commercial interests (Piggin 2015). Thus EiM not only positions health and exercise in the commercial market place through its choice of partners, it further raises concerns about the process of knowledge production underlying PAHP policies. So clearly aligning with industrial partners exposes the public to commercial exploitation. Incorporating gym and sportswear manufacturers into PAHP could be said to be akin to trusting food manufacturers to lead on public health dietary campaigns.

Conclusion: Implications for future physical activity policy and practice

This chapter has sought to question the appropriateness and implications of the claim that exercise is medicine. It has been argued that the literal sense that exercise is synonymous with a form of treatment or a pharmaceutical contains inherent problems related to the lack of self-reflection and, in particular, regulation. Zealously promoting exercise as a 'wonder drug' for the entire population to consume in ever-increasing quantities, without any regard for the clearly demonstrable side effects of (some types of) participation, capitalizes on the privileges of medical classification (i.e. enhanced social status) without embracing the ethical obligations that medical practice entails (see below). Secondly, I have suggested that in the broader sense of convergence of exercise and medicine, there are fundamental questions about jurisdictional legitimacy, the disempowerment of citizens and the blurring of the distinction between health and ill-health. The potential unintended impacts of the initiative are victim-blaming of the non-compliant and the reproduction of health inequalities. This takes place against a backdrop of medicine and exercise groups forging alliances such that public health campaigns promote certain commercial interests.

What are the policy and practical implications of this? If, as its advocates appear to believe, exercise *is* medicine, then it should be subject to standard medical ethical principles. In particular, EiM appears to have been produced without due regard for notions of patient autonomy (evident in the elements of compulsion) or informed choice (the failure to disclose the health consequences of different types of exercise). In forging alliances with the fitness industry and health insurers, the medical ethical principle of always and solely working in the interests of patients is also called into question. While it is the role of critical social scientists to point out that the extension of medical influence in society cannot simply be assumed to be benign, for the medical profession itself there are highly practical implications. The authority and influence of medicine in contemporary societies is fundamentally linked to the maintenance of these ethical principles (Freidson 1970). The neglect of medical ethical principles represents a key threat to medicine's social influence.

Secondly, inherent in the structure of the EiM initiative is a logic that will at best limit its impact and at worst lead to its self-defeat. Ironically a direct consequence of the success of EiM will be an increase in the prevalence of sports injury which, in turn, will reduce people's ability to exercise and therefore adhere to health advice. *A Clinician's Guide* makes brief mention of this: 'for most people, "too much too soon" . . . will lead to muscle pain and possible injury, as well as a greater likelihood of early quitting' (Phillips et al. 2009a:p.88). But there is evidence to suggest that this is a more tangible problem than EiM literature suggests. For instance, Andrew et al. (2014) have found that 'serious sport and active recreation injuries have large, negative, persistent impacts on participants' physical activity levels, independent of functional recovery'. For instance, a year after incurring a sports injury, just 40 to 65 per cent of patients had returned to sports participation and, of those who had not, relatively few compensated by replacing sport with less vigorous activities (e.g. walking). Return to sports participation was particularly poor amongst lower socio-economic groups.

Thirdly, therefore, any PAHP should be accompanied by a parallel strategy for the prevention and treatment of injury (Pollock and Kirkwood 2008), which is sensitive to social structural differences in access to medical treatment. This, in turn, must be accompanied by a rigorous and comprehensive cost-benefit assessment of the health outcomes of exercise which incorporate SRIs in their multiple forms, treated both within and outside of formal healthcare provision, assessed with due sensitivity to the essentially qualitative experience of illness. While governments tend to be disinterested in injuries that impact on sports participation because such injuries do not translate to an observable and easily measurable cost (Finch 2012), their policies will always have questionable foundations until such an evidence base is assembled. Unfortunately we currently see the extensive resourcing of research which will support PAHP, and a distinct disinterest in SRIs (Malcolm 2017). If exercise is medicine, there is an obligation to maximize its efficacy by making sufficient provision to cater for the inevitable, undesirable side effects of 'treatment'.

Note

1 The exception is in relation to cardiac complications, and in this respect a large proportion of potential exercisers are deemed to require medical or fitness professional supervision.

References

ACSM (2014) Exercise is Medicine Factsheet. www.exerciseismedicine.org/assets/page_documents/EIMFactSheet_2014.pdf. Accessed 11 September 2015.

AMRC (2015) *Exercise: The miracle cure and the role of the doctor in promoting it.* London: AMRC.

Andrew, N., Wolfe, R., Cameron, P. et al. (2014) The impact of sport and active recreation injuries on physical activity levels at 12 months post-injury, *Scandinavian Journal of Medicine and Science in Sports*, 24(2): 377–385.

Armstrong, D. (1995) The rise of surveillance medicine, *Sociology of Health and Illness*, 17(3): 393–404.

Aronowitz, R. (2009) The converged experience of risk and disease, *The Milbank Quarterly*, 87(2): 417–442.

Baum, F. and Fisher, M. (2014) Why behavioural health promotion endures despite its failure to reduce health inequalities, *Sociology of Health and Illness*, 36(2): 213–225.

Berryman, J. (2010) Exercise is medicine: A historical perspective, *Current Sports Medicine Reports*, 9(4): 1–7.

Bourdieu, P. (1978) Sport and social-class, *Social Science Information*, 17(6): 819–840.

Burrows, R., Nettleton, S. and Bunton, R. (1995) 'The sociology of health promotion: Health, risk and consumption under late-modernism', in R. Bunton, S. Nettleton and R. Burrows (eds.), *The sociology of health promotion: Critical analyses of consumption, lifestyle and risk*. London: Routledge.

Conrad, P. (1992) Medicalization and social control, *Annual Review of Sociology*, 18: 209–232.

Davis, J. (2006) How medicalization lost its way, *Society*, 43(6): 51–56.

DoH (2004) *At least five a week: Evidence of the impact of physical activity and its relationship with health.* London: Department of Health.

Edwards, S. and McNamee, M. (2006) Why sports medicine is not medicine, *Health Care Analysis*, 14(2): 103–109.

Egger, G. (1991) Sport injuries in Australia: Causes, cost and prevention, *Health Promotion Journal of Australia*, 1: 28–33.

Elias, N. and Dunning, E. (1986) *Quest of excitement: Sport and leisure in the civilizing process.* Oxford: Blackwell.

Elers, J., Pedersen, L. and Backer, V. (2011) Asthma in elite athletes, *Expert Review of Respiratory Medicine*, 5(3): 343–351.

Finch, C.F. (2012). Getting sports injury prevention on to public health agendas – addressing the shortfalls in current information sources, *British Journal of Sports Medicine,* 46(1): 70–74.

Freidson, E. (1970) *Profession of medicine: A study of the sociology of applied knowledge.* New York: Dodd, Mead & Co.

Horrocks, C. and Johnson, S. (2014) A socially situated approach to inform health and wellbeing, *Sociology of Health and Illness*, 36(2): 175–186.

Illich, I. (1975) *Medical nemesis.* London: Calder & Boyers.

Jonas, S. (2009a) 'Introduction: What this book is about', in S. Jonas and E. Phillips, *ACSM's Exercise is Medicine: A Clinician's Guide to Exercise Prescription*. Philadelphia: Lippincott, Williams and Wilkins, 1–12.

Jonas, S. (2009b) 'Choosing the activities, sport, or sports', in S. Jonas and E. Phillips, *ACSM's Exercise is Medicine: A Clinician's Guide to Exercise Prescription*. Philadelphia: Lippincott, Williams and Wilkins, 168–180.

Jonas, S. and Phillips, E. (2009) *ACSM's Exercise is Medicine: A clinician's guide to exercise prescription.* Philadelphia: Lippincott, Williams and Wilkins.

Kreiner, M. and Hunt, L. (2013) The pursuit of preventive care for chronic illness: Turning healthy people into chronic patients, *Sociology of Health and Illness*, 36(6): 870–884.

Kuijta, M., Inklaarb, H., Gouttebargea, V. and Frings-Dresena, M. (2012) Knee and ankle osteoarthritis in former elite soccer players: A systematic review of the recent literature, *Journal of Science and Medicine in Sport*, 15(6): 480–487.

Lupton, D. (1995) *The imperative of health: Public health and the regulated body.* London: Sage.

Malcolm, D. (2017) *Sport, medicine and health: The medicalization of sport?* London: Routledge.

McClaren, P. (1996) *A study of injuries sustained in sport and recreation in Ontario.* Unpublished report for the Ontario Ministry of Citizenship, Culture and Recreation.

McCutcheon, T., Curtis, J. and White, P. (1997) The socio-economic distribution of sport injuries: Multivariate analyses using Canadian national data, *Sociology of Sport Journal*, 14(1): 57–72.

Moore, L., Frost, J. and Britten, N. (2015) Context and complexity: The meaning of self-management for older adults with heart disease, *Sociology of Health and Illness*, 37(8): 1254–1269.

Mummery, W.K., Schofield, G. and Spence, J.C. (2002) The epidemiology of medically attended sport and recreation injuries in Queensland, *Journal of Science and Medicine in Sport*, 5(4): 307–320.

Nettleton, S. (2006) *The sociology of health and illness*. 2nd edition. Cambridge: Polity.

Neville, R.D. (2013) Exercise is Medicine: Some cautionary remarks in principle as well as in practice, *Medicine, Health Care and Philosophy*, 16(3): 615–622.

Nicholl, J.P., Coleman, P. and Williams, B.T. (1995) The epidemiology of sports and exercise related injury in the United Kingdom, *British Journal of Sports Medicine*, 29(4): 232–238.

Nike et al. (2012) *Designed to move: A physical activity action agenda*. Nike.

PHE (2014) *Everybody active, everyday: An evidence based approach to physical activity*. London: Public Health England.

Phillips, E.M. and Capell, J. (2009) 'Risk assessment and exercise screening', in S. Jonas and E. Phillips, *ACSM's Exercise is Medicine: A clinician's guide to exercise prescription*. Philadelphia: Lippincott, Williams and Wilkins, 31–47.

Phillips, E.M., Capell, J. and Jonas, S. (2009a) 'Getting started as a regular exerciser', in S. Jonas and E. Phillips, *ACSM's Exercise is Medicine: A clinician's guide to exercise prescription*. Philadelphia: Lippincott, Williams and Wilkins, 84–98.

Phillips, E.M., Capell, J. and Jonas, S. (2009b) 'Staying active', in S. Jonas and E. Phillips, *ACSM's Exercise is Medicine: A clinician's guide to exercise prescription*. Philadelphia: Lippincott, Williams and Wilkins, 134–150.

Piggin, J. (2015) Designed to move? Physical activity lobbying and the politics of productivity, *Health Education Journal*, 74(1): 1–12.

Pollock, A. (2014) *Tackling rugby: What every parent should know about injuries*. London: Verso.

Pollock, A. and Kirkwood, G. (2008) *Response to the Scottish Government's consultation on 'Glasgow 2014 – Delivering a Lasting Legacy for Scotland'*. Edinburgh: Centre for International Public Health Policy.

Sallis, R.E. (2009a) Exercise is Medicine and physicians need to prescribe it! *British Journal of Sports Medicine*, 43(1): 3–4.

Sallis, R.E. (2009b) 'Foreword', in S. Jonas and E. Phillips, *ACSM's Exercise is Medicine: A clinician's guide to exercise prescription*. Philadelphia: Lippincott, Williams and Wilkins, vii–viii.

Scarborough, P., Bhatnagar, P., Wickramasinghe, K., Allender, S., Foster, C. and Rayner, M. (2011) The economic burden of ill health due to diet, physical inactivity, smoking, alcohol and obesity in the UK: An update to 2006–07 NHS costs, *Journal of Public Health*, 33(4): 527–535.

Schneider, S., Seither, B., Tonges, S. and Schmitt, H. (2006) Sports injuries: Population based representative data on incidence, diagnosis, sequelae, and high risk groups, *British Journal of Sports Medicine*, 40(4): 334–339.

Smith-Maguire, J. (2008) *Fit for consumption: Sociology and the business of fitness*. London: Routledge.

van der Sluis, CK et al. (1998) Long-term physical, psychological and social consequences of severe injuries, *Injury*, 29(4): 281–285.

White, P. (2004) 'The costs of injury from sport, exercise and physical activity: A review of the evidence', in K. Young (ed.), *Sporting bodies, damaged selves*. Oxford: Elsevier Press.

WHO (2011) *Promoting sport and enhancing health in European Union countries: A policy content analysis to support action*. Copenhagen: World Health Organization (Europe).

Williams, S., Martin, P. and Gabe, J. (2011) The pharmaceuticalisation of society? A framework for analysis, *Sociology of Health and Illness*, 33(5): 710–725.

Zola, I. (1972) Medicine as an institution of social control, *Sociological Review*, 20(4): 487–504.

5

SPORT AND PHYSICAL ACTIVITY FOR HEALTH AND WELLBEING
Choice and competing outcomes

Paul Downward

Introduction

When sport and physical activity are bracketed together with economics, this is often within the context of discussing the cost-effectiveness of an intervention in an evaluation of its relative benefits. More generally health economics tends to focus on the demand for, and production of, health services, as well as the assessment of health outcomes of policy interventions, some of which might be connected with enhancing physical activity.[1] The current chapter is not concerned with such insights but, rather, adopts a more critical review of health and physical activity policy from the perspective of the core theoretical foundations of economics. The chapter aims to contribute to the Handbook by examining the role of sport as physical activity in the UK.

In this respect the current normative emphasis of sports policy, which seeks to promote physical activity in the UK, is presented in the following section. It is shown that policy is underpinned by economic concepts that stress the role of markets and individual choice. Policy intervention is thus identified as desirable only in the presence of market failures. The section then provides an examination of the paradoxes and tensions within current policy by identifying a conflation between health and wellbeing. The next section then provides an overview of the evidence that is used to support claims made in current sports policy but that an account of the existing evidence can be offered that is not consistent with market failure. Following this, the next section argues that the greatest wellbeing that is generated from sports participants lies potentially in activity that is connected more with social interactions than with higher intensity activity and the targeted health benefits. This is somewhat paradoxical in that these claims emerge from a theoretical position that focusses on individual behaviour. Nonetheless, it is shown that this reasoning has some resonance with current prescriptions for sports policy as identified by stakeholders in sport. The chapter draws upon previously published work by the author, but is original in drawing together insights from this research within this reflection.

Sports policy in the UK: The economic kernel

From a general economic perspective what activities constitute the specific labels of 'sport', 'recreation', 'exercise' or 'physical activity' are of less intrinsic concern than perhaps for those who research 'sport' from a policy or sociological perspective. Quite naturally in the context of policy or sociological study attention is drawn to the social construction of, and power relationships between, social activities and organisations in specifically defined social domains. In contrast, physical activity researchers are ultimately interested in any activities that can produce health benefits. In the limit physical activity 'is any movement in the body generated by the muscular-skeletal system and fuelled by energy expenditure' (WHO, 2004). Likewise economics focusses less on the specificity of domains and more upon the resource allocation that takes place in sport, a central component of which for participation in sport is the allocation of time. In this respect economics tends to make a distinction between obligated and non-obligated time, and thus the focus of the current chapter is upon sport as physical activity which is the engagement in activity that takes place voluntarily during leisure time. In this regard, the chapter shares Gratton and Taylor's (2000, p. 7) view that definitions of sport involve 'the criterion of general acceptance that an activity is sporting, e.g. by the media and sports agencies'. This general acceptance consequently implies that sport is measured through large-scale official data for public policy purposes. In the UK this occurs through the Active People Survey and Taking Part Surveys commissioned by Sport England and the DCMS (Department for Digital, Culture, Media and Sport - formerly Department for Culture, Media and Sport) respectively to monitor and to inform policy.[2] Both surveys began in 2005–06 and are collected on a rolling monthly basis, with waves published annually. The Active People Survey typically interviews app-roximately 160,000 individuals annually by landline call. Originally respondents were aged 16 years or older, but since 2012 children aged 14 years or older are surveyed. A very large number of sports activities and sub-sets of activities are investigated. The Taking Part Survey interviews about 15,000 individuals face to face over the age of 16 years old, though more recent waves also collect data on children from 2008–09. Approximately 67 sports activities are investigated along with arts, heritage and cultural activities. Naturally, different countries and cultures can recognise different activities as sport but may also monitor the same activities and they might be formal, as with participating in a competitive team sport like rugby or football operating under the auspices of strict governing body regulations, or informal activities such as a 'kick about' with friends or recreational bicycle ride or swim (see Downward et al., 2009).

Of course sport takes place within the economy not only through 'consumption of time' as participation of an informal and formal nature, but also comprises consumption through spectatorship of competition at events and in professional team sports (Downward et al., 2009). In the UK the policy emphasis for sport has embraced these varieties of engagement. Game Plan (2002, p.12) for example stressed the important of a 'twin track' approach to sport in which

government should set itself two overarching objectives:

- a major increase in participation in sport and physical activity, primarily because of the significant health benefits and to reduce the growing costs of inactivity;

and

- a sustainable improvement in success in international competition, particularly in the sports which matter most to the public, primarily because of the 'feelgood factor' associated with winning.

At the time it was argued that policy should focus on promoting grassroots participation to tackle barriers to participation; to prioritise which sports are funded at the highest level; that more caution should be adopted in hosting Mega sporting events and that organisational reform and focussing on what works as interventions was needed before government investment in sport. Leaving aside these arguments, it is important to note that the central public policy message of Game Plan (2002, p. 76), however, was that:

> There are benefits from sport which accrue to individuals, communities and the nation as a whole. However, this is not a sufficient argument for government intervention in the market for sport ... In the competition for scarce resources, however, sport must face up to the challenge of justifying, in more tangible ways, why public money should be invested in it. ... Government does not run sport – and nor should it. Government intervention, however, is legitimate where it remedies ...
>
> • Inefficiency. Private and voluntary provision may be inadequate in some way. This undersupply results in reductions in social welfare that might be avoided by government intervention.
> • Inequity. The government may wish to intervene to promote fairer access to all than would be otherwise achieved.

This suggests that the government should only be involved in the supply of sport when markets fail, with the corollary that when markets do not fail, which is implicitly assumed to be the normal situation, markets are efficient for society. This is a well-known proposition in welfare economics and reflects 'Pareto optimality'. This means that the price by which resources are exchanged captures the relative values of the resources to individuals (allocative efficiency), and that production is taking place at the lowest possible cost (productive efficiency) (Downward et al., 2009).

Current sport strategy (Sporting Future, 2015, p.6–7) essentially emphasises the same arguments, suggesting linking sport to:

• Harnessing the potential of sport for social good
• Prioritising long-term elite success in Olympic and Paralympic sports as well as non-Olympic sports
• Promoting the integrity of sport with new governance codes required for sports receiving public money

with 'the biggest gains and the best value for public investment ... found in addressing people who are least active ... and face common barriers to taking part' (Sporting Future, 2015, p.19). This is identified to be the case for females, black and ethnic minorities, those with a low income and the elderly. There is an assumption, therefore, that market failure is evident either through constraints on behaviour or simply because of inequitable access to opportunities.

Notwithstanding the current sport strategy, current international public policy generally has increasingly emphasised a need for the improvement of the health of individuals (Department of Health, 2004; WHO, 2010). Increases in sport and exercise have been identified in the UK and internationally (GAPA/PSPAH, 2012) as opportunities to contribute towards 'Health Enhancing Physical Activity' (HEPA) (Sport England, 2013), therefore, with a corresponding reduction in health care costs estimated to range between £2 billion (Game Plan, 2002) and £3 billion in the UK. There is, therefore, a generalised normative impetus that public resources are prioritised towards physical activity initiatives. It is argued in the UK, that policy

> guidelines provide recommendations on levels of physical activity which best support population level changes in health ... Action and investment is urgently

needed to increase population levels of physical activity in the UK in order to reap the wide reaching health, social and economic benefits.

BHF, 2013, p.2

The main difference in the new sports strategy in the UK from the past, therefore, is that the focus is not now on

how many people we could get to meet our definition of playing sport, and how may medals we could win. This approach is too simplistic.

Sporting Future, 2015, p.8

But on

five simple but fundamental outcomes: physical health, mental health, individual development, social and community development and economic development. It is these outcomes that will define who we fund, what we fund and where our priorities lie in the future.

Sporting Future, 2015, p.9

Significantly these outcomes are conflated with health. For example it is subsequently argued that

We are redefining what success looks like in sport by concentrating on five key outcomes: physical well-being, mental well-being, individual development, social and community development and economic development.

Sporting Future, 2015, p.10

The first two of these are physical health and mental health; that is stress, anxiety, confidence and self-esteem. The above discussion consequently raises the questions of:

1   What is the nature of sports participation and its structure?
2   What is the value of active leisure expressed as sport and exercise to individuals?
3   Is there a subsequent case to prioritise the promotion of activity of an intensity to generate health benefits versus activity that produces more general wellbeing benefits?

The next section addresses question 1, whilst questions 2 and 3 are addressed in subsequent sections.

Sports participation in the UK: Evidence and interpretation

An examination of the data from the major surveys of sports participation suggests some support for the claims made in Sporting Future (2015). Figure 5.1 shows that the proportion of sports participation in any sport rises with income cohorts.

Figure 5.2 also reflects this, showing that participation is higher overall for those in a higher National Statistics Socio-economic Classification (NS-SEC). The higher classification contains, for example, higher managerial and professional occupations compared to lower supervisory and routine occupations.

The data also reveal that there is an age gradient to participation. Figure 5.3 indicates that sports participation falls consistently with ageing.

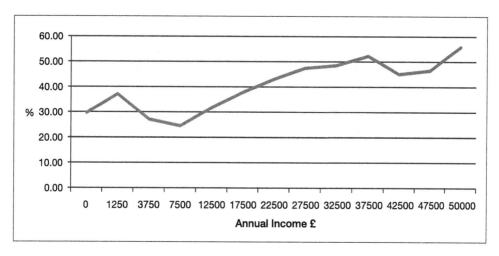

Figure 5.1　Participation in any sport in last four weeks: Taking Part Survey (16+) 2005–2013

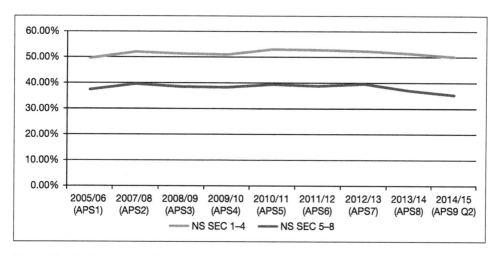

Figure 5.2　Participation rate in any sport: Active People Survey (16+)

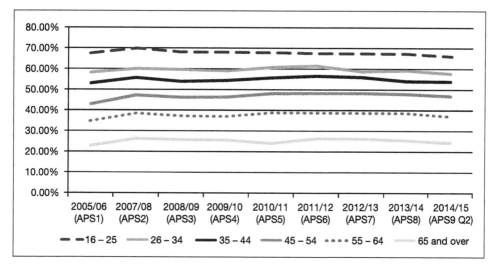

Figure 5.3　Participation rate in any sport: Active People Survey (16+)

Figure 5.4 also shows that more males undertake sport than females.

Figure 5.5 shows that the presence of children in the household raises participation but does not close the 'gender' gap.

The above outline of the evidence seemingly supports the claims made by Sporting Future (2015). However, an examination of black and ethnic minority participation, in Figure 5.6, suggests that the behaviours are not so different from the majority of the population.

More fundamentally, a case can be made that such structured behaviour is to be expected in society from an economic perspective, in which such behaviour is the outcome of a choice rather than reflecting a constraint. This can be illustrated with reference to economic theories of participation.

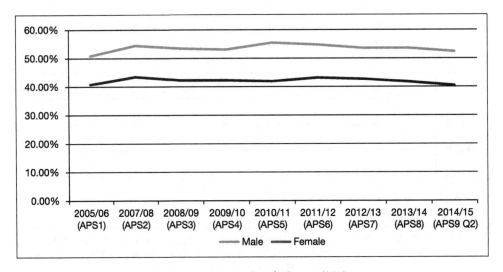

Figure 5.4 Participation rate in any sport: Active People Survey (16+)

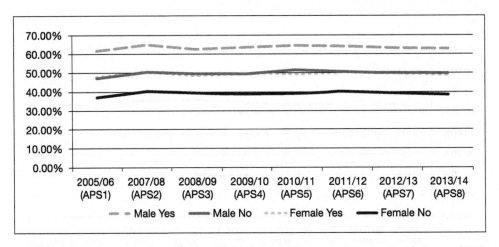

Figure 5.5 Participation rate in any sport (child in household yes or no): Active People Survey (16+)

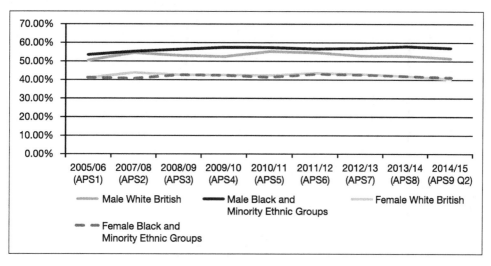

Figure 5.6 Participation rate in any sport: Active People Survey (16+)

The income-leisure trade-off model

The most rudimentary economic analysis of sports participation can be expressed in the income-leisure trade off economic model of behaviour (Gratton and Taylor, 2000; Downward et al., 2009). In this model it is argued that individuals seek to maximise their utility (U), or subjective wellbeing, by the possession of income (I) in order to buy goods and services, or from having leisure time (L) out of total time available (T), which could be used for sports participation. Formally the economist writes that the individual

Maximises $U(I,L)$ subject to $I=w(T-L)$ (1)

Where the wage rate (w) is the cost of time. The model is illustrated in Figure 5.7. Here the individual faces a constraint in that income needs to be earned at a prevailing wage-rate through work (i.e. obligated time), and this involves a reduction in leisure time. This is shown by the straight line on Figure 5.7. The model predicts that an individual will prefer some leisure time, and some income. This is because of the individual's preferences. These are represented by the indifference curves which measure given levels of utility – just as contour lines represent given levels of height – that increases as at least one of either income or leisure increases. The indifference curves capture the economic theoretical perspective that preferences are 'given', and that they are characterised by a set of properties (asymmetrical, non-satiated, strictly convex and transitive; see, for example, Samuelson, 1947) which produces a utility function in which (marginal) utility declines as increments of the same resource are successively consumed. This means that the rate at which people are prepared to exchange resources will vary depending on their relative utility i.e. value to them and this is represented by the declining slope of the indifference curves, the marginal rate of substitution (MRS), which is defined to be the rate at which an individual is prepared to substitute any two resources and leave their overall level of utility constant. As marginal utility declines with consumption this means that if an individual is endowed, say, with a

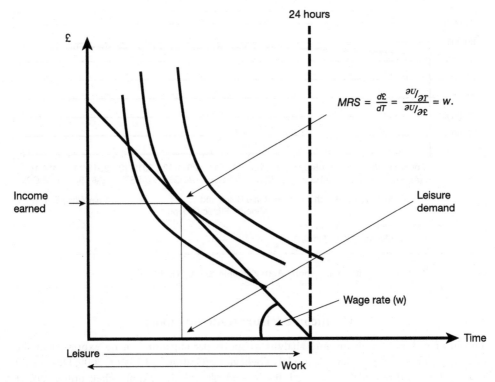

$$MRS = \frac{d\pounds}{dT} = \frac{\partial U / \partial T}{\partial U / \partial \pounds} = w.$$

Figure 5.7   The income-leisure trade-off model

relatively large leisure time and little income (i.e. they were 'cash poor but time rich') they would be prepared to substitute relatively more leisure to obtain income, than would be the case if they had relatively low leisure time and relatively higher income (i.e. they were 'cash rich but time poor'). It can be shown, therefore, that an individual is unlikely to choose to have only leisure or income and that, in general, a combination of the resources will be consumed because of the convexity of preferences, i.e. the indifference curves. Moreover, this consumption will take place where the individual maximises their utility when facing the income and time constraint where the MRS = w.

At this point the subjective value of the resources to the individual is correspondent to the current objective value of them, as presented by the wage rate in the labour market, and this is the highest possible level of utility that is attainable. This result is essential to underpinning Pareto optimality as it shows that individuals are allocating resources according to the values that they attach to them as individuals. It follows that if the wage rate increases, and more of both leisure and income are available to the individual, then they will choose to increase both as illustrated in Figure 5.8.[3] Clearly this prediction is consistent with Figures 5.1 and 5.2 in the latter case of which, higher professional occupations are likely to offer higher incomes and time available for leisure.

The remaining set of social behaviours, outlined in Figures 5.3 to 5.6, however, essentially need to be explained by the preferences of individuals. This is unsatisfactory because ethnicity and gender are represented as choices only in a problematic sense in as much that both physiological and identity criteria are relevant to defining these categories. Moreover, for changes in age to affect participation through preferences suggests that preferences are *not* given

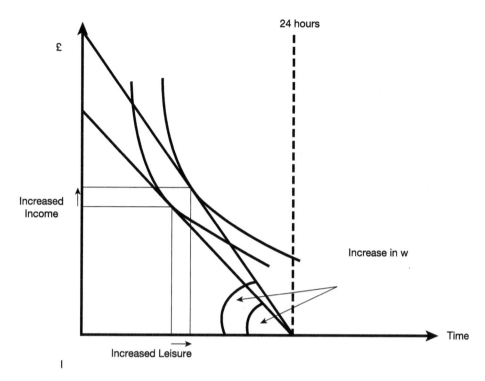

Figure 5.8 Increased participation from increased income

throughout the life course, which contradicts the assumptions of the model. One might argue that behaviours according to these social characteristics might help to determine the wage-rate. For example a gender pay gap might imply that females have lower relative rates of pay which supresses their leisure demand as well as income.[4] This is potentially plausible. It also might be the case that falling incomes with age – particularly as people retire – could explain the falling demand for leisure, but clearly problems with this account are that the model cannot then account for the increased leisure time that retirement brings simultaneously with the fall in income. Work cannot apply to a retiree unless one assumes that all pensioners engage in some part-time activity! Moreover, it is also clear that in middle age incomes are higher, typically, and yet the data suggests a smooth age gradient for declining sports participation. It is clear, therefore, that these additional arguments offer an unsatisfactory explanation because the theory does not actually outline the mechanisms by which behavioural change occurs.

The time allocation model

A better economic explanation is offered in the 'time allocation' framework first developed by Becker (1965). In this approach Becker argued that the resources that we consume are actually, in part, produced within households.

Consequently within the household resources (x) purchased from income are combined with time (t) to produce the goods that are finally consumed (Z). These goods thus have input resource mixes that are either 'goods' or 'time' intensive. Formally this means that the individual

Maximises $U(Z(x,t))$ subject to $Z(x,t)$ (2)

As Becker (1965, p. 98, emphasis added) writes,

> What, then, is the relation between our analysis, which treats all commodities sym-
> metrically and stresses only their differences in relative time and earning intensities, and
> the usual analysis, which distinguishes a commodity having special properties called
> 'leisure' from other more commonplace commodities? It is easily shown that the usual
> labour-leisure analysis can be looked upon as a special case of ours in which the cost
> of the commodity called leisure consists entirely of foregone earnings and the cost of
> other commodities entirely of goods.

This means that the economic cost of an activity is a composite cost comprising the prices
of goods and the opportunity cost of time. Moreover, as individuals invest in activity it might
be expected that skill acquisition will develop and lead to the consolidation of behaviours in
particular areas because of the development of human capital. Consequently the theory
suggests that males and females invest in different skill sets through their leisure choices, thus
accounting for, for example, differences in male and female sport participation rates. This
suggests that such differences are not about constraints but choice. For example it can be
shown that 65.9 per cent of theatregoers in the UK in the last 12 months were females
compared to 34.1 per cent males from the Taking Part Survey for 2013–14.

Becker's initial work was extended in two fundamental directions. The first of these is
through the work of Becker (1974) and Stigler and Becker (1977) who showed that the
individual might also invest in social capital, that is characteristics that were considered to
be desirable and that they might also develop consumption capital, that is skills in the
consumption of particular activities. This theoretical development suggests the potential for
'sporty' people to emerge *versus* 'non-sporty' people and that individuals participating in sport
are more likely to be multi-sport participants. The evidence supports these predictions.
Downward and Rasciute (2010) show that the number of sports undertaken by individuals
varies inversely with the number of other leisure activities undertaken by individuals based
on the Taking Part Survey for 2005. This is illustrated in Figure 5.9.

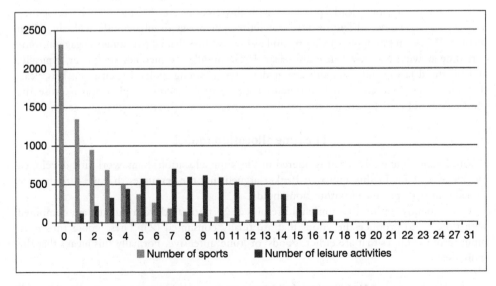

Figure 5.9   Number of sport and leisure activities: Taking Part Survey 2005

Significantly too, Downward and Rasciute (2010) also show that relatively high cost – that is goods and time intensive – activities like playing rugby and a musical instrument have relatively low participation rates at 0.8 per cent and 9.2 per cent respectively. Activities that are relatively less goods and time intensive however, like swimming and reading, have much higher participation rates at 29.8 per cent and 64.8 per cent respectively. Moreover, Downward and Riordan (2007) show that an individual's participation in a specific sport is likely to be enhanced not only by their own individual characteristics, but by their similarity to other groups of people, such as those predominantly engaged in leisure activities, those in recreational and keep-fit activities, and those in competitive and more technical sports, as indicative of social capital. The number of other sports participated in also increased the participation of a specific sport as indicative of consumption capital.

The second extension to the time allocation model is due to Grossman (1972), who argued that individuals possess a stock of inherited health capital. This will naturally depreciate with aging. Consequently individuals can choose to invest in health care to counter the depreciation. Undertaking sport and physical activity might then be viewed as an investment in health care. However, it might also flow from a desire to avoid reductions in health. Figure 5.10 shows that the specific age profile of a sport can vary with age and that more intense and competitive activities like outdoor football very rapidly reduce with age compared to activities such as swimming, which might be considered overall to be a more recreational and healthy-oriented pursuit. Significantly this extension to the model shows that the ageing relationship again can be understood to be an outcome of choice and, significantly, that health is not necessarily an outcome of sporting activity.

Health and wellbeing from sport

The previous sections have illustrated how economic analysis can account for the sports participation patterns as identified in the UK, and challenge the argument that the observed

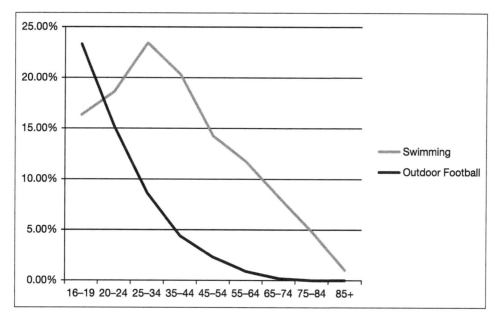

Figure 5.10   Sport participation with age: Taking Part Survey 2013–14

behaviour is the outcome of constraints that require targeting through policy. In the latter part of the previous section it was suggested that health is not necessarily an outcome of sporting participation. In this section this issue is investigated further and particularly the issue of health and wellbeing being presented as synonymous outcomes for policy.

To begin with it should be noted that there is no doubt that sport can improve physical health (Warburton et al., 2006), and that it has the potential to reduce depression and hence improve psychological mood (Chalder et al., 2012). The medical literature consequently presents ubiquitous findings supporting these claims and these draw upon randomised controlled trials of interventions, observational studies and large-scale analysis of correlates (Downward and Dawson, 2015). However, the focus upon one, often contrived, intervention in analysis is not the same thing as observing an individual's actual choices in the population which, as the economic analysis above suggests, reflects an individual allocating their resources to maximise their utility or wellbeing. The economic analysis of sport and its impacts on health and wellbeing consequently tends to focus on large-scale secondary datasets, such as those noted in the earlier section. Table 5.1 summarises some of the literature and its findings.

Table 5.1 The impact of sport participation on health: Economic studies

Author	Data	Type	Findings
Lechner (2009)	German Socio-economic panel	Causal (matching estimator)	Examines the effect of sports participation on illness preventing work (as an objective measure of health) as well as subjective single-scale statements of health. Positive impacts of sport on health are broadly identified, though there is less evidence of this for males for the subjective statements.
Rasciute and Downward (2010)	Taking Part Survey	Associational (Bivariate estimator)	Show that in the UK participation in sports as well as walking and cycling positively affects a single scale subjectively defined health measure.
Humphreys et al. (2014)	Canadian Community Health Survey	Causal (Bivariate estimator with instrumental variable)	Show that a series of binary measures of varying frequencies and intensities of physical activity affect the reported incidence of actual health conditions.
Sarma et al. (2015)	Canadian Community Health Survey	Causal (Bivariate estimator with instrumental variable)	Show that controlling for workplace physical activity some of the results of Humphreys et al. (2014) can be challenged with respect to diabetes, blood pressure and heart disease.
Downward et al. (2015)	Taking Part Data	Causal (Time-series estimator)	Increases in the level of health requires accelerating increases in sport participation. No feedback is revealed. Reductions in the level of health are brought about by increases in sports participation in early adulthood and that this gets reversed in middle age. However, a reduction in health re-emerges for older males compared to females.

In general it is shown that sport can improve health, though Downward et al. (2015) suggest that the effect can be negative for younger males and females, and older males.

The more important issue for economists to address, however, is to identify the greatest social welfare from sports participation. Economists have addressed this issue by examining the impact of sport on measures of subjective wellbeing that are seen to be proxies for utility (Frey, 2008). These measures and their reliability and validity are discussed fully in Stiglitz et al. (2008) and OECD (2013) and they are now incorporated in UK Official Statistics (ONS, 2014). Their analysis is also seen to be important for policy evaluation Fujiwara and Campbell (2011). Table 5.2 provides an overview of recent economic contributions. A clear examination of the table shows that sport increases subjective wellbeing, that is welfare. What is interesting too is that in papers such as Becchetti et al. (2008) and Downward and Rasciute (2010) collective activities contribute towards the individual's wellbeing and that sport undertaken in groups or teams particularly so. The tables also suggest, for example from considering Rasciute and Downward (2010), that health and wellbeing are not necessarily synonymous. A further issue raised by the research is that the effect of sport is measured in

Table 5.2 The impact of sport participation on subjective wellbeing: Economic studies

Author	Data	Type	Findings
Becchetti et al. (2008)	German Socio-economic panel	Associational	SWB increases with increasing frequency of attending social gatherings, attending cultural events, participation in sports, performing volunteer work and attending church or religious organizations.
Lechner (2009)	German Socio-economic panel	Causal (Matching estimator)	Significant and positive effects of sport participation upon the SWB of males but insignificant effects for females.
Rasciute and Downward (2010)	Taking Part Survey	Associational (Bivariate estimator)	Show that sports as well as walking *unlike* cycling positively affects SWB.
Downward and Rasciute (2011)	Taking Part Survey	Associational	Social interactions enhance effects as SWB larger for group and team sports.
Pawlowski et al. (2011)	International Social Survey	Causal (instrumental variable estimator)	SWB is increased with sports but the effects are larger for the more elderly.
Becchetti et al. (2011)	World Values Survey	Causal (Recursive bivariate model with instrumental variable)	SWB increases with time spent in collective leisure activity.
Huang and Humphreys (2012)	Behavioural Risk Factor Surveillance System	Causal (Instrumental variables)	A positive effect of sports participation on SWB for both males and females.
Becchetti et al. (2012)	German Socio-economic panel	Causal (Instrumental variables)	A positive relationship between SWB and social and leisure activities.
Dolan et al. (2014)	Eurobaramoter data	Causal (Instrumental variables)	Participation increases SWB.

these studies in a relatively crude way such as the engagement or not in sport generally over a certain, often unspecified period of time.[5] The intensity is not typically explored. In order to investigate the relative importance of health and wellbeing as an outcome from sport, therefore, Downward and Dawson (2015) examined data on the actual minutes of participation in 67 sports activities from the Taking Part Survey and measure sport in three ways: Any sport (the total minutes of any sport undertaken in the last four weeks); Low intensity (the total minutes of sports participation of less than 30 minutes once a week at moderate intensity); and 3x30mins (the total minutes of at least three sessions of 30 minutes of moderate intensity sport a week in the last four weeks). The aim was to measure sport that contributed to recommended guidelines for health, and that which did not, but would be of a more recreational and casual basis.

Figure 5.11 shows that sport of a more intense nature is less frequent than that of a less intense nature.

To measure the wellbeing effects the model that was estimated is implied in equation 3.

$$SWB_i = \beta_1 + \beta_2 Sport_i + \beta_3 Income_i + \beta_4 Confounding\ variables_i + \varepsilon_i \tag{3}$$

Where 'i' represents a given individual in the data, 'SWB' represents their level of subjective wellbeing, which is measured in the data as a score on a scale of 1 to 10, with 1 representing the individual being extremely unhappy with their life and 10 representing them being extremely happy, taking all things into consideration. 'Sport' is the minutes of participation in sport undertaken by an individual for any of the measures of sport just outlined. Income is the personal earnings of the individual in the last year before tax and other deductions and the confounding variables were included to control for observed factors that may influence SWB. These included age, gender, ethnicity and household composition, regional location, etc. ε_i is a random error term that reflects all of the unmeasured influences on the individuals SWB and the β_i are parameters to be estimated from the data. Each of these give the unit change in the

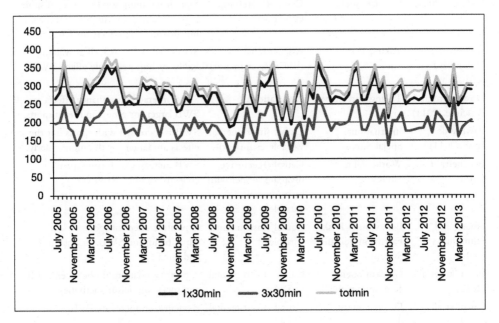

Figure 5.11 Sports participation

value of 'SWB' following a unit change in the respective variable. The sign of the parameter indicates the direction of the changes. Equation 3 is written to imply that changes in 'Sport', 'Income' and other confounding variables cause the changes in 'SWB'. In fact it is possible that 'SWB' could cause changes in 'Sport'. To allow for this, and to ensure that the casual influence of 'Sport' on 'SWB' is measured, the equation was estimated using an instrumental variable estimator, with the month of the survey and proximity to sports facilities used as instruments. Based on this analysis it is possible to calculate the values given in equation 4.

$$-\frac{dI_i}{dS_i} = \frac{\partial SWB_i / \partial Sport_i}{\partial SWB_i / \partial Income_i} = \frac{\beta_2}{\beta_3} \tag{4}$$

This equation represents how much income would need to increase/decrease to compensate for an increase/decrease in sports participation leaving overall wellbeing unchanged. It is a monetary valuation of the wellbeing associated with marginal variations in sports participation, and corresponds to the marginal rate of substitution between time and income. It was found that the marginal valuation placed on a minute of sport of the most intense nature was much greater than the others, which corresponds to its relative scarcity. However, when multiplied by the total minutes of activity at that level e.g. the wealth effect of overall time being allocated, then the total values were greater for the less intense activity. Prima facie this suggests that health and wellbeing through sport are not the same thing, and there is a case for examining the priority given to the promotion of higher intensity sport for health, if maximising social welfare is the objective of policy.

Implications for future physical activity policy and practice

There are a number of implications for future physical activity policy raised by this research and the economic perspective. The first is that it is not obvious that encouraging all individuals to undertake higher intensity activity for longer will have the desired effect often suggested by physical activity researchers. The nature of preferences in economic theory suggests that as activities become less scarce, then their marginal values will fall and thus there is no guarantee that an increase in such activity will create an overall gain in social welfare. This is an empirical question that will depend on the MRS in society. In general making simple linear extrapolations of outcomes is highly misleading. The second is that policy to promote health might be better served by 'stealth' and 'nudging' strategies in which sport is primarily promoted as fun. David Cameron actually remarks in Sporting Future (2015, p. 6) that 'Above all, sport is fun'. Such ideas already have some resonance with the Sport and Recreational Alliance, which suggests policy themes should reflect concepts like:[6]

- 'Game on' – The incorporation of playfulness into mainstream products, services and retail contexts.
- 'Healthy hedonism' – The increasing expectation that healthy behaviours should be fun.

A more radical economic perspective might be to continue to relax government intervention altogether and to recognise that individuals have to take responsibility for their wellbeing. As much as it is often argued that investing in physical activity can reduce health care costs through NHS savings, such savings (as externalities – that is costs and benefits that affect third parties in society) are predicated on the existence of the NHS. In the UK in the last 20 years 'nationalised' industries in energy, transport, telecommunications and even higher education have given way to market allocation to a degree. There is no reason to assume that health will continue to remain a nationalised industry other than through political pressure. What is important to take account of is that sport receives huge amounts of public funding and yet participation is stagnant. It may just be that most of the population is just not interested in it, despite its impact on health and wellbeing.

Conclusions

This chapter has shown that sports policy now has a role to play in a more general normative perspective of the need to promote physical activity in the UK. Current sports policy emphasises the need to encourage more participation from particular low participation groups. However, it is shown that current sports policy is underpinned by economic concepts that stress the role of markets and individual choice. Having reviewed the evidence on sports participation it is also shown, with reference to economic theory and research, that this behaviour can be understood as one of choice rather than constraint. The chapter argues, consequently, that the greatest wellbeing that is generated from sports participation lies potentially in activity that is connected more with social interactions than with higher intensity activity and the targeted health benefits. Sport and physical activity policy consequently needs to be reviewed.

Notes

1 The reader is encouraged, for example, to scroll through the contributions to, say, the *Journal of Physical Activity and Health*, and the *Journal of Health Economic*.
2 The Active People Survey has now been replaced by the Active Lives Survey as a direct result of the new Sports Strategy Sporting Future (2015). As discussed further below, this reflects a change in emphasis and the monitoring of different activities than has been traditionally monitored but which have, for example, health outcomes. Information on the surveys can be obtained from: www. sportengland.org/research/about-our-research/what-is-the-active-people-survey/ and the Taking Part Survey from: www.gov.uk/search?q=Taking+Part+Survey (both retrieved 15 February, 2016).
3 The final choice actually depends on the net outcome from the substitution and income effects. The former is the choice that would have taken place if the wage rate changed and there was no enhancement of income that is where the changed cost of time only is considered. The individual's choice would lie on their original indifference curve where the income-time constraint was tangential at a slope corresponding to the new wage rate. The convexity of preferences means that the substitution effect is always negative such that the demand for leisure time varies inversely with the cost of time i.e. w. The income effect would then be determined as the movement from this hypothetical choice to the final individual's choice recognising that access to resources has increased because of the wage rate.
4 See, for example, http://ec.europa.eu/justice/gender-equality/gender-pay-gap/index_en.htm (retrieved 19 February, 2016).
5 The Taking Part Survey asks about participation in the last four weeks prior to the interview. Other data sets such as the German Socio-economic panel or Eurobarometer data ask about participation in sport generally in a highly qualitative ordered way, in which the intervals do not correspond to specific gaps between frequency of engagement.
6 www.sportandrecreation.org.uk/webforms/future-trends (last retrieved 19 February, 2016).

References

Becchetti, A., Pelloni, A. and Rossetti, F. (2008). Relational goods, sociability, and happiness. *Kyklos*, 61(3), 343–363.
Becchetti, L., Trovato, G. and Londono Bedoya, D.A. (2011). Income, relational goods and happiness. *Applied Economics*, 43(3), 273–290.

Becchetti, L., Ricca, E.G. and Pelloni, A. (2012). The relationship between social leisure and life satisfaction: Causality and policy implications. *Social Indicators Research*, 108(3), 453–490.

Becker, G. (1965). A theory of the allocation of time. *Economic Journal*, 75(299), 493–517.

Becker, G. (1974). A theory of social interactions. *Journal of Political Economy*, 82(6), 1063–1091.

British Heart Foundation National Centre (2013). *Economic Costs of Physical Inactivity Evidence Briefing.* Loughborough: Loughborough University.

Chalder, M., Wiles, N.J., Campbell, J., Hollinghurst, S.P., Haase, A.M., Taylor, A.H., et al. (2012). Facilitated physical activity as a treatment for depressed adults: Randomised controlled trial. *British Medical Journal*, 344, DOI: 10.1136/bmj.e2758.

Department of Health (2004). At least five a week: Evidence on the impact of physical activity and its relationship to health. A report from the Chief Medical Officer. http://webarchive.nationalarchives. gov.uk/20130107105354/http://www.dh.gov.uk/en/Publicationsandstatistics/Publications/ PublicationsPolicyAndGuidance/DH_4080994(last retrieved 20 February, 2016).

Dolan, P., Kavetsos, G. and Vlaev, I. (2014). The happiness workout. *Social Indicators Research*, 119(3), 1363–1377.

Downward, P. and Dawson, P. (2015). Is it pleasure or health from leisure that we benefit from most? An analysis of well-being alternatives and implications for policy. *Social Indicators Research*, 126(1), 443–465, DOI 10.1007/s11205-015-0887-8.

Downward, P., Dawson, P. and Mills, T.C. (2015). Sports participation as an investment in (subjective) health: A time series analysis of the life course. *Journal of Public Health*, 38(4), e504–e510, DOI: 10.1093/pubmed/fdv164.

Downward, P.M., Dejonghe, T. and Dawson, A. (2009). *Sports Economics: Theory, Evidence and Policy.* London: Elsevier.

Downward, P.M. and Rasciute, S. (2010). The relative demands for sports and leisure in England. *European Sports Management Quarterly*, 10(2), 189–214.

Downward, P.M. and Riordan, J. (2007). Social interactions and the demand for sport: An economic analysis. *Contemporary Economic Policy*, 25(4), 518–537.

Frey, B. (2008). *Happiness: A Revolution in Economics.* Cambridge Mass.: MIT Press.

Fujiwara, D. and Campbell, R. (2011). *Valuation Techniques for Social Cost-Benefit Analysis.* London UK: HM Treasury.

Game Plan: A strategy for delivering government's sport and physical activity objectives (2002). DCMS/Strategy Unit.

Global Advocacy for Physical Activity (GAPA) the Advocacy Council of the International Society for Physical Activity and Health (ISPAH) (2012). NCD prevention: Investments that work for physical activity. *British Journal of Sports Medicine*, 46(8), 709–712.

Gratton, C. and Taylor, P. (2000). *Economics of Sport and Recreation.* London: E. and F.N. Spon.

Grossman, M. (1972). On the concept of health capital and the demand for health. *Journal of Political Economy*, 80(2), 223–255.

Huang, H. and Humphreys, B. (2012). Sports participation and happiness: Evidence from U.S. micro data. *Journal of Economic Psychology*, 33(4), 776–793.

Humphreys, B.R., McLeod, L. and Ruseski, J.E. (2014). Physical activity and health outcomes: Evidence from Canada. *Health Economics*, 23(1), 33–54.

Lechner M. (2009). Long-run labour market and health effects of individual sports activities. *Journal of Health Economics*, 28(4), 839–854.

OECD (2013). *OECD Guidelines on Measuring Subjective Well-being.* Paris: OECD Publishing.

ONS (2014). *Measuring National Well-Being: Life in the, UK, 2014.* London: UK Government.

Pawlowski, T., Downward, P. and Rasciute, S. (2011). Subjective well-being in European countries: On the age specific impact of physical activity. *European Review of Aging and Physical Activity*, 8(2), 93–102, DOI 10.1007/s11556-011-0085-x.

Rasciute, S. and Downward, P. (2010). Health or happiness? What is the impact of physical activity on the individual. *Kyklos*, 63(2), 256–270.

Samuelson, P.A. (1947). *Foundations of Economic Analysis.* Cambridge, MA: Harvard University Press.

Sarma, S., Devlin, R.A., Gilliland, J., Campbell, M.K. and Zaric, G.S. (2015). The effect of leisure-time physical activity on obesity, diabetes, high BP and heart disease among Canadians: Evidence from 2000/2001 to 2005/2006. *Health Economics*, 24(12), 1531–1547.

Sport England (2013). A summary of sports participation indicators. www.sportengland.org/ media/643832/summary-of-sport-participation-indicators.pdf (last retrieved 20 February, 2016).

Sporting Future: A New Strategy for an Active Nation (2015). HM government. www.gov.uk/government/uploads/system/uploads/attachment_data/file/486622/Sporting_Future_ACCESSIBLE.pdf (last retrieved 20 February, 2016).

Stigler, G. and Becker, G. (1977). De Gustibus Non Est Disputandum. *The American Economic Review*, 67(2), 76–90.

Stiglitz, J.E., Sen, A. and Fitoussi, J.P. (2008). Report by the Commission on the Measurement of Economic Performance and Social Progress. www.stiglitz-sen-fitoussi.fr/documents/rapport_anglais.pdf (last retrieved 20 February, 2016).

Warburton, D.E.R., Nicol, C.W. and Bredin, S.S.D. (2006). Health benefits of physical activity: The evidence. *Canadian Medical Association Journal*, 174(6), 801–809.

WHO (2004). Global strategy on diet, physical activity and health. www.who.int/dietphysicalactivity/strategy/eb11344/strategy_english_web.pdf (last retrieved 20 February, 2016).

WHO (2010). Global recommendations on physical activity for health. www.who.int/dietphysicalactivity/publications/9789241599979/en/index.html (last retrieved 20 February, 2016).

6

THE IMPERATIVE OF PHYSICAL ACTIVITY IN PUBLIC HEALTH POLICY AND PRACTICE

Louise Mansfield

Introduction

This chapter examines the interplay between the promotion and prescription of physical activity and public health. It discusses the historical development of the modern public health movement in which the imperative of physical activity has developed. Educative practices of public health and the significance of 19th century schooling are identified as developmental processes in the establishment of a modern public health movement through which the health and wellbeing benefits of physical activity have been championed. The chapter illustrates the ways that dominant public health discourses emphasising healthy lifestyle behaviours have ushered in a contemporary focus on the role of physical activity. In critiquing current policy agendas in public health that reinforce ideas about individual responsibility for physical activity, the chapter then considers alternative strategies for ensuring any potential benefits of physical activity for public health might be realised. Three overlapping strategies are presented: (1) an emphasis on community-based and participatory approaches to understanding inactivity, activity engagement and social diversity, (2) recognition of cross sector expertise and knowledge exchange in physical activity and public health and (3) a focus on collaborative partnership approaches to evaluation of physical activity programmes.

The historical context for physical activity in public health

The historical development of the public health movement worldwide has shaped the imperative of physical activity in health promotion and disease prevention. The precise historical trajectory of public health discourse, policy and practice, and the role of physical activity within it, differs between countries. There are worldwide inequities in health, in access and opportunities for physical activity for health, and disparities in the way public health broadly, and physical activity specifically, is promoted, accessed and experienced between social groups. However, the most well established public health systems, those characterised by state standards and governance, have emerged from three overlapping processes: (1) the growth of sanitary science led by reformers in 19th century Britain and Europe, (2) the prevalence of regimes of personal and public hygiene and (3) a contemporary or 'new' public health authority emphasising the role of health education and lifestyle behaviours in improving and protecting public health (Armstrong, 1993).

In Britain, one of the most significant developments in state commitment to promoting and protecting public health was the enactment of the 1848 Public Health Act, a government treatise engineered by the 19th century social reformer Sir Edwin Chadwick. The Act was underpinned by recognition that regular contraction and spread of infectious diseases amongst the lower social classes living in urban areas was the result of insanitary living conditions directly associated with inadequate or absent drainage and removal of waste and sewage. Moreover, the Act was predicated on the view that effective and sustained improvement in public health needed the proactive involvement of the state in monitoring disease, setting and guaranteeing public health standards and the provision of local government resources to deliver improvements (Sram and Ashton, 1998). Legislative measures to support state-sponsored approaches to public health were revolutionary in the mid-19th century. Yet they have a legacy in contemporary public health policy in terms of the involvement of central government, local communities and individuals in promoting and enhancing people's health and wellbeing (Hamlin and Sheard, 1998). In 1848, Chadwick's determination to progress from reactive strategies of disease control involving quarantine, burning of clothing and travel restrictions to state responsibility for addressing environmental threats to public health resulted in the supply of clean water and the efficient removal of sewage and waste. Debates prevail in the historical literature about the successes and flaws of the 1848 Public Health Act (Hamlin and Sheard, 1998). It has served as the foundation for systematic inquiry and data collection on health risks, disease prevalence and environmental health threats. Through the Act, technical solutions to environmental threats to public health were delivered. Moreover, government accountability, legislation and resource provision became established mechanisms for public health improvement. Yet, the welfare intentions of the 1848 Public Health Act were also characterised by doctrines of social control of the lower classes through practices of surveillance and government legislation (Lupton, 1995). These motifs remain in contemporary public health policy and practice broadly and in the promotion and prescription of physical activity for health more specifically.

Coupled with the recognition of the role of the state in monitoring and regulating public health, an intensifying medicalisation of public health shifted the discipline from one based on amateurism and superstition to a legitimate scientific, professional practice (Turner, 2008). From the late 19th century, the establishment of government-led legislative strategies for public health moved beyond environmental sanitation towards ideologies and practices of personal hygiene. The public health agenda twinned a continuing concern about environmental determinants of disease (e.g. dirt and squalor) with individual responsibility for personal cleanliness (e.g. hand washing and desisting from openly sneezing and coughing). Health became a personal moral duty, regulated by medical and state surveillance (Lupton, 1997). In several countries worldwide the concern with personal hygiene became coupled with the prioritisation of fitness in the population and physical activity emerged as a principal cultural context for health education in the service of medical and state regulation of public health.

Physical activity, education and the emergence of a public health movement

Histories of public health reveal that popular and academic knowledge of controlled physical exertion has always advocated the wider health benefits of active lifestyles (Turner, 2008; Featherstone et al., 1991). The modern public health movement, initially influenced by social reform and the sanitarian movement of the late 18th century developed during the early 19th century to focus on ignorance (particularly amongst the poor) as a cause of inadequate hygiene and ill health. Even in the late 17th and early 18th centuries, there was an educative role for medical professionals in promoting public health through physical activity. For example, the Aberdonian doctor George Cheyne (1671–1743) was especially influential in promoting the benefits of 'diet, moderation in drink, and light exercise for healthy living and mental stability' (Turner, 2008: 96).

The contribution of physical activity for mental and physical health and wellbeing are a recurrent theme in the development of the modern public health movement from the 19th century onwards. A doctrine characterised by medical and state regulation and restraint of health was advanced by a moral imperative towards teaching individual responsibility for health; an exercise in disciplining the appearance and functioning of one's body (Crawford, 1984; Waddington, 2000; Gard and Wright, 2005). Dominant standards of health, externally imposed by the medical professions, social reformers, indeed any arbiter of state health policy goals, became subjected to pedagogical processes of reflection, negotiation and internalisation. Health status emerged as a central measure of one's moral standing. Being active was not only associated with the learning of physical abilities. More broadly knowing about and taking part in physical activity represented a certain standard of health knowledge.

Through physical activity, people came to demonstrate an ability to care for and know their own bodies in accordance with two overlapping corporeal ideals: the active, fit, capable body, and the hygienic body. By this view, physical activity represents a therapeutic technology in the sense that it is a way in which 'good' habits are learned, internalised and taken on as unthinking habits of self-care. To be healthy remains symbolic of a robust moral disposition and a disciplined lifestyle, whereas to be unhealthy carries the stigma of moral weakness associated with sloth, gluttony and over-indulgent living (Shilling, 2012). At the start of the 19th century, education became an established means of ensuring public health improvements. Health education including a pedagogical focus on the contribution of physical activity to health remains a central feature of modern public health policy and practice.

The role of schools and schooling cannot be underestimated in the growing focus on educating the population about public health and the role of physical activity in health promotion throughout the 19th century. At this time, Boards of Education and Ministers for Health began to formalise policy goals towards the provision of physician-led health education (Lupton, 1997). The extant literature indicates that a health-hygiene-therapeutic technology has always been part of the established ideology of physical activity, exercise and sport in the schooling of boys and the education of men. What is also striking, however, is the evidence that the health promoting aspect of physical activity was particularly significant in the legitimation of female exercise for women in England during the nineteenth century (Hargreaves, 2002). Atkinson (1978) points out that considering medical opposition to any type of female education, the physical education curriculum for middle class English girls was radical in its defence of physical activity on the grounds of health. Such a position remained wedded to the development of stringent moral characteristics based on discipline and responsibility as it did for boys. Illustrating the legacy of earlier discourses of public health, health education at this time included teachings about hygiene, sanitation and ventilation.

In the latter half of the 19th century, the emphasis on corporeal control through schooling the body reflected the development of wider public health measures. The early modern public health movement was linked to capitalist ideals of productivity and the requirement of a healthy work force, and was largely aimed at combating the social diseases of the working class, such as typhoid, smallpox, tuberculosis and venereal disease (Lupton, 1997; Turner, 2008). Notions of physical fitness, cleanliness and hygiene already characterised ideas about working class male identity and physical exertion. And, notwithstanding the contradictory nature of physical activity for girls and women, by the end of the 19th century, the physical and mental health of middle class girls had come to be viewed as a serious problem that could be addressed through medical inspection, health education and physical exercise. Thus, the medical doctor and physical educationalist may be regarded as complementary professional personnel acting as agents of corporeal discipline and control (Atkinson, 1978), their work helping to shape men and women to conform with dominant expectations regarding productivity, morality and public health.

Modern public health discourse, lifestyle politics and the role of physical activity

In a contemporary sense, public health refers to a range of approaches in research, policy and practice which aim to prevent disease, promote health and prolong life in a population as a whole (WHO, 2007). Previous sections have articulated the long and complex history underpinning public health and physical activity for health. These continue to be dynamic political spheres involving the surveillance of populations, evidence-based policy and practice, evolving approaches to policymaking, policy implementation and policy enactment and diversity of interventions and programming. Public health (and the prescription and promotion of physical activity within it) now involves many different professionals delivering a multitude of initiatives in a wide range of settings, all of which are intended to contribute to the welfare of people (Douglas et al., 2009).

Increasing population rates of physical activity is a current priority area for public health policy in the UK and globally. The World Health Organization emphasises the significance of physical activity for worldwide public health through global recommendations focusing on prevention of non-communicable diseases (NCDs) (WHO, 2010). The UK's Department of Health has embedded these ideas in public health campaigns such as *Start Active, Stay Active* (DoH, 2011). Illustrating the continued dominance of medical evidence in policy and decision making about public health, these policy agendas stem from a range of scientific (physiologically based) studies and position statements showing that physical activity, of a regular and moderate kind, reduces risk of disease and improves health in relation to cardio-respiratory function, muscular strength and endurance, flexibility and body composition (Foster et al., 2005; Garber et al., 2011). There is also a developing literature on the psychological value of exercise for adults in improving mental health by reducing anxiety (Ströhle, 2009) and depression (Mammen and Faulkner, 2013), and moderating levels of stress and producing positive moods (Landers and Arent, 2001). In children and adolescents physical activity is associated with positive outcomes connected to depression, anxiety, self-esteem and cognitive function (Biddle and Asare, 2011). Such evidence, though, is not utilised in a politically neutral way in formulating public health policy and promoting physical activity for health.

Dominant narratives and 'common-sense' ideas about healthy bodies and active lifestyles prevail in the policy arena of physical activity (Waddington, 2000). Since the late 20th century, the ideology of lifestyle has been used as a vehicle for enhancing public health across the public and private spheres. The dominant motif in government health policy and the concomitant commercial market for health and fitness, in the UK, USA and Canada certainly, but in other countries worldwide, has been a focus on the idea that individual responsibility for health should be the basis for the health of the nation. The wider political milieu of new-right government thinking provided the catalyst for a reformed relationship between lifestyle, public health policy and culture during the 1980s in the UK, for example. In particular, debates about the sustainability of the welfare state led to the reassessment of the role of the state in intervening in and allocating resources to public health. Like the USA, the UK witnessed a shift in resource allocation from social expense to capital expense (largely based on corporate tax relief) with a parallel political appeal to the population to be self-reliant, self-disciplined and self-sacrificing (Howell and Ingham, 2001). As Howell and Ingham (2001) argue, the language of lifestyle and its associated practices (principally connected to diet, physical activity, smoking, alcohol consumption, drug use and sexual activity) captured the popular imagination serving to secure the internalisation of political ideology of individual responsibility for health. Health and illness were conflated with personal character, and public health problems were reduced to personal issues of lifestyle. Physical activity was arguably the centerpiece for articulating the ideology of personal responsibility, lifestyle and public health improvements. Howell and Ingham (2001: 331) explain this contention in terms of the politics of public health in the USA in the 1980s:

> Nowhere was this relationship between self-improvement and lifestyle more commonly articulated than on the exercise and fitness marketplace. Since the recognition of the jogging boom of the late 1970s we have witnessed the dramatic growth of a fitness and health industry that has embraced and promoted the relationship between exercise and character, responsibility and prevention in quite specific ways.

A politics of physical activity promotion that emphasises individual responsibility and lifestyle change is to be challenged. The idea that there is a ubiquitous 'Western' lifestyle, represented by general decline in healthy lifestyles, which somehow has the potential to make everyone unhealthy, is flawed (Gard and Wright, 2005). It is a rhetoric which masks the reality that different groups of people hold different values about, and orientations towards health and active living. Furthermore, as Waddington (2000) points out, a focus on individual responsibility for health presents the over-simplified idea that individual people have total control over their health and physical activity status. Illness, disease and inactivity are shaped by important socio-cultural dimensions, which are ignored in the conflation of health with self-control.

Contrary to public health messages in the UK, the provision of information and the acquisition of knowledge about health and the health benefits of physical activity do not necessarily lead to increased participation levels, even when people recognise a need for, or wish to choose a more active lifestyle. There are several significant barriers to engaging in physical activity, including poverty, challenges of time, (dis)ability, illness, lack of access to facilities and services and family/cultural restrictions. These characteristics of social life contribute to inequalities in physical activity and health which are not recognised in the contemporary focus on health as individual responsibility. If any of the potential health benefits of physical activity are to be realised, an alternative strategy for promoting and supporting the design and implementation of, access to and engagement with programmes is required. Below I suggest three overlapping strategies involving community-based and participatory approaches, cross sector knowledge exchange, and collaborative partnership working to evaluate the impact of physical activity projects, all of which eschew an overbearing emphasis on individual responsibility for physical activity and health. Rather, they focus on creating learning spaces and stimulating cross sector and stakeholder dialogue that may better enable people to engage in ethical and respectful social change in the promotion of, engagement in and evaluation of physical activity for health (Mansfield and Rich, 2013).

Community-based and participatory approaches to understanding physical activity for public health

There is evidence that community engagement interventions can have a positive impact on health behaviours (Brown et al., 2003). A variety of community approaches for health and wellbeing improvement can be employed that focus variously on developing communities through volunteering and peer roles, collaborations and partnerships and access to community resources (Wendel-Vos et al., 2009), as well as through empowering people, ensuring democratic decision making and addressing social exclusion (South, 2015). Community is commonly taken to refer to a group of people sharing common characteristics, interests and/ or attitudes. Yet, community is a contested concept characterised by theoretical, empirical and methodological continuity and contestation over time (Crow and Mah, 2012). Community defines the relationships, identities and interests that have the potential to bring people together and push people apart, by place, culture and/or activity. Understanding diversity and difference, and continuities and discontinuities in community contexts has the potential to support the development of relevant, accessible and effective physical activity for health programmes. Successful community-based health interventions are associated with extensive formative research, participatory strategies and a theoretical and practical focus on recognising the significance of social norms in understandings and practices of health (Merzel and D'afflitti, 2003). Such perspectives seek to account for the complexities of ecological factors that impact on health behaviours. A focus on social diversity and inequality is important in this regard. However, so too is an emphasis on identifying the complex relationships between local and national policy and practice and the public in understanding community contexts, needs and roles central to developing, implementing and evaluating projects for health and wellbeing improvements.

Several scholars have identified the significance of working within what can be broadly termed a participatory action research or community participatory action research framework in both UK and international development contexts. Whilst different in their precise objectives, methods and outcomes, such work reflects the common feature of participatory and community-based approaches which is to co-develop programmes of activity through the coproduction of knowledge about potential participants, delivery processes, evaluation strategies and dissemination work (see for example, Baum, 1995; McIntyre, 2007). Participatory methods are also wide-ranging although often draw from qualitative approaches enabling high degrees of involvement in community projects. Arguably, a point of convergence in participatory methods is the centrality of narrative inquiry in defining the meaning that people attach to their experiences; the lay knowledge that can inform community physical activity provision.

Whilst increasingly accepted as evidence, lay knowledge (the stories, narratives and experiential meaning that people articulate) is commonly omitted from, or utilised to support established discourses of provision in much current objectivist policy and practice in public health including the promotion and delivery of physical activity programmes. There are notable exceptions. For example, in the UK-based Health and Sport Engagement Project (Mansfield et al., 2015) participatory focus groups formed a central part of the planning phase with those who identified as inactive, for whom there were likely to be barriers to physical activity, and who were interested in becoming more physically active through community sport. This method represented public or lay involvement in the project and enabled researchers, delivery personnel and policy makers to listen to those who wished to take part in community sport. The methods allowed a deeper understanding of participants' views about inactivity, activity and local sport opportunities. In international development work in sport, Kay et al. (2015) outline a long-term partnership strategy for developing local research capacity between researchers and local project delivery teams on the Go Sisters girls' empowerment programme in Zambia. A community approach based on co-learning through participatory knowledge exchange workshops enabled the evaluation to be framed by culturally relevant understandings, localised knowledge and the pursuit of decolonisation in research. Bringing the expertise of the local delivery teams to the project improved the quality and integrity of the evaluation processes but also supported the growth of community sport projects by allowing delivery staff to better understand the successful and unsuccessful elements of their projects (Museke et al., 2015).

In arguing for community-based approaches to physical activity for public health in this chapter, a critical framework for analysis is emphasised. Community is almost always imagined in public health, for its positive connotations. In practice, communities are also characterised by tension, division, inequality and exclusion (Crow and Mah, 2012). Whilst it can be argued that shifting power and decision making to local community contexts can be a way to create more democratic, equitable models of physical activity for health provision, the fact that community collaborations can serve to protect the status quo and limit the role of diverse community-based leadership must be considered (Chavis, 2001). In developing understanding of what works, for whom, how and why in design, promotion and implementation, methods which explore the significance of the complex social lives of people living in communities cannot be underestimated. Participatory strategies which capture lay knowledge offer a way to embed sophisticated insights about physical activity experiences into the design and delivery of programmes. This represents a different, potentially alternative and certainly complementary approach to current individualised behaviour change interventions in which future physical activity levels are matched to current engagement levels of different target groups be that a stage of contemplation, preparation or action. Involving communities and the people for whom health services are designed has some potential for improving delivery and experience by genuinely listening to and working with potential users of public health services (Popay and Williams, 1996).

Cross sector expertise and knowledge exchange in physical activity for public health

The social, political and economic complexity of the modern public health movement and the diversity of people engaging in its services means that there is a need to harness multiple perspectives in design and implementation. The previous section explained the promise of working with potential participants to ensure physical activity provision is tailored to them, and to achieve success in engaging them. Equally significant is a focus on the managers, coordinators, commissioners, coaches, teachers and instructors involved in community programmes; those who represent a local workforce with extensive expertise in delivering a wide range of physical activities to diverse community groups. Their skills and knowledge can be invaluable in identifying participants, recruiting and retaining them and providing education about and promoting physical activity in local public health contexts; a role perhaps more commonly associated with health care in GP and health centre settings (PHE, 2014; NICE, 2013).

In the UK, physician-prescribed exercise referral or 'exercise on prescription' has become the default approach to delivering physical activity for public health outcomes (Morgan, 2005). In such schemes, the general practitioner (physician) or practice nurse offers expert health advice, identifies those at (health) risk from low levels of physical activity and prescribes a programme of physical activity (three to four months) usually delivered in leisure centre (gym-based) settings. Despite the absence of evidence about the effectiveness of such exercise referral schemes (Hillsdon et al., 2004), and the limits of exercise provision within the offer (gym-based exercise programmes dominate) they have been politicised as a panacea for public health problems (Dugdill et al., 2005). More recent attempts to examine the effectiveness of public health professionals in delivering complex physical activity interventions have identified the leading role of practice nurses in delivering effective behaviour change interventions (Boase et al., 2012). In complex physical activity interventions, involving walking, the practice nurse is positioned as skilled and knowledgeable about the significance of physical activity in public health and able to develop professional advisory-based relationships with patients in an effective technical, caring and educative role (Beighton et al., 2015). Still, major barriers remain in a continued focus on public health professionals delivering population level physical activity interventions. The limits of time in routine consultations reduces their role to an advisory rather than deeply supportive one, prescription is limited to short-term gym-based exercise programmes and they know little of the wide range of community-based physical activity programmes available to people. There is restricted scope for public health professionals to be able to prescribe extensive opportunities for engagement with physical activity that wholly suits the diverse needs and preferences of people in their appointments.

Professionals working in the community sport sector have a potential role in developing and delivering public health and wellbeing programmes that involve physical activity. Community coaches and instructors represent local physical activity experts who can offer valuable insights and act as a community resource in this regard. Not only are they well placed to design and deliver a range of physical activity including walking, dance, community games, cycling and more traditional sport, but they have considerable experience and understanding of adapting physical activities to people's diverse needs and wants. The local leisure and culture workforce engage in extensive and extended face-to-face contact with communities, sometimes daily, providing opportunities for continual support and expert advice on physical activity and public health.

Despite such potential, the expertise of the community-based sport and physical activity sector does not necessarily include formal training or detailed understanding of public health or the complexities of health in diverse community groups. There is a knowledge gap in both public health and sport/physical activity sector training. It remains the case that the training of those delivering community sport/physical activity emphasises the teaching of skills and competencies in a range of movement-based activities from sport to dance to meditative and therapeutic pursuits. Conversely, the training of those prescribing physical activity in public health is likely to be more focused on medical and clinical expertise and skill. Strategies focused on knowledge development and exchange between public health and community delivery organisations may serve to re-model the public health workforce towards a more collaborative cross sector framework. There is some evidence that local leisure organisations in the UK are investing in knowledge and skills development in their workforce and partnerships with the public health sector in understanding and delivering positive public health outcomes from physical activity programmes (Gillingwater, 2016; Mansfield et al., 2016). This includes opportunities for the workforce from both sectors to take part in skills auditing, knowledge and skills exchange events, and to signpost effectively to the services that each offers.

Sports coaches and other physical activity experts represent community assets (Griffiths and Armour, 2014) in the development of sport for health and wellbeing programmes.

Training them in understanding public health, targeting, recruiting and retaining people to wide-ranging opportunities for community-based physical activity for health and wellbeing can support the planning, design and delivery of projects. There are existing high-quality training courses and workshops delivered and accredited by professional public health organisations that can be employed in training a skilled and knowledgeable community sport and public health workforce. In the UK, the Royal Society for Public Health offers courses in understanding health improvement, Mental Health First Aid England teaches courses on both adult and youth mental health issues, The National Health Service e-learning service includes modules on dementia training and behaviour and lifestyle change. In addition, sport-delivery organisations (see for example www.efds.co.uk/; www.sportingequals.org.uk/) have developed a range of strategies for delivering and adapting programmes to make active lives possible for diverse communities. Bespoke knowledge exchange activities (town hall meetings, sandpit events and community-based seminars) also serve to develop effective partnerships between the sport and public health sectors for collaborative approaches to promoting and delivery physical activity in community settings.

Whilst the proposal in this chapter, for cross-sector working and knowledge exchange, represents a significant development from individualised prescription through exercise referral schemes, the widely held assumption that providing a suite of physical activity opportunities will automatically result in increased participation and positive health and wellbeing outcomes is flawed (Gould and Carson, 2008). Still little is known about when and under what conditions physical activity programmes will lead to public health improvements and indeed why provision does not necessarily lead to participation. The development of cross-sector approaches needs to capitalise on the scope to include rigorous approaches to monitoring and evaluation of community sport/physical activity for public health outcomes by developing research-policy-practice partnerships.

Partnership approaches to evaluation of physical activity programmes for public health

Evaluating projects with the people who make decisions about programme goals and deliver projects and with those who take part in physical activity offers a style of inquiry orientated towards an interplay between research and practice (Bradbury and Reason, 2003). There is an emphasis here on the development of collaborative partnerships between participants, community delivery experts, public health professionals and researchers (Minkler, 2005).

Evaluation partnerships involving different academic, managerial, delivery and citizen organisations are a fundamental feature of public health where evidence-based policy and practice has become a universally accepted strategy for determining priorities, organisational structures, service delivery and surveillance mechanisms (Petticrew et al., 2004). Evidence-based *practice* is directly drawn from evidence-based medicine which focuses on integrating clinical expertise with the best research evidence into decision making about patient care (Sackett et al., 1996). The key principles of any evidence-based strategy are effectiveness; the achievement and measurement of stated outcomes, and efficiency; delivery with minimum resource wastage (Thomas et al., 2010). Yet a focus on these tenets has led to the dominance of quantification of outcomes, an evaluation approach wedded to the management of cost such that evidence-based policy and practice has become the strategy for controlling health and health care costs. Successful interventions which are cost-effective are those deemed to be efficient.

The authority of objective measurement of effectiveness and efficiency in public health has produced and reproduced a knowledge economy defined narrowly by the status and generation of predominantly quantitative data on which to base decisions about health. Debates abound regarding the proliferation of quantitative measures of effectiveness. Allied to such discussions is a critique of the applicability of an established hierarchy of evidence for assessing the relevance, significance, rigour and quality of evidence on which to make decisions about health; one which ranks a range of study designs in order of internal validity and thus credibility (Petticrew and Roberts, 2003). Despite the trend towards evidence-based policy and practice, the enactment of it remains challenging as those charged with implementing it struggle to interpret and employ relevant methods with varying resource capacities. The direct impact of research in policy-practice relations is somewhat lacking (Phillips and Green, 2015; Petticrew et al., 2004). Three failings are identified (Black, 2001): (1) a failure of researchers to understand the environment of policy making and the policy making process; (2) a failure of funders to understand the complexities of research impact especially in relation to the time it takes for impact to be realised, and the iterative nature of impact; and (3) the failure of policy makers to be more involved in the inception, design and delivery of research projects. There is a need to develop communities of researchers, policy makers, practitioners and participants in the production, mobilisation and translation of evidence; communities which I have defined elsewhere as research-policy-practice partnerships (Mansfield, 2016). In community-based physical activity programmes, such partnerships cannot be thought of as a simple extension of the practices of normative evidence-based medicine because this would reinforce the failings identified above. Furthermore, it would rely on a narrow conceptualisation of evidence connected to study design, excluding a full consideration of methodological aptness and additional evidence types that can be legitimate in making policy and practice decisions in public health (Petticrew and Roberts, 2003; Rychetnik et al., 2002). Rather, an approach is needed that enables on-going consideration of the values, goals, methods and objectives of all actors in the partnership as well as recognition of a range of sources of knowledge and types of evidence that can contribute to decision making. Scrutiny of the processes by which evidence is produced and becomes legitimate is also needed. Such an approach may require levels of transparency not previously experienced in the community physical activity sector. Furthermore, there may well be challenges in the extent to which community delivery organisations are able to be 'open' to methods which challenge their modes of delivery, find no evidence to support their work, or which are perceived by them to potentially have a detrimental effect on current delivery. However, given the identified weak evidence base for understanding what works in community-based physical activity, for whom, when and under what conditions, more rigorous evaluation is required in this sphere.

Conclusion

Active lifestyle change approaches, focused solely on individualised responsibility, are central to the imperative of physical activity in public health. However, the emphasis is limited in achieving increased population levels of physical activity. It excludes proper attention to the social determinants of health that are central to understanding and addressing the context and reasons why people do and do not engage in physical activity. Such behavioural interventions will be constrained in their effectiveness relative to the material conditions in which people live. If the acclaimed health and wellbeing benefits of physical activity are to be realised more widely, policy and practice requires an approach that recognises and addresses the challenges and constraints of any physical activity intervention in light of the different, diverse and unequal circumstances that people face in their life and in their opportunities for, access to and experiences of physical activity. A focus on identifying the diverse physical activity needs of communities of participants, recognising the skills and knowledge of community physical activity and public health professionals and ensuring a rigorous research strategy in designing, implementing and evaluating community programmes has merit. Taking an approach that challenges the dominance and narrowness of rigid socio-political structures and ideologies of physical activity provision and evaluation, and lays the ground for alternative actions (Giroux, 2004), can serve to engender critical dialogue amongst stakeholder groups and public engagement for a more inclusive and potentially more effective physical activity sector. In this chapter, it is argued that such an approach is likely to involve community-based and participatory approaches, cross sector expertise and knowledge exchange, and collaborative partnership approaches to evaluation of physical activity programmes for public health.

References

Armstrong, D., 1993. Public health spaces and the fabrication of identity. *Sociology, 27*(3) pp.393–410.

Atkinson, P., 1978. Fitness, feminism and schooling. In: S. Delamont and L. Duffin, eds. *The nineteenth century woman: Her cultural and physical world*. London: Croom Helm, 92–134.

Baum, F., 1995. Researching public health: Behind the qualitative-quantitative methodological debate. *Social Science & Medicine, 40*(4), pp.459–468.

Beighton, C., Victor, C., Normansell, R., Cook, D., Kerry, S., Iliffe, S., Ussher, M., Whincup, P., Fox-Rushby, J., Woodcock, A. and Harris, T., 2015. 'It's not just about walking. . . . . it's the practice nurse that makes it work': A qualitative exploration of the views of practice nurses delivering complex physical activity interventions in primary care. *BMC Public Health, 15*(1), p.1236.

Biddle, S. J. and Asare, M., 2011. Physical activity and mental health in children and adolescents: A review of reviews. *British Journal of Sports Medicine*, 45(11), pp. 886–895.

Black, N., 2001. Evidence based policy: Proceed with care. *British Medical Journal, 323*(7307), p.275.

Boase, S., Kim, Y., Craven, A. and Cohn, S., 2012. Involving practice nurses in primary care research: The experience of multiple and competing demands. *Journal of Advanced Nursing, 68*(3), pp.590–599.

Bradbury H. and Reason, P., 2003. Action research an opportunity for revitalizing research purpose and practices. *Qualitative Social Work, 2*(2), pp.155–175.

Brown, W., Eakin, E., Mummery, K., et al., 2003. 10,000 steps Rockhampton: Establishing a multi-strategy physical activity promotion project in a community. *Journal of Physical Activity and Health, 3*(1), pp.1–14.

Chavis, D. M., 2001. The paradoxes and promise of community coalitions. *American Journal of Community Psychology, 29*(2), pp.309–320.

Crawford, R., 1984. A cultural account of 'health': Control, release, and the social body. In: J. McKinley, ed. *Issues in the political economy of health care*. New York and London: Tavistock, 60–103.

Crow, G. and Mah, A., 2012. Conceptualisations and meanings of 'community': The theory and operationalisation of a contested concept. In: *Report to the Arts and Humanities Research Council*. Swindon, UK: Art and Humanities Research Council.

DoH, 2011. *Start active, stay active: A report on physical activity from the four home countries' chief medical officers*, London: Crown Copyright.

Douglas, J., Earle, S., Handsley, S., Jones, L. J., Lloyd, C. E. and Spurr, S. eds., 2009. *A reader in promoting public health*. London: SAGE.

Dugdill, L., Graham, R.C. and McNair, F., 2005. Exercise referral: The public health panacea for physical activity promotion? A critical perspective of exercise referral schemes; their development and evaluation. *Ergonomics, 48*(11–14), pp.1390–1410.

Featherstone, M., Hepworth, M. and Turner, B. S. eds., 1991. *The body: Social process and cultural theory* (Vol. 7). London: SAGE.

Foster, C., Hillsdon, M., Thorogood, M., Kaur, A. and Wedatilake, T., 2005. Interventions for promoting physical activity. Cochrane Database of Systematic Reviews (1) CD003180 *The Cochrane Library*.

Garber, C., Blissner, B., Deschenes, M., Franklin, A., Lamonte, M., Lee, I., Nieman, D. and Swain, D., 2011. *ACSM Position Stand. Quantity and quality of exercise for developing and maintaining cardiorespiratory, musculoskeletal, and neuromotor fitness in apparently healthy adults: guidance for prescribing exercise*, USA: ACSM.

Gard, M. and Wright, J., 2005. *The obesity epidemic: Science, morality and ideology*. London: Routledge.

Gillingwater, C., 2016. Supporting positive health outcomes through leisure and culture trusts. *Perspectives in Public Health, 136*(5), pp. 262–263.

Giroux, H. A., 2004. Cultural studies, public pedagogy, and the responsibility of intellectuals. *Communication and Critical/Cultural Studies, 1*(1), pp.59–79.

Gould, D. and Carson, S., 2008. Life skills development through sport: Current status and future directions. *International Review of Sport and Exercise Psychology, 1*(1), pp.58–78.

Griffiths, M. and Armour, K., 2014. Volunteer sports coaches as community assets? A realist review of the research evidence. *International Journal of Sport Policy and Politics, 6*(3), pp.307–326.

Hamlin, C. and Sheard, J., 1998. Revolutions in public health 1848 and 1998. *British Medical Journal, 317*(7158), pp. 587–591.

Hargreaves, J., 2002. *Sporting females: Critical issues in the history and sociology of women's sport*. New York: Routledge.

Hillsdon, M., Foster, C., Naidoo, B. and Crombie, H., 2004. *The effectiveness of public health interventions for increasing physical activity among adults: A review of reviews*, London: Health Development Agency.

Howell, J. and Ingham, A., 2001. From social problem to personal issue: The language of lifestyle. *Cultural Studies, 15*(2), pp.326–351.

Kay, T., Mansfield, L. and Jeanes, R., 2015. Researching with GoSisters Zambia: Reciprocal learning in sport for development. In: L. Hayhurst, T. Kay and M. Chawansky, eds. *Beyond sport for development and peace – transnational perspectives on theory, policy and practice*. London: Routledge, 214–230.

Landers, D. M. and Arent, S. M., 2001. Physical activity and mental health. *Handbook of Sport Psychology, 2*, pp.740–765.

Lupton, D., 1995. *The imperative of health: Public health and the regulated body* (Vol. 90). London: SAGE.

Lupton, B., Fønnebø, V. and Søgaard, A., 2003. The Finnmark Intervention Study: Is it possible to change CVD risk factors by community-based intervention in an Arctic village in crisis? *Scandinavian Journal of Public Health, 31*(3), pp.178–186.

Mammen, G. and Faulkner, G., 2013. Physical activity and the prevention of depression: A systematic review of prospective studies. *American Journal of Preventive Medicine, 45*(5), pp.649–657.

Mansfield, L., 2016. Resourcefulness, reciprocity and reflexivity: The three Rs of partnership in sport for public health research. *International Journal of Sport Policy and Politics, 8*(4), pp.713–729.

Mansfield, L. and Rich, E., 2013. Public health pedagogy, border crossings and physical activity at every size. *Critical Public Health, 23*(3), pp.356–370.

Mansfield, L., Anokye, N., Fox-Rushby, J. and Kay, T., 2015. The Health and Sport Engagement (HASE) Intervention and Evaluation Project: Protocol for the design, outcome, process and economic evaluation of a complex community sport intervention to increase levels of physical activity. *BMJ Open, 5*(10), p.e009276.

Mansfield, L., Kay, T., Anokye, N. and Fox-Rushby, J., 2016. *The Health and Sport Engagement (HASE) intervention and evaluation project: The design, delivery and evaluation of a complex community sport intervention for improving physical activity, health and wellbeing. Volume 1: Evaluation of the Design and Delivery of the HASE project*. Report for Sport England – Get Health Get Active. Brunel University, London: Sport England.

McIntyre, A., 2007. *Participatory action research* (Vol. 52). London: SAGE.

Merzel, C. and D'afflitti, J., 2003. Reconsidering community-based health promotion: Promise, performance, and potential. *American Journal of Public Health, 93*(4), pp.557–574.

Minkler, M., 2005. Community-based research partnerships: Challenges and opportunities. *Journal of Urban Health, 82*(2), pp.ii3–12.

Morgan, O., 2005. Approaches to increase physical activity: Reviewing the evidence for exercise-referral schemes. *Public Health, 119*(5), pp.361–370.

Museke, S., Namukanga, A. and Palmer-Felgate, S., 2015. Reflection on researching with GoSisters Zambia: Reciprocal learning in sport for development. In: L. Hayhurst, T. Kay, and M. Chawansky, eds. *Beyond sport for development and peace – Transnational perspectives on theory, policy and practice*. London: Routledge, 230–237.

NICE, 2013. National Institute for Health and Care Excellence. Physical activity: brief advice for adults in primary care. NICE public health guidance 44.

Petticrew, M. and Roberts, H., 2003. Evidence, hierarchies, and typologies: Horses for courses. *Journal of Epidemiology and Community Health*, *57*(7), pp.527–529.

Petticrew, M., Whitehead, M., Macintyre, S.J., Graham, H. and Egan, M., 2004. Evidence for public health policy on inequalities: 1: The reality according to policymakers. *Journal of Epidemiology and Community Health*, *58*(10), pp.811–816.

PHE, 2014. *Public Health England: Everybody active, everyday: An evidence-based approach to physical activity*, London: Public Health England.

Phillips, G. and Green, J., 2015. Working for the public health: Politics, localism and epistemologies of practice. *Sociology of Health & Illness*, *37*(4), pp.491–505.

Popay, J. and Williams, G., 1996. Public health research and lay knowledge. *Social Science & Medicine*, *42*(5), pp.759–768.

Rychetnik, L., Frommer, M., Hawe, P. and Shiell, A., 2002. Criteria for evaluating evidence on public health interventions. *Journal of Epidemiology and Community Health*, *56*(2), pp.119–127.

Sackett, D., Rosenberg, W., Gray, J., Haynes, R. and Richardson, W., 1996. Evidence based medicine: What it is and what it isn't. *BMJ: British Medical Journal*, *312*(7023), p.71.

Shilling, C., 2012. *The body and social theory*. London: SAGE.

South, J., 2015. A guide to community-centred approaches for health and wellbeing. Public Health England and NHS England.

Sram, I. and Ashton, J., 1998. Millennium report to Sir Edwin Chadwick. *BMJ: British Medical Journal*, *317*(7158), p.592.

Ströhle, A., 2009. Physical activity, exercise, depression and anxiety disorders. *Journal of Neural Transmission*, *116*(6), pp.777–784.

Thomas, M., Burth, M. and Parkes, J., 2010. The emergence of evidence-based practice. In: J. McCarthy and P. Rose, eds. *Values-based health and social care: Beyond evidence-based practice*. London: SAGE, 3–25.

Turner, B. S., 2008. *The body and society: Explorations in social theory*. London: SAGE.

Waddington, I., 2000. *Sport, health and drugs: A critical sociological perspective*. London: Taylor & Francis.

Wendel-Vos, G., Dutman, A., Verschuren, W., et al., 2009. Lifestyle factors of a five-year community-intervention program: The Hartslag Limburg intervention. *American Journal of Preventative Medicine*, *37*(1), pp.50–56.

World Health Organization (WHO), 2007. *The world health report 2007 – A safer future: global public health security in the 21st century*. Geneva: WHO.

World Health Organization (WHO), 2010. *Global recommendations on physical activity for health*. Geneva: WHO.

THEME B INTRODUCTION
Evidence and policy

The mantra of 'evidence-based policy' has gained contemporary currency in political discourse because it implies that decisions about what to do and what to fund are based not on the ideologies or whims of politicians or political parties, but on evidence bases collated, appraised and interpreted by experts. However, the route from evidence to policy is not as smooth as one might imagine it to be. There are different bodies of evidence, and the discipline-bound nature of scientific and social-scientific practice means that those generating and promoting such evidence bases rarely look beyond the evidence that their discipline has generated. In fact, the route from evidence to policy may mean that disciplines are disincentivised from collaborating, instead competing for influence over policy and seeking to demonstrate that 'their' discipline and practices have the greatest impact.

In this second theme of the Handbook, these various evidence bases and the influence, warranted or not, that they wield on policy are explored. Bodies of biomedical, social science and behavioural evidence are set out, as are the ways in which such bodies of evidence are translated into policy and their perceived successes measured.

The first chapter in this theme, written by Mike Weed, focuses on the way in which biomedical evidence has been interpreted to inform one of the most foundational elements of physical activity policy worldwide, guideline recommendations for physical activity participation. Exploring audiences for such guidelines, Weed contends that, regardless of intention, physical activity guidelines are direct public health interventions. Within this context, he shows that those interpreting biomedical evidence have failed to consider evidence outside their discipline, and have made un-evidenced assumptions about what is an achievable target for the less and least active as well as value judgements about what populations will value as a significant health benefit. This leads Weed to conclude that physical activity guidelines are an un-evidenced intervention that may have the potential to cause net harm to population health.

Retaining the focus on physical activity guidelines, Tess Kay picks up some of the themes in Weed's chapter, arguing that physical activity policy suffers from a failure to consider social science evidence. In particular, Kay argues that physical activity guidelines do not consider evidence about the structural causes of health inequalities and the ways in which people's health can be constrained by their social situation, instead focusing solely on individual responsibility to adopt healthy behaviours. Consequently, Kay concludes that without incorporating social science evidence, guideline recommendations cannot effectively serve those parts of the population that have been shown to be at the greatest risk of ill-health and thus where the greatest public health benefit can be gained.

Focusing on the link between behavioural evidence and physical activity policy, Fiona Gillison and Fay Beck consider how far physical activity policies based on individual responsibility can go in supporting people's motivation and self-efficacy, and opportunities that exist for social support. In exploring the potential of different physical activity policy types, including exercise referral and financial incentives, they discuss the problems of intervening in a society where physical activity can easily be avoided and in which, for the most part, physical activity requires active 'opting in'.

In exploring policies utilising social marketing approaches, Jessica Lee, Benjamin Williams and Bernadette Sebar attempt a deep dive into the chain of evidence that underpins social marketing campaigns and the way in which such evidence is translated for policy. In particular, they note that commonly accepted scientific evidence on the risks of physical activity and its links with obesity is more complex than is assumed as well as contradictory. They note that with the move from complex evidence to simplified policy each translation imbues policy with more values and less evidence, and that it is the needs and goals of the developers of policies at each stage that become progressively prominent.

Finally under this theme, Dale Esliger, Andrew Kingsnorth and Lauren Sherar explore the ways in which physical activity can be measured to estimate prevalence and detect trends, identify factors correlated with physical activity and evaluate the efficacy and effectiveness of interventions. Clearly, each of these measurement types have a different purpose, from establishing the extent to which physical (in)activity is a problem and justifying the need for action, through informing what action might be taken, to understanding whether such actions have been successful. They note the need to develop best practices in the measurement of physical activity, and this complements the wider disciplinary evidence bases for physical activity.

7

THE INTERPRETATION AND MISINTERPRETATION OF BIOMEDICAL EVIDENCE TO INFORM PHYSICAL ACTIVITY GUIDELINES

Mike Weed

Introduction

There is a clear international consensus regarding the biomedical evidence for the efficacy of physical activity in conferring a range of health benefits and reducing all-cause mortality risk (Kokkinos & Myers, 2010; Woodcock et al., 2011), and this has led national governments to produce guidelines for physical activity levels for their populations (Department of Health [DoH], 2011a; Department of Health Australia [DoHA], 2013; United States Department of Health and Human Services [USDHHS], 2008), and to the production of global recommendations on physical activity for health by the World Health Organization (WHO, 2010a). It is broadly accepted that there is a dose-response relationship between physical activity levels and all-cause mortality (Physical Activity Guidelines Advisory Committee [PAGAC], 2008; Wen et al., 2011), and that the dose-response curve is inverse curvilinear, with the greatest benefits existing with a move from nothing to something and there being diminishing returns later in the curve. The core common recommendation across WHO (2010a), USA (USDHHS, 2008), UK (DoH, 2011a), and Australian (DoHA, 2013) guidelines is that 150 minutes of moderate intensity exercise per week provides substantial health benefits for adults. In addition, guidelines variously state that 300 minutes provides additional and more extensive health benefits (USDHHS, 2008; WHO, 2010a), that any physical activity is better than none (DoHA, 2013; USDHHS, 2008), and that adults should aim to be active daily (DoH, 2011a), together with a range of further recommendations for other groups and at other exercise intensities.[1]

However, while a clear consensus exists regarding evidence for the *efficacy* of physical activity in conferring heath benefits, there is less evidence for the *effectiveness* of physical activity guidelines as a public health intervention. Furthermore, in the USA, UK, and Australia, from just over half to as low as one third of populations achieve guideline levels of physical activity (Australian Bureau of Statistics, 2013; Centers for Disease Control and Prevention, 2014; Scholes & Mindell, 2013). Some guidelines suggest (at least in places) that the public may not be an intended audience (DoH, 2011a; USDHHS, 2008; WHO, 2010a), thus questioning whether guidelines should be considered a public health intervention, but the WHO definition of public health as "all organized measures [to] . . . promote health . . . among the population as a whole" (WHO, 2010b) suggests they should be so considered.

This chapter seeks to evaluate the way in which biomedical evidence for the efficacy of physical activity in conferring a range of health benefits and reducing all-cause mortality risk has been interpreted to set physical activity guideline recommendations around the world. It also explores how far such biomedical evidence has been misinterpreted to infer that because there is evidence for the efficacy of physical activity in conferring health benefits, there is also evidence for the effectiveness of current physical activity guidelines in improving population physical activity levels. Finally, the chapter considers the possibility that, when compared against the opportunity cost of alternative guidelines, current guidelines may result in harm to population health, and notes that such considerations cannot be explored if the evidence base is limited to biomedical evidence. First, however, the chapter considers whether physical activity guidelines should be considered to be a public health intervention.

Are physical activity guidelines a public health intervention?

The Nuffield Council on Bioethics (2007) has developed a public health intervention ladder that includes, towards the top of the ladder, interventions that restrict choice through regulation, such as a ban on smoking in public places, through interventions that seek to guide choice using incentives, such as tax breaks for the purchase of bicycles to be used to travel to work, to those at the bottom of the ladder that seek to inform choice through the provision of information. These universal information provision interventions are also recognised and endorsed by Public Health England (Newton, 2013), and if physical activity guidelines are used directly to inform and educate the public about their health, then clearly they should be considered a public health intervention.

Setting aside the WHO (2010a) guidelines which, quite legitimately, cite national-level policy-makers as the primary target audience, the national guidelines vary in the audiences they identify. The evidence report underpinning the Australian guidelines made a clear recommendation that "a set of resources, targeted to multiple audiences and users, should be developed and be available at the same time as the formal launch of the guide-lines" (Brown et al., 2012, p. 100), and the final guidelines for adults directly address the public in the first person (DoHA, 2013). The USA guidelines (USDHHS, 2008) note that they are "intended to be a primary source of information for policy makers, physical educators, health providers, and the public" (p. ii), and that "messages contained in these guidelines should be dissemina-ted to the public" (p. 6). However, the UK guidelines (DoH, 2011a) state that they are "intended for professionals, practitioners and policy-makers concerned with formulating and implementing policies and programmes" (p. ii), and that the document "does not and indeed cannot set out the specific messages we need to reach communities across the UK with diverse needs, lifestyles and attitudes to activity" (pp. 3–4) and that there "needs to be careful and planned translation of these guidelines into appropriate messages for the public" (p. 46). This suggests that the Australian and USA guidelines should be considered direct public health interventions as the public is explicitly identified as an intended direct audience, but in the UK, the public is explicitly excluded as an intended direct audience and the stated intention of the guidelines is to inform policy and practice.

However, regardless of the stated intention for policy-makers and practitioners to undertake careful and planned translation into appropriate messages to be communicated to the public, the use of the guidelines in practice in the UK is somewhat different. The National Health Service (NHS) publishes NHS Choices, a government website intended to be used by the general public, with a stated purpose to "provide a comprehensive health information service to help put you in control of your healthcare . . . it helps you make choices about your health, [and] decisions about your lifestyle, such as smoking, drinking and exercise".[2] The website repeats verbatim the recommendation from the UK guideline document regarding 150 minutes of moderate intensity activity and being active daily, prefacing it with the statement that to stay healthy adults must be active at this level and frequency.[3]

The launch of the UK guidelines was accompanied with a press release that, once again, repeated verbatim the 150-minute recommendation, but added that there is "a renewed focus on being active everyday" and "more emphasis on vigorous activity" (DoH, 2011b). This led to widespread press coverage of the 150-minute recommendation, but also of "concerns that activities like walking or cycling alone are insufficient" and that "[p]eople should be pushing themselves" and "should take up vigorous games . . . because moderate exercise is not enough" (Adams, 2011). Beyond government, translation for local campaigns tends to uprate messages, with one local authority's "5 × 30 move more" campaign noting that the "Department of Health have recommended that in order to go from a sedentary to an active lifestyle you should *take up* 5 sessions of 30 minutes of exercise every week" (emphasis added).[4]

It appears, therefore, that although the UK guidelines clearly state that they are "intended for professionals, practitioners and policymakers" (DoH, 2011a, p. ii), in every practical sense, the guidelines are being treated and implemented as a direct public health intervention by government, the media, and local practitioners. While this is clearly an unintended outcome, it is both naive and irresponsible to fail to consider, acknowledge, and accept that in practice, and regardless of intent, the guidelines have become a direct public health intervention.

The efficacy of physical activity in conferring health benefits: Biomedical evidence

Efficacy evidence relates to the performance of an intervention under ideal and controlled conditions (Singal et al., 2014). For physical activity guidelines, ideal conditions are that members of the public would adopt and adhere to recommended guideline levels. Consequently, efficacy evidence is concerned with the health benefits physical activity confers at various levels. In this respect, all four guideline documents agree that 150 minutes of moderate intensity activity confers substantial health benefits (DoH, 2011a; DoHA, 2013; USDHHS, 2008; WHO, 2010a), and it is this 150-minute level that is the core recommendation in each of the guidelines.

The evidence for 150 minutes is most recently summarised in the report underpinning the Australian guidelines (Brown et al., 2012), which uses an all-cause mortality curve adapted from Powell et al. (2011), which was itself adapted from the report underpinning the USA recommendations (PAGAC, 2008). Given that the UK guidelines (DoH, 2011a) highlight the US report as a primary source, all of the national guidelines are using the same summary all-cause mortality curve. The all-cause mortality curve was developed using data from 11 prospective cohort studies published between 1995 and 2006 (Carlsson et al., 2006; Fried et al., 1998; Janssen & Jolliffe, 2006; Kujala et al., 1998; Lan et al., 2006; Lee et al., 1995; Lee & Paffenbarger, 2000; Rockhill et al., 2001; Sundquist et al., 2004; Tanasescu et al., 2003; Trolle-Lagerros et al., 2005) that assessed at least five levels of physical activity, with 268,962 observations of individuals aged 25 and over and a total of 18,075 deaths.

The Australian commentary (Brown et al., 2012) on this all-cause mortality curve is that there is a steep initial slope, there is no obvious lower threshold for benefit, there is no obvious optimal amount, and there is no obvious upper threshold. However, the report notes that there are significant benefits from levels of activity below 150 minutes, but that these "have largely been ignored in public health recommendations" (p. 84). In fact, in the unsmoothed version of the summary all-cause mortality curve (PAGAC, 2008; Powell et al., 2011), the steep initial slope appears to abate at 90 minutes a week, where an all-cause mortality risk reduction of 20 per cent is conferred (compared to a baseline of 30 minutes or less activity per week). At 150 minutes, an all-cause mortality risk reduction of around 25 per cent is suggested, with a 27 per cent risk reduction shown at a specific data point at 180 minutes. This shows clear diminishing returns in terms of all-cause mortality risk reduction from 90 minutes of moderate intensity exercise per week, although protection against additional conditions such as some cancers is added with a more than three-fold increase in activity to around 300 minutes per week (Brown et al., 2012), where the all-cause mortality risk reduction is around 35 per cent. The interpretation of this evidence in the Australian report (Brown et al., 2012) is that the "optimal range" in terms of benefits secured versus effort invested is between 150 and 300 minutes, for which the all-cause mortality risk reduction is from 25 per cent to 35 per cent. This is the central justification for the ubiquitous guideline that 150 minutes provides substantial health benefits. However, this view of what constitutes substantial health benefits is but one interpretation of the evidence, which also shows that a 40 per cent drop in active minutes from 150 to 90 minutes would result in only a 20 per cent loss in all-cause mortality risk reduction from 25 per cent to 20 per cent.

It is also acknowledged that there is increasing evidence that a lower risk of all-cause mortality and lower incidence of coronary heart disease is conferred at levels of no more than one hour of moderate intensity activity per week (Brown et al., 2012; PAGAC, 2008). Furthermore, summary reports, papers, and guidelines (Brown et al., 2012; DoH, 2011a; PAGAC, 2008; Powell et al., 2011) universally explicitly acknowledge that there are significant proportions of the population that are at the lowest end of the activity spectrum, and that the steep initial slope of the all-cause mortality curve that provides rapid improvement with a movement from nothing to something will bring both substantial health benefits to those individuals and the greatest public health benefit, and this is further supported by more recent evidence (De Souto Barreto, 2015; Moore et al., 2012; Sparling, 2015). However, it is difficult to estimate a specific all-cause mortality risk reduction at levels below 90 minutes because published guideline levels often provide the threshold levels for studies (Moore et al., 2012; PAGAC, 2008) and thus "research on the value of activity outside these parameters has been limited" (Powell et al., 2011). Of the 73 studies that provided the evidence base for the USA report (PAGAC, 2008), 59 studied three or more levels of physical activity, but only 12 studied five or more, and across these 59 studies, the lowest activity level studied mostly falls between 60 and 90 minutes. Therefore, although it is clear that there is an all-cause mortality benefit at 60 minutes (Brown et al., 2012; PAGAC, 2008; Powell et al., 2011), the magnitude of that benefit is less clear, and the baseline comparator in the unsmoothed version of the curve is 30 minutes activity or less rather than zero.[5] Nevertheless, the smoothed version of the all-cause mortality curve (Brown et al., 2012) suggests that 60 minutes of activity confers an all-cause mortality risk reduction of 18 per cent compared to a zero baseline, which translates to a circa 15 per cent risk reduction compared to the baseline of 30 minutes or less used in the unsmoothed curve (Leitzmann et al., 2007; PAGAC, 2008; Powell et al., 2011).

Given both the lack of evidence relating to the impact of specific low doses of moderate intensity physical activity and the acknowledged individual and public health benefits that could be realised by increasing activity at these levels, it is surprising that there are not more widespread calls for research on such low doses. Particularly surprising is that the US report (PAGAC, 2008), in listing research needs in relation to all-cause mortality, suggests that "[s]tudies are needed to determine the point (if any) on the dose–response curve at which no further reduction in all-cause mortality occurs", but makes no mention of a need to determine all-cause mortality reductions at low doses of activity.

In summary, the biomedical efficacy evidence cited to inform the three national guidelines suggests all-cause mortality risk reductions of 15 per cent at 60 minutes of moderate intensity activity per week, 20 per cent at 90 minutes, 25 per cent at 150 minutes, 27 per cent at 180 minutes, and 35 per cent at 300 minutes, compared to a baseline of 30 minutes activity or less.

The effectiveness of guidelines in increasing physical activity levels: The limits of biomedical evidence

Effectiveness evidence relates to the performance of an intervention under "real world" conditions, and considers issues such as provider acceptance and target audience compliance (Singal et al., 2014). For physical activity guidelines, key real-world conditions to consider are: firstly, the likelihood that target audiences – in general, the public; specifically, the least active – will adopt and adhere to recommended guideline levels; secondly, in the UK case, how far practitioners will recognise and accept the stipulated need to translate guidelines for public consumption (DoH, 2011a). Effectiveness evidence goes beyond the biomedical evidence for the health benefits of recommended levels of physical activity to consider the external validity of recommending those levels in the real world (Rothwell, 2005). Given that the biomedical efficacy evidence shows no obvious optimal amount of physical activity (Brown et al., 2012), rather an inverse curvilinear scale, it might be expected that effectiveness evidence would inform what level should be recommended to achieve the greatest public health benefit. However, no effectiveness evidence is cited either in the guideline documents (DoH, 2011a; DoHA, 2013; USDHHS, 2008; WHO, 2010a) or in the documents that provide their stated underlying evidence bases (Brown et al., 2012; Kesaniemi et al., 2010; O'Donovan et al., 2010; PAGAC, 2008; Warburton et al., 2010; WHO, 2010b). While the lack of direct effectiveness evidence (Sparling, 2015) could be offered as an explanation for this omission, evidence does exist on compliance with other public health guidelines (Blackwell et al., 2008; May et al., 1999) and, indeed, on compliance with physical activity guidelines (Pate et al., 2002; Rafferty et al., 2002; Tucker et al., 2011), which could provide insights into the potential effectiveness of guideline recommendations. Evidence is also available on the communication and reception of science-based health recommendations (Fineberg & Rowe, 1998; Jaime & Lock, 2009; Rowe, 2002), or such evidence could be commissioned from consumer panel research (Pollard, 2002). But no such evidence is cited in the guidelines or their supporting documents, nor is the issue of potential effectiveness recognised or discussed.

The report underpinning the Australian guidelines (Brown et al., 2012) notes that the universally recommended 150-minute threshold is "somewhat arbitrary" (p. 84), but is an "achievable quantum" (p. 80) or "minimal . . . realistic behavioural target for the general population" (p. 84). No evidence is given for these assertions other than the recognition of a convention that "most countries provide a recommended minimum target . . . [and] this minimal target is accepted as being about 150 minutes" (p. 84). However, recent evidence on compliance with the 150-minute recommendation in the USA showed that, while self-reports suggested compliance of 62 per cent among US adults, objective accelerometry measures demonstrated that compliance was far lower at 9.6 per cent in the same sample of

3,082 adults (Tucker et al., 2011). This is, of course, just one study, but neither this study, published 18 months before the Australian report, nor any other study on compliance or effectiveness, was used to reach the conclusion that the 150 minutes convention is an achievable quantum or a minimal realistic behavioural target.

All three national guidelines recommend 150 minutes as providing substantial health benefits (DoH, 2011a; DoHA, 2013; USDHHS, 2008). However, there is no evidence to support the value judgement that populations will consider a 25 per cent all-cause mortality risk reduction (conferred at 150 minutes) rather than a 20 per cent risk reduction (at 90 minutes), or even a circa 15 per cent risk reduction (at 60 minutes) to be a substantial health benefit. In fact, if the aim is to set guidelines at a level "representing a balance of benefit, compared with the effort required to do it" (Brown et al., 2012, p. 84), then the objective efficacy evidence would suggest recommending 90 minutes, as this is the point after which the steep initial slope of all-cause mortality risk reduction abates to deliver diminishing returns (PAGAC, 2008; Powell et al., 2011).

In summary, neither the guidelines nor their stated underlying evidence bases cite evidence for effectiveness or potential effectiveness. Instead, unsupported value judgements are made about what populations will value as a substantial health benefit, and un-evidenced assumptions and assertions, based on nothing more than convention, are made about what represents a realistic behavioural target for the general population.

Effectiveness, comparative effectiveness, and harm

The sole reliance on biomedical evidence to formulate physical activity guidelines, and indeed on what appears to be a rather arbitrary interpretation of that evidence, calls into question the extent to which the universally recommended level of 150 minutes of moderate physical activity per week might legitimately be considered to be evidence-based. Firstly, although there is clear biomedical evidence that 150 minutes is efficacious in delivering an all-cause mortality risk reduction of 25 per cent, the decision to recommend 150 minutes is not based on evidence, but on a value judgement that a 25 per cent risk reduction represents a substantial health benefit, and that risk reductions of 20 per cent (conferred at 90 minutes) or even 15 per cent (conferred at 60 minutes) do not. Secondly, an objective consideration of the biomedical efficacy evidence suggests recommending 90 minutes, as this is the point on the all-cause mortality curve after which there are diminishing returns on additional time spent active. Thirdly, because it is beyond the limits of biomedical evidence, no evidence other than convention is provided for the assertion that 150 minutes represents a realistic behavioural target for the general population. In fact, evidence on objectively measured compliance in the USA, UK, and Canada across a combined sample of over 12,500 adults demonstrates that only 10–15 per cent of adults achieve the recommended 150 minutes, thus suggesting that it is not an achievable target (Centers for Disease Control and Prevention [CDC], 2006; Garriguet & Colley, 2014; Rafferty et al., 2002; Tucker et al., 2011). Finally, no evidence is cited for the effectiveness of a recommendation of 150 minutes in increasing physical activity levels, nor is evidence for the potential effectiveness of a recommendation at this level considered. Collectively, these insights suggest that physical activity guidelines are an un-evidenced public health intervention.

Analyses in the UK have concluded that public health interventions "are likely to be ineffective or lack evidence to establish effectiveness" (Katikireddi et al., 2011, p. 3), and that un-evidenced public health interventions "are experiments on the public and can be as damaging (in terms of unintended effects and opportunity cost) as unevaluated new drugs or surgical procedures" (House of Commons Health Committee, 2009, p. 115). Furthermore, "[s]uch wanton large-scale experimentation is unethical, and needs to be superseded by a more rigorous culture of piloting, evaluating and using the results to inform policy" (House of Commons Health Committee, 2009, p. 115). In respect of physical activity guidelines in the UK, there is no evidence of any evaluation of effectiveness that meets the standards government sets for itself (HM Treasury, 2011a, 2011b, 2013; National Audit Office, 2013), nor of those set out by the then newly appointed Secretary of State for Health in 2010 that "public health services must meet tougher tests of evidence and evaluation . . . We must only support effective interventions that deliver proven benefits" (Lansley, 2010, para. 104, 106).

Largely because they consider only biomedical evidence, and also because such evidence is interpreted in a rather arbitrary way, physical activity guidelines, in the UK and elsewhere, do not meet these standards of evidence or ethics, and the potential for harm from unintended effects and opportunity cost are not considered. In terms of the former, unintended effects relate to whether guidelines perceived to be "challenging goals will cause the public to reject the guidelines as unrealistic" (Brawley & Latimer, 2007, p. S181) and thus discourage them from trying in the first place (Bethancourt et al., 2014; Couch et al., 2015; Moore et al., 2012; Sparling, 2015), which raises the prospect that the guidelines may cause actual harm by being less effective than doing nothing. Opportunity costs relate to the possibility that recommendations at alternative levels may result in greater health benefits at a population level. Given that the biomedical evidence shows a dose-response relationship in which there is no obvious lower threshold for benefit, no obvious optimal amount, and no obvious upper threshold (Brown et al., 2012), a consideration of the comparative effectiveness of different recommendation levels is surely warranted.

Comparative effectiveness evidence is concerned with the relative benefits and harms of alternative interventions (Sox & Greenfield, 2009). This includes the relative or net harm of interventions in comparison to the opportunity cost of not implementing alternatives (House of Commons Health Committee, 2009). Therefore, in terms of physical activity guidelines would, for example, a recommendation at 60 or 90 minutes deliver sufficiently greater compliance than the circa 10–15 per cent compliance delivered by the current recommendation at 150 minutes (CDC, 2006; Garriguet & Colley, 2014; Rafferty et al., 2002; Tucker et al., 2011) to be more effective in delivering health benefits at a population level despite lower efficacy in reducing all-cause mortality? Neither existing objective compliance evidence (CDC, 2006; Garriguet & Colley, 2014; Rafferty et al., 2002; Tucker et al., 2011) nor the dose-response nature of biomedical evidence (Brown et al., 2012) provides evidence to suggest that a recommendation at 150 minutes is more effective in delivering population health outcomes than potential alternative recommendations at 60 or 90 minutes. This raises the real possibility that, in terms of comparative effectiveness (Sox & Greenfield, 2009), current guidelines are inflicting net harm on the population in comparison to the opportunity cost of not implementing alternatives (House of Commons Health Committee, 2009). This is not to say that there is evidence that alternatives would be more effective but, equally, nor is there evidence that they would not. The key issue is that such possibilities have not been considered or evaluated, and this is both unethical (House of Commons Health Committee, 2009) and negligent.

Conclusion

Physical activity guidelines are recognised as a public health intervention in Australia (DoHA, 2013) and the USA (USDHHS, 2008), and the implementation and use of the guidelines in the UK show that, despite intent, they have become a direct public health intervention there, and to consider them otherwise would be both naïve and irresponsible. All three national guidelines, and the WHO global guidelines, draw on the same evidence base of efficacy evidence. However, no attempt has been made to move beyond biomedical evidence to explore evidence for effectiveness, nor to consider potential effectiveness, and un-evidenced value judgements have been made about what represents a substantial health benefit and an achievable behavioural target. These value judgements, together with the failure to consider effectiveness, have led to an interpretation of the biomedical evidence that appears to overestimate at 150 minutes the amount of physical activity required for health benefits. Ultimately, this calls into question the claim that the guidelines are evidence-based.

Clearly, one outcome of the way in which physical activity guidelines have been developed with reference only to biomedical evidence, alongside the way in which that evidence has been interpreted, is that there has been a sub-optimal policy process which appears to have led to a sub-optimal policy. However, a further more significant outcome is that the failure of this sub-optimal policy process to consider both unintended effects and the potential comparative effectiveness of alternative recommendations raises the real prospect that the current guidelines may be resulting in actual and net harm to population health.

Notes

1 While the universal "headline recommendation" is for 150 minutes at moderate intensity, guidelines also include a recommendation that 75 minutes at vigorous intensity, or an equivalent combination of moderate and vigorous intensities, will confer the same health benefits as 150 minutes moderate intensity. Guidelines also provide separate recommendations for children (5–18), and increasingly toddlers (<5), and further advice for older adults (>65).
2 www.nhs.uk/aboutNHSChoices/aboutnhschoices/Aboutus/Pages/Introduction.aspx (accessed: 17 October 2014).
3 www.nhs.uk/Livewell/fitness/Pages/physical-activity-guidelines-for-adults.aspx (accessed: 17 October 2014).
4 www.brighterliving.org.uk/?page_id=51 (accessed: 17 October 2014).
5 A baseline of zero is taken across all the cited guidelines, reports, and studies to mean zero additional activity of at least moderate intensity over and above all sedentary and light-intensity activities of daily life.

References

Adams, S. (2011, July 11). Take up volleyball, says department of health. *The Telegraph*.
Australian Bureau of Statistics. (2013). Let's get physical: How do adult Australians measure up? *Perspectives on Sport*, 6(2).
Bethancourt, H. J., Rosenberg, D. E., Beatty, T., & Arterburn, D. E. (2014). Barriers to and facilitators of physical activity program use among older adults. *Clinical Medicine Research*, 12(1–2), 10–20.
Blackwell, D. L., Martinez, M. E., & Gentleman, J. F. (2008). Women's compliance with public health guidelines for mammograms and pap tests in Canada and the United States. *Women's Health Issues*, 18(2), 85–99.
Brawley, L. R., & Latimer, A. E. (2007). Physical activity guides for Canadians: Messaging strategies, realistic expectations for change, and evaluation. *Applied Physiology, Nutrition and Metabolism*, 32(Suppl. 2E), S170–S184.
Brown, W. J., Bauman, A. E., Bull, F. C., & Burton, N. W. (2012). *Development of evidence-based physical activity recommendations for adults*. Canberra: Department of Health.
Carlsson, S., Andersson, T., Wolk, A., & Ahlbom, A. (2006). Low physical activity and mortality in women: Baseline lifestyle and health as alternative explanations. *Scandinavian Journal of Public Health*, 34(5), 480–487.
Centers for Disease Control and Prevention (CDC). (2006). National health and nutrition examination survey data 2005–2006. Atlanta, GA. Retrieved January 1, 2016, from www.cdc.gov/nchs/nhanes/search/nhanes05_06.aspx.

Centers for Disease Control and Prevention (CDC). (2014). State indicator report on physical activity. Atlanta, GA. Retrieved January 23, 2016, from http://cdc.gov/physicalactivity/downloads/pa_state_indicator_report_2014.pdf

Couch, D., Han, G.-S., Robinson, P., & Komesaroff, P. (2015). Public health surveillance and the media: A dyad of panoptic and synoptic social control. *Health Psychology & Behavioural Medicine*, 3(1), 128–141.

Department of Health (DoH). (2011a). *Start active, stay active: A report on physical activity from the four home countries' Chief Medical Officers*. London.

Department of Health (DoH). (2011b). Press release: UK-wide advice on activity and fitness levels. London. Retrieved October 17, 2014, from http://webarchive.nationalarchives.gov.uk/+/www.dh.gov.uk/en/MediaCentre/Pressreleases/DH_128211.

Department of Health Australia (DoHA). (2013). *Make your move – sit less – be active for life! – Australia's physical activity & sedentary behaviour guidelines for adults*. Canberra.

De Souto Barreto, P. (2015). Global health agenda on non-communicable diseases: Has WHO set a smart goal for physical activity? *British Medical Journal*, 350, article no. h23.

Fineberg, H. V., & Rowe, S. B. (1998). Improving public understanding: Guidelines for communicating emerging science on nutrition, food safety, and health for journalists, scientists, and other communicators. *Journal of the National Cancer Institute*, 90(3), 194–199.

Fried, L. P., Kronmal, R. A., Newman, A. B., Bild, D. E., Mittelmark, M. B., Polak, J. F., & Gardin, J. M. (1998). Risk factors for 5-year mortality in older adults: The cardiovascular health study. *Journal of the American Medical Association*, 279(8), 585–592.

Garriguet, D., & Colley, R. C. (2014). A comparison of self-reported leisure-time physical activity and measured moderate-to-vigorous physical activity in adolescents and adults. *Health Reports*, 25(7), 3–11.

Global Advocacy Council for Physical Activity/International Society for Physical Activity and Health. (2010). The Toronto charter for physical activity: A global call to action. Retrieved September 1, 2017, from www.globalpa.org.uk

HM Treasury. (2011a). *The green book: Appraisal and evaluation in central government*. London.

HM Treasury. (2011b). *The Magenta book: Guidance for evaluation*. London.

HM Treasury. (2013). *Managing public money*. London.

House of Commons Health Committee. (2009). *Health inequalities: Third report of session 2008–09– Volume I*. London: The Stationery Office.

Jaime, P. C., & Lock, K. (2009). Do school based food and nutrition policies improve diet and reduce obesity? *Preventative Medicine*, 48(1), 45–53.

Janssen, I., & Jolliffe, C. J. (2006). Influence of physical activity on mortality in elderly with coronary artery disease. *Medicine and Science in Sport and Exercise*, 38(3), 418–417.

Katikireddi, S. V., Higgins, M., Bond, L., Bonell, C., & Macintyre, S. (2011). How evidence based is English public health policy? *British Medical Journal*, 343, article no. d7310.

Kesaniemi, I., Riddoch, C. J., Reeder, B., Blair, S. N., & Sorensen, T. (2010). Advancing the future of physical activity guidelines in Canada: An independent expert panel interpretation of the evidence. *International Journal of Behavioural Nutrition and Physical Activity*, 7, article no. 41.

Kokkinos, P., & Myers, J. (2010). Exercise and physical activity: Clinical outcomes and applications. *Circulation*, 122(16), 1637–1648.

Kujala, U. M., Kaprio, J., Sarna, S., & Koskenvuo, M. (1998). Relationship of leisure-time physical activity and mortality: The Finnish twin cohort. *Journal of the American Medical Association*, 279(6), 440–444.

Lan, T. Y., Chang, H. Y., & Tai, T. Y. (2006). Relationship between components of leisure physical activity and mortality in Taiwanese older adults. *Preventative Medicine*, 43(1), 36–41.

Lansley, A. (2010). Secretary of state for health speech to the UK faculty of public health conference: A new approach to public health. London: Department of Health. Retrieved November 24, 2014, from http://webarchive.nationalarchives.gov.uk/+/www.dh.gov.uk/en/MediaCentre/Speeches/DH_117280.

Lee, I. M., Hsieh, C. C., & Paffenbarger, R. S. Jr. (1995). Exercise intensity and longevity in men. The Harvard Alumni Health Study. *Journal of the American Medical Association*, 273(15), 1179–1184.

Lee, I. M., & Paffenbarger, R. S. Jr. (2000). Associations of light, moderate, and vigorous intensity physical activity with longevity. The Harvard Alumni Health Study. *American Journal of Epidemiology*, 151(3), 293–299.

Leitzmann, M. F., Park, Y., Blair, A., Ballard-Barbash, R., Mouw, T., Hollenbeck, A. R., & Schatzkin, A. (2007). Physical activity recommendations and decreased risk of mortality. *Archives of Internal Medicine*, 167(22), 2453–2460.

May, D. S., Kiefe, C. I., Funkhouser, E., & Fouad, M. N. (1999). Compliance with mammography guidelines: Physician recommendation and patient adherence. *Preventative Medicine*, 28(4), 386–394.

Moore, S. C., Patel, A. V., Matthews, C. E., Berrington de Gonzalez, A., Park, Y., Katki, H. A., Linet, M. A., Weiderpass, E., Visvanathan, K., Helzlsouer, K. J., Thun, M., Gapstur, S. M., Hartge, P., & Lee, I.-M. (2012). Leisure time physical activity of moderate to vigorous intensity and mortality: A large pooled cohort analysis. *PLoS Med*, 9(11), article no. e1001335.

National Audit Office. (2013). *Evaluation in government*. London: NAO Communications.

Newton, J. (2013). Public health matters: Information as an intervention. London: Public Health England. Retrieved January 4, 2016, from https://publichealthmatters.blog.gov.uk/2013/09/25/information-as-an-intervention/.

Nuffield Council on Bioethics. (2007). *Public health: Ethical issues*. London.

O'Donovan, G., Blazevich, A. J., Boreham, C., Cooper, A. R., Crank, H., Ekelund, U., Fox KR, Gately P, Giles-Corti B, Gill JM, Hamer M, McDermott I, Murphy M, Mutrie N, Reilly JJ, Saxton JM, & Stamatakis, E. (2010). The ABC of physical activity for health: A consensus statement from the British Association of Sport and Exercise Sciences. *Journal of Sports Science*, 28(6), 531–591.

Pate, R. R., Freedson, P. S., Sallis, J. F., Taylor, W. C., Sirard, J., Trost, S. G., & Dowda, M. (2002). Compliance with physical activity guidelines: Prevalence in a population of children and youth. *Annals of Epidemiology*, 12(5), 303–308.

Physical Activity Guidelines Advisory Committee. (2008). *Physical activity guidelines advisory committee report*. Washington, DC: DHHS.

Pollard, W. E. (2002). *Use of consumer panel survey data for public health communication planning: An evaluation of survey results*. Proceedings of the American Statistical Association Joint Statistical Meeting – section on Health Policy Statistics (pp. 2720–2724). Alexandria, VA: ASA.

Powell, K. E., Paluch, A. E., & Blair, S. N. (2011). Physical activity for health: What kind? How much? How intense? On top of what? *Annual Review of Public Health*, 32, 349–365.

Rafferty, A. P., Reeves, M. J., McGee, H. B., & Pivarnik, J. M. (2002). Physical activity patterns among walkers and compliance with public health recommendations. *Medicine and Science in Sport and Exercise*, 34(8), 1255–1261.

Rockhill, B., Willett, W. C., Manson, J. E., Leitzmann, M. F., Stampfer, M. J., Hunter, D. J., & Colditz, G. A. (2001). Physical activity and mortality: A prospective study among women. *American Journal of Public Health*, 91(4), 578–583.

Rothwell, P. M. (2005). External validity of randomized controlled trials: "To whom do the results of this trial apply?" *The Lancet*, 365(9453), 82–93.

Rowe, S. B. (2002). Communicating science-based food and nutrition information. *The Journal of Nutrition*, 132(8), 2481S–2482S.

Scholes, S., & Mindell, J. (2013). *Physical activity in adults. Health Survey for England – 2012*. London: Health and Social Care Information Centre.

Singal, A. G., Higgins, P. D. R., & Waljee, A. K. (2014). A primer on effectiveness and efficacy trials. *Clinical and Translational Gastroenterology*, 5, article no. e45.

Sox, H. C., & Greenfield, S. (2009). Comparative effectiveness research: A report from the institute of medicine. *Annals of Internal Medicine*, 151(3), 203–205.

Sparling, P. B. (2015). Recommendations for physical activity in older adults. *British Medical Journal*, 350, article no. h100.

Sundquist, K., Qvist, J., Sundquist, J., & Johansson, S. E. (2004). Frequent and occasional physical activity in the elderly: A 12-year follow-up study of mortality. *American Journal of Preventative Medicine*, 27(1), 22–27.

Tanasescu, M., Leitzmann, M. F., Rimm, E. B., & Hu, F. B. (2003). Physical activity in relation to cardiovascular disease and total mortality among men with type 2 diabetes. *Circulation*, 107(19), 2435–2439.

Trolle-Lagros, Y., Mucci, L. A., Kumle, M., Braaten, T., Weiderpass, E., Hsieh, C. C., Sandin S, Lagiou P, Trichopoulos D, Lund E, Adami, H. O. (2005). Physical activity as a determinant of mortality in women. *Epidemiology*, 16(6), 780–785.

Tucker, J. M., Welk, G. J., & Beyler, N. K. (2011). Physical activity in U.S. adults: Compliance with the physical activity guidelines for Americans. *American Journal of Preventative Medicine*, 40(4), 454–461.

United States Department of Health and Human Services. (2008). *Physical activity guidelines for Americans*. Washington, DC: Author.

Warburton, D. E. R., Charlesworth, S., Ivey, A., Nettlefold, L., & Bredin, S. S. D. (2010). A systematic review of the evidence for Canada's physical activity guidelines for adults. *International Journal of Behavioural Nutrition and Physical Activity*, 7, article no. 39.

Wen, C. P., Wai, J. P. M., Tsai, M. K., Yang, Y. C., Cheng, T. Y. D., Lee, M. C., . . . Wu, X. (2011). Minimum amount of physical activity for reduced mortality and extended life expectancy: A prospective cohort study. *The Lancet*, 378(9798), 1244–1253.

Woodcock, J., Franco, O. H., Orsini, N., & Roberts, I. (2011). Non-vigorous physical activity and all-cause mortality: Systematic review and meta-analysis of cohort studies. *International Journal of Epidemiology*, 40(1), 121–138.

World Health Organization. (2010a). *Global recommendations on physical activity for health*. Geneva.

World Health Organization. (2010b). *Public health*. Geneva. Retrieved October 14, 2014, from www.who.int/trade/glossary/story076/en/.

8

ONLY CONNECT

How social science can improve physical activity guidance

Tess Kay

Introduction

This chapter examines how international efforts to promote physical activity intersect with another universal health challenge – global health inequalities. Inequitable health outcomes are a worldwide phenomenon: in all countries, whether high, medium or low income, the risk of physical and mental ill-health is higher for poorer groups than for affluent members of the same nation (World Health Organization (WHO), 2008a). The majority of this unequal disease burden arises from Non Communicable Diseases (NCDs), which disproportionately impact low income groups. In theory this means that physical activity, recognised internationally for its capacity to moderate the risk of NCDs (WHO, 2009), is a potential tool for reducing health inequalities. In practice, however, many of the social structural trends that fuel inequalities – including population ageing, rapid unplanned urbanisation and globalisation (WHO, 2008a, 2008b) – are also the source of obstacles to individuals pursuing active lifestyles. These structural challenges have gone largely unrecognised, however, in the development of national and transnational PA guidance in which individual behaviour change is presented as the key to increasing population levels of physical activity (e.g. WHO, 2010; WHO European Regional Office, 2015; U.S. Department of Health and Human Services, 2008; Australian Government Department of Health, 2014). This is the omission that this chapter addresses.

The analysis here examines these issues through a UK lens. In England, addressing health inequalities is a public policy objective and a legal duty under the Health and Social Care Act (2012). In all four UK countries, however, PA policy is uninformed by social science evidence on the social determinants that underpin health inequalities. The resulting guidance fails to address the situations of those at the lower end of the social gradient, who have above-average risk of ill-health, and potentially most to gain by becoming more active. The UK case is therefore illustrative of how over-reliance on individually focused health behaviourist theories produce PA policies that neglect the influence of social structural processes on people's health behaviour. Addressing this gap requires a paradigm shift, in which structural influences on physical activity and inactivity are as fully recognised as behavioural factors. This requires significant changes in the scope and content of the evidence base underpinning PA policy, and corresponding changes to the knowledge community which produces it.

The focus for the chapter is the UK PA guidance contained in the *Start Active Stay Active* report (Department of Health, 2011). The *Start Active Stay Active* (hereinafter "SASA") report makes recommendations for the UK population on the health implications of being physically active, inactive and sedentary, and is underpinned by a robust and authoritative evidence base. In translating this evidence into guidance for PA policy and practice for "everyday life" situations, however, the report's credibility becomes more questionable. Unlike most population-wide social policies, the SASA guidance makes no use of social science data to inform this, thus excluding statistical data on population characteristics, trends and diversity, and empirical research into the complex and constrained contexts which foster inactivity. While the content of the SASA recommendations on PA have high scientific quality, the efforts to connect these to the social world do not. The purpose of this chapter is therefore to consider the value of incorporating social science theories and research into the evidence base informing PA policy.

The chapter first sets the scene by briefly reflecting on the strong tradition of social science contributions to social policy – including the resistance often encountered, especially in health-related fields. The main body of the chapter then explores this resistance in relation to PA policy, as illustrated by the SASA report. It outlines the approach adopted by the Start Active Stay Active expert review groups, examines the omission of social science knowledge and highlights the narrow theoretical underpinning of PA policy that fosters this. It further suggests that current omissions arise not from a dearth of evidence, but rather from the failure of PA expert communities to make use of it. The chapter introduces alternative approaches to analysing population health that address social structural influences, and advocates their use in the area of PA. It concludes by making recommendations for measures to diversify the knowledge base, connect PA policy with the wider public health debate around health inequalities, and produce more informed PA guidance.

Social science, public policy and public health

Social scientists have a long tradition of informing social policy. When the modern welfare state was established in the UK in the 1950s, social enquiry burgeoned as researchers strove to throw light on the issues facing post-war Britain. Over the following decades seminal texts on patterns of social change and disadvantage emerged which highlighted the persistence of acute poverty (Abel-Smith and Townsend, 1965) and informed social welfare and planning. Among the work of this time was Young and Willmott's (1957) research into *Family and Kinship in East London*, which examined how post-war rehousing policy impacted a tight-knit urban working class community and drove new family ideologies and practices. Acknowledged as one of the most influential sociological studies of the twentieth century, it revealed an everyday world which policy-making elites were too distanced from to comprehend. In doing so it demonstrated both the need for systematic research to capture the realities of an increasingly complex and diverse society, and the capacity of social science to do so.

Social scientists are therefore long accustomed to providing analysis for policy, and have methodologies that facilitate these aims. These include direct engagement with the social world in everyday settings; inclusive and participatory approaches for working with research participants whose accounts may otherwise go unheard; and partnership approaches that promote collaborative knowledge production. Social science might therefore be expected to play a prominent role in informing physical activity policy, but instead has been largely side-lined through a knowledge production process underpinned by the conventions and practices of the natural sciences. Within the academy, this long-standing tension in public health has most recently been exacerbated by the international "impact agenda" (Kay, 2016a), which favours "'hard', quantitative experimental studies and computational models" that have "clear, measurable and attributable short-term impacts (most commonly, incorporation into guidelines)" (Greenhalgh & Fahy, 2015, p. 7). This is problematic for health policy research where impact is inherently less linear, more complex and multi-stakeholder, and thus harder to demonstrate than the impact of biomedical studies. The impact agenda may therefore be reinforcing barriers that discourage the use of social science in public health. This reinforces the importance of establishing social scientists as members of the expert community producing PA guidance.

The primacy of the natural sciences is evident in the SASA report on physical activity (Department of Health, 2011). Compiled by expert working groups that met from 2009 to 2011, the report was jointly produced by the UK's four "Home Countries" – England, Scotland, Wales and Northern Ireland. Its purpose was to update and synthesise available evidence on physical activity and develop guidance from it. Its opening sections emphasised its scope, scientific quality and value for policy and practice. They described the "evidence for action" as "compelling", and asserted with some confidence that "we know enough now to act on physical activity" (Department of Health, 2011, p. 8) .

Social scientists might not share this confidence. In a period when the politics of austerity featured daily in national and international media – especially during the UK 2010 general election campaign – the SASA report made no reference at all to poverty, social isolation or material hardship, or to the long-established association between social and economic stratification and health inequalities. The internationally recognised evidence on the structural influences that shape health inequalities was not alluded to: individuals were portrayed as unconstrained, with plentiful opportunities to be active in their everyday lives. This view of the characteristics, circumstances and lifestyles of the UK population was both narrow and uninformed – and while the report's analyses of the health benefits of physical activity were determinedly evidence-based, its representations of the population were not. The SASA expert working groups thus appeared guilty of a common weakness in health behaviour research – assuming a normative view of the individual, and offering guidance that was "more reflective of the characteristics of those who produced it than those to whom it might apply" (Burke et al., 2009, p. 59S). Subsequent UK policy statements concerning sport-related PA (DCMS, 2015; Sport England, 2016), which are more specifically underpinned by behaviour change theory, continue this focus on decontextualised individuals, compromising both the relevance and practical utility of guidance in this field.

These limitations can be addressed through a wider evidence base in which appropriate social science knowledge is included. As we will see below, such evidence is plentiful and accessible, yet neither recognised nor used by the PA community. This raises the question of who controls the definition of evidence, and what evidence is acceptable to whom (Morse, 2006). The inclusion of social science knowledge would mean redefining what constitutes "expertise" in physical activity, and expanding the knowledge community to reflect this – "horizontally", to include a wider array of disciplines, and "vertically" to include the expertise of practitioners and lay people. The next sections now use the development of the SASA report as a vehicle for looking more closely at how this might be done.

Locating physical activity in everyday life

The UK *Start Active, Stay Active* report is a 60-page document on "physical activity for health" which drew on a wide evidence base on to establish "a UK-wide consensus on the amount of physical activity we should all aim to do at each stage of our lives" (Department of Health, 2011, p. 6). The report adopts a life course approach, emphasises the importance of physical activity for all ages and, for the first time in the UK, provides age-appropriate guidance on the amount and intensity of PA required to achieve health benefits. This is presented in four chapters addressing four phases – "early years" (under-5s), "children and young people" (5–18 years), "adults" (19–64 years) and "older adults" (65+ years). The report also details the methodology adopted to produce the guidelines, including the evidence base used and the work undertaken by the five expert sub-groups – one for each of the four age groups, and a fifth focused on sedentary behaviour. Membership overlapped between groups.

The four age group chapters set out the developmental and health characteristics of the relevant age group, present the guidelines for recommended levels and types of PA and provide a summary of the scientific evidence on which they are based. Each then offers a section on "Understanding the guidelines", which discusses how the guidance may translate into practice. Each of these sections contains two or three ~200 word "boxed" examples of physical activity being incorporated in daily life of an individual of the relevant age group. There are ten examples, populated by 15 adults and eight children, which vary in their content and detail – for example, some mention employment status while others do not.

The inclusion of the examples recognises the importance of contextualising individuals' behaviour. As the report is intended as the "first link" in a communication chain to policy makers, practitioners and ultimately the public, the examples have potential utility in illustrating how individuals at different points in the life course can incorporate physical activity into their lifestyles. All ten emphasise opportunity and capability – individuals appear almost wholly unconstrained, with excellent access to facilities and environments for physical activity; those with disabilities find ways to overcome them; older adults in particular defy stereotypes of ageing by leading energetic, busy lives. Although the two examples of older adults are research based, the remainder are not attributed to sources. All ten offer deliberately upbeat descriptions of individuals' living conditions and of their opportunities to be active.

While this positivity has value, it raises questions about how adequately the situations of less favoured groups in the population are addressed – or more fundamentally, whether they are in fact recognised. The population sectors with most to gain from becoming more active are those with the poorest health status – those with whom health professionals are most likely to work. In fact, given the significance of physical activity to redressing health inequalities, we might expect low-income and marginalised groups to be a primary focus for PA guidance. Exposure to stressors in the social and physical environment is known to be associated with both short-term changes in physiology, perceptions and behaviour, and longer-term risk of adverse outcomes including cardiovascular disease, diabetes and anxiety disorders (Thompson, 2015, p.18). Between 2009 and 2011, the period during which the SASA report was produced, 2.5 million children were classed as living in poverty, along with 5.6 million working-age adults (Brewer et al., 2011). This equates to one-in-five children (19.7%), and nearly one-in-six working age adults (16%); a further ~23 per cent of pensioners (2.6 million people) were also in poverty. Evidence on the effects of material deprivation on health has a long tradition in the UK and internationally (e.g. Haan et al., 1987; Wilson et al., 2004; Weaver et al. 2014; in Thompson, 2015, p. 18), especially in periods of economic downturn or policy priority (the inter-war depression; mass unemployment in the 1980s; child poverty in the 1990s; post-2008 austerity), and includes research into income poverty, food insecurity, low quality housing and poor living environments. Among this work are also bodies of research addressing the complex and interrelated effects of deprivation on particular population groups, including women, lone parents, minority ethnic communities and adults in older age.

Failure to address these social structural processes limits the likely effectiveness of health policies. As Bambra warns, policies are unlikely to succeed when they "attempt to tackle health inequalities by trying to 'empower' people or encouraging them to feel happier, more confident or more responsible, without necessarily addressing the key, underlying issues" (Bambra et al., 2011, p. 403). Marmot is more specific, arguing that diverse social factors are *more influential* on individuals than those more obviously and directly associated with health, including health behaviour, genetic makeup and access to health care services (Marmot, 2010b). It is therefore unhelpful that the SASA report gives no attention to the factors often experienced by those in the lower reaches of the social gradient, such as low income, job insecurity, poor quality housing, limited access to public services and unattractive or insecure neighbourhoods.

The fact that PA experts in the UK failed to address social factors is particularly notable. When the SASA review group first convened in 2009 the national discussion on health inequalities was already three decades old and strongly established in the public and policy domains. It had been launched thirty years previously by the Black Report (Black, 1980) and reinvigorated in 1998 by the first of three "New Labour" governments through the Acheson Inquiry into Health Inequalities (Acheson, 1998). More recently, Sir Michael Marmot had been commissioned to lead the *Strategic Review of Health Inequalities in England* (2008–2010), whose report *Fair society, healthy lives* (Marmot, 2010a) was published to wide public exposure in 2010, during the period when the SASA working groups were meeting. Despite this, the UK's guidance to increase levels of physical activity failed to engage with debates around health inequalities and gave no consideration to the social processes affecting health behaviour.

If PA interventions are to address the multiple influences that affect individuals, they need to be underpinned by theories that incorporate these factors. Although not used in the SASA report, such theories are available and well-established in health behaviour research, in social ecological models of health (SEMs). SEMs therefore appear to allow the social factors that PA guidance omits to be directly addressed. The chapter now considers their content and operationalisation in more detail.

Addressing the social: Recognising structural influences on health behaviour

This section of the chapter reprises the arguments put forward in Kay's (2016b) recent review of the potential for physical activity guidance to draw on the conceptual models associated with the social determinants of health framework. Kay's analysis examines how SEMs developed by health behaviourists conceptualise "social" influences on health very differently from frameworks developed by social scientists.

First proposed by McLeroy et al. (1988), SEMs bring together two core concepts: that individuals interact with external and contextual influences, and that these occur at multiple "levels". McLeroy et al.'s initial SEM identified five levels at which influence occurred (intrapersonal, interpersonal, organisational, community and public policy). Despite this broad approach, it nonetheless omitted key social structural variables, leading Winch (2012, n.p.) to later comment that "it is not clear where culture, social class, racism, gender, economics/ employment are supposed to fit, or if they fit anywhere". Later variants include Stokols (1992, 1996; six levels of influence); Glanz, Sallis, Saelens and Frank (2005; four); Story et al. (2008; four); and Sallis (2009; six). These versions incorporate more social variables, including gender, age, race/ethnicity and SES.

In theory SEMs provide frameworks that identify multiple levels of social and physical environments and encourage intervention at these different levels. Yet in practice this multi-level approach has rarely been in evidence. Golden and Earp (2012) found that fewer than 10 per cent of the interventions they reviewed were based on SEMs. The great majority were instead underpinned by other widely accepted theoretical approaches which were "rooted in utility concepts from psychology and focus[ed] on changing individual motivations to stimulate behavior change". They concluded that in practice, "the predominant theories in the literature we reviewed continue to have an individual orientation". Even when SEMs were used to guide interventions, they seldom resulted in a comprehensive strategy intended to address multiple levels of influence; instead, they commonly focused on one or two types, most often individual levels – inter-and inter-personal. Collective and structural factors were rarely addressed.

The failure to address "higher level" factors partly reflects the difficulty of doing so in tangible ways. Golden and Earp suggest that targeting structural factors "is likely more challenging than adapting intrapersonal- and interpersonal-level programs", and that there are particular difficulties in translating theories about "higher level social and behavioural change" into practical action at intervention level (Golden and Earp, 2012, p. 370). Burke et al. (2009) suggest however that the failure is not simply a failure of application, but reflects a more fundamental theoretical feature: that although SEMs purport to address multi-level social influences, in reality they remain rooted in individual theories. They conclude that SEMs are undermined by their reliance on these pre-existing health behaviour theories and constructs for intervention at each level (Burke et al., 2009, p. 61S). Kay's (2016b) critique draws particular attention to the failure of SEMs to recognise that characteristics that SEMs categorise as "individual" – such as gender, culture and social class – embody structural properties and transmit social processes.

The *Social Determinants of Health* framework for conceptualising structural influences on physical activity

There are alternatives to social ecological models for theorising how health behaviour is influenced by factors beyond the individual. For physical activity specialists, there may be particular value in approaches that encourage the situation of the least advantaged sectors of the population will be addressed. One such approach is the Social Determinants of Health (SDH) framework, which addresses the social gradient of health and, like SEMs, has multiple variants.

SDH frameworks draw on a lengthy tradition. As Irwin and Scali (2007) note, "Analysts have long observed that social and environmental factors decisively influence people's health" (Irwin and Scali, 2007, p. 236). This thinking underpinned the health movements of the nineteenth century, which sought to alleviate the impacts of industrialisation on the working and living conditions of the poor. In the modern era, the focus on social determinants traces back to the emergence of community health approaches in the 1960s and 1970s, with the modern health inequalities agenda gaining particular momentum in the post-Thatcher era in the1990s and 2000s. More recently the SDH framework has provided the theoretical underpinning for the World Health Organization's Commission on the Social Determinants of Health (CSDH; cf. *Closing the gap in a generation*; WHO, 2008a), the UK Marmot Review (*Fair society, healthy lives*, 2010), and the European Commission's Commission on *Health inequalities in the EU* (2013).

The core premise of SDH frameworks is that individuals' health outcomes are influenced by a range of social structural factors which reflect the wider organisation of power and resources in society. The resulting inequalities underpin more immediate health "determinants", which are the range of interacting factors that shape health and well-being. These include material circumstances, the social environment, psychosocial factors and biological factors, which are "in turn . . . influenced by social position, itself shaped by education, occupation, income, gender, ethnicity and race" (Marmot, 2010b, p. 11). Serious health inequalities do not, therefore, arise by chance, or as a result of individual behaviour or characteristics; rather, "Social and economic differences in health status reflect, and are caused by, social and economic inequalities in society" (Marmot 2010b, p.12). Addressing health inequalities means addressing social structural factors, making it important that the means for doing so are incorporated in health policy, guidance and interventions.

The conceptualisation of social determinants of health that underpins the work led by Marmot strongly emphasises the concept of "social position" as playing a central role in determining health inequalities (Solar and Irwin, 2010, p. 4–5). The resulting SDH framework recognises three forms of "mechanism" which interact with each other to influence exposure to health risk (Figure 8.1). The three mechanisms consist of two categories of "structural determinants" (*context,* and *social positioning*) which produce structural health inequalities, which give rise to a third category (*intermediary determinants*) which influence individuals' specific health outcomes:

- The first category of determinants operate at the level of "context", and include "all social and political mechanisms that generate, configure and maintain social hierarchies" (Solar and Irwin, 2010, p. 5), including the labour market, the educational system and the welfare state.
- The second category are those that influence "social positioning"; they are closely connected with *context* as they emerge from socioeconomic and political institutions to produce stratification and social class divisions which define individual socioeconomic position within hierarchies of power, prestige and access to resources. They include income, education, occupation, social class, gender and race/ethnicity. In identifying these, the framework therefore demonstrates the connection between high level contextual factors, and the resources and characteristics that position an individual in society.
- The final category consists of *intermediary determinants of health*. Intermediary determinants are reflective of people's place within social hierarchies, and influence their material circumstances. The main intermediary determinants are material circumstances, psychosocial circumstances and behavioural and/or biological factors. Based on their social position, individuals experience differences in exposure and vulnerability to health-compromising conditions. The health system itself is recognised as a social determinant at this level, allowing many of the provision factors addressed in SEMs – such as availability of programmes and facilities – to be included.

In its use of different "levels" of influencing factors, the SDH approach therefore bears similarities to the "multi-level" approach used in SEMs. Whereas SEMs centre the individual and work up/outward to wider influences, the SDH framework does the opposite, encouraging analysis that begins at the structural level, and from there works towards the factors directly experienced by individuals. In this sense SDH approaches might almost be said to invert that taken by SEMs, by foregrounding the influence of the social.

It should be evident that SDH frameworks have considerable common ground with SEMs. The two approaches address similar factors at individual, household, community and policy levels, albeit in different configurations, and there are few factors named in one approach that could not be included in the other. The SDH framework is however

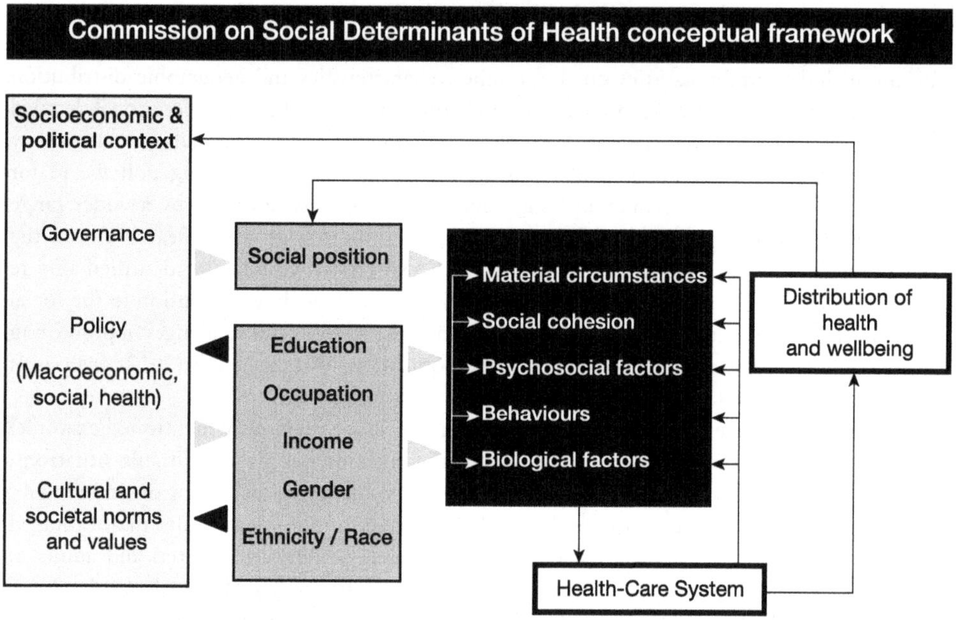

Figure 8.1 Conceptualising the social determinants of health

Source: Adapted from Solar, O. and Irwin, A., 2010. *A conceptual framework for action on the social determinants of health*. Geneva: World Health Organization.

distinguished by the explicit coherence across its three categories: any factor referred to in one domain can be linked to corresponding elements in the other two. This contrasts with SMEs where, as noted, characteristics such as gender and ethnicity appear only as individual factors and their structural properties are not addressed.

Frameworks which explicitly address social conditions can offer benefits to PA policy, practice and analysis. At the aggregate level, they recognise and direct attention to those in hardship, acknowledging the significance of constraining influences and barriers which are not of an individual's own making. This is why it is important for PA policy to also be informed by the evidence on the social determinants of health and their effect on people's capacities to behave in healthy ways. Doing so provides a valuable counterbalance to a narrow focus on individual agency that depicts inactive people as behaving "badly". Inevitably, this broader conceptualisation requires an equivalent evidence base, and the remaining sections consider how this might be achieved.

Diversifying the evidence base

Research into physical activity and health inequalities provides opportunities for social scientists to continue their tradition of influence beyond academia, aligning also with the modern impact agenda. Arguably physical activity policy *requires* a social science sensibility, to address the social structural processes that underpin health inequalities. It is therefore useful to consider whether the omission of health inequalities in PA guidance to date arises from the dearth of evidence available, or from a failure to access it.

Even a cursory review of the situation in the UK suggests that in social democracies where welfare provision is underpinned by evidence-based social planning, high quality, relevant data is readily available. At the descriptive level, large-scale, long-term population statistics describe the diverse and changing characteristics of national populations (e.g. ONS, 2013, 2015). These typically include current statistics on the number, characteristics and geographic distribution of the population, trend data on patterns of population change, and include occasional detailed analyses of data on priority social policy issues, such as population ageing. Such data are widely used by central and local government and the health sector for informing policy and for planning and monitoring resource allocation and service delivery, and also by a wider range of user groups including commercial companies, special interest groups, researchers and the general public. The use of such data to inform the SASA report would have identified a more diverse population than the one represented, and is likely to have drawn attention to the social gradient in health, encouraging greater consideration of the benefits and challenges of promoting physical activity to less advantaged sectors of the population. Wright et al.'s (2012) analysis of deprived youth in the London Olympic boroughs does exactly this.

Relevant analytical evidence is also easily obtainable: as the previously mentioned examples illustrated, numerous studies have investigated the lives of people in difficult situations, providing empirical accounts of the impact of poverty and other hardships on individuals' capacity for health behaviour. Among this is a lengthy tradition of research into disadvantaged groups accessing sport, e.g. projects to promote physical activity to children and adults in school (e.g. Hills and Croston, 2012) and community settings (e.g. Edwards et al., 2015; Mansfield et al., 2015), give access and voice to marginalised groups (e.g. Smith et al., 2015), and engage disaffected youth (Hills et al., 2013; Hills and Maitland, 2014). More recently the focus has narrowed more specifically to work focused on the health agenda, resulting in a range of publicly accessible accounts of barriers and facilitators to getting inactive people active through sport (e.g. Mansfield et al., 2016).

The failure of the SASA report to draw on such evidence is therefore noteworthy. The work of the SASA expert groups was virtually concurrent with the most extensive and high profile review of health inequalities ever undertaken in a UK country – the Strategic Review of Health Inequalities in England, led by Sir Michael Marmot. Marmot's Review was commissioned in November 2008, and SASA a few weeks later, and for more than a year the two ran in parallel until the Marmot Review was published in February 2010, a year before the SASA expert groups completed their work and published theirs (in July 2011). Some of the debate surrounding health inequalities might therefore have been expected to inform and perhaps influence the SASA analysis and guidance. Yet this did not happen, and more detailed examination of the complete separation of these virtually contemporaneous reviews provides useful insights into the gap between the two bodies of knowledge.

For the separation is indeed complete: there is no mention of health inequalities in the SASA report. The 2010 Marmot Review is not referred to, and nor is the equivalent work from the World Health Organization that immediately preceded it. Yet when Marmot's report *Fair society, healthy lives* (Marmot, 2010a) was published in 2010, to extensive public exposure, writing of the SASA report had yet to begin (Department of Health, Annex A, pp. 50–52) (Table 8.1). Furthermore, the Marmot Review team had adopted a high-profile, outward-facing approach throughout their work, engaging with a diverse swathe of actors across the health and welfare sectors. This included publishing a draft version of the report in summer 2009 and conducting a substantial online consultation on it – a process which attracted more than 6,000 visits and 135 institutional and individual responses. The launch of the final report in February 2010 featured prominently in television, radio, newspaper and online reporting – and this was reprised a year later, in February 2011, when the first anniversary of the Review was marked with the publication of an empirically based analysis

Table 8.1 Timeline of the work undertaken by the Marmot and SASA working groups

Producing Fair Society, Healthy Lives – *the Marmot Review of health inequalities in England*		*Producing* Start Active, Stay Active – *the UK guidance on PA*	
November 2008	Review of health inequalities in England commissioned	Winter 2008–09	PA guidance commissioned
January 2009	3 sub-groups undertake tasks and report		
Jun–Aug 2009	Draft Review released; web-based consultation	June 2009	4 sub-groups undertake tasks and report
September 2009		October 2009	Scientific meeting of stakeholders
February 2010	*Fair Society, Healthy Lives* published	Dec–Jan 2009–10	Web-based consultation
		May 2010	
		September 2010	Group convened to author guidelines
		July 2011	*Start Active, Stay Active* PA guidance published

of health indicators in England. This too was accompanied by extensive media coverage – a continuation of the strategy of keeping health inequalities visible across diverse outlets that variously reached the research community, politicians, policy makers and the public. Over the two years these included news reporting (BBC online and television news, *The Guardian*, *The Daily Mail*, *Northern Ireland News* and multiple regional news outlets), feature interviews and programmes (BBC Radio 4; Panorama (a prime time current affairs programme)), the medical and health sector (*Health Services* journal, *GP Magazine*, *British Medical Association*, *Men's Health Forum*), peer reviewed journals (*BMJ*) and popular magazines (*New Scientist*).

The closeness in timing between the Marmot Review and SASA reviews could hardly have offered greater and more immediate opportunities for the PA expert community to be aware of and informed by its analysis. That this did not happen reflects the narrow terms of reference bounding its work and highlights the need for disrupting established notions of the scope of this field. The onus is likely to be on social scientists to overcome this by overcoming the disciplinary divide and gaining entry to an established expert community – and challenging also its conceptions of what constitutes expert knowledge.

Only connect: Bridging PA knowledge communities

To become influential in physical activity policy, social scientists need to establish the value of their work in a field of enquiry in which it is often held in low regard. This can be especially the case in health-related research where hierarchies of evidence position experimental designs as the "gold standard" and judge many of the research designs through which social science contributions are made as being of poor quality. Resistance to qualitative research is particularly common, and this resistance is especially problematic in the area of PA as it dismisses approaches that have considerable potential to improve PA policy. As Veltri, Lim & Miller (2014) observe, qualitative social science research includes a commitment to viewing phenomena from the perspective of those being studied, thus giving the subjects of research a "voice", and makes use of non-standardised, semi-structured or unstructured methods that are sensitive to the social context of enquiry (Veltri et al., 2014, p .1). Studies such as Mansfield et al. 2016 demonstrate how effectively qualitative research extends understanding of physical (in)activity beyond the individualised focus of behaviour change theories, by both contextualising individuals in their social setting and examining their physical activity in the context of their wider lifestyle.

In advocating for the value of social science to PA policy, social scientists can point to its use in other policy fields (Kay, 2016a). One of the most persuasive examples may be the methods used by the Marmot Review itself. On the surface, there were considerable similarities with the methodologies adopted by the SASA review groups: both combined scientific review of research evidence with stakeholder engagement and each also undertook a web-based consultation at an interim stage in their work. Differences are nonetheless also apparent, the most notable being the more diverse range of scientific evidence used by the Marmot Review, including extensive social science data. There are also differences in the consultation and stakeholder engagement activities, in which the Marmot Review Group adopted a broader approach than the SASA expert groups. In comparison to the SASA consultation, which gave particular emphasis to the scientific and policy communities, the Marmot Review engaged with more diverse stakeholders. This included commissioning qualitative work to explored perceptions of inequalities and potential solutions with deprived groups including single parents, people with mental health problems from black and minority ethnic backgrounds and people with low-level stress and mental health problems. Its stakeholder engagement therefore reached well beyond the health sector, through multiple additional activities:

> Running alongside the Review were numerous meetings, discussions and consultations, presentations and seminars with community groups, health sector representatives, housing associations and organisations, the Local Government Association, IDeA (the Improvement and Development Agency for local government), health care organisations, regional government, other government departments, local public health and local government leaders, Primary Care Trusts, third sector and other delivery organisations, and the public.

This approach illustrates a further dimension of the potential contributions that the social sciences offer PA policy. The Marmot Review not only indicates the value of a multidisciplinary evidence base, but also demonstrates an inclusive approach to how expertise is defined, in whom it resides and what therefore counts as knowledge. In this it resonates with Mansfield's call, in her seminal paper on research partnerships in sport for public health: that knowledge in sport, health and physical activity should to be generated through "communities of researchers, policymakers, practitioners and participants" joining together in the "production, mobilisation and translation of evidence" (Mansfield, 2016, p. 718).

Conclusions

Promoting PA at population level requires guidance that resonates widely: the challenge is to provide this without the requirement for such broad relevance producing over-simplified, normative messaging. PA policy itself needs to give more attention to population complexity and diversity, accompanied by corresponding broadening of the evidence base. Social science has a major contribution to make to improved understanding of the challenges around PA by centring the structural influences that influence health behaviour. While not wholly negating behaviour change perspectives, this recognises their limits and assigns them a secondary role.

Guidance derived from such approaches would be characterised by:

- *Theoretical underpinning* in which social determinants of health perspectives replace behaviour change theories as the primary basis of PA guidance. Foregrounding the social processes that produce inequality in this way addresses the key omission in current PA guidance: that high levels of physical inactivity are associated with structural trends such as urbanisation and population ageing (cf.WHO ref) that materially influence individuals' living circumstances but lie outside their control. These "problems" are not of individuals' sole making, and their "solution" does not lie with them alone.
- *Policy guidance* that recognises that individuals are exposed to constraining factors and that these can reduce both their opportunity and their *capacity* to be active. The use of social determinants of health perspectives to inform PA policy would identify these barriers to activity and recognise the need to address them. The importance attributed to changing the "culture" surrounding PA (as advocated by some national agencies, e.g. Public Health England, 2014) would be reduced to a secondary role, as a support to strategies that directly address constraints.
- *Practitioner guidance* that takes the specific needs of potential users and the constraints affecting them as the basis for designing and delivering interventions that respond to local situations and use contextualised local knowledge to address them.
- *Public health messaging* which acknowledges that becoming active can be difficult, recognises the obstacles that inactive people may need to overcome and admits and supports efforts that may be needed to achieve this.

Generic messages to "be more active" have limited value to practitioners confronting the specific needs of diverse and complex populations and seeking strategies to support them. Individuals are indeed individual – diverse in their characteristics, biographies and everyday circumstances. The evidence base underpinning PA policy and practice needs to reflect this, and this chapter has provided an illustration of how this has been done in other areas of public health. Drawing on this, it advocates developing a broader expert community for physical activity that crosses disciplinary boundaries and professional sectors, and incorporates lay knowledge. Such collaborations may assist in connecting social science theory more explicitly to the everyday (Golden and Earp, 2012), and allow the structural processes influencing health to be addressed in PA policy. In time the PA expert community may also recognise that the "link between social conditions and health is not a footnote to the 'real' concerns with health but should become the main focus" (Marmot, 2010b, p.4).

References

Abel-Smith, B. and Townsend, P., 1965. *The poor and the poorest: A new analysis of the Ministry of Labour's family expenditure surveys of 1953–54 and 1960.* London: Bell.

Acheson, D. (Chairman), 1998. *Independent enquiry into inequalities in health.* London: The Stationery Office.

Australian Government Department of Health, 2014. *Australia's physical activity and sedentary behaviour guidelines for adults*. Commonwealth of Australia: Canberra.

Bambra, C., Smith, K. E., Garthwaite, K., Joyce, K. E. and Hunter, D. J., 2011. A labour of Sisyphus? Public policy and health inequalities research from the Black and Acheson Reports to the Marmot Review. *Journal of Epidemiology and Community Health*, 65, 399–406.

Black, D. (Chair), 1980. *Inequalities in health*. London: DHSS.

Brewer, M., Browne, J. and Joyce, R., 2011. *Child and working-age poverty from 2010 to 2020, Commentary 121*. London: Institute for Fiscal Studies.

Burke, N., Joseph, G., Pasick, R. J. and Barker, J. C., 2009. Theorizing social context: Rethinking behavioral theory. *Health Education & Behavior*, 36(Suppl. 1), 55S–70S.

DCMS, 2015. *Sporting future: A new strategy for an active nation*. London: Crown Copyright.

Department of Health, 2011. *Start active, stay active: A report on physical activity from the four home countries' Chief Medical Officers*. London: HMSO.

Edwards, G., Grubb, B., Power, A. and Serle, N., 2015. *Moving the goal posts: Poverty and access to sport for young people. CASE report 95*. London: London School of Economics.

European Commission, 2013. *Health inequalities in the EU – Final report of a consortium. Consortium lead: Sir Michael Marmot*. Available from: http://ec.europa.eu/health/social_determinants/docs/healthine qualitiesineu_2013_en.pdf.

Glanz, K., Sallis, J.F., Saelens, B.E. and Frank, L.D., 2005. Healthy nutrition environments: Concepts and measures. *American Journal of Health Promotion*, 19, 330–333.

Golden, S. D. and Earp, J. A. L., 2012. Social ecological approaches to individuals and their contexts: Twenty years of health education & behavior health promotion interventions. *Health Education & Behavior*, 39(3), 364–372.

Greenhalgh, T. and Fahy, N., 2015. Research impact in the community-based health sciences: An analysis of 162 case studies from the 2014 UK Research Excellence Framework. *BMC Medicine*, 13(232), DOI: 10.1186/s12916-015-0467-4.

Haan, N., Kaplan, G.A. and Camacho, T., 1987. Poverty and health: Prospective evidence from the Alameda County Study. *American Journal of Epidemiology*. 125, 989–998.

Hills, L., Bradford, S. and Johnston, C., 2013. *Building a participation legacy from the London 2012 Olympic and Paralympic games in disadvantaged areas. Report for StreetGames*. London: Brunel University London.

Hills, L. A. and Croston, A., 2012. "It should be better all together": Exploring strategies for "undoing" gender in coeducational physical education. *Sport Education and Society*, 17(5), 591–605. doi:10.108 0/13573322.2011.553215.

Hills, L. and Maitland, A., 2014. Research-based knowledge utilization in a community sport evaluation: A case study. *International Journal of Public Sector Management*, 27(2), 165–172.

Irwin, A. and Scali, E., 2007. Action on the social determinants of health: A historical perspective. *Glob Public Health*, 2(3), 235–256.

Kay, T. A., 2016a. Bodies of knowledge: Connecting the evidence bases on physical activity and health inequalities. *International Journal of Sport Policy and Politics*, 8(4), 539–557.

Kay, T.A., 2016b. Knowledge, not numbers: The value and place of qualitative research in sport, exercise and health. In Smith, B. and Sarkes, A. (eds) *Handbook on Qualitative Research in Sport and Exercise*. London: Routledge

Mansfield, L., 2016. Resourcefulness, reciprocity and reflexivity: The three Rs of partnership in sport for public health research. *International Journal of Sport Policy and Politics*, 8(4), 713–729, DOI: 10.1080/19406940.2016.1220409.

Mansfield, L., Anokye, N., Fox-Rushby, J. and Kay, T., 2015. The Health and Sport Engagement (HASE) Intervention and Evaluation Project: Protocol for the design, outcome, process and economic evaluation of a complex community sport intervention to increase levels of physical activity. *BMJ Open*, 5(10), e009276–e009276.

Mansfield, L. and Kay, T. A. with Anokye, N. and Fox-Rushby, J., 2016. The Health and Sport Engagement (HASE) intervention and evaluation project: The design, delivery and evaluation of a complex community sport intervention for improving physical activity, health and wellbeing. Volume 1: Evaluation of the Design and Delivery of the HASE project. Unpublished report to Sport England. London: Brunel University London.

Marmot, M., 2010a. *The Marmot Review: Fair society, healthy lives: A strategic review of health inequalities in England post-2010*. Marmot Review Final Report. London: University College London.

Marmot, M., 2010b. *The Marmot Review: Fair society, healthy lives: A strategic review of health inequalities in England post-2010*. Marmot Review Executive Summary. London: University College London.

McLeroy, K. R., Bibeau, D., Steckler, A. and Glanz ,K., 1988. An ecological perspective on Health Promotion Programs. *Health Education Quarterly*, 15(4), 351–377.

Morse, J., 2006. The politics of evidence. *Qualitative Health Research*, 16(3), 395–404, DOI: 10.1177/1049732305285482.

ONS, 2013. *Life expectancy at birth and at age 65 for local areas in England and Wales: 2009–11*. London: HMSO.

ONS, 2015. *Families and households, 2015*. London: HMSO.

Public Health England, 2014. *Everybody active, every day. An evidence-based approach to physical activity*. London: Public Health England.

Sallis, J. F., 2009. *Using research to create a less obesogenic world*. Presentation to the Texas Obesity Research Center, April 9. Accessed on 9th December 2015 at http://sallis.ucsd.edu/Documents/Pubs_documents/Slides_HoustonObesity_040909.pdf.

Smith, B., Tomasone, J. R., Latimer-Cheung, A. E. and Martin Ginis, K. A., 2015. Narrative as a knowledge translation tool for facilitating impact: Translating physical activity knowledge to disabled people and health professionals. *Health Psychology*, 34(4), 303–313.

Solar, O. and Irwin, A., 2010. *A conceptual framework for action on the social determinants of health*. Geneva: World Health Organization.

Sport England, 2016. *Towards and active nation. Strategy 2016–2021*. London: Sport England.

Stokols, D., 1992. Establishing and maintaining healthy environments: Toward a social ecology of health promotion. *American Psychologist*, 47(1), 6–22.

Stokols, D., 1996. Translating social ecological theory into guidelines for community health promotion. *American Journal of Health Promotion*, 10, 282–298.

Story, M., Kaphingst, K., Robinson-O'Brien, R. and Glanz, K., 2008. Creating healthy food and eating environments: Policy and environmental approaches. *Annual Review of Public Health*, 29, 253–72.

Thompson, R. A., 2015. Relationships, regulation, and early development. *Handbook of Child Psychology and Developmental Science*. 3(6), 1–46.

U.S. Department of Health and Human Services, 2008. *Physical Activity Guidelines for Americans*. ODPHP Publication No. U0036. Washington (DC): U.S. Department of Health and Human Services.

Veltri, G. A., Lim, J. and Miller, R., 2014. More than meets the eye: The contribution of qualitative research to evidence-based policy-making. *Innovation: The European Journal of Social Science Research*, 27(1), 1–4, DOI: 10.1080/13511610.2013.806211.

Weaver, R. R., Lemonde, M., Payman, N. and Goodman, W.M., 2014. Health capabilities and diabetes self-management: The impact of economic, social, and cultural resources. *Social Science and Medicine*, 102, 58–68.

WHO, 2008a. *Closing the gap in a generation: Health equity through action on the social determinants of health*. Commission on Social Determinants of Health Report. Geneva: World Health Organization.

WHO, 2008b. *Closing the gap in a generation: Health equity through action on the social determinants of health*. Commission on Social Determinants of Health Executive Summary. Geneva: World Health Organization.

WHO, 2009. *Global health risks: Mortality and burden of disease attributable to selected major risks*. Geneva: World Health Organization.

WHO, 2010. *Global recommendations on physical activity for health*. Geneva: World Health Organization.

WHO European Regional Office, 2015. *Physical activity strategy for the WHO European Region 2016–2025*. Copenhagen: World Health Organization European Regional Office.

Wilson, K., Elliot, S., Law, M., Eyles, J., Jerrett, M. and Keller-Olaman, S., 2004. Linking perceptions of neighbourhood to health in Hamilton, Canada. *Journal of Epidemiology and Community Health*, 58, 192–198.

Winch, P., 2012. Ecological models and multilevel interventions: Health Behavior Change at the Individual, Household and Community Levels. John Hopkins University. Accessed on 9th November 2015 at http://ocw.jhsph.edu/courses/healthbehaviorchange/PDFs/C14_2011.pdf

Wright, C., Lodge, H. and Jacobson, B., 2012. *Child's play? The antenatal to adolescent health legacy in the Olympic boroughs*. London: London Health Observatory.

Young, M. and Willmott, P., 1957. *Family and kinship in East London*. London: Routledge and Kegan Paul.

9

THE USE OF BEHAVIOURAL EVIDENCE IN PHYSICAL ACTIVITY POLICY

Fiona Gillison and Fay Beck

Physical activity is vital for the health and well-being of people of all ages. It has been shown to reduce the risks of developing chronic disease and reverse some disease processes (Lee et al., 2012), to contribute to the maintenance of a healthy body weight (Swift et al., 2014), and to promote positive health and well-being (Penedo and Dahn, 2005, Biddle and Asare, 2011). Despite these potential benefits, around 30 per cent of the world's adults are physically inactive, rising to over 40 per cent in many high-income nations (Hallal et al., 2012). Over 80 per cent of children fail to achieve the recommended 60 minutes of moderate to vigorous physical activity per day (Hallal et al., 2012). Global and regional strategies have been in place for some years to provide guidance to governments in establishing policies to promote physical activity (World Health Organization [WHO], 2013, 2015), however no country has yet succeeded in achieving a trajectory of increasing participation. Should we conclude that the policy approaches we have tried so far are ineffective, and that we need to look for alternatives? Or is it possible that the intended approaches are sound, but require improvement in their design and/or implementation in order to reach their full potential? This chapter aims to explore these two questions by examining examples of existing physical activity policies in the light of 'best practice' within behavioural theory and behavioural science research.

The examples of policy that we will review are drawn from the WHO European Physical Activity Strategy, which incorporates a range of policy approaches operating at the individual, community, cultural, political and environmental levels (WHO, 2015, Heath et al., 2012). It is widely agreed that to bring about community-wide and lasting effects on health behaviours we need to incorporate policies of different types, operating at different levels, and which simultaneously target the different determinants of the behaviour that we aim to promote (Jebb et al., 2013, Butland et al., 2007). Findings from other behavioural domains where policy action is more advanced, such as tobacco control, can provide a useful worked example of what a comprehensive set of policies should include (West, 2007, WHO, 2008). For example, the MPOWER framework for tobacco control identifies the contribution of six distinct policy approaches: 1) routine monitoring and surveillance of behaviour, 2) health protection, 3) offering support, 4) health messaging, 5) legislative approaches and 6) financial or economic approaches (WHO, 2008). The examples of policy that we will focus on in this chapter address the four MPOWER categories that are most applicable to behavioural theory and a physical activity setting: *monitoring and surveillance*, through the UK National Child

Measurement Programme (NCMP), *offering support*, through the provision of brief advice in primary care and exercise referral services, *health messaging*, through social marketing and workplace campaigns to promote active transport and *financial or economic approaches*, through the provision of incentives. We acknowledge that physical activity policies may not fit neatly into the MPOWER categories, but it nonetheless provides a guide to the breadth of initiatives likely to be required to promote population-level behaviour change.

The aim of this chapter is to consider the use of behavioural evidence within physical activity policy. However, to do this comprehensively we also need to consider the use of behavioural theory. Evidence and theory are necessarily intertwined; well-established theories are derived from evidence, they provide a means of integrating different sources of evidence in a systematic way and can be tested against evidence to assess their utility. Theory is also important in helping us to understand why people act in the ways that they do (i.e., mechanisms of effect), which may provide insight into public responses to policy (i.e., why some policies or initiatives gain support and momentum, and why others fail). This understanding is also useful when attempting to translate successful approaches from one domain or setting to another, which is often conducted to meet requirements for evidence-based policies in settings where bespoke evidence is lacking. Using theory can help by providing a model of the psychological (and other) processes that underpin the success of a policy or intervention, and thus which also need to be targeted in any adapted versions, albeit usually through different techniques. That is, theory can help to identify what the core elements of a policy are that we need to retain in order to claim that our adaptation is still 'evidence-based'. Within this chapter we will therefore outline some key theories relevant to promoting physical activity within behavioural science research, and discuss how and where these theories could be, and have been, applied within physical activity policies. This analysis is a complex process; theory may be implicit in the content of a policy, but also in who it targets, when and how. Thus, the five illustrative examples incorporated within the chapter are included to provide a more in-depth analysis of the different ways in which we can assess a policy's alignment with theory and evidence.

Behavioural theory applied to physical activity

Theories of behaviour change provide structure for exploring and understanding the mechanisms through which people change and maintain their health behaviours (Michie et al., 2008). They help to identify what needs to change in the way a person thinks, feels or experiences the world around them in order to engage in health behaviours, and thus can suggest where interventions and policies are best targeted. While a poorly designed or implemented intervention will be poor quality whether based on theory or not, the use of behavioural theory is argued to produce research evidence of higher quality and usability (Craig et al., 2008, Michie et al., 2008), achieving this by:

- encouraging researchers to set out explicit, testable models of the processes underpinning behaviour change (i.e., causal pathways), extending our focus from establishing *whether* or not things work, to *how* they work (Schaalma and Kok, 2009),
- the use of standardised definitions of constructs and terms to facilitate direct comparisons between studies, and thus the more meaningful aggregation of data from multiple studies for meta-analysis (Michie, 2008, Gardner et al., 2010) and
- the identification of behaviour change techniques that can be systematically mapped to theoretical pathways of action in the translation of research into practice (Kok et al., 2004).

Evidence from systematic reviews supports the contention that behaviour change interventions based on theory are more effective than those that are not (Gardner et al., 2010, Webb et al., 2010, Prestwich et al., 2014, Horodyska et al., 2015). However, there are a large number of behavioural theories to choose from, each of which may be more or less effective depending on the setting, population or type of behaviour we wish to influence. While choosing a theory may thus appear a daunting task, there is considerable overlap between the constructs that are identified across theories, and indeed most, if not all, comprehensive theories of behaviour change converge to support the importance of three psychosocial determinants in driving health behaviours and behaviour change: self-efficacy, social support and motivation (Schwarzer and Luszczynska, 2008, Michie et al., 2011, Greaves et al., 2011, Olander et al., 2013, Amireault et al., 2013). Thus, we will focus on these three elements in exploring the theoretical content of physical activity policies.

Self-efficacy

Self-efficacy is a core construct of Social Cognitive Theory, the most commonly applied theory within physical activity research (Bandura, 1998). It is also an important component of other well-known frameworks such as the Transtheoretical Model (often referred to as the Stages of Change model by health practitioners; Prochaska and Velicer, 1997). Self-efficacy can be defined as a person's belief in their ability to carry out a particular task or challenge (Bandura, 1998), and is a very specific belief, relating to the particular type of behaviour on the specific occasion under consideration rather than a general sense of confidence. As such, the detail of how physical activity is described and marketed within policies can make a big difference to the level of self-efficacy people feel towards it. Self-efficacy is important on the basis that people are unlikely to initiate an action if they have little belief that they will be able to achieve it (Schwarzer and Luszczynska, 2008; Michie et al., 2011). The results of systematic reviews suggest that self-efficacy towards physical activity can be enhanced by: facilitating vicarious experiences (i.e., providing opportunities to observe people similar to oneself successfully carrying out an activity); the provision of personal feedback (e.g., through self-monitoring techniques; Ashford et al., 2010); the provision of instruction, facilitating action planning and providing reinforcement for being active (Williams and French, 2011). Policies may operate at a population or individual level, but in either case can be scrutinised for the degree to which they are supportive of people's self-efficacy for physical activity; for example policy may directly aim to boost self-efficacy as in the case of providing behavioural support services, or indirectly by reducing perceived barriers to an active lifestyle, such as through creating more supportive physical environments.

Social support

Social support is a broad set of factors ranging from interpersonal influences such as emotional support and encouragement, instrumental support (e.g., providing transport to sports activities for children; van Sluijs et al., 2007) and having people to exercise with, to community and societal level factors such as social norms and social cohesion (i.e., coming together with others in communities that promote the adoption of physical activity) (McNeill et al., 2006). Social norms are challenging to create through policy, as they rely on both actual change (e.g., prevalence) in addition to perceptions of change (e.g., visibility), but may nonetheless be an important target. For example, in the smoking domain, social norms for *not* smoking (rather than smoking) in many countries shifted very slowly after decades-long comprehensive policy approaches towards tobacco control. Not only did the shift in norms help to increase public acceptance of policy intervention (e.g., even among smokers there was very little opposition to smoke free legislation; Borland et al., 2006), but individual smoking behaviours were also influenced. Contrary to critics' fears for the unanticipated effects of smoke-free legislation, smoking in the home (particularly in the presence of children) actually decreased following the ban of smoking in public places, suggesting the legislation had strengthened smokers' recognition and endorsement of the rationale for reducing exposure of non-smokers to second hand smoke (Phillips et al., 2007, Akhtar et al., 2009). Similar positive effects of social norms have also been observed in the physical activity domain, such that when physical activity becomes highly visible within a community (i.e., people report seeing others walking and cycling frequently), this perceived norm for activity is predictive of increased physical activity over and above the effects of direct social support from friends and family (Ball et al., 2010). However, even with the addition of considerable infrastructure, increases in the critical mass of active walkers and cyclers are difficult to achieve (Goodman et al., 2013), and people report their attempts to be active are often undermined by those around them who are inactive (Whale et al., 2014).

Motivation

Many theories of motivation are available providing different emphases on the determining characteristics of our motivation to improve our health behaviours. Common examples include: protection motivation theory (PMT; Rogers, 1975) which models the motivating mechanisms of threat and coping appraisals (i.e., responding to 'fear appeals'); the health belief model (HBM; Conner and Norman, 1996) that is grounded in assumptions of people choosing to act or not to act as a result of their attitudes and beliefs (e.g., perceptions of susceptibility, severity, potential benefits and barriers); and the trans-theoretical model, which draws on theories of psychotherapy to describe a model of progressive stages of readiness to change and the processes driving people's progression through these stages (Prochaska and Velicer, 1997). While providing useful frameworks for studying phenomena, theories such as these have been criticised for being of limited use in helping to understand and influence motivation in relation to physical activity in particular, where the link between the behaviour and health outcomes are typically not well defined or understood: For example, many people who are inactive do not feel an imminent health threat or believe their behaviour is risky (i.e., limited relevance for fear appeal within PMT and perceived severity within the HBM), and they may perceive more barriers or threats (e.g., discomfort, lack of time or enjoyment, injury risk) than advantages to becoming active (i.e., limiting the perceived benefits within the HBM). Further, such theories are criticised as providing a simplistic view based on the assumption that people make rational and planned decisions based on coherent attitudes, leading to relatively stable and predictable states of motivation.

No theory is perfect in helping to understand any behaviour, but one that perhaps provides a more comprehensive view of people's multiple and changing motives for physical activity is self-determination theory (SDT) (Ryan and Deci, 2000a). SDT is a macro-theory of human motivation that incorporates many theoretical perspectives, conceptualising motivation as something that is dynamic, influenced by both internal and external factors, and reflective of people's ability to hold multiple competing motives at any one time. SDT has been shown to be useful in the design of physical activity interventions (e.g., Teixeira et al., 2012, Fortier et al., 2012), and importantly for the focus of this chapter, also provides insight into how policy effects could influence individual behaviour (Moller et al., 2006). Within SDT, motivation is framed as a continuum, ranging from more controlled types of regulation (i.e., with low self-determination) at one end, to high quality, autonomous motivation at the other (Ryan and Deci, 2000a). Autonomous motivation is associated with positive behavioural and affective outcomes, such as long-term behavioural engagement, greater effort and enjoyment, whereas controlled motivation is associated with only the temporary or short-term behavioural engagement, and poorer well-being, effort and enjoyment (Teixeira et al., 2012, Ryan et al., 2008). Controlled types of motivation include occasions when we act purely in response to overt controls, such as to gain rewards or avoid punishment (e.g., payment, legal requirements), or when we act in response to internalised controls, such as to avoid feeling guilt or shame, or to impress and please others. Conversely, autonomous motivation reflects a greater sense of volition, when our behaviour is more aligned with our personal values. For example, and in increasing order of self-determination, people may take exercise autonomously because they personally endorse and value the outcomes of an activity (e.g., health or fitness benefits), because it reflects their identity and sense of self (i.e., 'being fit and active is part of who I am') or for the sheer pleasure and enjoyment of doing so (intrinsic motivation) (see Standage and Ryan, 2012 for a comprehensive review of the application of SDT in the physical activity setting).

So how can we design policies and interventions that promote autonomous motivation? A key component of any autonomy supportive approach is acknowledging (and respecting) the views of the people we are trying to influence, and ensuring that they perceive a meaningful rationale for changing their behaviour (Deci et al., 1994). Research suggests that there is at least some public recognition of the need for policies to promote physical activity (Emm et al., 2013, Brownson et al., 2001, Oliver and Lee, 2005), and thus that there is already acceptance of a meaningful 'rationale' for some level of government intervention. However, we all too often assume that people are motivated to change for the same reasons that are pertinent to health professionals and policy makers (e.g., future health and financial benefits), but this may not be the case. For example, retired adults report a range of motives for being active from seeking a daily sense of challenge and purpose, to enjoyment and seeking social affiliation, whereas health outcomes may appear only as a welcome but secondary by-product; for some older adults improved fitness can even be a disincentive if it distances them from their less able peers (Beck et al., 2010). Similarly, people adopting active forms of commuting may do so for cost and convenience and be unmoved by the rationale to do so for health benefits (Hansen and Nielsen, 2014). However, it is upholding people's sense of their own volition and freedom to choose that is of greatest importance in promoting autonomous motivation. Even if the public largely agree with the values driving policy initiatives, feeling that an activity is no longer one's own choice but as a result of 'complying' with instructions can undermine existing autonomous motivation and lead to psychological reactance (i.e., perceiving the message as a threat to personal freedom, and responding with anger and/or commitment to take the opposite course of action; Quick and Considine, 2008). Behaviour may be reduced to below the level observed prior to intervention if a new policy initiative generates a sense of reactance (Paul-Ebhohimhen and Avenell, 2008).

Two policy examples, financial incentives and the National Child Measurement Programme (NCMP), provide an illustration of how an understanding of SDT could help to improve policy design. The case of incentives also highlights some of the challenges and limitations of attempting to translate policies supported by evidence from one context to another, and shows how theory could help to identify alternative techniques to achieve the same ends:

Policy Example 1: Financial policies to support physical activity: The use of incentives

In other health domains (such as smoking cessation), the most effective policy in shaping behaviour is taxation (West, 2007). However, this type of punitive economic approach is primarily appropriate for reducing the behaviours that we wish people to do less of, whereas behaviours that require active engagement are better shaped by incentives (Petry, 2000). Incentives can be an attractive approach as they unarguably show positive short-term outcomes (Finkelstein et al., 2008), however in practice, financial incentives in particular are rarely associated with long-term positive outcomes such as sustained physical activity (Strohacker et al., 2014). For example, in a trial to promote physical activity to children in Singapore, participants were rewarded with a ~£15 toy store voucher for reaching agreed step-count goals (8,000 steps on 15 days/month, assessed by pedometers), and entry into a prize draw for continued attendance (Ngo et al., 2014). The impact on step count was initially positive, with steps increasing from 8,763 at baseline to 9,394 at their peak five months later. However, attendance at physical activity sessions was low (43% in the first month, 25% at five months and 6% at nine months), and any initial benefit facilitated by incentives was not sustained; steps dropped back to baseline levels within nine months. Similar findings have been found with payment schedules to college students; incentives increased gym attendance over a three month period, but attendance dropped to below baseline levels within a couple of months of the withdrawal of the incentive (Pope and Harvey, 2015). From an SDT perspective, such findings are consistent with the undermining effect of rewards on autonomous motivation, as we come to feel our behaviour as directed by the values of someone else (the incentiviser) and no longer our own (Moller et al., 2013). So while financial incentives may be enough to get us through the door of a leisure centre a couple of times and to support behaviours that do not require persistence (e.g., attending screening), the controlled motivation that results is insufficient to sustain long-term behaviour changes such as the adoption of regular physical activity (Haskell et al., 2007).

Despite the evidence against using monetary incentives, not all forms of incentive are perceived to be controlling (Cerasoli et al., 2014). It is worth exploring alternative types of incentive, as if we can identify incentives that are not perceived to be coercive, people may benefit from their strong initial 'stimulus' effect, prompting the first steps towards long-term behaviour change. The provision of informational feedback shows promise as one such type of incentive, as it is effectively a form of praise grounded in objective information about a person's level of achievement rather than someone else's values, and thus has been found to be supportive of autonomous motivation (Ryan and Deci, 2000b, Patrick and Canevello, 2011). From the perspective of population-level approach, an advantage of this form of incentive is that it is easily facilitated by mobile technology through providing real-time feedback of personalised information such as step counts, and the automated delivery of rewards/praise in response to goal achievement (Zuckerman and Gal-Oz, 2014, Turner-McGrievy et al., 2013). The commercial expertise in designing engaging interfaces on which most computerised systems draw also means that using an app or website for feedback purposes can be fun in itself, and thus appealing to more autonomous (intrinsic) motives for their use (Zuckerman and Gal-Oz, 2014). Apps and Internet-based resources endorsing 'self-help' approaches to physical activity promotion are already widely endorsed by UK policy makers (e.g., NHS apps library, NHS, 2015, myPace, Barnett et al., 2015). While the motivation to continue to use such apps and web-based programmes to support behaviour change may not always be long-lived, if these tools can serve the purpose of prompting the initial uptake of behaviour for sufficiently long to become part of a person's routine, then they are clearly a useful component of a comprehensive policy approach.

Little research has been conducted in identifying other types of incentives that could be perceived as endorsements of a person's choices, rather than coercive means of directing their behaviour. Given how strongly evidence supports taxation to reduce unhealthy behaviours at a policy level, research is warranted to explore the motivational effects of the related approach of providing subsidies (already evident in practices such as policies to provide free swimming for children, or workplace gym/cycle subsidy schemes), investigating whether subsidies in this setting are perceived by recipients to be controlling or autonomously supportive prompts towards physical activity.

Policy Example 2: Monitoring and surveillance policy related to physical activity: The UK National Child Measurement Programme (NCMP)

The use of monitoring and surveillance policies is also interesting from an SDT perspective, as they provide inherent challenges to perceptions of autonomy and control; the act of monitoring is one that is done to a person rather than with or for them. While not exclusively relating to physical activity, the NCMP was initially introduced as a surveillance programme to monitor obesity rates among primary school children, and the data it generates has been used to provide justification for national investment in, and prioritisation of, the promotion of physical activity for children. Most public health teams have chosen to feed back their NCMP measurements to parents of overweight children (Mooney et al., 2010) as a means of improving parental awareness of childhood overweight (Jeffery et al., 2005). However, the receipt of this feedback has created strong reactance from some parents (Grimmett et al., 2008, Statham et al., 2011, Gillison et al., 2014), and anecdotal evidence from school nurses and public health teams indicates that the uptake of child weight management programmes and other forms of support offered to parents within NCMP letters has been minimal. Research conducted with parents indicates that such negative reactions result from a combination of factors including: the lack of perceived legitimacy of school nurses to measure and report this information (i.e., an infringement of a family's perceived autonomy), a lack of self-efficacy to effect change (what to do if children refuse to be more active, or are already perceived to be as active as possible within the family's limitations?) and as parents' primary concerns for their child's health relate more to their psychological well-being than their weight alone (Gillison et al., 2014, Syrad et al., 2014). The issue of childhood obesity may represent a particularly sensitive area, but nonetheless this example provides insight into how surveillance programmes are often perceived, and suggests that if we are to use them as a springboard to try to encourage individual action then further steps first need to be taken to minimise perceptions of unwarranted intrusion into family autonomy that can lead to reactance. Theories of health communication may be helpful in designing more acceptable implementation plans, for example, reactance can be reduced and support for autonomy strengthened when people feel a greater sense of self-worth, stronger self-efficacy to make the required changes, and when alternative viewpoints are acknowledged and respected (Byrne and Niederdeppe, 2011).

Integrating behavioural theories into policy design

So far, we have argued that theory can be useful in understanding people's responses to policy intervention, providing examples critiqued through the lens of SDT. But how can we identify effective strategies that promote all three highlighted psychosocial determinants of physical activity (i.e., motivation, self-efficacy and social support) to incorporate within physical activity promoting policies? On-going work led by UK researchers has been conducted to try to facilitate this process, by defining specific, identifiable behaviour change techniques within published interventions and linking these to the theoretical constructs that they aim to target (Craig et al., 2008, Michie and Prestwich, 2010, Michie et al., 2005). The result to date is a comprehensive taxonomy of behaviour change techniques, providing standard descriptions of frequently used strategies (BCT taxonomy; Michie et al., 2013).[1] For example, the techniques of 'self-monitoring' (Nietfeld et al., 2006), 'goal setting' and 'modelling' are linked to promoting self-efficacy (Bandura, 2004), and the technique 'provide information about the health-behaviour link' is linked to motivation through strengthening one's rationale to change (Deci et al., 1994). Use of the taxonomy enables researchers to engage in a more transparent design process and build interventions, services and policies that can be clearly described as a set of hypothesised 'active ingredients'. While it is acknowledged that in reality strategies are likely to interact and operate in concert with others rather than to confer independent effects (Peters et al., 2015), the standardisation of terms allows us to identify what a given intervention (which could be a policy) includes. Describing interventions in this way allows us to compare the outcomes of studies containing specific techniques to assess their performance across studies. In this way, a meta-regression exploring the effect of specific behaviour change techniques in healthy eating and physical activity interventions found particular support for self-monitoring in promoting change (Michie et al., 2009), and as a result this technique has experienced a renaissance in its popularity and is included in most new services and interventions (NICE, 2014). Such a swift and comprehensive response is perhaps testament to the appetite for direct evidence as to what works in physical activity promotion from policy makers. The following two examples demonstrate how taxonomies of theoretically informed behaviour change techniques can help us to more objectively assess the degree to which policies to provide individual support are informed by behavioural theory and evidence in both their content, and the determinants of behaviour change that they target.

Policy Example 3: Offering support through exercise referral schemes

A common element of physical activity policy across the UK is the provision of exercise referral services for people at high cardio-vascular risk. The National Institute for Health and Care Excellence (NICE) has raised concerns over the efficacy of such schemes (NICE, 2006), reflecting findings from the research literature that the overall effect of services on physical activity is minimal (Pavey et al., 2011). However, in recognition that some schemes *do* work, deconstructing the active behaviour change content of effective schemes may help to identify what strategies underpin their efficacy and could thus be rolled out to improve less successful services. A starting point for this process lies in identifying the constituent behaviour change techniques within service protocols, in the same way that has been done in research trials, allowing them to be scrutinised in relation to the broader behaviour change literature (Beck et al., 2016, Murphy et al., 2012). By scrutinising behaviour change techniques within services and their outcomes (i.e., evaluating the efficacy of processes of change) rather than simply their impact on behaviour, we are better able to target adaptations and service improvements. That is, if a process evaluation identifies that a service successfully enhances self-efficacy but fails to enhance motivation, improvements may be more productively made through additional or alternative motivational strategies rather than adding further techniques to bolster self-efficacy.

Two independent studies have used taxonomies of behaviour change techniques to try to identify what type of behavioural support is routinely delivered through exercise referral services (Beck et al., 2016, Murphy et al., 2012). In each case, the research teams conducted structured observations of standard services to identify what behaviour change strategies were present during consultations as opposed to those written within a protocol. The process was conducted with a view to identifying potential gaps in the behavioural support provided, and suggesting additional or alternative strategies to bridge these. Both studies reported unexpectedly large inconsistencies in the behaviour change techniques delivered; whether as a result of limited time, skills or other factors, clients attending the same service often received very different behavioural support from each other, and often different support from that set out in the intended service protocol. Such insight is informative in directing service improvements, for example if exercise referral advisors are failing to deliver a complete protocol through lack of time, structural changes to the service may be a priority (more staff, longer appointments), whereas if deviation from the protocol results from a lack of skills, resources may be better invested in training (Beck et al., 2016). While it has yet to be formally tested whether the recommendations generated by such an approach would result in more effective exercise referral services, it does provide greater insight into how we can align evidence to practice to make sure that future evaluations of the implementation of a given policy on service provision represent a fair assessment of that service operating to its full potential. If other services are equally mixed in the support they provide, this suggests that a single policy such as the provision of exercise referral services does not in reality relate to the provision of a homogenous type of intervention or support, and undermines the conclusions of meta-analyses that work on the assumption of the comparability of trials reported under the same name.

Policy Example 4: Offering support through brief advice within primary care

The provision of brief advice within primary care provides a second example of the importance of evaluating the implementation of policies before concluding on their potential for efficacy. The provision of brief advice in primary care is a core physical activity policy within the UK (NICE, 2006), US (Moyer and Force, 2012) and across Europe (Oja et al., 2010). In this setting, brief advice is defined as the provision of information (e.g., on the risks of inactivity), encouragement to change and direction of where to seek further help, following an 'ask, advise, assist' structure. Brief advice is not designed or intended to provide a full programme of behavioural support to help people to make long term changes, but to prompt people to consider change who may not otherwise consider it (or who are not eligible for more intensive behavioural support services), and signpost them to sources of further support. Thus, it represents the first step in supporting the development of a person's motivation, through the provision of personally referenced information and communication of personal risks and benefits.

Relating this to theory, such an approach is certainly a useful part of a wider supportive environment for physical activity; we know that people are more likely to act on health risk information when this is communicated by a person in a respected position (e.g., O'Malley et al., 2004, Becker and Roblin, 2008), and when that information is personalised (Broekhuizen et al., 2012). One of the key limitations of health messaging is that many people within the community ignore health messages as they do not believe they apply to them. We could therefore hypothesise that if brief advice increases a person's awareness of their personal health risk, it could act as a 'prime' making them more receptive to the existing generic information, support and advice available elsewhere in their environment, and thus heighten the effect of these complementary campaigns. However, this hypothesis of a priming effect needs investigation. Evaluations of the efficacy of opportunistic brief advice show a small but significant positive effect on physical activity (Lawlor and Hanratty, 2001, Anokye et al., 2014, Campbell et al., 2012), suggesting that it does appear to encourage people to move towards taking action. Given its low costs and potentially wide reach, the impact of even this small size of effect on national physical activity levels could be considerable.

Organisational and community level approaches to physical activity promotion

Policies to facilitate the provision of interpersonal support for behaviour change provided through brief advice and exercise referral schemes are an important part of a comprehensive policy approach, particularly when targeted at people with heightened health risk. However, broader approaches reaching whole communities are necessary to bring about the population-level shift in activity levels necessary to make an impact on any nation's health. Given that physical activity has been largely 'designed out' of daily life for most people in high-income nations (e.g., through motorised transport, and the mechanisation of manual occupations and domestic chores), we need to include policies that establish long-lasting support for physical activity to ensure that those who are active are supported in their efforts to remain so. Health messaging and social marketing can help to form part of this positive environment: in the UK for example, the NHS launched a Change 4 Life campaign in 2009, comprising social marketing delivered at a national level, with encouragement for further implementation at a local level, both supported by a comprehensive interactive website that could be used to develop personal physical activity (and other health behaviour) plans (Department of Health [DoH], 2009). The initiative incorporates numerous behaviour change techniques and has a strong emphasis on appropriate tailoring to different audiences (DoH, 2009). However, efficacy cannot be assumed on this basis alone; an early RCT evaluation of one module within the campaign ('How are the kids?') found that while a six-month intervention to provide materials to parents was successful in raising awareness of the initiative, it did not improve parental attitudes towards promoting more physical activity to their children (Croker et al., 2012). Further, the campaign had an unintended negative outcome by reducing the perceived importance of physical activity among parents in higher socio-economic groups (Croker et al., 2012). The authors of the study evaluating the efficacy of the programme cited the lack of parental interest and engagement with the materials as a reason for failure, potentially as the materials were perceived to have little personal relevance. In effect, this example demonstrates that just as physical changes to the environment are necessary but not sufficient to encourage communities to use them (Giles-Corti, 2006), neither is the provision of information and tailorable online resources sufficient to support individual behaviour change.

A further example of the promotion of physical activity to communities that can be targeted at a local, organisational or national level, and through approaches ranging from social marketing, traditional health messaging, to multi-faceted work-place interventions, is the promotion of active transport.

Policy Example 5: Health messaging policy related to physical activity: Promoting active transport

Active transport represents a potentially important focus for health messaging campaigns, as it is relevant to both school children and most ambulant adults (whether in relation to travel to work or for leisure) and has been shown to increase overall physical activity to a meaningful degree (Heath et al., 2012). The promotion of active transport is endorsed within UK physical activity policy (NICE, 2006). The type of physical activity (i.e., cycling or walking) and the level of energy expenditure required is familiar to most people, so it is easier to form positive predictions of one's self-efficacy to achieve it than for some other more intensive exercise options. There are also a broad range of potential motives for, and benefits from, active transport that could contribute to a meaningful rationale for taking part for a wide range of people (e.g., health and fitness, journey time and predictability, environmental impact, enjoyment, cost savings). However, active transport presents a further advantage; when an activity is regularly enacted in response to a similar prompt or cue within the environment (i.e., preparing to go to work or school), there is potential for that behaviour to become a habit (Verplanken and Melkevik, 2008). Habits are defined as 'learned sequences of acts that have become automatic responses to specific cues, and are functional in obtaining certain goals or end states' (Verplanken and Aarts, 1999). That is, behaviours that we perform with little conscious awareness or self-regulatory effort (Verplanken and Orbell, 2003). Habits are an efficient means of driving frequent behaviours as they bypass conscious decision making by operating as a cue-response behavioural pattern. As such, when a behaviour (or in the case of physical activity, the decision to act; Phillips and Gardner, 2015) becomes a habit rather than an activity requiring deliberation, it is less likely to be disrupted by the challenges encountered in our day to day environment, such as if the weather is bad, if we're feeling tired or have a more attractive offer. Furthermore, observational research shows that active transport is associated with habitual processes both in adults (Gardner et al., 2011) and children (Murtagh et al., 2012).

Habit theory thus suggests that in principle, policies to promote physical activity through active transport would have the potential to promote long term change through promoting habit formation, and that this will be true to the degree to which they support the consolidation of a cue-response relationship between preparation for work or school and physically active travel choices. The behaviour change technique termed implementation intentions (or if-then plans, setting out specific actions to be undertaken in response to very specific cues) has been shown through experimental research to help people to create new habits. However, habit formation first requires the repetition of the behaviour to enable the physical activity pattern to be established, and thus support for the same psychosocial determinants of behaviour that are important for other forms of physical activity are equally important in this setting (i.e., self-efficacy, motivation and social support). Work-place schemes are well placed to do this, through providing proximal and locally relevant forms of both environmental and social support (e.g., Audrey et al., 2015, Wen et al., 2005). For example, positive effects have been reported to using posters depicting actual employees within a company using modes of active transport to get to work, alongside testimonials of why they choose to travel in this way (e.g., for environmental reasons, better predictability, mood enhancement, etc.) (Wen et al., 2005). The posters thus incorporated the techniques of *modelling* to promote self-efficacy for change, creating *social norms* among work colleagues, and (across a series of posters) the provision of alternative rationales for active travel in order to promote autonomous motivation. Thus, active transport policies reflect behavioural theory through the way in which they link physical activity to daily routines with the potential to foster habits, and through harnessing the potential from within existing social groups to provide the social support that theory and evidence suggests to be crucial in promoting the uptake and continuation of health behaviours.

Critical reflections on the application of behavioural theory to physical activity policy

A number of limitations are useful to consider in setting realistic expectations of what behavioural theory can contribute to the enhancement of physical activity policy. First, the use of theory is not a guaranteed route to policy success; theoretical approaches commonly improve the transparency and quality of design, but poor understanding of the needs of the target group(s), poor specification and poor implementation of behaviour change techniques will still lead to poor quality policies regardless of reference to theory. Conversely, policies designed by well-informed experts without reference to theory could be successful; our argument is simply that referring to theory enhances our ability to build meaningfully on past work to incorporate evidence and increase the chances of positive outcomes. There is growing awareness among policy makers of the evidence base surrounding behaviour change techniques, in recognition of the advantages of behaviour change theory. For example, NICE has published generic guidelines on individual approaches to behaviour change across a range of health behaviours that draws specifically on this literature (NICE, 2014), providing a resource for all commissioners and personnel involved in initiatives to promote health behaviour change. However, while this represents a clear and encouraging example of how behavioural theory can become embedded as standard practice within policy design, the quality of behavioural support will still depend on sound implementation. Implementation is influenced both by available resources and infrastructure, including the articulation of different policies within communities that maximise people's perceptions of a clear and consistent message (e.g., 'move more'). The skills of the staff charged with providing face-to-face behavioural support are also important in the translation of theoretically informed behavioural science to practice. This has perhaps not received sufficient attention to date; we are expecting people with limited training in behaviour change to deliver complex combinations of behaviour change techniques in short amounts of time. While evidence suggests that we can teach people from health professional and allied-health backgrounds to adopt more autonomy supportive styles (e.g., in the provision of autonomy support; Williams and Deci, 2001, Rouse et al., 2011), to do so with little basic understanding of theory, techniques and the rationale for changing their own practice is a lot to ask.

Finally, it remains the case that despite strong observational evidence confirming the association between the theoretical psychosocial determinants of behaviour and health behaviours themselves (Amireault et al., 2013), most physical activity interventions are relatively short term (i.e., ≤ one year). As such, the evidence that these initial interventions bring about long-term maintenance of physical activity is less convincing. At present, while behavioural science can recommend an 'end-point' towards which policy can be directed, the research base for behavioural maintenance is relatively young and these recommendations are likely to change. Furthermore, we have yet to provide the proven tools with which to reach all of these end points.

Implications for future physical activity policy and practice

In drawing the discussions within this chapter together, we come back to the questions posed at the outset: are current policy approaches well informed by behavioural science but ineffective, or are the approaches sound but in need of better implementation? Through exploring the examples of five physical activity-related policies, we have attempted to highlight the importance of considering both the target of a policy and its content in addressing these points. In terms of the targets of physical activity policies, we reflected on the degree to which policies are oriented to facilitate the provision of social support, and support for people's self-efficacy and motivation to be active. A number of the policy examples discussed were consistent with support for these determinants; for example the availability of behavioural support through exercise referral services (Policy Example 3) may enhance self-efficacy through helping people to perceive they have access to the specialist assistance they need to get active, and the promotion of active transport (Policy Example 5) could be argued to support self-efficacy by endorsing a simple, cheap type of physical activity of achievable (low-to-moderate) intensity that can be regularly accommodated into daily life, in addition to facilitating opportunities for social support from colleagues/friends. We also identified where policies appear to work in opposition to theory, for example through the potential for financial incentives (Policy Example 1) and the use of monitoring programmes to identify people at risk (Policy Example 2) to undermine people's autonomous motivation for change, and cause them to react against perceptions of external control. Assessing the degree to which the content of physical activity policies are consistent with behavioural evidence was more challenging, as what is intended by a policy may not relate to what is delivered in practice, and there may be wide variations in what aspects of support which should be available is implemented or accessed. This was most clearly demonstrated by the evaluations of exercise referral services (Policy Example 3). This research highlighted that variations in the practice of exercise referral staff meant that the support given to clients within the same service (and in theory according to the same protocol) included very different sets of behaviour change techniques, and thus levels or types of behavioural support that were not directly comparable. Such findings emphasise how the task of ensuring that policies are informed by behavioural evidence does not stop at the design phase, but needs to extend to implementation.

So what should a well-designed and implemented policy look like? Physical activity is an effortful and often functionally unnecessary part of daily life, requiring motivation and the self-efficacy to direct and sustain one's behaviour in the face of attractive sedentary alternatives. Exerting the self-control required to adopt behaviours over a prolonged period is not usually sustainable (Vohs et al., 2008), so policies need to ensure that once people have made the effort to incorporate physical activity into their lives the social and physical environment around them supports these to continue. In order to foster long-term participation, policies need to provide support for autonomy through emphasising choice rather than imposing requirements or using coercion, to acknowledge and strengthen the rationale people perceive for being active, and ensure that policies are informed by consultations with the communities they aim to influence, taking on board their priorities, preferences and attitudes towards physical activity (Moller et al., 2006). Without acceptance from target communities, policies risk unintended negative consequences through people reacting against them, and without acceptance from those who will be asked to deliver policies, they risk failing through poor implementation. Similarly, policies need to increase perceptions of self-efficacy for change. Different strategies may be more or less appropriate in different settings, but providing vicarious examples of the successful adoption of physical activity (i.e., modelling) and the resources to obtain personalised feedback and self-monitor progress present a good starting point. Self-efficacy can also be enhanced by the simple knowledge that achievable levels of physical activity will be of benefit and that support is available, so raising awareness of what services are already provided in a given community could also help to move people towards action. Finally, given the importance of social support in promoting physical activity (Greaves et al., 2011), policies to encourage proximal social support (e.g., co-participation with friends and family, and positive social environments within exercise settings), and more distal supports (e.g., normalising physical activity and encouraging community-level social cohesion) could play an important role in both promoting the uptake, and longer-term maintenance of active lifestyles.

Note

1 Valuable evidence syntheses have also been conducted that contribute to our knowledge base without adhering to the categories set out in the taxonomy of behaviour change on which we draw in this chapter, but we stick to this method for simplicity.

References

Akhtar, P. C., Haw, S. J., Currie, D. B., Zachary, R. & Currie, C. E. 2009. Smoking restrictions in the home and secondhand smoke exposure among primary schoolchildren before and after introduction of the Scottish smoke-free legislation. *Tobacco Control, 18*, 409–415.

Amireault, S., Godin, G. & Vézina-Im, L.-A. 2013. Determinants of physical activity maintenance: A systematic review and meta-analyses. *Health Psychology Review, 7*(1), 55–91.

Anokye, N. K., Lord, J. & Fox-Rushby, J. 2014. Is brief advice in primary care a cost-effective way to promote physical activity? *British Journal of Sports Medicine, 48*, 202–206.

Ashford, S., Edmunds, J. & French, D. P. 2010. What is the best way to change self-efficacy to promote lifestyle and recreational physical activity? A systematic review with meta-analysis. *British Journal of Health Psychology, 15*, 265–288.

Audrey, S., Cooper, A. R., Hollingworth, W., Metcalfe, C., Procter, S., Davis, A. & Rodgers, S. E. 2015. Study protocol: The effectiveness and cost effectiveness of an employer-led intervention to increase walking during the daily commute: The Travel to Work randomised controlled trial. *BMC Public Health, 15*(1), 154.

Ball, K., Jeffery, R. W., Abbott, G., Mcnaughton, S. A. & Crawford, D. 2010. Is healthy behavior contagious: Associations of social norms with physical activity and healthy eating. *International Journal of Behavioral Nutrition and Physical Activity, 7*, 86.

Bandura, A. 1998. Health promotion from the perspective of social cognitive theory. *Psychology and Health, 13*, 623–649.

Bandura, A. 2004. Health promotion by social cognitive means. *Health Education & Behavior, 31*(2), 143–164.

Barnett, J., Harricharan, M., Fletcher, D., Gilchrist, B. & Coughlan, J. 2015. myPace: An integrative health platform for supporting weight loss and maintenance behaviors. *IEEE Journal of Biomedical and Health Informatics, 19*(1), 109–116.

Beck, F., Gillison, F. & Standage, M. 2010. A theoretical investigation of the development of physical activity habits in retirement. *British Journal of Health Psychology, 15*(3), 663–679.

Beck, F. E., Gillison, F. B., Koseva, M. D., Standage, M., Brodrick, J. L., Graham, C. & Young, H. 2016. The systematic identification of content and delivery style of an exercise intervention. *Psychology and Health 31*(5), 602–621.

Becker, E. R. & Roblin, D. W. 2008. Translating primary care practice climate into patient activation: The role of patient trust in physician. *Medical Care, 46*(8), 795–805.

Biddle, S. J. & Asare, M. 2011. Physical activity and mental health in children and adolescents: A review of reviews. *British Journal of Sports Medicine, 45*, 886–895.

Borland, R., Yong, H.-H., Siahpush, M., Hyland, A., Campbell, S., Hastings, G., Cummings, K. M. & Fong, G. T. 2006. Support for and reported compliance with smoke-free restaurants and bars by smokers in four countries: Findings from the International Tobacco Control (ITC) Four Country Survey. *Tobacco Control, 15*, iii34–iii41.

Broekhuizen, K., Kroeze, W., Van Poppel, M. N., Oenema, A. & Brug, J. 2012. A systematic review of randomized controlled trials on the effectiveness of computer-tailored physical activity and dietary behavior promotion programs: An update. *Annals of Behavioral Medicine, 44*(2), 259–286.

Brownson, R. C., Baker, E. A., Housemann, R. A., Brennan, L. K. & Bacak, S. J. 2001. Environmental and policy determinants of physical activity in the United States. *American Journal of Public Health, 91*(12), 1995–2003.

Butland, B., Jebb, S. A., Kopelman, P., Mcpherson, K., Thomas, S., Mardell, J. & Parry, V. 2007. Foresight. *Tackling obesities: Future choices – project report.* London, UK: Government Office for Science.

Byrne, S. & Niederdeppe, J. 2011. Unintended consequences of obesity prevention messages. In: Cawley, J. (ed.) *The Oxford Handbook of the Social Science of Obesity.* Oxford: Oxford University Press.

Campbell, F., Blank, L., Messina, J. & Al., E. 2012. *National Institute for Health and Clinical Excellence (NICE) public health intervention guidance physical activity: BA for adults in primary care. Review of effectiveness evidence.* London: NICE.

Cerasoli, C. P., Nicklin, J. M. & Ford, M. T. 2014. Intrinsic motivation and extrinsic incentives jointly predict performance: A 40-year meta-analysis. *Psychological Bulletin, 140*(4), 980–1008.

Conner, M. & Norman, P. 1996. *Predicting health behavior. Search and practice with social cognition models.* Ballmore, Buckingham: Open University Press.

Craig, P., Dieppe, P., Macintyre, S., Michie, S., Nazareth, I. & Petticrew, M. 2008. Developing and evaluating complex interventions: The new Medical Research Council guidance. *BMJ, 337,* a1655.

Croker, H., Lucas, R. & Wardle, J. 2012. Cluster-randomised trial to evaluate the 'Change for Life' mass media/social marketing campaign in the UK. *BMC Public Health, 12,* 404.

Deci, E. L., Eghrari, H., Patrick, B. C. & Leone, D. R. 1994. Facilitating internalization: The self-determination theory perspective. *Journal of Personality, 62*(1), 119–142.

Department of Health (DoH). 2009. *Change4Life Marketing Strategy.* London: UK Department of Health.

Emm, L. G., Gillison, F. B. & Juszczyk, D. 2013. Support for obesity-related policy and its association with motivation for weight control. *Psychology, Public Policy, and Law, 19*(3), 321–330.

Finkelstein, E. A., Brown, D. S., Brown, D. R. & Buchner, D. M. 2008. A randomized study of financial incentives to increase physical activity among sedentary older adults. *Preventive Medicine, 47*(2), 182–187.

Fortier, M. S., Duda, J. L., Guerin, E. & Teixeira, P. J. 2012. Promoting physical activity: Development and testing of self-determination theory-based interventions. *International Journal of Behavioral Nutrition and Physical Activity, 9,* 20.

Gardner, B., De Bruijn, G. J. & Lally, P. 2011. A systematic review and meta-analysis of applications of the Self-Report Habit Index to nutrition and physical activity behaviours. *Annals of Behavioral Medicine, 42,* 174–187.

Gardner, B., Whittington, C., Mcateer, J., Eccles, M. P. & Michie, S. 2010. Using theory to synthesise evidence from behaviour change interventions: The example of audit and feedback. *Social Science and Medicine, 70*(10), 1618–1625.

Giles-Corti, B. 2006. People or places: What should be the target? *Journal of Science and Medicine in Sport, 9*(5), 357–366.

Gillison, F., Beck, F. & Lewitt, J. 2014. Exploring the basis for parents' negative reactions to being informed that their child is overweight. *Public Health Nutrition, 17*(5), 987–997.

Goodman, A., Sahlqvist, S., Ogilvie, D. & iConnect Consortium. 2013. Who uses new walking and cycling infrastructure and how? Longitudinal results from the UK iConnect study. *Preventive Medicine, 57*(5), 518–524.

Greaves, C. J., Sheppard, K. E., Abraham, C., Hardeman, W., Roden, M., Evans, P. H., Schwarz, P. & Grp, I. S. 2011. Systematic review of reviews of intervention components associated with increased effectiveness in dietary and physical activity interventions. *BMC Public Health, 11,* 119.

Grimmett, C., Croker, H., Carnell, S. & Wardle, J. 2008. Telling parents their child's weight status: Psychological impact of a weight-screening program. *Pediatrics, 122*(3), e682–e688.

Hallal, P. C., Andersen, L. B., Bull, F. C., Guthold, R., Haskell, W., Ekelund, U. & Group, L. P. A. S. W. 2012. Global physical activity levels: Surveillance progress, pitfalls, and prospects. *The Lancet, 380*(9838), 247–257.

Hansen, K. B. & Nielsen, T. A. S. 2014. Exploring characteristics and motives of long distance commuter cyclists. *Transport Policy, 35,* 57–63.

Haskell, W. L., Lee, I.-M., Pate, R. R., Powell, K. E., Blair, S. N., Franklin, B. A., Macera, C. A., Heath, G. W., Thompson, P. D. & Bauman, A. 2007. Physical activity and public health: Updated recommendation for adults from the American College of Sports Medicine and the American Heart Association. *Circulation, 116,* 1081.

Heath, G. W., Parra, D. C., Sarmiento, O. L., Andersen, L. B., Owen, N., Goenka, S., Montes, F., Brownson, R. C. & Group, L. P. A. S. W. 2012. Evidence-based intervention in physical activity: Lessons from around the world. *The Lancet, 380*(9838), 272–281.

Horodyska, K., Luszczynska, A., Van Den Berg, M., Hendriksen, M., Roos, G., De Bourdeaudhuij, I. & Brug, J. 2015. Good practice characteristics of diet and physical activity interventions and policies: An umbrella review. *BMC Public Health*, *15*, 19.

Jebb, S. A., Aveyard, P. N. & Hawkes, C. 2013. The evolution of policy and actions to tackle obesity in England. *Obesity Reviews*, *14*(Suppl 2), 42–59.

Jeffery, A. N., Voss, L. D., Metcalf, B. S., Alba, S. & Wilkin, T. J. 2005. Parents' awareness of overweight in themselves and their children: Cross sectional study within a cohort (EarlyBird 21). *BMJ*, *330*(7481), 23–24.

Kok, G., Schaalma, H., Ruiter, R. A., Van Empelen, P. & Brug, J. 2004. Intervention mapping: Protocol for applying health psychology theory to prevention programmes. *Journal of Health Psychology*, *9*(1), 85–98.

Lawlor, D. & Hanratty, B. 2001. The effect of physical activity advice given in routine primary care consultations: A systematic review. *Journal of Public Health*, *23*(3), 219–226.

Lee, I. M., Shiroma, E. J., Lobelo, F., Puska, P., Blair, S. N., Katzmarzyk, P. T. & The Lancet Physical Activity Series Working Group. 2012. Effect of physical inactivity on major non-communicable diseases worldwide: An analysis of burden of disease and life expectancy. *The Lancet*, *380*(9838), 219–229.

McNeill, L. H., Kreuter, M. W. & Subramanian, S. 2006. Social environment and physical activity: A review of concepts and evidence. *Social Science & Medicine*, *63*(4), 1011–1022.

Michie, S. 2008. Designing and implementing behaviour change interventions to improve population health. *Journal of Health Services Research Policy*, *13*(Suppl 3), 64–69.

Michie, S. & Prestwich, A. 2010. Are interventions theory-based? Development of a theory coding scheme. *Health Psychology*, *29*(1), 1–8.

Michie, S., Abraham, C., Whittington, C., Mcateer, J. & Gupta, S. 2009. Effective techniques in healthy eating and physical activity interventions: A meta-regression. *Health Psychology*, *28*(6), 690–701.

Michie, S., Johnston, M., Abraham, C., Lawton, R., Parker, D. & Walker, A. 2005. Making psychological theory useful for implementing evidence based practice: A consensus approach. *Qual Saf Health Care*, *14*(1), 26–33.

Michie, S., Johnston, M., Francis, J., Hardeman, W. & Eccles, M. 2008. From theory to intervention: Mapping theoretically derived behavioural determinants to behaviour change techniques. *Applied Psychology*, *57*(4), 660–680.

Michie, S., Richardson, M., Johnston, M., Abraham, C., Francis, J., Hardeman, W., Eccles, M. P., Cane, J. & Wood, C. E. 2013. The behavior change technique taxonomy (v1) of 93 hierarchically clustered techniques: Building an international consensus for the reporting of behavior change interventions. *Annals of Behavioral Medicine*, *46*(1), 81–95.

Michie, S., Van Stralen, M. M. & West, R. 2011. The behaviour change wheel: A new method for characterising and designing behaviour change interventions. *Implementation Science*, *6*, 42.

Moller, A. C., Buscemi, C. P., Mcfadden, H. G., Hedeker, D. & Spring, B. 2013. Financial motivation undermines potential enjoyment in an intensive diet and activity intervention. *Journal of Behavioral Medicine*, *37*(5), 819–827.

Moller, A. C., Ryan, R. M. & Deci, E. L. 2006. Self-determination theory and public policy: Improving the quality of consumer decisions without using coercion. *Journal of Public Policy and Marketing*, *25*(1), 104–116.

Mooney, A., Statham, J., Boddy, J. & Smith, M. 2010. The National Child Measurement Programme: Early experiences of routine feedback to parents of children's height and weight. London: University of Sussex, Institute of Education.

Moyer, V. A. & Force, U. S. P. S. T. 2012. Behavioral counseling interventions to promote a healthful diet and physical activity for cardiovascular disease prevention in adults: U.S. Preventive Services Task Force recommendation statement. *Annals of Internal Medicine*, *157*(5), 367–371.

Murphy, S. M., Edwards, R. T., Williams, N., Raisanen, L., Moore, G., Linck, P., Hounsome, N., Din, N. U. & Moore, L. 2012. An evaluation of the effectiveness and cost effectiveness of the National Exercise Referral Scheme in Wales, UK: A randomised controlled trial of a public health policy initiative. *Journal of Epidemiology and Community Health*, *66*(8), 745–753.

Murtagh, S., Rowe, D. A., Elliott, M. A., Mcminn, D. & Nelson, N. M. 2012. Predicting active school travel: The role of planned behavior and habit strength. *International Journal of Behavioral Nutrition and Physical Activity*, *9*, 65.

National Health Service. 2015. *NHS Choices Tools Library* [Online]. UK: NHS. Available: www.nhs.uk/tools/pages/toolslibrary.aspx.

National Institute for Health and Care Excellence (NICE) 2006. Four commonly used methods to increase physical activity: Brief interventions in primary care, exercise referral schemes, pedometers and community based exercise programmes for walking and cycling. London, UK: NICE.

National Institute for Health and Care Excellence (NICE). 2014. *Behaviour change: Individual approaches.* London, UK: NICE.

Ngo, C. S., Pan, C. W., Finkelstein, E. A., Lee, C. F., Wong, I. B., Ong, J., Ang, M., Wong, T. Y. & Saw, S. M. 2014. A cluster randomised controlled trial evaluating an incentive-based outdoor physical activity programme to increase outdoor time and prevent myopia in children. *Ophthalmic and Physiological Optics, 34*(3), 362–368.

Nietfeld, J. L., Cao, L. & Osborne, J. W. 2006. The effect of distributed monitoring exercises and feedback on performance, monitoring accuracy, and self-efficacy. *Metacognition and Learning, 1,* 159–179.

Oja, P., Bull, F. C., Fogelholm, M. & Martin, B. W. 2010. Physical activity recommendations for health: What should Europe do? *BMC Public Health, 10*(10), 10.

Olander, E. K., Fletcher, H., Williams, S., Atkinson, L., Turner, A. & French, D. P. 2013. What are the most effective techniques in changing obese individuals' physical activity self-efficacy and behaviour: A systematic review and meta-analysis. *International Journal of Behavioral Nutrition and Physical Activity, 10,* 29.

Oliver, J. E. & Lee, T. 2005. Public opinion and the politics of obesity in America. *Journal of Health Politics, Policy and Law, 30*(5), 923–954.

O'Malley, A. S., Sheppard, V. B., Schwartz, M. & Mandelblatt, J. 2004. The role of trust in use of preventive services among low-income African-American women. *Preventive Medicine, 38*(6), 777–785.

Patrick, H. & Canevello, A. 2011. Methodological overview of a self-determination theory-based computerized intervention to promote leisure-time physical activity. *Psychology of Sport and Exercise, 12*(1), 13–19.

Paul-Ebhohimhen, V. & Avenell, A. 2008. Systematic review of the use of financial incentives in treatments for obesity and overweight. *Obesity Reviews, 9*(4), 355–367.

Pavey, T. G., Anokye, N., Taylor, A. H., Trueman, P., Moxham, T., Fox, K. R., Hillsdon, M., Green, C., Campbell, J. L., Foster, C., Mutrie, N., Searle, J. & Taylor, R. S. 2011. The clinical effectiveness and cost-effectiveness of exercise referral schemes: A systematic review and economic evaluation. *Health Technology Assessment, 15*(44), i–xii, 1–254.

Penedo, F. J. & Dahn, J. R. 2005. Exercise and well-being: A review of mental and physical health benefits associated with physical activity. *Current Opinion in Psychiatry, 18*(2), 189–193.

Peters, G. J., De Bruin, M. & Crutzen, R. 2015. Everything should be as simple as possible, but no simpler: Towards a protocol for accumulating evidence regarding the active content of health behaviour change interventions. *Health Psychology Review, 9*(1), 1–14.

Petry, N. M. 2000. A comprehensive guide to the application of contingency management procedures in clinical settings. *Drug and Alcohol Dependence, 58,* 9–25.

Phillips, L. A. & Gardner, B. 2015. Habitual exercise instigation (vs. execution) predicts healthy adults' exercise frequency. *Health Psychology.* Advance online publication. http://dx.doi.org/10.1037/hea0000249.

Phillips, R., Amos, A., Ritchie, D., Cunningham-Burley, S. & Martin, C. 2007. Smoking in the home after the smoke-free legislation in Scotland: Qualitative study. *BMJ, 335*(7619), 553.

Pope, L. & Harvey, J. 2015. The impact of incentives on intrinsic and extrinsic motives for fitness-center attendance in college first-year students. *American Journal of Health Promotion, 29*(3), 192–199.

Prestwich, A., Sniehotta, F. F., Whittington, C., Dombrowski, S. U., Rogers, L. & Michie, S. 2014. Does theory influence the effectiveness of health behavior interventions? Meta-analysis. *Health Psychology, 33*(5), 465–474.

Prochaska, J. O. & Velicer, W. F. 1997. The transtheoretical model of health behavior change. *American Journal Of Health Promotion, 12*(1), 38–48.

Quick, B. L. & Considine, J. R. 2008. Examining the use of forceful language when designing exercise persuasive messages for adults: A test of conceptualizing reactance arousal as a two-step process. *Health Communication, 23*(5), 483–491.

Rogers, R. W. 1975. A protection motivation theory of fear appeals and attitude change. *Journal of Psychology, 91,* 93–114.

Rouse, P. C., Ntoumanis, N., Duda, J. L., Jolly, K. & Williams, G. C. 2011. In the beginning: role of autonomy support on the motivation, mental health and intentions of participants entering an exercise referral scheme. *Psychology & Health*, *26*(6), 729–749.

Ryan, R. M. & Deci, E. L. 2000a. Self-determination theory and the facilitation of intrinsic motivation, social development, and well-being. *American Psychologist*, *55*(1), 68–78.

Ryan, R. M. & Deci, E. L. 2000b. Intrinsic and extrinsic motivations: Classic definitions and new directions. *Contemporary Educational Psychology*, *25*(1), 54–67.

Ryan, R. M., Patrick, H., Deci, E. L. & Williams, G. C. 2008. Facilitating health behaviour change and its maintenance: Interventions based on self-determination theory. *European Health Psychologist*, *10*, 2–5.

Schaalma, H. & Kok, G. 2009. Decoding health education interventions: The times are a-changin'. *Psychology and Health*, *24*(1), 5–9.

Schwarzer, R. & Luszczynska, A. 2008. How to overcome health-compromising behaviors: The health action process approach. *European Psychologist*, *13*(2), 141–151.

Standage, M. & Ryan, R. M. 2012. Self-determination theory and exercise motivation: Facilitating self-regulatory processes to support and maintain health and well-being. *In*: Roberts, G. C. and Treasure, D. C. (eds.) *Advances in Motivation in Sport and Exercise, 3rd Edition*. Champaign, U.S.A.: Human Kinetics, pp. 233–270.

Statham, J., Mooney, A., Boddy, J. & Cage, M. 2011. Taking stock: A rapid review of the National Child Measurement Programme. Available at http://eprints.ioe.ac.uk/6743/1/Statham2011Taking%28Report%29.pdf.

Strohacker, K., Galarraga, O. & Williams, D. M. 2014. The impact of incentives on exercise behavior: A systematic review of randomized controlled trials. *Annals of Behavioral Medicine*, *48*(1), 92–99.

Swift, D. L., Johannsen, N. M., Lavie, C. J., Earnest, C. P. & Church, T. S. 2014. The role of exercise and physical activity in weight loss and maintenance. *Progress in Cardiovascular Diseases*, *56*(4), 441–447.

Syrad, H., Falconer, C., Cooke, L., Saxena, S., Kessel, A., Viner, R., Kinra, S., Wardle, J. & Croker, H. 2014. 'Health and happiness is more important than weight': A qualitative investigation of the views of parents receiving written feedback on their child's weight as part of the National Child Measurement Programme. *Journal of Human Nutrition and Dietetics*, *28*, 47–55.

Teixeira, P. J., Carraca, E. V., Markland, D., Silva, M. N. & Ryan, R. M. 2012. Exercise, physical activity, and self-determination theory: A systematic review. *International Journal of Behavioral Nutrition and Physical Activity*, *9*, 78.

Turner-McGrievy, G. M., Beets, M. W., Moore, J. B., Kaczynski, A. T., Barr-Anderson, D. J. & Tate, D. F. 2013. Comparison of traditional versus mobile app self-monitoring of physical activity and dietary intake among overweight adults participating in an mHealth weight loss program. *Journal of the American Medical Informatics Association*, *20*(3), 513–518.

Van Sluijs, E. M., Mcminn, A. M. & Griffin, S. J. 2007. Effectiveness of interventions to promote physical activity in children and adolescents: Systematic review of controlled trials. *BMJ*, *335*(7622), 703.

Verplanken, B. & Aarts, H. 1999. Habit, attitude, and planned behaviour: Is habit an empty construct or an interesting case of goal-directed automaticity? *European Review of Social Psychology*, *10*, 101–134.

Verplanken, B. & Melkevik, O. 2008. Predicting habit: The case of physical exercise. *Psychology of Sport and Exercise*, *9*(1), 15–26.

Verplanken, B. & Orbell, S. 2003. Reflections on past behavior: A self-report index of habit strength. *Journal of Applied Social Psychology*, *33*(6), 1313–1330.

Vohs, K. D., Baumeister, R. F., Schmeichel, B. J., Twenge, J. M., Nelson, N. M., & Tice, D. M. May 2008. Making choices impairs subsequent self-control: A limited-resource account of decision making, self-regulation, and active initiative. *Journal of Personality and Social Psychology*, *94*(5), 883–898.

Webb, T. L., Sniehotta, F. F. & Michie, S. 2010. Using theories of behaviour change to inform interventions for addictive behaviours. *Addiction*, *105*(11), 1879–1892.

Wen, L. M., Orr, N., Bindon, J. & Rissel, C. 2005. Promoting active transport in a workplace setting: Evaluation of a pilot study in Australia. *Health Promotion International*, *20*(2), 123–133.

West, R. 2007. What lessons can be learned from tobacco control for combating the growing prevalence of obesity? *Obesity Reviews*, *8*(Suppl 1), 145–150.

Whale, K., Gillison, F. B., & Smith, P. C. (2014). 'Are you still on that stupid diet?': Women's experiences of societal pressure and support regarding weight loss, and attitudes towards health policy intervention. *Journal of Health Psychology, 19*(12), 1536–1546.

Williams, G. C. & Deci, E. L. 2001. Activating patients for smoking cessation through physician autonomy support. *Medical Care, 39*(8), 813–823.

Williams, S. & French, D. 2011. What are the most effective intervention techniques for changing physical activity self-efficacy and physical activity behaviour – and are they the same? *Health Education Research, 26*(2), 308–322.

World Health Organization. 2008. *WHO report on the global tobacco epidemic, 2008: The MPOWER package*. Geneva: World Health Organization.

World Health Organization. 2013. *Global action plan for the prevention and control of noncommunicable diseases*. Geneva: World Health Organization.

World Health Organization. 2015. *Physical activity strategy for the WHO European Region 2016–2025*. Geneva: World Health Organization.

Zuckerman, O. & Gal-Oz, A. 2014. Deconstructing gamification: Evaluating the effectiveness of continuous measurement, virtual rewards, and social comparison for promoting physical activity. *Personal and Ubiquitous Computing, 18*, 1705–1719.

10

TRACING TRANSLATIONS

The journey from evidence to policy to physical activity promotion campaigns

Jessica Lee, Benjamin Williams and Bernadette Sebar

Introduction: Why trace translations?

The slogans of physical activity promotion campaigns have become ubiquitous the world over, "Find your 30", "Shape Up America!", "Swap sitting for moving", "Move more live longer". Such campaigns make big claims about the expected outcomes for individuals and populations, "the first major nation to reverse the rising tide of obesity", "reduce morbidity and mortality due to lifestyle related chronic disease". In recent times, these claims have been backed by unprecedented levels of public funding. As such, there is a lot at stake when it comes to policy that promotes physical activity to gain health. Given the high stakes, governments and health promotion agencies profess to employing evidence-based policy/ practice. Indeed, evidence-based policy is the expected standard in health policy and practice. Evidence-based policy at its most simple has come to be understood as "the use of evidence to make decisions about groups of patients or populations" (Muir Gray 2004, p. 988). Finding a clear and comprehensive definition of evidence-based policy is difficult however, as the meaning is seen to be self-explanatory (Marston & Watts 2003).

While the concept of evidence-based policy in physical activity promotion is taken for granted, the process by which it is undertaken is rarely explored nor critiqued. Given the proposed outcomes for population health and government health budgets and the funds being spent to achieve them, there is a strong rationale to investigate the process by which they are informed and produced. In this chapter we review literature on the place of evidence-based policy and its foundations in evidence-based medicine and provide an overview of the critique of the limitations of the narrow set of standards that evidence-based policy has come to represent. To investigate the process in action we engage semiotic analysis tools adapted from studies in science and technology for the purpose of studying the translation of evidence into policy into practice. We apply these tools to examine the translation of evidence in three health promotion campaigns that focus on increasing physical activity along with healthy nutrition, Change4Life (UK), Measure Up (Australia), Healthier.Happier (Queensland, Australia). It is evident from our study that concerns in the literature regarding the types of knowledge regarded as evidence are warranted, and that inherent in the process of translation that there are gains and losses. Thus, it is important that in the process of translating evidence into policy and practice where there is a lot to be gained and lost by governments and populations alike, that the process is undertaken thoughtfully.

Background

This section draws on literature from critical studies of evidence-based medicine (EBM) and evidence-based policy. Evidence-based policy as we know it today in physical activity and health promotion has its roots in EBM. As such, there are multiple debates and tensions in this area that have arisen as decision making in policy and practice have evolved. In this section we provide a brief overview of the history of EBM and evidence-based policy and highlight the main tensions that have informed the basis of our exploration of tracing translations across physical activity policy and promotion campaigns.

From the EBM example of the Cochrane Collaboration that compiles and stores systematic reviews of randomised controlled trials (RCTs) in the area of health care have sprung the equivalent in evidence-based policy such as the Campbell Collaboration in the UK and the USA's Coalition for Evidence Based Policy (now known as the Laura and John Arnold Foundation) (Marston & Watts 2003). The rationale for these evidence-based policy organisations is rooted in EBM, which, it is argued, "has produced extraordinary advances in health over the past 50 years" due to the focus on "scientifically rigorous evidence" (Coalition for Evidence-Based Policy 2016, para. 1). By contrast, it was suggested that in most areas of social policy "government programs were implemented with little regard to evidence, costing billions of dollars yet failing to address critical social problems" (Coalition for Evidence-Based Policy 2016, para. 1). Despite being shed in such a positive light by the USA's Coalition for Evidence-Based Policy, throughout the evolution of EBM, researchers have observed that while it initially met with an enthusiastic reception, EBM itself also generated considerable controversy (Mykhalovskiy & Weir 2004). Such controversy continues to raise debate in both EBM and evidence-based policy arenas.

Indeed, while the basis of EBM is in the systematic review of RCTs, therein also lies some of its greatest critiques. Reliance on a traditional "hierarchy of evidence" (e.g. Brighton, Bhandari, Tornetta & Felson 2003) tends to pay little attention to, or exclude the sociocultural, qualitative, and humanist forms of evidence. As such, the types of evidence informing policy and practice serves to ignore the stories of individuals and populations and the meaning of their experiences (Frankford cited in Mykhalovskiy & Weir 2004). It has been further suggested that EBM focuses on the fate of individuals to the exclusion of the social and environmental factors (Mykhalovskiy & Weir 2004) that shape health behaviours and risk for disease. This understanding of evidence is explicitly positivist by eliminating culture, contexts, and the subjects of knowledge production from consideration (Goldenberg 2006).

The term "evidence-based" in EBM and evidence-based practice in health and other sciences is typically taken to stand for "the empirically adequate standard of reasonable practice and a means for increasing certainty" (Goldenberg 2006, p. 2623). It is often used as a catch phrase for *scientific, scholarly, rational* (Marston & Watts 2003). In this vein it is proposed that the use of evidence provides the conceptual warrant for belief or action in policy making and practice (Goodman 2003). The evidence resulting from scientific enquiry is assumed to be "facts" about the world and therefore justifies the title *scientific* evidence (Goldenberg 2006, p. 2623). However, critics argue that the apparent obviousness of EBM can and should be challenged on the grounds of how "evidence" has been problematised, that is, in the seemingly unproblematic nature of evidence as noted above. Goldenberg (2006) suggests that the appeal to the authority of evidence that characterises evidence-based practices does not increase objectivity but rather obscures the subjective elements. As such, EBM has been described as an "ideological resource that the medical profession uses to buttress its authority" (Denny cited in Mykhalovskiy & Weir 2004) and its transferability into the human services (including health promotion) is questionable (Marston & Watts 2003, p. 1061).

Given the largely positivist approach to EBM and evidence based policy, one of the main tensions is the contentiousness of what counts as evidence. DeVasto (2015), following the work of Annemarie Mol, refers to this contention by posing the question, "Who gets to sit at the table?" In health policy and practice the predominant form of evidence is top-down, privileging expert, scientific, or generalisable knowledge to the exclusion of "lay knowledge" (Springett, Owens & Callaghan 2007). Again the critique is raised that such approaches to evidence-based practice decontextualise knowledge by ignoring everyday reality (Springett et al. 2007). In the case of health promotion, lay expertise (if utilised) tends to be applied at the delivery stage to contextualise a devised intervention rather than being valued at the development stage as sources of experiential and practical knowledge (Springett et al. 2007). As such, it is proposed that the greatest risk in overlooking or deprioritising lay or sociocultural knowledge in health promotion is an actual increase in the levels of health inequalities.

> The failure to understand and take into account and value different knowledge systems and cultures and to situate lifestyle issues in a broader context has led to the differential impact of public health interventions in favour of less disadvantaged groups, actually increasing the levels of health inequalities.
>
> *Springett et al. 2007, p. 244*

DeVasto (2015) argues that, "scientific knowledge is like any other form of knowledge; it is socially constructed, and thus, does not have special access to the truth" (p. 2) and researchers in science and technology studies endeavour to overcome science's elitist position and authority, to achieve a more democratic approach to policy and decision making.

However, as DeVasto (2015) suggests, it is important to examine *how* policy decision making is conducted rather than focussing only on who should be present. While current debates in evidence-based policy discourse concern the relative value of research and other kinds of evidence as inputs into policy, this chapter is also concerned with the process of translation. In particular, what is gained and lost in moving from evidence to policy and then to physical activity promotion campaign. Due to the tensions outlined above and the political model of policy-making (where evidence is just one input in the policy process), it is not possible to draw simple or linear relationships between "evidence" and policy outcomes (Marston & Watts 2003). Therefore, in this chapter we aim to open the Pandora's box that is three physical activity promotion campaigns to explore the complex process of the translation of evidence into physical activity promotion campaign. There are many aspects that could be explored in this process. We are focussing on the government texts which prioritises language and discourse as it is recognised that policy problems and solutions arise from these representations. To frame the scope of our exploration we draw on the tools of science and technology studies which position claims about the nature of the social world as based on "assembled sets of assumptions about the relationship between the lived world and its human inhabitants" (Marston & Watts 2003, p. 158).

The aim of this chapter is to trace the translations from evidence to policy to practice. Therefore, the following questions are addressed:

1 What sort of evidence informs the policy documents and campaign materials, and how is it used?

2 What is gained and lost as the evidence is translated and with what consequences?

Analysing translations

We answered these questions using a method adapted from studies of science and technology. This approach comprised a set of semiotic tools for studying translation. Researchers who draw on this perspective understand translation as the process of shifting an entity from one time, location, or form to another by making connections and creating equivalences (Brown 2002). According to this school of thought, complete fidelity can never be achieved because perfect equivalence can never be established. Thus, some aspects of the displaced entity are retained in every translation, while others are unavoidably lost or modified (Law 2002). Thinking in this way helped us study translations of evidence in physical activity policies by sensitising us to the range of entities deemed pertinent to a given policy, the connections made and the relationships assumed between these entities, and the changes these entities underwent along the way.

We used this sensibility to investigate translations of evidence in three public health campaigns targeting obesity: the British Government's Change4Life program, the Australian Government's Measure Up initiative, and the Queensland Government's Healthier.Happier. strategy. Rather than dissecting all the evidence that informed these campaigns, we limited our analysis to each campaign's use of evidence when discussing physical activity and sedentary behaviour. Besides its use in the campaign materials, we also examined how evidence was used in the key scientific and technical documents that informed the campaigns. This collection consisted of the Healthy Weight, Healthy Lives cross-government strategy and consumer insight summary (Cross-Government Obesity Unit, Department of Health [DoH] and Department of Children, Schools and Families [DCSF] 2008, DoH and DCSF 2008), the consumer insight report that informed the Measure Up initiative (Blue Moon 2007), and the Queensland Chief Health Officer's fourth report on the health of Queenslanders (Queensland Health 2012).

The first series of translations we analysed in these materials was the authors' (of the government documents) use of modalities. In studies of scientific literature, a modality is a statement that modifies or qualifies some other statement in one of two directions (Latour 1987). A positive modality accepts the original statement's facticity by using it to propose or justify subsequent actions. That is to say, a positive modality translates the original statement by connecting and equating the original "factual" claim with the resulting action. In contrast, a negative modality highlights controversy about the original statement's facticity either by attacking its veracity or defending it against criticism. In other words, a negative modality translates both the original statement and the statements used to support or contradict it. By analysing the use of modalities in this way, we were able to trace the fate of the statements each campaign was based on and identify what was lost, gained, and retained through these translations.

To study the translations produced by the authors' (of the government texts) use of modalities, we deployed two specific techniques. The first method was an examination of the authors' citation practices. We completed this aspect of the investigation by counting the citations used by the authors and by studying the context of each citation (Latour 1987). To study a citation's context, we looked at how the citation was being used to support a given statement. We noted the author of the cited source and the focus of the claim it was used to lend weight to. We also attended to the kinds of statements the authors did not support with citations. The second method was an analysis of the authors' inductions. By induction, we mean the ways an author makes claims about their own or others' data. According to Latour (1987), successfully composing a scientific or technical document involves stacking claims such that each layer convincingly adds something to those that preceded it through interpretation and generalisation. So, whenever data or a citation was used to support a claim in the documents, we noted the empirical basis of the claim and the kind of interpretation or generalisation this use entailed.

The second, related group of translations we analysed was the character of the actor-worlds constructed in the campaign materials and the documents that informed them. In studies of science and technology, the idea of an actor-world describes the universe that a given claim or device is designed to operate in or requires to function properly (Callon 1986). It defines the entities that comprise this world, their roles, their relationships, their sizes, their histories, and their futures. To investigate the actor-worlds constructed by the materials, we studied how the authors' diagnoses of sedentary behaviour as a significant social problem and their proposals about how to solve it. Specifically, we focused on the entities they identified as participating in the problem or its solution, the contributions that these entities make, the nature of the relationships between the entities, and the historical trajectories the authors placed them in. By analysing the character of these actor-worlds, we were able to trace how the authors sought to connect, displace, and enrol ideas, data, people, objects, and so on into their efforts to address obesity.

The campaigns

The campaigns analysed in this chapter were chosen for two reasons. First, the three campaigns are inter-related and can be seen as a progression over time starting with Change4Life (2009), then Measure Up (2010), and finally Healthier.Happier. (2013). Change4Life is considered the starting point, as it is cited as contributing to the design of the Measure Up campaign, particularly the animated characters and "swap it" messages (Blue Moon 2010). Furthermore, the Healthier.Happier. campaign is informed by the same formative research as Measure Up and also utilises the Change4Life "swap it" recommendations (Manager, Preventive Health Branch, Queensland Health 2015, pers. comm., 30 January). Second, together the three campaigns represent national campaigns (Change4Life and Measure Up, England and Australia respectively) and a state campaign (Healthier.Happier from Queensland, Australia). Each campaign is described below detailing the background, main messages, and documents analysed.

Change4Life

Reflecting the main tenets of contemporary mass media health promotion campaigns, Change4Life proposed ambitious results, was backed by unprecedented public funding, and claimed to be evidence based. Established in 2009, the aim of Change4Life was for England "to be the first major nation to reverse the rising tide of obesity and overweight in the population . . . by 2020 we aim to reduce the proportion of overweight and obese children to 2000 levels" (Cross-Government Obesity Unit, DoH and DCSF 2008, v). This ambition, said to be "on a scale never previously witnessed" (DoH 2009, 6), was initially supported by £75 million for the social marketing campaign. The "evidence-based marketing programme" seeks to "empower parents in making changes to their children's diet and levels of physical activity" (Cross-Government Obesity Unit, DoH and DCSF 2008, xii).

The documents analysed for this study are Healthy Weight, Healthy Lives: A cross government strategy for England (Cross-Government Obesity Unit, DoH and DCSF 2008) and Healthy Weight, Healthy Lives: Consumer insight summary (DoH and DCSF 2008). These two documents contain the background research that informs the rationale for the campaign and the consultation with target communities. They are both publicly available from the Change4Life website.

Measure Up

There was a $500 million dollar budget for the Australian Better Health Initiative (ABHI) of which the Measure Up campaign was a significant component. In a similar vein as Change4Life, the Australian Measure Up campaign, launched in October 2008, sought to decrease the prevalence of chronic diseases in Australia via changing perceptions of who was actually at risk. The formative research identified that most people conceptually accepted the link between lifestyle and chronic disease but were not aware of their own susceptibility. Therefore one of the major aims was to raise awareness of personal risk beyond the risks of smoking and being morbidly obese. The campaign drew on two major theoretical assumptions. First that raising awareness would lead to behaviour change if this awareness raising was coupled with messages of "why" change is necessary and "how" to make those changes. The second assumption was the uncontested link between (unhealthy) weight and chronic disease. While the research acknowledged that the relationship between diet, weight, and exercise is more complex than between smoking and health (p. 64), the key strategy for Phase One of the campaign was encouraging the public to measure their waistlines in order to raise awareness of personal susceptibility of chronic disease. Men were considered at risk of chronic disease if their waistlines were bigger than 94cms and women 80cms (p. 29).

The documents analysed for the study include two formative research reports conducted for each phase of the Measure Up campaign: *Diet, Exercise and Weight* (Blue Moon 2007) and *Measure Up Phase Two* (Blue Moon 2010).

Healthier.Happier.

The Healthier.Happier. campaign is a Queensland Government initiative that launched in 2013. As with the campaigns outlined above, Healthier.Happier. aimed to improve health outcomes by addressing nutrition and exercise. Also featuring in this campaign is the focus on the individual responsibility to reduce obesity, "The first phase . . . aimed to personalise the issue of obesity of all Queenslanders", while the second phase focussed on achieving behaviour change through making small changes in people's everyday lives. The key difference in the Healthier.Happier. campaign, compared to its predecessors above, is that it employed an m-health approach. The first phase of the campaign was supported by a Health and Fitness Age calculator which was initially launched on the campaign website. This tool allowed users to enter details of their weight, nutrition, and physical activity habits and were then provided with a "Health and Fitness Age". The intention then was that users would compare their Health and Fitness age to their chronological age as motivation for making changes to their physical activity and nutrition behaviour. The second phase was supported by a mobile app that acted like a "personal trainer in your pocket" that allowed for recording of physical activity and nutrition behaviour as well as providing reminder alerts and health and fitness tips. A positive, encouraging, and supportive approach informed all facets of the campaign, comprising TV, online, outdoor, and press advertising. The documents analysed for the study included two letters to stakeholders produced by the Queensland Health Preventive Health Unit and the Fourth Report of the Chief Health Officer of Queensland (Queensland Health 2012).

In the overviews of the three campaigns provided here it is evident that there are similarities in their focus on chronic disease and (by proxy) obesity, their emphasis on individual responsibility, and the solution of "swapping" "risky" lifestyle choices for "healthier" ones. Indeed, the Measure Up and Healthier.Happier. campaigns both cite Change4Life as motive for their approaches and messages. The Healthier.Happier. campaign stands somewhat apart from the other two however, in that aspects of the campaign were not made public, such as the background research informing the campaign (hence the different type of documents analysed for this study) and the amount of funding.

Tracing the evidence

The methodological and theoretical sensibilities offer a framework for unpacking the process of translation as it is enacted in three examples of physical activity promotion campaigns. The three campaigns all claim to have taken an "evidence-based" approach. This section presents an analysis of the translation of evidence across the three campaigns and is structured according to the overall questions addressed in this chapter around the types of evidence that inform the policy documents and how that evidence is used, and the gains and losses as this evidence is translated.

Types of evidence: Allies and citation contexts

Across the three campaigns, overwhelmingly the sources of evidence were "in-house", produced by or for government agencies. The formative research for the Measure Up campaign (Blue Moon 2007) for example, relies heavily on research commissioned by the Australian Department of Health and Aging produced for concept testing of health promotion messages for smoking, nutrition, alcohol, physical activity, and obesity (SNAP-O) (Blue Moon 2006). Other evidence cited to support claims about health trends and responses includes the Cancer Council website ("Stay in Shape" and "Move your body" pages), factsheets on the Australian Department of Health and Aging website, and a newspaper article published in the Weekend Australian. There was a complete absence of "scientific" or peer-reviewed evidence.

The Chief Health Officer's (CHO) report (Queensland Health 2012) played a major role in informing the conception of the Healthier.Happier campaign. Another in-house government document, the Queensland Health epidemiology department report on "measured obesity" (Queensland Department of Health 2013), played a lesser role. The CHO report describes the state of Queensland's health (e.g. burden of disease, rates of healthy and health risk behaviours) and targets for change. More than half (68%) of the sources of evidence cited are from government sources (including state, national, and international governments) or reports and fact sheets from health related organisations and councils (e.g. Cancer Council, Diabetes Australia). Similarly, the Healthy Weight, Healthy Lives report (Cross-Government Obesity Unit, DoH and DCSF 2008) that informed the Change4Life campaign cited a majority (55%) of government sources. While government and health organisation reports have their place, the issue with such a heavy reliance on them to inform behaviour change campaigns is that they represent a singular approach to gathering knowledge biased by government agendas without engaging with debates in scholarly literature, they often do not invite a range of stakeholders to the table, and close off the important contribution of certain types of evidence such as qualitative, sociological research.

Where sources were cited to fortify "facts" the context of the citation was noteworthy. Citations were used liberally to support descriptive facts such as those relating to the state of population health albeit with a heavy reliance on certain types of knowledge as discussed above. However, where positive modalities were utilised in a prescriptive fashion, citations were perfunctory or general statements about commonly used approaches to behaviour change (e.g. trans-theoretical model of behavior change). In other words, where campaign strategies were prescribed to address a particular health problem or lack of community health knowledge, there was little justification for those specific actions. For example, following the consumer insight summary that informed Change4Life (DoH and DCSF 2008) the final section outlined implications for local program design. The first sentence of this section reads, "The findings from the research programme led us to the conclusion that there is a need for a national mass engagement campaign to 'reframe' the issue of childhood obesity" (p. 53). There are no citations to support the suggestion that a mass engagement campaign has been successful previously for such a complex endeavour. There is a complete absence of supporting evidence of any kind in this section that describes the design of the campaign which for physical activity includes, "encourage active out of home play", "get families walking", and "develop active communities". The literature base evaluating physical activity interventions certainly exists with varying degrees of success, however, this evidence is not cited.

Across the government policy documents informing the three campaigns there were many positive modalities that followed the citation of "facts" garnered from government sources. The most common of these positive modalities in all the texts analysed was the acceptance of an existing and escalating "obesity epidemic" as the impetus for the campaigns promoting physical activity (and healthy nutrition). Other more subtle examples included the claim that "many people underestimated their personal susceptibility to chronic conditions" therefore, the campaign must focus on raising "appreciation of 'why' change is a priority" (Blue Moon 2007, p. 5): "parents do not associate themselves or their families with the terminology of 'being obese' or 'being fat'" therefore, "the campaign will seek to 'reframe' the issue of obesity so that families begin to personalise the issues of poor diet and low physical activity" (DoH and DCSF 2008, pp. 7–8).

It is notable that no negative modalities were recorded from the documents analysed. There are many uncertainties in health knowledge not least concerning the complex relationship between physical activity, weight status, and chronic disease (e.g. Sui et al. 2007; Despres 2012). However, no controversies nor acknowledgement of uncertainties were presented in any of the policy or campaign texts. This demonstrates the singular perspective from which the evidence is presented in order to make a more compelling case.

To the contrary, there were many examples of taken for granted knowledge that seemingly were so indisputable that they did not require the support of any kind of evidence. Latour (1987) refers to such statements "devoid of any trace of ownership, construction, time and place" (p. 23) as a *black box*. A black box is formed when knowledge becomes "fact" or accepted and less controversial. The analogy with a black box arises from the basis that when knowledge becomes accepted as fact its inner workings are no longer open for scrutiny or debate because they have been accepted by both the scientific community and broader community. It is perhaps because of the black box that evidence-based policy itself has become the taken for granted synonym for scientific, scholarly, and rational. Indeed, Latour (1987, p. 304) claims, "when a matter of fact is settled, one need focus only on its inputs and outputs and not on its internal complexity". Thus suggesting, we need not interrogate the inner workings of evidence-based policy itself as it is already the accepted standard for health policy making.

The most obvious black box in the policy documents for all three of the physical activity promotion campaigns is the taken for granted relationship between overweight and obesity and poor health outcomes (see also Lupton 2014). While overweight and obesity statistics are supported by local and national epidemiological reports, it is accepted as inevitable that increased burden on the health system will result. For example, the *Healthy Weight, Healthy*

Lives document (Cross-Government Obesity Unit, DoH and DCSF 2008, p. xi) starts its executive summary with

> Britain is in the grip of an epidemic. Almost two-thirds of adults and a third of children are either overweight or obese [references the Health Survey for England]. . . . This matters because of the severe impact being overweight or obese can have on an individual's health – both are associated with an increasing risk of diabetes, cancer, and heart and liver disease among others – and the risks get worse the more overweight people become.

In the quote above, it is evident that rates of overweight and obesity are supported by statistical sources, but the relationship to the stated chronic diseases and the increasing risk as people become more overweight is black boxed, taken as a fact that requires no evidence to fortify the claim.

Furthermore, the cause of overweight and obesity is also a black box in each of the informing documents for the three campaigns. Both the Change4Life and Measure Up documents explicitly implicate an imbalance between "energy in" and "energy out" (Cross-Government Obesity Unit, DoH and DCSF 2008, xi; Queensland Health 2012, p. 67). A black box in a policy document is often used as a rationale for certain action or strategy, known as a positive modality. As such, "No evidence claim underpinning evidence-based policy arguments can be considered detached, value free, and neutral" (Marston & Watts 2003, p. 157). In this way, we observe the translation process as a layering of inductions – from fact, to positive modality, to campaign message.

How the evidence is used: Modalities and inductions

We can now begin to follow the inductions from fact to fact, from the obesity epidemic, caused by "energy in, energy out", to the solution – "Halting the obesity epidemic is about individual behaviour and responsibility, how people choose to live their lives, what they eat and how much physical activity they do" (Cross-Government Obesity Unit, DoH and DCSF 2008, p. xi). Thus, physical (in)activity being accepted as a cause of the obesity epidemic by its involvement in the "energy out" process becomes a target for change in the resulting campaign. The leap from a black box as a fact within the evidence to campaign action was most clear in the Measure Up campaign informing documents that begin with the aim to "reduce morbidity and mortality caused by lifestyle related chronic diseases" (Blue Moon 2007, p. 4) and results in a campaign that focuses on encouraging the population to measure their waist/hip ratio. "The link" between lifestyle and chronic diseases is mentioned a number of times, however with no elucidation of what that link actually is and the complexities concerned.

Gains and losses in the translation process: Inductions

In the translating of evidence into policy and campaign strategy using modalities and inductions, something new is gained. At the same time however, something else is lost. As demonstrated in the previous example of the Measure Up campaign, the complexity in the relationship between lifestyle behaviours and chronic disease as acknowledged in the scientific literature is lost. A similar pattern is noted in the Change4Life campaign where consumer insight (DoH and DCSF 2008) provides a nuanced and in-depth understanding of the social determinants of physical activity that is not incorporated into the campaign messages. For example, insights from parents from diverse cultural backgrounds present different understandings of health, physical activity, and body shape such as, "Improving health was not a compelling reason to exercise, especially for older Black African women, who believed that 'big is beautiful'" (DoH and DCSF 2008, p. 38); "Time spent going to church together is also an activity, not just jumping around. It should not be purely physical" (African father, DoH and DCSF 2008, p. 65). In the process of translation, the rich evidence around the meanings of health and physical activity in the lives of the target populations gets simplified and complexity is lost in an attempt to create a simple one-size-fits-all campaign.

Furthermore, with the loss of complexity in understanding the many and varied experiences of health and physical activity, a more personalised responsibility is gained. That is, the responsibility for behaviour change is shifted from complex social and physical environments to individuals (Lupton 2014). This kind of induction can be seen on the Change4Life website which states

> For adults, it can seem hard to fit activity into a busy schedule. Working and looking after the rest of the family and the home can mean there isn't much free time. And sometimes activity can seem expensive too – but it doesn't have to be.

This statement acknowledges the complexity of people's lives and the difficulty in choosing to change one's physical activity behaviour. The listed suggestions for action however are simplistic and do not account for any of the previously mentioned complexity, such as, "Take up an active hobby, get active for free, plan ahead for PA". In the loss of agency, an easier "sell" and the ability to make more generalised claims is gained.

Distributions of agency

As we explained earlier, every technology (such as in this case, a health promotion campaign) has inscribed into it the kind of universe in which it is intended to function (Callon 1986; see also Akrich 1992). This actor-world, as it is known, defines the elements that compose the technology, as well as their functions, associations, dimensions, and historical trajectories. In this way, the existence of a technology is bound up with its actor-world. Without its actor-world, a technology does not and could not exist. Thus, the success of a technology depends upon the ability of its designers (in this case, policy makers and campaign designers) to enrol the necessary elements and then prevent them from escaping the logic of the actor-world they have been enlisted into (something they are always at risk of doing). That is, a physical activity promotion campaign is designed to function in a particular "perfect world" context which assumes roles of other actors (community members) and technologies. This theory allows us to examine government texts and policies and their resulting physical activity promotion campaigns as "actors" in a network, as "an actant can literally be anything provided it is granted to be the source of action" (Latour 1996, p. 373).

This way of thinking about the world is thoroughly and rigorously relational (Law 1992; see also Law 2009; Law & Mol 1995; Mol 2010). Applying a semiotic conception of relatedness to both the material and the discursive dimensions of reality, it says that entities have the identities and competencies they do because of their relationships and interactions with other entities. With the ability to shift the action of other entities in some way (Akrich & Latour 1992), agency is therefore understood as an effect of networks of relations. What we are concerned with below are the competencies inscribed in the materials we analysed, the way these competencies are distributed among the elements that make up the respective actor-worlds (Latour 1992), and the changes that these competencies and distributions do and do not undergo in the movement from government documents to campaign materials. To do so, we treated these materials as technologies qua, *"ways of doing something"* (Boulding as cited in Franklin, 1999, p. 6, original emphasis).

One notable dimension of the actor-worlds inscribed in the analysed materials concerns the civic relation between the state and its citizens. Here, there was very little change between the distribution of competencies in the shift between the actor-worlds of the informing documents and the actor-worlds of the campaign materials. All the materials we analysed were heavily inscribed with a logic of choice (Mol 2008). In other words, as the following quote illustrates, they were characterised as autonomous individuals who possessed the ability to choose how physically active they were:

> Halting the obesity epidemic is about individual behaviour and responsibility: how people choose to live their lives, what they eat and how much physical activity they do.
>
> *Cross-Government Obesity Unit, DoH and DCSF 2008, p. xi*

These individuals were also endowed with the ability to directly affect the health and prosperity of the collectives they belong to:

> Queenslanders would be healthier if they were to eat well, be active, prevent weight gain, not smoke, take care that alcohol consumption doesn't exceed guidelines, be sun safe, invest in good oral healthcare, practise safe sex, keep up with recommended immunisation and screening schedules and look after their mental health. The result would be less chronic disease, less pressure on health services and systems and the state would be wealthier through improved productivity.
>
> *Queensland Health 2012, p. i*

The state, for its part in this relation, was endowed with the ability to create conditions that promoted and facilitated its citizens' ability to do so without, however, directly impinging on their freedom to make healthy lifestyle choices:

> The campaign is for all Australians and aims to provide them with the tools and understanding to make healthy lifestyle choices. . . . The long term objectives of the campaign are: to encourage Australians to make and sustain changes to their behaviour, such as increased physical activity and healthier eating behaviours.
>
> *Australian Department of Health and Aging 2011, para. 13*

In this way, these three campaigns and their informing documents translate a similar civic logic to those studied by others researching physical activity policies (e.g. Macdonald, Wright & Abbott 2010; McGannon & Mauws 2002; Powell & Gard 2015).

A related dimension of the actor-worlds we analysed was the ways agency was distributed between people and their environment. In this instance, there were marked changes in the shift from the informing documents to the campaign materials. In the actor-worlds of the former, both people and their environment were inscribed with the capacity to shift action regarding physical activity and sedentary behaviour.

> Much has been published on the determinants of health and it is well recognised that health is influenced by a complex interplay of societal, environmental, socioeconomic, biological and lifestyle factors.
>
> *Queensland Health, 2012, p. 9*

Yet, in the actor-worlds of the campaign, the agency of the environment is diminished and the people are endowed with the most significant forms of agency (i.e., just choose to make changes), when it comes to being more physically active.

> The creative for the second phase of the *Healthier. Happier.* campaign has the core message "small changes can make a difference" . . . From this, four key messages have been developed: add fruit and vegetables to your meals; have smaller portion sizes; cut back on sugary drinks; less sitting and more moving.
>
> *Queensland Health Preventive Health Unit, Stakeholder Letter, 28 March 2014, p. 1*

This shift seems to sit uneasily with the previous observation about the competencies of the citizen in the actor-worlds of the informing documents. Indeed, this tension between two competing models of human behaviour appeared again and again as we traced the distribution of agency within the informing documents and the campaign materials.

From this analysis of the actor-worlds built by government texts, physical activity policy and campaigns, we have highlighted how roles of the citizen, the environment, and the state are defined and distributed. Through the process of translation of evidence, the importance of social, environmental, political, and demographic "actors" have been lost while a focus on individual responsibility and simplicity of message have been gained. The mis-match in the agency afforded to individuals between the government texts and the resulting campaigns is potentially significant in understanding the success (or lack thereof) of physical activity behaviour change campaigns.

Conclusion

In this chapter we sought to trace the translations from evidence to policy to practice across three physical activity promotion campaigns. To do so we utilised a methodology adapted from studies of science and technology to examine questions of sources of evidence and its uses, and gains and losses resulting from the process of translation. This is an important endeavour given the expected standard of evidence-based policy and the large budgets supporting physical activity promotion campaigns. Furthermore, the acceptance of evidence-based policy disregards the critiques around "who gets invited to the table" and the "black box" surrounding this process.

We cannot be naive to think that the evidence will remain the same through the different stages in development of campaign messages and strategies. However, what is gained and lost becomes important when so much money is being spent on campaigns and when we place so much faith in evidence-based practice.

If we think about translation in this way there is no avoiding that something will be lost, something will change, and something will be gained. In the analysis reported in this chapter we found that the most prominent source of evidence was in-house government documents that were used to support "facts" about prevalence of health behaviours and chronic diseases but not for the strategies enacted in the campaigns. There was also much that was taken for granted such as first, the acceptance of the relationship between body weight (overweight and obesity) and chronic disease, and second, the unquestioned cause of obesity being energy imbalance which implicated physical activity as a target behaviour in health promotion campaigns.

Throughout this process what was gained was a certainty and acceptance of simplicity in the causes of health issues and their solutions. The inductions utilised in building this case on the basis of energy imbalance resulted in the responsibility for behaviour change lying squarely with individuals – an approach often critiqued in academic literature. This was despite at least some evidence in the policy documents related to all three campaigns that acknowledged the complexity of physical activity as a health behaviour (particularly from the perspectives of the target audience) and its relationship with chronic disease.

As such, we are led to consider the robustness of these translations. Compared to what is lost, are the gains worth it? The political dimension of evidence-based policy and practice is also highlighted. It is clear that the campaigns were not solely led by the evidence given what was lost in the final strategies. Science and politics are inextricably linked. If this is the case, as advocates for physical activity participation, what changes are we happy with?

In this chapter we have provided a valuable critique of evidence-based policy and practice in physical activity promotion campaigns. In doing so, we have opened the black box to consider the steps in the process, not just the end product. We highlighted that lay understandings of physical activity and health were lost in the translation of evidence into policy and then to campaign. This represents a loss of valuable knowledge that decontextualises physical activity behaviours in order to gain a simple, one-size-fits-all campaign, which ultimately may increase inequalities in health as proposed by Springett and colleagues (2007). Potentially then, if we are facing another unsuccessful public physical activity promotion campaign, a lot of money is also set to be lost from health budgets. Ultimately, we can never have perfectly faithful translations but we do have to be thoughtful about how the process of translation is carried out.

References

Akrich, M. (1992). The de-scription of technical objects. In W. E. Bijker & J. Law (Eds.), *Shaping technology/building society: Studies in sociotechnical change* (pp. 205–224). Cambridge, MA: The MIT Press.

Akrich, M. & Latour, B. (1992). A summary of a convenient vocabulary for the semiotics of human and nonhuman assemblies. In W. E. Bijker & J. Law (Eds.), *Shaping technology/building society: Studies in sociotechnical change* (pp. 259–264). Cambridge, MA: The MIT Press.

Australian Department of Health and Aging. (2011). *Measure Up – About the Measure Up Campaign*, viewed 29 April 2011, http://measureup.gov.au/internet/abhi/publishing.nsf/Content/About.

Blue Moon. (2006). *SNAP-O Concept Testing*, Sydney, NSW.

Blue Moon (for the Australian Department of Health and Aging). (2007). *Australian Better Health Initiative: Diet, Exercise and Weight Developmental Communications Research*, Sydney, NSW.

Blue Moon (for the Australian Department of Health and Aging). (2010). *Measure Up Phase Two: Qualitative Formative Research Report*, Sydney, NSW.

Brighton, B., Bhandari, M., Tornetta, P. & Felson, D. T. (2003). Hierarchy of evidence: From case reports to randomized controlled trials. *Clinical Orthopaedics and Related Research*, *413*, 19–24.

Brown, M. (2002). Michel Serres: Science, translation and the logic of the parasite. *Theory, Culture & Society*, *19*(3), 1–27. doi: 10.1177/0263276402019003001.

Callon, M. (1986). The sociology of an actor-network: The case of the electric vehicle. In M. Callon, J. Law & A. Rip (Eds.), *Mapping the dynamics of science and technology: Sociology of science in the real world* (pp. 19–34). London: Macmillan.

Change4Life. (2009). *Change4Life 'Activity'* [television commercial], viewed 5 February 2016, www.youtube.com/watch?v=kfCC3Sjz8Dk.

Coalition for Evidence-Based Policy. (2016). Viewed 5 February 2016, http://coalition4evidence.org/.

Cross-Government Obesity Unit, Department of Health [DoH] and Department of Children, Schools and Families [DCSF]. (2008). *Healthy Weight, Healthy Lives: A Cross-Government Strategy for England*, London, UK.

Department of Health. (2009). *Change4Life Marketing Strategy*, London, UK.

Department of Health and the Department for Children, Schools and Families (DoH and DCSF). (2008). *Healthy Weight, Healthy Lives: Consumer Insight Summary*, London, UK.

Despres, J-P. (2012). Body fat distribution and risk of cardiovascular disease: An update. *Circulation, 126*(10), 1301–1313.

DeVasto, D., (2015). Being expert: L'Aquila and issues of inclusion in science-policy decision making. *Social Epistemology, 30*(4), 1–26.

Franklin, U. M. (1999). *The real world of technology* (revised ed.). Toronto, Canada: Anansi Press.

Goldenberg, M.J. (2006). On evidence and evidence-based medicine: Lessons from the philosophy of science. *Social Science & Medicine, 62*(11), 2621–2632.

Goodman K. W. (2003). *Ethics and evidence-based medicine: Fallibility and responsibility in clinical science,* Cambridge, Cambridge University Press.

Latour, B. (1992). Where are the missing masses? The sociology of a few mundane artifacts. In W. E. Bijker & J. Law (Eds.), *Shaping technology/building society: Studies in sociotechnical change* (pp. 225–258). Cambridge, MA: The MIT Press.

Latour, B. (1987). *Science in action: How to follow scientists and engineers through society.* Cambridge, MA: Harvard University Press.

Latour, B. (1996). On Actor-Network Theory: A Few Clarifications. *Soziale Welt, 47*(4), 369–381.

Law, J. (1992). Notes on the theory of the actor-network: Ordering, strategy, and heterogeneity. *Systems Practice, 5*(4), 379–393. doi: 10.1007/BF01059830.

Law, J. (2002). *Aircraft stories: Decentering the object in technoscience.* Durham, NC: Duke University Press.

Law, J. (2009). Actor network theory and material semiotics. In B. Turner (Ed.), *The new Blackwell companion to social theory* (pp. 141–158). Malden, MA: Wiley-Blackwell.

Law, J. & Mol, A. (1995). Notes on materiality and sociality. *The Sociological Review, 43*(2), 274–294. doi: 10.1111/j.1467-954X.1995.tb00604.x.

Lupton, D. (2014). "How do you measure up?" Assumptions about "obesity" and health-related behaviors and beliefs in two Australian "obesity" prevention campaigns. *Fat Studies, 3*(1), 32–44. doi: 10.1080/21604851.2013.784050.

Macdonald, D., Wright, J. & Abbott, R. (2010). Anxieties and aspirations: The making of active, informed citizens. In J. Wright & D. Macdonald (Eds.), *Young people, physical activity and the everyday* (pp. 121–135). London and New York: Routledge,

Marston, G. & Watts, R. (2003). Tampering with the evidence: A critical appraisal of evidence-based policy making. *The Drawing Board: An Australian Review of Public Affairs, 3*(3), 143–163.

McGannon, K. R. & Mauws, M. K. (2002). Exploring the exercise adherence problem: An integration of ethnomethodological and poststructuralist perspectives. *Sociology of Sport Journal, 19*(1), 67–89.

Mol, A. (2008). *The logic of care: Health and the problem of patient choice.* New York, NY: Routledge.

Mol, A. (2010). Actor-network theory: Sensitive terms and enduring tensions. *Kölner Zeitschrift für Soziologie und Sozialpsychologie, 50*(1), 253–269.

Muir Gray, J. A. (2004). Evidence based policy making [editorial]. *BMJ, 329*(7473), 988–989.

Mykhalovskiy, E. & Weir, L. (2004). The problem of evidence-based medicine: Directions for social science. *Social Science & Medicine, 59*(5), 1059–1069.

Powell, D. & Gard, M., (2015). The governmentality of childhood obesity: Coca-Cola, public health and primary schools. *Discourse: Studies in the Cultural Politics of Education, 36*(6), 854–867.

Queensland Department of Health. (2013). *Measured obesity in Queensland 2011–12,* viewed 5 February 2016, www.health.qld.gov.au/publications/research-reports/population-health/measured-obesity. pdf.

Queensland Health. (2012). *The health of Queenslanders 2012: Advancing good health,* Fourth report of the Chief Health Officer Queensland, viewed 5 February 2016, www.health.qld.gov.au/cho_report/2012/documents/2012-cho-report-all.pdf.

Queensland Health Preventive Health Unit. (2014). *Stakeholder letter,* 28 October 2013.

Springett, J., Owens, C. & Callaghan, J. (2007). The challenge of combining 'lay' knowledge with 'evidence-based' practice in health promotion: Fag Ends Smoking Cessation Service. *Critical Public Health, 17*(3), 243–256.

Sui, X., LaMonte, M. J., Laditka, J. N., Hardin, J. W., Chase, N., Hooker, S. P. & Blair, S. N. (2007). Cardiorespiratory fitness and adiposity as mortality predictors in older adults, *JAMA, 289*(21), 133–146.

11

MEASURING PHYSICAL ACTIVITY

Dale Esliger, Andrew Kingsnorth and Lauren Sherar

Introduction

The concept of measurement has evolved over time from being overly focused on quantification in and of itself, to a broader focus on the elicitation of information about the phenomena being measured and making that information meaningful and usable (Ferris 2004). In the case of physical activity, if one were to use a classical measurement system paradigm (Sydenham 1985), the following questions would need to be posed and answered:

i)   What knowledge of physical activity is sought?
ii) What specific physical activity measurands (i.e., entity) need to be measured?
iii) What should the performance specification of the physical activity measurands be?
iv) How are the resultant measured physical activity data to be used?

This concept of measurement can be described further by understanding that from a starting point, simple data evolves towards information (i.e., increases cognitive content), then on to knowledge, then on to wisdom and ultimately on to its highest form in the continuum, intelligence (Sydenham 2003). Unfortunately, the most challenging step in the measurement process is the decision of what to measure. The sign hanging over Albert Einstein's office door at Princeton captures this sentiment particularly well, it reads: Not everything that counts can be counted, and not everything that can be counted counts. It is clear that the decision of what to measure (i.e., what data to collect) needs to be well informed in order to facilitate the task of translating data into much sought after knowledge and further up the continuum to intelligence.

There are some common motivations for measuring physical activity for policy purposes; including but not limited to: monitoring prevalence/surveillance (epidemiological research), understanding correlates/determinants of physical activity, and measuring the effectiveness and impacts of small (local) and national health promotion programmes/policy changes in an effort to link it to a health/economic/societal outcome(s). Although policy makers often have quite tailored needs to fulfil a specific requirement, interestingly they also have a vested interest and may have a part to play in advocating for good quality measurement tools. Broad health promotion and policy initiatives often require a diverse and strong evidence base, which is largely dependent on the appropriateness and quality of data collection tools used by others. The choice of measurement tool will depend on a number of factors, including the aforementioned, but also the target population and the practicality of the data collection. This chapter strives to take the reader through the common measurement tools available and finishes with some general recommendations for policy relevant research.

Definition of physical activity

In the field of physical activity, the decision of what to measure is made even more difficult because the exposure is complex and multidimensional (LaPorte, Montoye et al. 1985) and researchers often use different terms to define the underlying dimensions. For example, exercise physiologists often define physical activity as "any bodily movement produced by skeletal muscles that results in caloric expenditure" (Caspersen 1989); however, this is often incorrectly used interchangeably with other terms such as "exercise" in the literature. Additionally, others stress the importance of sub-dimensions of physical activity—frequency, intensity, duration, mode, and context to define the behaviour (Haskell 2001, Kesaniemi, Danforth et al. 2001, Montoye 2000). Frequency is defined as the number of bouts of activity per time period (e.g., day, week, month, etc.). Intensity is the effort associated with the physical activity (e.g., light, moderate, vigorous) and is usually expressed in terms of energy expenditure, and duration refers to the time spent in physical activity (e.g., minutes, hours). Together, the product of frequency, intensity, and duration yields the volume of physical activity or dose. The mode of physical activity helps describe what type of activity is being performed (e.g., walking, running, swimming, gardening), and finally, the physical activity context refers to the practice of categorizing one's physical activity according to identifiable portions of daily life (e.g., leisure-time, occupational, transportation-related physical activity). To ensure consistency, this section of the book chapter we will be referring to physical activity as per the Caspersen 1989 definition.

Measuring physical activity

In addition to understanding the sub-dimensions of physical activity, one must understand the relationship between physical activity and energy expenditure. This is particularly important in terms of understanding the dose-response relationship between physical activity and health. As outlined in Figure 11.1, the global construct representing the exposure variable within the activity-health paradigm is best defined as "movement", with two dimensions: physical activity (the behaviour) and energy expenditure (the physiological response to the behaviour) (Lamonte, Ainsworth 2001). Assessments of physical activity behaviour include, among others, direct observation, physical activity diaries, recall questionnaires, pedometers, and accelerometers. Assessments of energy expenditure include, among other methods, calorimetry, labelled isotope methods, and energy intake. The choice of method often varies considerably by the specifications of the research, resources available and the training required. Therefore the following sections will focus on physical activity behaviour and act as a summary of the main behavioural methods and their methodological implications for policy relevant research.

Self-report methods

The most common method of measuring population-level physical activity is through self-report measures, such as diaries/logs, surveys, questionnaires, or interviews. These measures

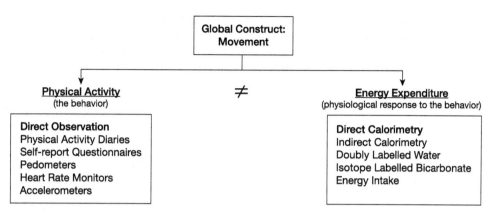

Figure 11.1 A conceptual model of the relationship between movement, physical activity, and energy expenditure, as well as various measurement methods.

Source: Adapted from Lamonte, Ainsworth 2001

Note: Bold typeface indicates the method is often considered a criterion method.

are popular due to their feasibility/practicality, low cost, low participant burden, and general acceptance (Strath, Kaminsky et al. 2013). Selecting a self-report tool that is culturally and cognitively appropriate is a key priority for policy makers and practitioners. Some of the common methods will be described in the following section in terms of their application for measuring physical activity; however, for useful recommendations to improve the accuracy of self-reported physical activity we point the reading to the following paper (Ainsworth, Caspersen et al. 2012).

Questionnaires

Physical activity questionnaires are often classified as global questionnaires, short term recall questionnaires and quantitative history recall questionnaires (Ainsworth, Cahalin et al. 2015). Global questionnaires tend to be short (usually comprised of one to four items), simple and quick to administer and thus have little participant burden. They are frequently used in large, multifaceted surveys where physical activity is only a small part. Respondents comment on their activity (either in total or on a specific domain) in quite general terms. Because of their brevity, global questionnaires are limited in their ability to collect detailed information, such as frequency of active commuting, but when categorical indicators, such as exercising regularly or rating of physical activity relative to peers is sufficient, then this type of questionnaire may be appropriate. Examples of global questionnaires include a single item measure designed to capture an assessment of physical activity against the national recommendation at that time of at least 30 min of moderate-to-vigorous physical activity (MVPA) on five or more days of the week. The question simply asked about the number of days in which respondents have accumulated ≥30 min of MVPA (Milton, Clemes et al. 2013).

Another popular tool, especially for policy relevant research purposes because of its perceived simplicity and low cost, is the short term recall questionnaire. These questionnaires usually range from 7–20 questions/items and ask participants to recall, over the past seven days or past month, on the frequency, intensity, duration of activities. The questions can focus on the number of minutes in different intensities (such as time in light or MVPA) on the whole, or will focus in on specific domains of physical activity, such as occupational physical activity, leisure time physical activity or active transportation. Summative scores (based on the frequency, intensity, and duration) are usually expressed as time (hours/minutes) of physical activity time or presented as a combination of the intensity and duration as MET hours or MET-minutes. Correlations between questionnaire physical activity data and more accurate or criterion measures may be slightly higher in questionnaires asking about the previous seven days compared with those asking about a usual week (van Poppel, Chinapaw et al. 2010).

Quantitative history recall questionnaire is where participants are asked to recall their physical activity over a longer period of time (e.g., one year, ten years, across a lifetime). The questionnaire is much longer (i.e., can include up to 60 questions) (Ainsworth, Cahalin et al. 2015) and thus inappropriate often for large epidemiological studies. Also, because of the length of recall and cognitive burden, often these questionnaires are interviewer assisted/led. The scoring of these questionnaires is similar to the short-term recall. Strengths of these questionnaires include the information rich, historic data. However, accurately recalling past physical activity behaviours is an obvious limitation/challenge (Shephard 2003, Smith, Cronin et al. 2013).

Logs/Diaries

Physical activity logs are where discrete activities are recorded during the day. These can include checklists of specific activities that are completed at set times during the day (e.g., every 15 minutes) or at the end of the day. For example, a checklist may ask participants to rate the intensity of their activity (from 1 to 9). Overall scores are calculated by assigning a MET value to each intensity level and multiplying the MET value by the epoch. Logs can be simple to administer and do not suffer from long recall. Physical activity diaries collect more detailed information about aspects of physical activity. Information could include duration and intensities of activities, postures while performing activities, co-existence of behaviours, etc. The summary variables of logs and diaries are similar to that from questionnaires. An advantage of a diary is the rich data that can be gleaned, and physical activity logs or diaries have been found to be more accurate than recall questionnaires (Irwin, Ainsworth et al. 2001); however, log/diary completion is burdensome to participants; diary interpretation is burdensome to investigators; diary records may not reflect long-term physical activity patterns; and, diary use may alter one's physical activity habits by acting as a motivational tool (i.e., subject reactivity) (Timperio, Salmon et al. 2004). The traditional paper-pen method of completing logs and diaries has, in some cases, been replaced with computer-assisted technology such as smartphone (Dunton, Liao et al. 2011, Dunton, Whalen et al. 2005, Atienza, Oliveira et al. 2006), which make the recording easier for the participant and the scoring easier for the researcher.

Although self-report methods are useful for gaining insight into the physical activity levels of populations, they risk overestimating and/or underestimating true physical activity energy expenditure (Prince, Adamo et al. 2008). Individuals, for instance, may find it difficult to average behaviour durations and/or frequencies over specific time frames such as the past week or month (Ainsworth, Caspersen et al. 2012). That said, as previously mentioned, some global assessments administered by telephone, questionnaire, or interview seek only categorical information, such as participation in regular exercise or self-rating of physical activity relative to peers. The self-report methods of recalling intensity, frequency, and duration of bouts of activity are considered problematic, especially in certain populations, such as children who are less time conscious than adults and tend to engage in physical activity in intermittent or sporadic bouts with varied intensities rather than consistent patterns (Rowlands, Eston 2007, Bailey, Olson et al. 1995). Not only is reliability compromised by recall difficulties but also the validity of measures may be affected in children or adults who feel compelled to respond in a certain way (Jago, Baranowski et al. 2007, Motl, McAuley et al. 2005). Warnecke and colleagues (1997) attributed the over reporting of physical activity in these situations to what he called social desirability (Warnecke, Johnson et al. 1997). It seems that society has come to know that being physically active, like eating a well-balanced diet, is the socially desirable "thing to do". Furthermore, comparisons between self-reports with direct measures, such as accelerometers, have shown that subjective error is not systematic but random, making attempts to correct for self-report–direct measure differences problematic (Prince, Adamo et al. 2008).

A major improvement in questionnaire assessment of physical activity was the inclusion of household sources of activity (e.g., gardening, cleaning), which can be the primary context for physical activity among some groups (e.g., stay at home parents, retirees, etc.) (Dong, Block et al. 2004). In addition, some types of questionnaires include sources of physical activity common/important among certain ethnic/cultural groups. However, efforts to understand how various population subgroups interpret certain constructs used in physical activity questionnaires, such as leisure time activity or moderate physical activity, are limited. The ease of use of self-reported tools may be an advantage for policy purposes as large numbers of people can be sampled, using traditional or online methods. However, any conclusions reached by using these methods will have to acknowledge the potential bias attributed to self-report, something which should also be considered when any subsequent policy decisions are being made.

Qualitative methods

Qualitative methodologies are used to gain a greater understanding of the in-depth experience of individuals in the field of physical activity where quantitative methods may be too limiting to investigate people and their situations (Eisner 1997). These methods can be an important component of research driving policies and/or as part of a process evaluation of an intervention. Qualitative methodology focuses on the subjective experience of the individual, thereby providing a richness of information to the field of physical activity. Methodologies include open ended questionnaires, interviews, and focus groups, among others and can garner subjective data on physical activity. A detailed description of these methodologies is beyond the scope of this chapter but we point the reader towards this excellent resource (Jones, Brown et al. 2012).

Objective measurement methods

In contrast to the subjective methods outlined in the previous sections, objective methods of physical activity measurement have only recently started to be used on a large scale due to commercialization of sensor technologies in both the research and consumer sectors. Whilst it is posited that the measurement of physical activity by objective means is considered to capture a more accurate representation of behaviour, they are still poor at determining the mode and/or context, which to many is equally important to the quantification of the volumetric dose of physical activity. The following section provides a brief overview of the current objective methods available to measure physical activity both in small laboratory studies and large population samples.

Direct observation techniques

Direct observation as a measurement technique is often used in free-living situations to directly monitor and describe what is taking place in the physical activity environment. Often used for children and in a school setting because of their limited ability to accurately recall physical activity (Anderssen, Jacobs et al. 1995), most utilized methods for direct observation in a defined space such as a school playground or park include the System for Observing Fitness Instruction Time (SOFIT) (McKenzie, Sallis et al. 1991) and the System for Observing Play and Leisure Activity in Youth (SOPLAY) (McKenzie, Marshall et al. 2000).

Direct observation systems are often developed for target populations in specific settings and include the following characteristics: a well-defined observation strategy to sample activities per unit of time, a list of activity categories to code movement types, a list of associated variables that may influence behaviour (e.g., context, teacher behaviour, environmental settings), supplemental methods to record concurrent levels of energy expenditure, data entry procedures (e.g., pencil and paper, computer, or tablets), and detailed scoring schemes used to summarize the data (Pettee, Storti et al. 2009). Whilst able to give accurate details and contextual information of physical activity, the disadvantages of this technique include:

- High expense (i.e., researcher burden) necessary for data collection and scoring (Montoye, Kemper et al. 1996), as sufficient training is necessary to ensure between-observer and within-observer agreement.
- Subject reactivity as the presence of the observer may disrupt or change regular physical activity patterns, decreasing the reliability and validity of the data.

As a result of these limitations, direct observation is typically confined to studies that are smaller and conducted in distinct settings over a shorter period of time. For a more comprehensive description of the various methods available the reader is referred to McKenzie (2010).

Pedometers

Evidence suggests that step-based ambulation accounts for the majority of physical activity energy expenditure (Bassett, Cureton et al. 2000), thus step counts provide an objective measure capturing a significant portion of daily physical activity. Pedometers are small match-box sized, battery operated waist, ankle, or foot-worn sensors that can vary in function and offer additional features in the technology used to detect step based movement. Common versions include a spring-levered mechanism that counts steps when sufficient vertical force causes the arm to complete an electrical circuit and newer piezo-electric version that counts the amount of "zero crossings" from the peaks in acceleration to calculate steps (Tudor-Locke, Bassett et al. 2011). As an easily digestible unit, step based targets such as 10,000 steps per day have been suggested as an important target to reach daily. Whilst the actual number was based on a Japanese manufacturer's pedometer product slogan which translates to "10,000 step meter" (Tudor-Locke, Hatano et al. 2008), the target has actually been found to be effective in increasing physical activity in community settings (De Cocker, De Bourdeaudhuij et al. 2007).

Research indicates that pedometers can offer distinct advantages over self-report methods as a form of physical activity monitoring (Freak-Poli, Cumpston et al. 2013). For example, physical activity questionnaires typically ask individuals to recall the distance that they walk on a daily basis (Ainsworth, Leon et al. 1993). Individuals often have trouble remembering or may lack perception of distance and therefore provide inaccurate reports of the distance actually walked on a daily basis (Welk 2002). Pedometers can overcome this by providing a proxy measure of physical activity in the form of steps, something which can be compared between individuals and periods of time.

Although pedometers can provide a volumetric index of physical activity and are reasonably accurate at counting steps, they cannot discriminate between steps accumulated in walking, running, or stair climbing and therefore compromise measures of physical activity intensity (Bassett, Strath 2002). In an effort to provide information on activity intensity some pedometer manufacturers have developed models that measure time-stamped step counts (e.g., Lifecorder EX, New Lifestyles). These new generation digital pedometers use steps accumulated per unit time to estimate intensity level. For policy purposes, pedometers could be a relatively cheap way of evaluating the success of an intervention or activity levels on a population level. However, the use of steps as a measurement outcome could be considered limited, and researchers are now more interested in additional information, such as time spent in physical activity intensities. The advancement of technology, in particular the accelerometer, has facilitated this transition and will be looked at in the next section.

Accelerometers

Accelerometers are small electronic devices that are one of the most commonly used devices for assessing free-living physical activity (Welk 2002). Able to measure the levels of accelerations in three orthogonal planes (anteroposterior, mediolateral, and vertical) (Chen, Bassett 2005), they were first developed for use in industry for applications such as aeroplanes (Walter 2007). Worn on the waist, upper arm, hip, wrist, and/or ankle, accelerometers are now used in large representative surveillance studies such as the National Health and Nutritional Examination Survey (NHANES) (Troiano, Berrigan et al. 2008), Canadian Health Measures Survey (CHMS) (Tremblay, Connor Gorber 2007), the Health Survey for England (HSE) (Craig, Mindell et al. 2009), and the UK Biobank (UK Biobank).

To equate accelerometric data into levels of physical activity, the raw acceleration is converted into an activity "count" over a user-defined time period of measurement that can vary from one second to several minutes or more (i.e., epoch). These activity counts provide an objective assessment of movement intensity, with greater accelerations producing greater counts. However, because counts are tallied in proprietary, manufacturer-specific units, they only allow the comparison of data among similar accelerometer models. In practice, these "counts" are further converted into more physiologically relevant units, usually based on energy expended per unit time, that have been developed using laboratory protocols. To date, the most popular method used to calibrate accelerometer count data into time spent in physical activity is some form of count to intensity (i.e., energy expenditure) prediction equation that is often used to generate intensity cut-points.

Increasingly a popular choice for researchers, commercial suppliers have responded by producing a number of different models and greatly increasing the functionality of these measurement tools (see Troiano, McClain et al. 2014 for a comprehensive review). Depending on the number of planes that the accelerometers measure, they can be classified as uniaxial (one), biaxial (two), or triaxial (three). Compared to uniaxial sensors, triaxial accelerometers theoretically provide a more comprehensive assessment of body movements; triaxial accelerometers have been shown to have higher correlations with measured energy expenditure in adults and children than uniaxial accelerometers in some but not all studies (Chen, Bassett 2005, Van Hees, Slootmaker et al. 2009, Westerterp 2009). Although the technological evolution of the field has been beneficial, it has made it more difficult for end users to choose the best accelerometer model for their purposes. Unfortunately the notion of a "one size fits all" accelerometer is highly unlikely because monitor selection depends on the application for which it is intended (Bassett 2000, Sanders, Loveday et al. 2016).

Those involved in the use of accelerometers or those dealing with accelerometric data must understand that the interpretations of these data are severely complicated by the methodological and analytical decisions that are required to be made before and after data collection. For instance the large availability of several differing cut-point ranges to define physical activity categories can yield markedly different results for the same data (Strath, Bassett et al. 2003). A discussion of appropriate cut-points is beyond the scope of this book chapter; however the lack of consensus, both within and between accelerometer models, remains a major barrier to data interpretation (Ward, Evenson et al. 2005). Other decisions or limitations that the user needs to be aware of include:

- Deployment challenges: the cost and the potential for the loss of devices, participant burden and adherence, wear position, and the training required.
- Analytical decisions: how to deal with different cutpoints, epoch lengths, non-wear, and sleep.
- Sources of error: technical (spurious data) and human (incorrect deployment and reactivity).
- Applicability: the choice of sensor and validity of measurement.

The intricacies of research grade devices are certainly a barrier to the use for policy/public health work, where an accelerometer expert might not always be to hand. Preliminary research into consumer products, such as the Nike Fuel band and the FitBit, have concluded that some monitors can provide reasonably accurate estimations of energy expenditure (Lee, Kim et al. 2014, Bai, Welk et al. 2015). Although premature to conclude that current research devices could be substituted by commercial devices, if developments in consumer grade technology and the "fitness tracker" market continues to grow, we may see more "plug and go" user-friendly devices for evaluation and wide scale monitoring purposes in the future. This may be particularly relevant if the desire for self-monitoring (the quantified self) continues momentum. Perhaps the future is to collate the multiple, on-going streams of data that are being collected by the public in the real world, rather than imposing artificial evaluation measures.

The developments in the consumer market have also initiated a trend of shifting accelerometer wear from the waist to the wrist to aid in compliance and ease of wear in certain populations such as obese individuals. Nonetheless as the seminal work in this area has solely been conducted on sensors that have been deployed closer to the centre of mass (waist), the ambulatory "noise" introduced by wearing the devices nearer the extremities is far yet to be understood, and more research is needed before these devices can be advocated.

Whilst accelerometers present a steep learning curve related to the understanding of the technology and the behaviour intended being measured, their deep analytical information provides great potential to unearth complex relationships such as patterns and types of behavioural profiles. This information can be used in conjunction with health outcomes to build associations on a specific sample and nationally representative levels. Therefore those investigating physical activity behaviours for policy should consider using accelerometers as an objective assessment in conjunction with other measurement methods, if resources allow.

Heart rate monitoring

Temporal heart rate data provides rich profiling information on frequency, intensity, and duration of physical activity. Obtaining measures of heart rate (e.g., beats per minute) provides direct temporal evidence of the physiological response attributable to physical activity (Armstrong 1998, Welk, Corbin et al. 2000). Based on the assumption that a linear relationship exists between oxygen uptake (O2) and heart rate (Wilmore, Haskell 1971) one can estimate physical activity energy expenditure. However, this method is plagued with high levels of individual variability, with errors in energy expenditure ranging from 20–50 per cent (Livingstone, Prentice et al. 1990). A large portion of the variability can be attributed to differences in age, gender, and fitness levels between individuals.

Further imprecision in the estimate of energy expenditure from heart rate can be attributed to attenuation in the O2–heart rate relationship during low and very high intensity activities (Acheson, Campbell et al. 1980). Other known confounders have been shown to skew heart rate while having minimal and, at times, variable impact on O2 (e.g., body temperature, size of the active muscle mass (upper vs. lower body), type of exercise (static vs. dynamic), stress, certain medications, fatigue, body position, hydration status, consumption of stimulants such as nicotine or caffeine (Acheson, Campbell et al. 1980, Livingstone 1997, Maas, Kok et al. 1989, Montoye, Kemper et al. 1996, Montoye, Taylor 1984, Parker, Hurley et al. 1989). Yet another challenge presented by heart rate monitoring is the fact that heart rate suffers from a temporal lag in response to the initiation or cessation of physical activity (Strath, Swartz et al. 2000), making it more difficult to assess concurrent validity with other measurement methods.

The physical activity compendium estimates the amount of energy expenditure or metabolic cost of undertaking certain activities (Ainsworth, Haskell et al. 2011). It has been argued that these estimates may have some methodological implications that may reduce their applicability directly to certain types of physical behaviours (Costa, Ogilvie et al. 2015). By monitoring the direct cost of certain activities within a physical activity protocol, the predictive quality of these relationships may be increased. Many research and commercial devices can measure heart rate, a popular method being electrodes embedded into a strap worn on the chest. Whilst able to provide estimations of energy expenditure, heart rate monitoring can be a burden to the user, is costly, and may not be feasible for large scale surveillance protocols. That said, new heart rate sensors that measure heart rate through Photoplethysmography (PPG) technology are entering the wearables market. PPG is a non-invasive optical technique used to measure blood volume change in micro-vascular beds of tissue (Alzahrani, Hu et al. 2015). These new sensor paradigms (i.e., using light rather than the heart's electrical signal) have reduced the obtrusiveness of measuring heart rate given that users no longer need to wear a chest strap as PPG sensors can be built into regular wrist watches. Going forward it is likely that heart rate will become a routine vital sign to measure in wearable sensors in addition to movement behaviours.

Multiple sensors

Multiple sensor systems by design hold an advantage over singular systems by incorporating many common elements together, reducing the burden relayed onto the participants. The first iterations of multiple systems entailed attaching multiple sensors to the body trunk and extremities. The Intelligent Device for Energy Expenditure and Activity (IDEEA) system captures body and limb motions through five biaxial accelerometer sensors attached to the chest, thighs, and feet (Zhang, Werner et al. 2003, Zhang, Pi-Sunyer et al. 2004). Using an artificial neural network to recognize 32 types of activities such as jumping, walking, and running, stair climbing and descending, IDEEA correctly identified posture and limb movement and gait 98 per cent of the time.

More recently, devices have taken a physiological multisensory approach rather than focusing on predicting physical activity through extremity pattern recognition. The rapid advancement of technology has enabled information such as accelerometry to be accompanied with galvanic skin response, respiration, global positioning systems (GPS), speed, distance, posture, and skin temperature. Due to the rapid advancement, a list of technologies would likely be out of date by publication; however current multi sensor technologies include the Zephyr Bioharness (Zephyr Technology Corporation, USA), SenseWear Armband (BodyMedia, USA), and the Actiheart (CamNtech, UK). Multisensory platforms however require complex sophisticated data processing techniques and have not been extensively validated in large and varying population samples. For these reasons, the measurement of physical activity using these platforms is perhaps constrained to small samples and validation protocols at this moment in time.

Conclusion

Accurate measurements of physical activity are crucial to our understanding of the activity-health relationship, estimating population prevalence, identifying correlates, detecting trends, and evaluating the efficacy of interventions (Dollman, Okely et al. 2009). Unfortunately, the exposure assessments in physical activity epidemiology are often crude which can contribute to inconsistent results among studies (Lagerros 2009, Lagerros, Lagiou 2007). Unfortunately, most large studies of physical activity, including most national population surveillance programs, rely almost exclusively on "simple" exposure measures such as those obtained from physical activity questionnaires (Katzmarzyk, Tremblay 2007). Although questionnaires have been sufficient to demonstrate crude associations with disease end-points, uncertainties exist about the subjective nature of the data, which dimension of physical activity is being assessed, and the degree to which the assessment is valid (Adams, Matthews et al. 2005, Rennie, Wareham 1998, Sallis, Saelens 2000, Schmidt, Cleland et al. 2008, Shephard 2003, Wareham, Rennie 1998).

This review of the various methods of measuring physical activity, and physical activity associated energy expenditure, highlights the fact that each measurement method varies in accuracy, feasibility (especially in large studies of free-living populations), cost, and reactivity (i.e., likelihood of influencing the activity they are designed to measure) (LaPorte, Montoye et al. 1985). This review should also convey the fact that the physical activity constructs one wants to quantify will have a direct influence on the selection of the method or tool used to measure it. Also, all methods do not measure all the constructs, nor do they measure the individual constructs equally well (see Table 11.1). Having said this, Table 11.1 does highlight the fact that accelerometers deliver as much capability as indirect calorimetry with the added benefit of being much less obtrusive. However, for some research applications where activity mode and/or context are important, accelerometry would need to be supplemented with another measurement method such as a questionnaire or some other sensor modality that can provide context/location information (see Loveday, Sherar et al. 2015 for a comprehensive review).

Effective population measurement of physical activity allows for the: 1) baseline prevalence of physical activity to be assessed, 2) tracking of physical activity throughout the lifespan, 3) identification of subgroups at high risk, 4) assessment of trends over time for the tracking of provincial/national targets, 5) evaluation of interventions, policies, and programs, 6) analysis

Table 11.1 Listing of physical activity measurement methods by constructs each instrument is capable of assessing

Method	Frequency	Intensity	Duration	Mode	Context	Energy Expenditure
Diary	Y	Y	Y	Y	Y	N
Questionnaire	Y	Y	Y	Y	Y	N
Accelerometer	Y*	Y*	Y*	N	N	Y*
Heart rate monitor	Y*	Y*	Y*	N	N	N
Pedometer	N	N	N	N	N	Y*
Observation	Y	Y	Y	Y	Y	N
Doubly labelled water	N	N	N	N	N	Y
Indirect calorimetry	Y*	Y*	Y*	N	N	Y
Caloric intake	N	N	N	N	N	Y

Y = yes, can assess that aspect of physical activity; N = no, cannot assess that aspect of physical activity; asterisk (*) denotes that this information is available for only some models of this type of instrument.

Notes: i) This is not an exhaustive list of the methods available to measure physical activity, nor is it a complete list of the constructs of physical activity; ii) Adapted from Mahar, Rowe (2002).

of systemic changes in counselling and environmental design, 7) determination of dose-response and measurement issues, 8) budgeting of public health resources, 9) development of population-specific physical activity interventions (Macera, Pratt 2000). We would suggest that objective monitoring is necessary to obtain accurate prevalence figures (including baseline, tracking, and identifying people/subgroups at risk; 1–5 listed above). This could include a range of tools from pedometers to accelerometers and would be dependent on the type and quality of evidence required. When examining dose-response (7), it is essential to have accurate and objective data, which at this time point would likely come from accelerometers (for in the field) or lab based techniques such as indirect calorimetry. When evaluating complex programmes/policies and development of interventions (8–9) it is likely that a number of tools – including self-report questionnaires (for context) and objective sensors (for behaviour) – are required.

In summary, Bull and Bauman (2011) put forward a number of thought provoking reasons to explain why inactivity, despite being the fourth leading risk factor for the prevention of NCD, receives little policy attention and resourcing proportionate to its importance. They stated that a leading reason for this is because: "Physical inactivity cannot be measured reliably to provide valid estimates of risk" (Bull, Bauman 2011). We would argue that, albeit challenging, valid tools are available to measure physical inactivity accurately at a population level. Nonetheless, it does require a wide scale recognition of the importance and need for high quality measurement, and a commitment to furthering the field of "measurement" for wide scale surveillance in innovative ways.

References

Acheson, K.J., Campbell, I.T., Edholm, O.G., Miller, D.S. and Stock, M.J., 1980. The measurement of daily energy expenditure – An evaluation of some techniques. *The American Journal of Clinical Nutrition*, 33(5), pp. 1155–1164.

Adams, S.A., Matthews, C.E., Ebbeling, C.B., Moore, C.G., Cunningham, J.E., Fulton, J. and Hebert, J.R., 2005. The effect of social desirability and social approval on self-reports of physical activity. *American Journal of Epidemiology*, 161(4), pp. 389–398.

Ainsworth, B., Cahalin, L., Buman, M. and Ross, R., 2015. The current state of physical activity assessment tools. *Progress in Cardiovascular Diseases,* 57(4), pp. 387–395.

Ainsworth, B.E., Caspersen, C.J., Matthews, C.E., Masse, L.C., Baranowski, T. and Zhu, W., 2012. Recommendations to improve the accuracy of estimates of physical activity derived from self report. *Journal of Physical Activity & Health,* 9(Suppl 1), pp. S76–84.

Ainsworth, B.E., Haskell, W.L., Herrmann, S.D., Meckes, N., Bassett, D.R.Jr, Tudor-Locke, C., Greer, J.L., Vezina, J., Whitt-Glover, M.C. and Leon, A.S., 2011. 2011 Compendium of Physical Activities: A second update of codes and MET values. *Medicine and Science in Sports and Exercise,* 43(8), pp. 1575–1581.

Ainsworth, B.E., Leon, A.S., Richardson, M.T., Jacobs, D.R. and Paffenbarger, R.S., Jr, 1993. Accuracy of the college alumnus physical activity questionnaire. *Journal of Clinical Epidemiology,* 46(12), pp. 1403–1411.

Alzahrani, A., Hu, S., Azorin-Peris, V., Barrett, L., Esliger, D., Hayes, M., Akbare, S., Achart, J. and Kuoch, S., 2015. A multi-channel opto-electronic sensor to accurately monitor heart rate against motion artefact during exercise. *Sensors (Basel, Switzerland),* 15(10), pp. 25681–25702.

Anderssen, N., Jacobs, D.R., Jr, Aas, H. and Jakobsen, R., 1995. Do adolescents and parents report each other's physical activity accurately? *Scandinavian Journal of Medicine & Science in Sports,* 5(5), pp. 302–307.

Armstrong, N., 1998. Young people's physical activity patterns as assessed by heart rate monitoring. *Journal of Sports Sciences,* 16 Suppl, pp. S9–16.

Atienza, A.A., Oliveira, B., Fogg, B.J. and King, A.C., 2006. Using electronic diaries to examine physical activity and other health behaviors of adults age 50+. *Journal of Aging and Physical Activity,* 14(2), pp. 192–202.

Bai, Y., Welk, G.J., Nam, Y.H., Lee, J.A., Lee, J.M., Kim, Y. et al., 2015. Comparison of consumer and research monitors under semistructured settings. *Medicine and Science in Sports and Exercise,* 48(1), pp. 151–158.

Bailey, R.C., Olson, J., Pepper, S.L., Porszasz, J., Barstow, T.J. and Cooper, D.M., 1995. The level and tempo of children's physical activities: An observational study. *Medicine and Science in Sports and Exercise,* 27(7), pp. 1033–1041.

Bassett D.R. and Strath, S.J., 2002. Use of pedometers to assess physical activity. In: Welk, G.J., editor. *Physical Activity Assessments for Health-Related Research.* Champaign, IL: Human Kinetics, 163–177.

Bassett, D.R., Jr, 2000. Validity and reliability issues in objective monitoring of physical activity. *Research Quarterly for Exercise and Sport,* 71(Suppl 2), pp. 30–36.

Bassett, D.R., Jr, Cureton, A.L. and Ainsworth, B.E., 2000. Measurement of daily walking distance-questionnaire versus pedometer. *Medicine and Science in Sports and Exercise,* 32(5), pp. 1018–1023.

Bull, F.C. and Bauman, A.E., 2011. Physical inactivity: The "Cinderella" risk factor for noncommunicable disease prevention. *Journal of Health Communication,* 16(Suppl2), pp. 13–26.

Caspersen, C.J., 1989. Physical activity epidemiology: Concepts, methods, and applications to exercise science. *Exercise and Sport Sciences Reviews,* 17, pp. 423–473.

Chen, K.Y. and Bassett, D.R., Jr, 2005. The technology of accelerometry-based activity monitors: Current and future. *Medicine and Science in Sports and Exercise,* 37(11 Suppl), pp. S490–500.

Costa, S., Ogilvie, D., Dalton, A., Westgate, K., Brage, S. and Panter, J., 2015. Quantifying the physical activity energy expenditure of commuters using a combination of global positioning system and combined heart rate and movement sensors. *Preventive Medicine,* 81, pp. 339–344.

Craig, R., Mindell, J. and Hirani, V., 2008. *Health Survey for England 2008. Vol. 1: Physical Activity and Fitness.* Leeds: NHS Information Centre for Health and Social Care.

De Cocker, K.A., De Bourdeaudhuij, I.M., Brown, W.J. and Cardon, G.M., 2007. Effects of "10,000 steps Ghent": A whole-community intervention. *American Journal of Preventive Medicine,* 33(6), pp. 455–463.

Dollman, J., Okely, A.D., Hardy, L., Timperio, A., Salmon, J. and Hills, A.P., 2009. A hitchhiker's guide to assessing young people's physical activity: Deciding what method to use. *Journal of Science and Medicine in Sport / Sports Medicine Australia,* 12(5), pp. 518–525.

Dong, L., Block, G. and Mandel, S., 2004. Activities contributing to total energy expenditure in the United States: Results from the NHAPS study. *The International Journal of Behavioral Nutrition and Physical Activity,* 1(1), pp. 4.

Dunton, G.F., Liao, Y., Intille, S.S., Spruijt-Metz, D. and Pentz, M., 2011. Investigating children's physical activity and sedentary behavior using ecological momentary assessment with mobile phones. *Obesity (Silver Spring, Md.),* 19(6), pp. 1205–1212.

Dunton, G.F., Whalen, C.K., Jamner, L.D., Henker, B. and Floro, J.N., 2005. Using ecologic momentary assessment to measure physical activity during adolescence. *American Journal of Preventive Medicine*, 29(4), pp. 281–287.

Eisner, E.W., 1997. The new frontier in qualitative research methodology. *Qualitative Inquiry*, 3(3), pp. 259–273.

Ferris, T.L., 2004. A new definition of measurement. *Measurement*, 36(1), pp. 101–109.

Freak-Poli, R.L., Cumpston, M., Peeters, A. and Clemes, S.A., 2013. Workplace pedometer interventions for increasing physical activity. *The Cochrane Database of Systematic Reviews*, 4, pp. CD009209.

Haskell, W.L., 2001. What to look for in assessing responsiveness to exercise in a health context. *Medicine and Science in Sports and Exercise*, 33(6 Suppl), pp. S454–S458; discussion S493–S494.

Irwin, M.L., Ainsworth, B.E. and Conway, J.M., 2001. Estimation of energy expenditure from physical activity measures: Determinants of accuracy. *Obesity Research*, 9(9), pp. 517–525.

Jago, R., Baranowski, T., Baranowski, J.C., Cullen, K.W. and Thompson, D.I., 2007. Social desirability is associated with some physical activity, psychosocial variables and sedentary behavior but not self-reported physical activity among adolescent males. *Health Education Research*, 22(3), pp. 438–449.

Jones, I., Brown, L. and Holloway, I., 2012. *Qualitative research in sport and physical activity*. UK: Sage.

Katzmarzyk, P.T. and Tremblay, M.S., 2007. Limitations of Canada's physical activity data: Implications for monitoring trends. *Canadian Journal of Public Health = Revue canadienne de sante publique*, 98(Suppl 2), pp. S185–194.

Kesaniemi, Y.K., Danforth, E., Jr, Jensen, M.D., Kopelman, P.G., Lefebvre, P. and Reeder, B.A., 2001. Dose-response issues concerning physical activity and health: An evidence-based symposium. *Medicine and Science in Sports and Exercise*, 33(6 Suppl), pp. S351–358.

Lagerros, Y.T., 2009. Physical activity – the more we measure, the more we know how to measure. *European Journal of Epidemiology*, 24(3), pp. 119–122.

Lagerros, Y.T. and Lagiou, P., 2007. Assessment of physical activity and energy expenditure in epidemiological research of chronic diseases. *European Journal of Epidemiology*, 22(6), pp. 353–362.

Lamonte, M.J. and Ainsworth, B.E., 2001. Quantifying energy expenditure and physical activity in the context of dose response. *Medicine and Science in Sports and Exercise*, 33(6 Suppl), pp. S370–378; discussion S419–420.

LaPorte, R.E., Montoye, H.J. and Caspersen, C.J., 1985. Assessment of physical activity in epidemiologic research: Problems and prospects. *Public Health Reports (Washington, D.C.: 1974)*, 100(2), pp. 131–146.

Lee, J.M., Kim, Y. and Welk, G.L., 2014. Validity of consumer-based physical activity monitors. Medicine and Science in Sports and Exercise, 46(9), pp. 1840–1848.

Livingstone, M.B., 1997. Heart-rate monitoring: The answer for assessing energy expenditure and physical activity in population studies? *The British Journal of Nutrition*, 78(6), pp. 869–871.

Livingstone, M.B., Prentice, A.M., Coward, W.A., Ceesay, S.M., Strain, J.J., McKenna, P.G., Nevin, G.B., Barker, M.E. and Hickey, R.J., 1990. Simultaneous measurement of free-living energy expenditure by the doubly labeled water method and heart-rate monitoring. *The American Journal of Clinical Nutrition*, 52(1), pp. 59–65.

Loveday, A., Sherar, L.B., Sanders, J.P., Sanderson, P.W. and Esliger, D.W., 2015. Technologies that assess the location of physical activity and sedentary behavior: A systematic review. *Journal of Medical Internet Research*, 17(8), pp. e192.

Maas, S., Kok, M.L., Westra, H.G. and Kemper, H.C., 1989. The validity of the use of heart rate in estimating oxygen consumption in static and in combined static/dynamic exercise. *Ergonomics*, 32(2), pp. 141–148.

Macera, C.A. and Pratt, M., 2000. Public health surveillance of physical activity. *Research Quarterly for Exercise and Sport*, 71(2 Suppl), pp. S97–103.

Mahar, M.T. and Rowe, D.A., 2002. Construct validity in physical activity research. In: Welk, G.J., editor. *Physical Activity Assessments for Health-Related Research*. Champaign, IL: Human Kinetics, 51–72.

McKenzie, T.L., 2010. 2009 CH McCloy lecture seeing is believing: Observing physical activity and its contexts. *Research Quarterly for Exercise and Sport*, 81(2), pp. 113–122.

McKenzie, T.L., Marshall, S.J., Sallis, J.F. and Conway, T.L., 2000. Leisure-time physical activity in school environments: An observational study using SOPLAY. *Preventive Medicine*, 30(1), pp. 70–77.

McKenzie, T.L., Sallis, J. and Nader, P., 1991. System for observing fitness instruction time. *Journal of Teaching in Physical Education*, 11, pp. 195–205.

Milton, K., Clemes, S. and Bull, F., 2013. Can a single question provide an accurate measure of physical activity? *British Journal of Sports Medicine,* 47(1), pp. 44–48.

Montoye, H.J., 2000. Introduction: Evaluation of some measurements of physical activity and energy expenditure. *Medicine and Science in Sports and Exercise,* 32(9 Suppl), pp. S439–441.

Montoye, H.J., Kemper, H.C., Saris, W.H. and Washburn, R.A., 1996. *Measuring physical activity and energy expenditure.* Champaign, IL: Human Kinetics.

Montoye, H.J. and Taylor, H.L., 1984. Measurement of physical activity in population studies: A review. *Human Biology,* 56(2), pp. 195–216.

Motl, R.W., McAuley, E. and Distefano, C., 2005. Is social desirability associated with self-reported physical activity? *Preventive Medicine,* 40(6), pp. 735–739.

Parker, S.B., Hurley, B.F., Hanlon, D.P. and Vaccaro, P., 1989. Failure of target heart rate to accurately monitor intensity during aerobic dance. *Medicine and Science in Sports and Exercise,* 21(2), pp. 230–234.

Pettee, K.K., Storti, K.L., Ainsworth, B.E. and Kriska, A.M., 2009. Measurement of physical activity and inactivity in epidemiologic studies. In: Lee, I-M., editor. *Epidemiological Methods in Physical Activity Studies.* New York: Oxford University Press, 15–33.

Prince, S.A., Adamo, K.B., Hamel, M.E., Hardt, J., Connor Gorber, S. and Tremblay, M., 2008. A comparison of direct versus self-report measures for assessing physical activity in adults: A systematic review. *The International Journal of Behavioral Nutrition and Physical Activity,* 6(5), pp. 56.

Rennie, K.L. and Wareham, N.J., 1998. The validation of physical activity instruments for measuring energy expenditure: problems and pitfalls. *Public Health Nutrition,* 1(4), pp. 265–271.

Rowlands, A.V. and Eston, R.G., 2007. The measurement and interpretation of children's physical activity. *Journal of Sports Science & Medicine,* 6(3), pp. 270–276.

Sallis, J.F. and Saelens, B.E., 2000. Assessment of physical activity by self-report: Status, limitations, and future directions. *Research Quarterly for Exercise and Sport,* 71(Suppl 2), pp. 1–14.

Sanders, J.P., Loveday, A., Pearson, N., Edwardson, C., Yates, T., Biddle, S.J. and Esliger, D.W., 2016. Devices for self-monitoring sedentary time or physical activity: A scoping review. *Journal of Medical Internet Research,* 18(5), pp. e90.

Schmidt, M.D., Cleland, V.J., Thomson, R.J., Dwyer, T. and Venn, A.J., 2008. A comparison of subjective and objective measures of physical activity and fitness in identifying associations with cardiometabolic risk factors. *Annals of Epidemiology,* 18(5), pp. 378–386.

Shephard, R.J., 2003. Limits to the measurement of habitual physical activity by questionnaires. *British Journal of Sports Medicine,* 37(3), pp. 197–206; discussion 206.

Smith, A.W., Cronin, K.A., Bowles, H., Willis, G., Jacobs, D.R., Jr, Ballard-Barbash, R. and Troiano, R.P., 2013. Reproducibility of physical activity recall over fifteen years: Longitudinal evidence from the CARDIA study. *BMC Public Health,* 28(13), pp. 180.

Strath, S.J., Bassett, D.R., Jr and Swartz, A.M., 2003. Comparison of MTI accelerometer cut-points for predicting time spent in physical activity. *International Journal of Sports Medicine,* 24(4), pp. 298–303.

Strath, S.J., Kaminsky, L.A., Ainsworth, B.E., Ekelund, U., Freedson, P.S., Gary, R.A., Richardson, C.R., Smith, D.T., Swartz, A.M. and American Heart Association Physical Activity Committee of the Council on Lifestyle and Cardiometabolic Health and Cardiovascular, Exercise, Cardiac Rehabilitation and Prevention Committee of the Council on Clinical Cardiology, and Council, 2013. Guide to the assessment of physical activity: Clinical and research applications: A scientific statement from the American Heart Association. *Circulation,* 128(20), pp. 2259–2279.

Strath, S.J., Swartz, A.M., Bassett, D.R., Jr, O'Brien, W.L., King, G.A. and Ainsworth, B.E., 2000. Evaluation of heart rate as a method for assessing moderate intensity physical activity. *Medicine and Science in Sports and Exercise,* 32(9 Suppl), pp. S465–470.

Sydenham, P., 1985. Structured understanding of the measurement process: Part 1: Holistic view of the measurement system. *Measurement,* 3(3), pp. 115–120.

Sydenham, P.H., 2003. Relationship between measurement, knowledge and advancement. *Measurement,* 34(1), pp. 3–16.

Timperio, A., Salmon, J., Rosenberg, M. and Bull, F.C., 2004. Do logbooks influence recall of physical activity in validation studies? *Medicine and Science in Sports and Exercise,* 36(7), pp. 1181–1186.

Tremblay, M.S. and Connor Gorber, S., 2007. Canadian health measures survey: Brief overview. *Canadian Journal of Public Health = Revue canadienne de santé publique,* 98(6), pp. 453–456.

Troiano, R.P., Berrigan, D., Dodd, K.W., Masse, L.C., Tilert, T. and Mcdowell, M., 2008. Physical activity in the United States measured by accelerometer. *Medicine and Science in Sports and Exercise,* 40(1), pp. 181.

Troiano, R.P., McClain, J.J., Brychta, R.J. and Chen, K.Y., 2014. Evolution of accelerometer methods for physical activity research. *British Journal of Sports Medicine,* 48(13), pp. 1019–1023.

Tudor-Locke, C., Bassett, D.R., Shipe, M.F. and Mcclain, J.J., 2011. Pedometry methods for assessing free-living adults. *Journal of Physical Activity & Health,* 8(3), pp. 445–453.

Tudor-Locke, C., Hatano, Y., Pangrazi, R.P. and Kang, M., 2008. Revisiting "how many steps are enough?". *Medicine and Science in Sports and Exercise,* 40(7), pp. S537.

UK Biobank, UK Biobank. Available: www.ukbiobank.ac.uk/ [03, 2016].

Van Hees, V.T., Slootmaker, S.M., De Groot, G., Van Mechelen, W. and Van Lummel, R.C., 2009. Reproducibility of a triaxial seismic accelerometer (DynaPort). *Medicine and Science in Sports and Exercise,* 41(4), pp. 810–817.

Van Poppel, M.N., Chinapaw, M.J., Mokkink, L.B., Van Mechelen, W. and Terwee, C.B., 2010. Physical activity questionnaires for adults: A systematic review of measurement properties. *Sports Medicine (Auckland, N.Z.),* 40(7), pp. 565–600.

Walter, P.L., 2007. The history of the accelerometer: 1920s-1996-prologue and epilogue, 2006. *Sound & Vibration,* 41(1), pp. 84–90.

Ward, D.S., Evenson, K.R., Vaughn, A., Rodgers, A.B. and Troiano, R.P., 2005. Accelerometer use in physical activity: Best practices and research recommendations. *Medicine and Science in Sports and Exercise,* 37(Suppl 11), pp. S582–88.

Wareham, N.J. and Rennie, K.L., 1998. The assessment of physical activity in individuals and populations: Why try to be more precise about how physical activity is assessed? *International Journal of Obesity and Related Metabolic Disorders: Journal of the International Association for the Study of Obesity,* 22(Suppl 2), pp. S30–38.

Warnecke, R.B., Johnson, T.P., Chavez, N., Sudman, S., O'Rourke, D.P., Lacey, L. and Horm, J., 1997. Improving question wording in surveys of culturally diverse populations. *Annals of Epidemiology,* 7(5), pp. 334–342.

Welk, G., 2002. *Physical activity assessments for health-related research.* USA: Human Kinetics.

Welk, G.J., Corbin, C.B. and Dale, D., 2000. Measurement issues in the assessment of physical activity in children. *Research Quarterly for Exercise and Sport,* 71(2 Suppl), pp. S59–73.

Westerterp, K.R., 2009. Assessment of physical activity: A critical appraisal. *European Journal of Applied Physiology,* 105(6), pp. 823–828.

Wilmore, J.H. and Haskell, W.L., 1971. Use of the heart rate-energy expenditure relationship in the individualized prescription of exercise. *The American Journal of Clinical Nutrition,* 24(9), pp. 1186–1192.

Zhang, K., Pi-Sunyer, F.X. and Boozer, C.N., 2004. Improving energy expenditure estimation for physical activity. *Medicine and Science in Sports and Exercise,* 36(5), pp. 883–889.

Zhang, K., Werner, P., Sun, M., Pi-Sunyer, F.X. and Boozer, C.N., 2003. Measurement of human daily physical activity. *Obesity Research,* 11(1), pp. 33–40.

THEME C INTRODUCTION
Policy communities and physical activity

The third theme in the Handbook focuses on policy communities in physical activity. Notwithstanding diverse and competing conceptualisations about policy communities they can usefully be understood as sets of actors who coalesce around, and shape, policy making about an issue – in this case physical activity. Physical activity policy communities contribute to enhancing, challenging and indeed undermining the policy making process. A key aim in analysing policy communities in these chapters is to understand who makes decisions about physical activity, how those decisions are made and in whose interests. There is no scope within a single theme to address all policy communities in the physical activity sector. The selected chapters nevertheless illustrate the complex network of actors and relationships, beyond state-bureaucratic ones, that characterise multiple types of policy community with common and competing interests and diverse and unequal influences on policy making about physical activity.

The first chapter by Guy Faulkner and Markus Duncan focuses on the significance of physical activity in the treatment and prevention of depression. Faulkner and Duncan explain that despite the evidence for exercise as therapy, the prescription and promotion of exercise programmes for preventing and treating depression is limited. There appears to be a knowledge-practice gap between the mental health professional and physical activity delivery communities. The chapter concludes that policy making in both mental health and physical activity spheres needs to recognise the evidence for the benefits of exercise and develop knowledge exchange between the communities to ensure the full potential of physical activity is realised in policy making and promotion of population level mental health.

The next two chapters address issues of the environment and physical activity in different contexts. The reprint of Hugh Barton, Michael Horswell and Paul Millar's paper has been included for its examination of UK urban planning policy in relation to the promotion of neighbourhood active travel for public health. Barton and colleagues argue that despite political and policy prioritisation, the extent to which planning can reshape the environment to change physical activity behaviours is complex and contested. In their study of four English cities, the pattern of use of local facilities and the degree to which people engage in active travel to access them is variable. Distance and 'walkability' is identified as a key factor in reducing car use, but local variations in patterns then depend on the type of facility being accessed, social grouping and the specific character of the location and place. It appears that individual attitudes to active travel do not predict behaviours but that community values about some behaviours such as walking and bike use are important in understanding dispositions to engage in active travel. The views of local people should inform decision making about active travel in neighbourhood policy communities. Barbara Humberstone, Heather Prince and Lois Mansfield turn attention from urban to rural environments in a discussion about policy and practice of the outdoors and physical activity. Highlighting the significance of nature-based practices in creating learning opportunities for physical activity, health and wellbeing, the authors examine the challenges that arise in developing sustainable use of the natural environment for outdoor recreation. There is a long history of tension and conflict in the use and misuse of land and waterscapes for physical activity. Humberstone, Prince and Mansfield propose a pedagogical approach, instilled in school-based education strategies, to create spaces for learning about the natural environment, sustainable practices of outdoor recreation and the promotion of an environmental ethic of physical activity.

Examining the interplay between sport and physical activity policy communities in the UK, Pippa Chapman's chapter highlights a history of difference and convergence in decision making agendas. Chapman emphasises that the UK sport policy agenda has always been based on the twin objectives of promoting elite performance and mass participation. Such participation and performance goals present different opportunities and outcomes for using sport to promote population level rises in physical activity. She highlights that advocacy of elite sport as a means of inspiring people to take part in physical activity in the UK and worldwide remains political rhetoric. Moreover, whilst the mass participation policy agenda has always been about encouraging people to take part, it has more recently been aligned with policy goals for increasing physical activity for public health. For Chapman, this signals a contemporary convergence between sport, physical activity and health sector communities in terms of the promotion of health and wellbeing. However, it creates challenges to the sport sector through policy taking approaches which serve to weaken the policy agenda for some sports in some contexts.

The final two chapters examine policy communities involved in the education of children and young people through physical activity. Stephanie Alexander examines the establishment of 'active play' interventions for children through physical activity policy in Canada. Alexander argues that rather than child's play being promoted for play's sake, policy and strategy in Canada fixes play to the production of the disciplined, healthy, happy, good Canadian citizen. Play strategies involve the surveillance and monitoring of children's play by adults and indeed by the children themselves. For Alexander, play has become a highly regulated physical activity through which children learn established messages about health, moral values and Canadian citizenship. Andy Smith, Ken Green and Miranda Thurston provide a critical expose of the ways that schools and teachers are increasingly responsible for a range of physical activity, health and wellbeing outcomes, especially through the delivery of physical education. This chapter sets out the policy context for promoting education as a context for increasing levels of physical activity and examines the role of physical education in this regard. Smith and colleagues discuss the limits of such policy agendas for promoting life-long participation in physical activity through school-based approaches. The chapter illustrates that education, schooling and physical education are one part of a young person's life that may have both enabling and constraining effects on physical activity in the short and long term. More influential are family relationships and the social determinants of physical activity which remain diverse and unequal in the UK and worldwide.

12

PHYSICAL ACTIVITY AND MENTAL HEALTH

A focus on depression

Guy Faulkner and Markus Duncan

There is a compelling and extensive body of literature supporting the role of physical activity in enhancing and maintaining physical health. Over the last decade there has been rapid growth in research findings concerning the mental health benefits of physical activity. The journal *Mental Health and Physical Activity* is dedicated to the topic while 2013 saw the publication of the most comprehensive synthesis to date on the subject (Ekkekakis 2013a). The collective body of evidence presents a strong case that physical activity similarly helps enhance and maintain many dimensions of mental health. As Boreham and Riddoch (2003, p. 24) neatly encapsulated, "from the cradle to the grave, regular physical activity appears to be an essential ingredient for human well-being".

What is mental health?

The terms mental health and mental illness are commonly differentiated as they are not mutually exclusive. Mental health has been defined as a state of well-being in which the individual realizes his or her own potential, can cope with the normal stresses of life, can work productively and fruitfully, and is able to make a contribution to her or his own community (WHO 2001). In contrast, mental illness is any health condition characterized by alterations in thinking, mood, or behaviour (or some combination thereof) associated with distress and/or impaired functioning (United States Department of Health and Human Services 1999); common examples include depression or anxiety. Referred to as a two continua model of mental illness and mental health, the model holds that both are related, but distinct dimensions: one continuum indicates the presence or absence of mental health, the other the presence or absence of mental illness (Westerhof & Keyes 2010). This has important implications. First, it allows the possibility of being diagnosed as having a mental illness but still having the capacity to achieve positive mental health. As such it justifies the promotion of mental health to individuals with a mental illness rather than just considering treatment or prevention. Second, mental health problems such as subclinical levels of depression or anxiety can affect us all without necessarily becoming a clinical, diagnosed condition. Consequently, mental health promotion has the capacity to improve the quality of life of clinical and non-clinical populations alike (Faulkner, Trinh, & Arbour-Nicitopoulos 2015). Mental health promotion might be seen as a form of inoculation to prevent or alleviate poor mental health.

Physical activity promotion as mental health promotion

Physical activity promotion has a number of positive attributes that make it an attractive approach to promoting mental health. First, it could be a cost-effective alternative for those preferring not to use medication or who cannot access therapy. For example, non-drug treatments such as cognitive behavioural therapy can be costly and difficult to access. Although not without methodological limitations, the Fraser Institute in Canada publishes reports on waiting times for psychiatric treatment. This consists of two components: waiting after being referred by a general practitioner before consultation with a psychiatrist, and then waiting to receive treatment after the first consultation with a psychiatrist. For Canada as a whole, the total waiting time in 2009 was estimated at 16.8 weeks (Esmail 2009). In the UK, the national average waiting time from referral to treatment (psychological therapies) is approximately 5 weeks although there is also considerable national variation with some having median waits of 3 months or longer (Health and Social Care Information Centre 2014).

Second, physical activity is associated with negligible deleterious side-effects. Compare this to concerns about antidepressant medication. A well-publicized systematic review (Sharma et al. 2016) reported that the risk of suicidality and aggression doubled in children and adolescents taking antidepressants (selective serotonin and serotonin-norepinephrine reuptake inhibitors). Third, physical activity is an effective method for improving important aspects of physical health thus the promotion of physical activity for mental health can be seen as a "win-win" situation with both mental and physical health benefits accruing (Faulkner, Hefferon, & Mutrie 2015). Fourth, given the scope of the burden of poor mental health, there is the need for population-based promotion, prevention, and treatment strategies. Attempts are already made to promote physical activity at a population level, for example, through social marketing campaigns developed by public health agencies and the development and dissemination of physical activity guidelines. Arguably, physical activity is a scalable, population level intervention for promoting mental health unlike pharmacotherapy and counselling (Faulkner, Trinh, & Arbour-Nicitopoulos 2015).

Given that a comprehensive review of existing research on physical activity and mental health is beyond the scope of a single chapter, the purpose of this chapter is to focus on the case for physical activity as a strategy to prevent and treat depression. A brief overview of potential mechanisms will be provided before a focus on implications for policy and practice of the existing evidence. In examining the case of depression, it is important to acknowledge that physical activity has a vital role to play in promoting positive mental health beyond a focus on mental illness.

A focus on depression

Depression is a common mental illness that is prevalent globally. It is estimated that 350 million people are currently affected by depression and by the year 2020, it is predicted to be the leading cause of disability worldwide (Ferrari et al. 2013; WHO 2012). This projection is concerning given the impact of depression on overall health and well-being. Depression is associated with a range of symptoms including low energy, lack of interest, low self-worth; poor sleeping patterns and appetite; and overwhelming feelings of sadness and anxiety (WHO 2012). Kessler and Bromet (2013) reviewed international data summarizing other psychosocial and secondary disorders linked with depression and these included reduced role functioning (e.g., low marital and work performance quality) and an elevated risk of chronic secondary disorders such as cancer, cardiovascular disease, and diabetes.

The adverse health effects of depression extend beyond the individual. As a result of lost work productivity and health care costs, the incremental economic burden of depression has risen from $83.1 billion to $210.5 billion between the years 2000 and 2010 in the United States (Greenberg et al. 2015). With the high prevalence of depression and its burden on health and the economy, there is an urgent need to halt these growing trends. Hence, the World Health Organization (2012) declared that preventing depression is an area that warrants urgent attention. One modifiable health behavior shown to prevent the onset of depression is physical activity.

Physical activity as prevention

Mammen and Faulkner (2013) reviewed studies with a longitudinal design examining relationships between physical activity and depression over at least two time intervals. A total of 25 of the 30 studies found a significant, inverse relationship between baseline physical activity and follow-up depression, suggesting that physical activity is preventive in the onset of depression. Given the different ways physical activity was measured in the reviewed studies, a clear dose-response relationship between physical activity and reduced depression was not readily apparent. However, there was evidence that any level of physical activity, including low levels, can prevent future depression. Further, everyday activities such as walking appear to confer a benefit. Meeting the recommended levels of physical activity, established for physical health benefits, appears equally appropriate for preventing depression. Data from the studies also suggest for individuals who are currently active to sustain their physical activity habits and those who are inactive to initiate a physically active lifestyle to help reduce the odds of developing depression.

Such studies involve large numbers of people and measure physical activity status prior to the incidence of depression. In one example, Lucas and colleagues (2011) conducted a prospective analysis involving 49,821 US women from the Nurses' Health Study who were free from depressive symptoms at baseline (1996). Physical activity was self-reported in 1992, 1994, 1996, 1998, and 2000. Having clinical depression was defined as reporting either a new physician's diagnosis of depression or beginning regular use of antidepressant medication. After controlling for a range of potential covariates such as socioeconomic status and physical limitations, there was an inverse age-adjusted dose-response relation between duration of physical activity and depression risk. Depression risk decreased with increasing time spent walking daily at an 'average pace' (<20 min/day, relative risk (RR) = 0.94; 20–40 min/day, RR = 0.94; ≥40 min/day, RR = 0.80) or brisk/very brisk pace (<20 min/day, RR = 0.95; 20–40 min/day, RR = 0.88; ≥40 min/day, RR = 0.83).

Although these findings are consistent, they cannot rule out the potential for self-selection and other forms of measurement bias. It is possible that individuals who are more physically active represent a selection of people who happened to have greater education, be of higher socioeconomic status, or social support networks that made them less likely to develop depression, irrespective of their participation in physical activity. However, even when these studies take account of a wide range of possible confounding factors in the statistical modelling (e.g., disability, body mass index, smoking, alcohol, and socioeconomic status), the relationship between physical activity and a decreased risk of depression remains. Despite consistency in the literature regarding a protective function of physical activity, some caution is required given that there may be a number of other factors, such as genetic variations (De Moor et al. 2008), that predict both physical activity and depression and these may not have been fully accounted for in the reviewed studies (Mammen & Faulkner 2013).

Exercise as treatment

Intervention literature for clinical depression emerged in the late 1970s (e.g., Greist et al. 1979) and 80s (e.g., McCann & Holmes 1984). In the case of treatment the focus has been on the impact of exercise – physical activity that is structured, often supervised, and undertaken with the aim of maintaining or improving physical fitness or health. An influential Cochrane review conducted by Cooney and colleagues (2013) identified 39 randomized controlled trials (RCTs) and a meta-analysis of these studies showed a moderate effect size (−0.62 (95% confidence interval (CI) −0.81 to −0.42)), for exercise versus no treatment control conditions. Pooled data from eight trials (377 participants) reporting long-term follow-up data found a small effect for exercise (standardized mean difference (SMD) −0.33, 95% CI from −0.63 to −0.03). For the six trials considered to be at low risk of methodological bias, a further analysis showed a small clinical effect in favour of exercise, which did not reach statistical significance (SMD −0.18, 95% CI from −0.47 to 0.11). This latter analysis has been critiqued given questionable inclusion and exclusion criteria (Ekkekakis 2015). Three of the six studies did not include adequate comparators (e.g., compared different doses of exercise). With the analysis restricted to three high-quality trials, the pooled SMD was significantly different from zero (SMD −0.33, 95% CI from −0.59 to −0.07).

Seven trials in the Cochrane review compared exercise with psychological therapy (189 participants), and found no significant difference (SMD −0.03, 95% CI from −0.32 to 0.26). Four trials (n = 300) compared exercise with pharmacological treatment and found no significant difference (SMD −0.11, −0.34, 0.12). In the most well-cited example, the effects of aerobic exercise were compared to sertraline (Zoloft) treatment among 156 older adults with depression (Blumenthal et al. 1999). Participants were randomized to either aerobic exercise (three times per week at 70–85% of their heart rate reserve), sertraline (an antidepressant), or combined sertraline and exercise for 16 weeks. After 16 weeks of treatment, patients in all three groups exhibited significant reductions in depressive symptoms. Notably patients responded more quickly in the medication group. After 10 months, remitted participants (those who no longer met diagnostic criteria for depression) in the exercise group had significantly lower relapse rates than participants in the medication group (Babyak et al. 2000).

Remarkably, Cooney et al. (2013), concluded that exercise appears to be no more effective than psychological or pharmacological therapies. A more suitable conclusion is that exercise appears to be as effective as psychological or pharmacological therapies, and is another evidence-based option for patients and treatment providers to consider. Other meta-analyses consistently report similar findings. Silveira et al. (2013) combined data from 10 RCTs and identified a 0.61 (95% CI from −0.88 to −0.33) standard deviation reduction in the exercise intervention group compared to the control group. Danielsson et al. (2013) reported that aerobic exercise had a similar and positive effect to antidepressants in two trials. Josefsson, Lindwall, and Archer (2014) found an overall effect size of 0.77 (n = 13; 95% CI from −1.14, −0.41) in favour of exercise compared to control conditions. Rosenbaum et al. (2014) reported a large effect of physical activity on depressive symptoms (n = 20; SMD 0.80). The effect for trials with higher methodological quality was smaller than that for trials with lower quality (SMD 0.39 vs 1.35) although this difference was not statistically significant. Another recent meta-analysis determined that the control groups used in many exercise and depression RCTs experienced large and significant improvements in depressive symptoms and these improvements were approximately double that reported in antidepressant meta-analyses (Stubbs et al. 2016). Accordingly, demonstrating a "strong" antidepressant effect of exercise has been challenging thus far.

As with any research endeavour questions always remain. There are methodological limitations to the existing research that largely reflect the behavioural nature of exercise interventions. Treatment blinding is impossible and there is likely a self-selection bias where study participants are choosing to participate in an exercise intervention for the treatment of depression. Further research is required as to what conditions and for whom exercise is most likely to help. In terms of dosage, one review (Stanton & Reaburn 2014) examined the dose characteristics of five RCTs that reported a significant treatment effect of exercise in the treatment of depression. They concluded that the exercise dose should likely use supervised aerobic exercise, and occur three times weekly at moderate intensity for a minimum of nine weeks in the treatment of depression. A similar dosage was recommended in an additional systematic review (Nyström et al. 2015).

How does exercise reduce depression?

As per the Bradford-Hill criteria (Hill 1965) for making a case for causality, it is important to understand potential mechanisms of the antidepressant effect of exercise. Several plausible biological and psychosocial mechanisms have been proposed for the efficacy of exercise in treating depression. The primary biological mechanisms that have been suggested can be broadly categorized as changes in 1) neurochemistry or 2) neuroplasticity. Changes in brain neurochemistry refer to altering the amount of neurotransmitters available in the synapses between neurons, and is the primary target of psychiatric medications. Neuroplasticity on the other hand is the creation of new neurons (neurogenesis) and new connections between neurons (synaptogenesis), and is a relatively novel mechanism that has been proposed.

Much of the understanding behind the biological mechanisms that may improve depression symptoms stems from a knowledge of the pharmacodynamic effects of antidepressant medications (Nutt 2008). The most common types of antidepressants are serotonin reuptake inhibitors (SSRIs) and tricyclic antidepressants (TCAs), which primarily increase the amount of serotonin in the brain, an important chemical for mood regulation. Similar to these medications exercise has also been shown to increase serotonin availability, which may explain its anti-depressant effects. It is well established that in animals, an acute bout of exercise is consistently shown to increase both hippocampal (a key brain region in depression) (Meeusen et al. 1996; Wilson & Marsden 1996) and whole brain serotonin concentration (see Meeusen & De Meirleir 1995). In humans where directly measuring serotonin in the brain is not possible, acute bouts of exercise increase free tryptophan (the amino acid precursor of serotonin) in the blood, which is a marker of serotonin production in the brain (Melancon, Lorrain, & Dionne 2012; Nybo et al. 2003). Additionally, exercise also seems to increase the availability of norepinephrine and dopamine, which are other neurotransmitters that have been implicated in depression (Alsuwaidan et al. 2009). Overall, it seems that exercise, like antidepressants, tends to increase the amount of serotonin available and other mood regulating neurotransmitters, which may be one way that exercise improves depression symptoms.

In addition to changing brain chemistry, antidepressants also increase neuroplasticity in the hippocampus and other mood related areas of the brain (Sahay & Hen 2007). Increases in neurogenesis and synaptogenesis have been identified in animals in response to administering antidepressants (Sahay & Hen 2007; Mahar et al. 2014). At least one study has shown that neurogenesis mediates the improvement of depression-like symptoms in a mouse model (Hill, Sahay, & Hen 2015).

Similarly, imaging studies of humans have shown increases in brain volume in the dentate gyrus and hippocampus (Boldrini et al. 2012; Mahar et al. 2014). Exercise appears to induce the same proliferation of neurons, at least in animal models (Chen 2013). In humans the results are mixed. Only one study has attempted to examine neural growth among patients with depression in response to exercise, and found no change in any of the markers of growth (Krogh et al. 2014). However, other studies have shown growth is possible in response to exercise (Pajonk et al. 2010; Erickson et al. 2011), and thus it should not be discounted as a potential mechanism given the evidence from antidepressant medication.

Overall, it appears that exercise may induce the same physiological changes as antidepressants, which may explain the benefits of exercise for symptoms of depression. As neurochemistry is constantly changing in response to external stimuli, this may be more responsible for acute effects of exercise on depression. In order to reap long-term benefits via these mechanisms, patients must undertake physical activity on a regular basis, similar to a typical prescription for an anti-depressant. On the other-hand, changes in brain anatomy are the result of a cascade of signals and develops over time. Therefore it is reasonable to hypothesize that this mechanism may be responsible for maintenance of remission and prevention. However, in keeping with the "use it or lose it" principle of neurology (Millington 2012), a regular dose of exercise is likely warranted to maintain any beneficial changes in brain anatomy over time. As a result, regardless of which biological mechanisms may be at work, regular physical activity is advisable.

While it may be argued from a reductionist perspective that psychosocial mechanisms may also fundamentally represent biological changes in neurochemistry and neuroanatomy, these changes are likely to be myriad, difficult to attribute directly to exercise, and spread throughout the brain. Several psychosocial mechanisms have been proposed including improvements in self-evaluations (e.g., self esteem), distraction from negative thoughts, and affect regulation (whereby patients are able to manage their current feeling state by engaging in acute bouts of exercise as they feel they need to) (Craft 2013). Correspondingly, depression is characterized by negative self-evaluation, rumination on negative thoughts, persistent depressed mood, and is often brought on or worsened by stress (American Psychiatric Association 2013). While the distractibility of PA is debatable, and likely highly dependent on context and ability of the participant (Craft 2013), the ability of exercise to improve self-evaluations (Spence, McGannon, & Poon 2005) and improve affect after an acute dose (Ekkekakis, Parfitt, & Petruzzello 2011) is well established. Despite this, relatively little research has examined whether these factors mediate the changes in depression as a result of physical activity.

Notably, one study has examined whether changes in coping self-efficacy – a component of self-evaluation – and distraction were related to changes in depression during an exercise intervention (Craft 2005). After controlling for baseline levels, increases in self-efficacy were correlated with lower depression levels, while distraction was not; ultimately, this led the author to conclude that there was stronger support for self-efficacy as a mechanism for treating depression than distraction.

As well, studies have shown that while acute bouts of exercise can improve affect among people with major depression (Bartholomew, Morrison, & Ciccolo 2005), it would be difficult from a practical perspective to examine whether brief improvements during single bouts of exercise translate into long-term reduction of symptoms. However, a recent self-report cross-sectional study of young adults found that moderate intensity exercise moderated depression symptoms among people with high levels of life stress (Maio, Sabiston, & O'Loughlin 2015), indicating that physical activity may help reduce depression by moderating stress – a negative emotion. Due to the limited research in this area, the psychosocial mechanisms proposed remain plausible factors in the use of exercise to treat depression. Just as there is a wide range of medications available with slightly differing mechanisms of action, it is reasonable to consider that when physical activity works for depression, it may not be working in the same way for every individual. However, unlike medication, where the pharmacodynamics are well documented, and the mechanism is thereby presumed, the mechanisms behind the benefit of exercise are less definitive. The implications of this for legitimizing the role of exercise as a treatment for depression are unknown.

Exercise as therapy: Little to argue against it!

There is a relatively large and consistent body of literature that indicates being physically active prevents depression and that exercise can alleviate depressive symptoms. The effect appears comparable to other therapeutic approaches including medication. Also, there is a range of plausible mechanisms that explain why physical activity may have an antidepressant effect. From a population-health perspective, promoting physical activity may serve as a valuable mental health promotion strategy in reducing the risk of developing depression (Mammen & Faulkner 2013). Exercise also appears, on the surface at least, to be a cheap, safe, and accessible option for treating depression. Yet, how likely is someone seeking help for depression to be prescribed exercise as treatment?

One way to address this question is to consider national guidelines for the treatment of depression. We reviewed evidence based treatment guidelines for clinical depression in Canada, the United Kingdom (UK), the United States (US), and Australia and New Zealand (ANZ) (Malhi et al. 2015; National Collaborating Centre for Mental Health and National Institute for Health and Clinical Excellence, 2010; Ravindran et al. 2009; Work Group On Major Depressive Disorder 2010). Table 12.1 provides an overview of the guidelines. All four guidelines recommend exercise for the treatment of mild to moderate depression, at least as an adjunct, although each guideline varies in the nature of their endorsement of exercise.

While currently being revised, the Canadian Network for Mood and Anxiety Treatments (CANMAT) Clinical guidelines (Ravindran et al. 2009) for the management of major depressive disorder (MDD) in adults considers exercise within the portfolio of complementary and alternative medicine treatments. These include strategies such as light therapy, acupuncture, nutraceutical therapies (e.g., omega-3 fatty acids), and herbal therapies (e.g., St. John's Wort). Being categorized as such might conceivably signal to clinicians and the general public that exercise is not *mainstream* and possibly not even *medical treatment*. In terms of the specific guidelines regarding exercise, it was concluded that there was *Level 2* evidence for the benefit of exercise as adjunct to medications in mild to moderate MDD, but not as *monotherapy*. Level 2 evidence is defined as "at least 1 RCT with adequate sample size and/or meta-analysis with wide confidence intervals" (see Ravindran et al., 2009, p. S55). It is not clear how these conclusions were drawn given the number of appropriately sized RCTs and meta-analyses actually cited by the authors in reaching these conclusions – including two large RCTs demonstrating an antidepressant effect equal to medication. Such a lukewarm endorsement regarding the evidence for exercise in the context of depression suggests broader barriers to the acceptance and promotion of exercise as a credible treatment option for depression.

The US guidelines mention exercise in the "choice of initial treatment modality" subsection dealing with treating the acute phase of depression (Work Group On Major Depressive Disorder 2010). While exercise is recommended both as monotherapy and adjunct for acute treatment, in the guidelines it is simultaneously overlooked as a treatment by not being provided a distinct section like pharmacotherapy, psychotherapy, or

Table 12.1 Summary of recommendations for physical activity in depression treatment guidelines

Document Details			Treatment						Prevention	
Country	Year	Document Name	Severity: Sub-threshold	Severity: Mild to Moderate	Severity: Severe	Comorbidities	Dosage	How to Discuss or Prescribe	Depression in General Population	Relapse
Australia & New Zealand	2015	RANZCP Clinical Practice Guidelines for Mood Disorders	+ ★	+ ★	+ [Adjunct]★	+ General Health & Well-being + Physical Comorbidities + All people with depression	National Guidelines[1,2]: Most days of the week >150min MPA or >75min VPA /week	Active Encouragement; Motivation more challenging in Severe Depression	+	+
Canada	2009	CANMAT Clinical Guidelines – Complementary and Alternative Medicine Treatments	0	+ Second line treatment: + Adjunct to medications, – Monotherapy	0	0	8–20 weeks 3x/week 30–60min/session	0	0	+
United Kingdom (UK)	2010	NICE UK Guidelines	+ Monotherapy	+ Monotherapy	0	+ Sleep hygiene	Groups with competent support practitioner; 10–14 weeks 3x/week 45–60min/session	0	0	0
United States of America	2010	APA Practice Guidelines for the Treatment of Patients with MDD (3rd Edition)	+	+ Monotherapy	+ Adjunct	+ Weight & BMI + Overall health	Based on patient preferences and adherence	Face-to-face education, books, pamphlets, & trusted web sites provided by physician	+	0

Notes: + = Supports, – = Discourages, 0 = No statement. RANZCP = Royal Australia and New Zealand College of Psychiatrists, CANMAT = Canadian Network for Mood and Anxiety Treatments, NICE = National Institute for Health and Care Excellence, APA = American Psychiatric Association, MDD = Major Depressive Disorder, MPA = Moderate Physical Activity, VPA = Vigorous Physical Activity,

★ = No explicit recommendation on using physical activity (PA) as monotherapy or adjunct therapy based on severity, however guidelines state "motivating more severely depressed patients to engage [in PA] is a challenge" implying PA likely to be used as an adjunct in severe depression.

[1] (Brown et al. 2012).

[2] (Ministry of Health 2015).

complementary and alternative therapies such as St. John's Wort or light therapy. Specifically, while these other therapies receive an assessment of the level of evidence similar to the CANMAT guidelines, exercise does not receive a formal review of research quality despite relevant studies being cited throughout the document. Rather the evidence for exercise is briefly reviewed in the subsection: Provide Education to the Patient and the Family stating that "data generally support at least a modest improvement in mood symptoms for patients with major depressive disorder who engage in aerobic exercise . . . or resistance training" (p. 29). There is also brief mention that physical activity may reduce the prevalence of depressive symptoms in the general population. Despite the recommendations that exercise be considered for treatment, and may be useful in prevention, it is not included in a summary figure of treatment modalities on page 31. The wording used to describe exercise as a treatment modality is also notable: "if a patient with mild depression wishes to try exercise alone for several weeks as a first intervention, there is little to argue against it . . ." (p. 30). So true! Such a statement can be interpreted in a number of ways. One is that exercise is not a credible first choice strategy to be recommended by a mental health professional. These same guidelines also provide dosage recommendations for physicians to provide patients and suggest that the optimal regimen for physical activity is one that patients will follow. Educational brochures and pamphlets are suggested for discussing physical activity with patients.

In its stepped-care approach, the UK guidelines explicitly include physical activity as one of three low intensity psychosocial treatment options for people with persistent subthreshold depressive symptoms or mild to moderate depression (National Collaborating Centre for Mental Health and National Institute for Health and Clinical Excellence, 2010). These include individual guided self-help based on the principles of cognitive behavioural therapy (CBT), computerized cognitive behavioural therapy (CCBT), or a structured group physical activity programme. Such programmes should be delivered in groups with support from a competent practitioner and consist typically of three sessions per week of moderate duration (45 minutes to 1 hour) over 10 to 14 weeks (average 12 weeks). There is no mention of physical activity protecting against depression in the general population.

The most recent guidelines from Australia and New Zealand (Malhi et al. 2015) classify physical activity as a healthy lifestyle intervention along with diet and smoking cessation. Like the US guidelines, the new ANZ guidelines make recommendations for physical activity in each treatment category identified in Table 12.1. Specifically, recommendations include that physical activity can be used to prevent worsening of symptoms in sub-threshold depression and that physical activity has demonstrated to be an effective treatment, at least as an adjunct, for all levels of depression. There is, however, no explicit statement about when it would be appropriate to consider physical activity as a monotherapy, just that it may be more difficult to motivate individuals with more severe depression. Taken together the guidelines advocate for promoting physical activity for all patients with depression or depressive symptoms. Furthermore, the guidelines advocate a physical activity dose consistent with public health guidelines to promote overall health and well-being.

In addition to recognizing the efficacy in treating depression, the ANZ guidelines recommend physical activity for both preventing depression in the general population, citing the Mammen and Faulkner (2013) review, as well as preventing relapse for patients in the maintenance phase of treatment. As can be expected from the most recently released guidelines, the ANZ guidelines represent the most up-to-date collection of research on the use of physical activity to treat depression, and, much like the UK guidelines, have explicitly identified exercise as a therapeutic option.

Overall, Canadian, UK, US, and ANZ guidelines for treating depression all mention a role for exercise although the North American guidelines are more cautious. Importantly, only the UK guidelines suggest that exercise programmes be undertaken with the support of a trained professional. However, no guideline provides any information as to whom patients could or should be referred to in order to receive adequate support for engaging in exercise (e.g., registered kinesiologists or occupational therapists). Any elaboration of the potential role of physical activity protecting against depression is scant although this is not necessarily surprising given the treatment focus of the guidelines.

Implications for future physical activity policy and practice

A range of factors may speculatively explain why there is such caution in recommending the consideration of exercise as a treatment option. Little focused attention has been given to this potential gap between evidence and practice. One qualitative study explored perceptions of twenty-one course directors of clinical psychology programmes in the United Kingdom (Faulkner & Biddle 2001). While participants were broadly positive regarding physical activity there was little, if any, mention of its role as a treatment strategy within curricula. At that time at least, mental health professionals were likely not receiving any exposure to the research evidence concerning exercise and little training for implementation. It is also likely that a process for knowledge exchange between researchers conducting exercise and depression research and practitioners was, and still remains, not well established. As a result, exercise as a treatment may be peripheral to how mental health professionals are being trained to treat individuals with depression. An incompatibility of exercise with traditional models of understanding and treating depression may still remain for many (Faulkner & Biddle 2001). Disciplinary territorialism also likely plays a role in that "exercise" is considered the mandate of "other" professionals. As commented by one director (Faulkner & Biddle 2001, p. 441), "exercise does not appear as a 'terribly glamorous solution', neither 'clever enough' nor 'psychologically based enough'". As another continued,

> I think there's an issue almost of legitimacy, like you've done all this training with quite sophisticated models and interventions and psychological work, and you're asking people to go out for a run. It's almost too simple.
>
> *p. 441*

Such simplicity needs to be contextualized in light of the difficulty for many, not just individuals with depression, in initiating and sustaining physical activity participation.

It is likely that such perspectives may have modified since the time of publication. With increasing acknowledgement of the physical health consequences of mental illnesses such as schizophrenia and depression, either directly or associated with medication side-effects, there has been growing recognition of the urgent need to address the physical health needs of individuals with mental illness (Ward, White, & Druss 2015). Yet again such recognition may see exercise considered as one component of a healthy lifestyle to be supported rather than a treatment in and of itself. More concerted knowledge translation efforts may be needed to integrate evidence regarding exercise into training curricula for mental health professionals. A final concern is likely a pragmatic one.

Specifically, is there a structure in place for referring individuals to supervised exercise programmes that includes exercise counselling by qualified practitioners? As highlighted by the UK NICE guidelines, it is recommended that individuals participate in structured group programmes supervised by a competent support practitioner. Recent meta-analyses also consistently demonstrate that interventions that are structured and supervised demonstrate stronger effects, while dropout is minimized in studies delivered by health care professionals with specific training in exercise prescription (Stubbs et al. 2016). Interventions are currently less successful when less structure and supervision is provided.

One well-publicized RCT in the UK reported that the addition of a facilitated physical activity intervention to usual care did not improve depression outcome or reduce use of antidepressants compared with usual care alone (Chalder et al. 2012). This was an ambitious trial examining whether physical activity counselling, rather than a supervised and structured exercise intervention, could alleviate depression. The intervention programme comprised an initial hour long face to face assessment session followed by two short telephone contacts, then a further face-to-face meeting for half an hour. Over the course of six to eight months, the physical activity facilitator offered up to eight further telephone contacts and one more face-to-face half hour meeting. Ekkekakis (2013b) has presented an extensive critique of this study. Two points warrant attention. First, there was no evidence that the differences in physical activity between the groups changed over the duration of the study. Interpreting the results to suggest that physical activity did not improve depression outcomes is incorrect – the intervention was unsuccessful in increasing physical activity to a level significantly greater than in the control condition. Presumably this must be a necessary precursor to showing a treatment effect. Second, the intervention was delivered by non-specialists with minimal training, and was based on a physical activity counselling model. The pragmatic nature of the trial is to be applauded but it may be that unsupervised, physical activity interventions are likely not sufficient to support behaviour change for many individuals seeking help for treatment.

Given this possibility and likely cost there are clear policy implications of this possibility. Both physical activity and mental health professionals have important roles to play in establishing inter-professional dialogue and collaborating in developing structures of referral to supervised and structured exercise interventions. For example, qualified exercise professionals should be incorporated into mental health care treatment teams. The recent Blueprint for an Active Britain (2015, p. 66) highlights one relevant policy recommendation in this regard:

> Every person who has a mental health diagnosis should have access to a named physical activity intervention in line with NICE guidance, based upon proven evidence-based behavioural interventions such as motivational interviewing.

It is likely that policies will need to be established that make this a reality and that provide support and guidance for mental health professionals in applying the evidence concerning exercise and depression. Without policies facilitating the creation of such structures it will not be possible to make exercise, an evidence-based treatment option, more accessible to more individuals seeking help for depression. In tandem with this will be the need for more research focusing on how to integrate exercise treatment within existing systems of care, and assessing the cost-effectiveness of exercise provision in real world settings.

Given the significant burden of depression on the individual, family, and health care system, more attention is needed in examining how depression might be prevented and how more individuals with depression can access structured and supervised exercise interventions. From a policy perspective, greater recognition should be given to the mental health benefits of physical activity within both physical activity and mental health initiatives. From a mental health promotion perspective specifically, evidence suggests that promoting any level of physical activity could be an important strategy for the prevention of future depression in addition to an already impressive list of physical and mental health benefits accrued through a physically active lifestyle. The full potential of physical activity as a mental health promotion strategy at a population level has yet to be determined.

References

Alsuwaidan, MT, Kucyi, A, Law, CW, & McIntyre, RS 2009, 'Exercise and bipolar disorder: A review of neurobiological mediators', *Neuromolecular Medicine,* vol. 11, no. 4, pp. 328–36.

American Psychiatric Association 2013, *Diagnostic and statistical manual of mentaldisorders (DSM-5®),* American Psychiatric Association, Arlington, VA.

Babyak, M, Blumenthal, JA, Herman, S, Khatri, P, Doraiswamy, M, Moore, K, Craighead, E, Baldewicz, TT, & Krishnan, KR 2000, 'Exercise treatment for major depression: Maintenance of therapeutic benefit at 10 months', *Psychosomatic Medicine,* vol. 62, no. 5, pp. 633–8.

Bartholomew, JB, Morrison, D, & Ciccolo, JT 2005, 'Effects of acute exercise on mood and well-being in patients with major depressive disorder', *Medicine and Science in Sports and Exercise,* vol. 37, no. 12, pp. 2032–7.

Blueprint for an Active Britain 2015, *UKActive's blueprint for an active Britain,* viewed on 10 March 2016, www.ukactive.com/downloads/managed/ukactivs_Blueprint_for_an_Active_Britain_-_online.pdf.

Blumenthal, JA, Babyak, MA, Moore, KA, Craighead, E, Herman, S, Khatri, P, Waugh, R, Napolitano, MA, Forman, LM, Appelbaum, M, Doraiswamy, PM, & Krishnan, KR 1999, 'Effects of exercise training on older patients with major depression', *Archives of Internal Medicine,* vol. 159, no. 19, pp. 2349–56.

Boldrini, M, Hen, R, Underwood, MD, Rosoklija, GB, Dwork, AJ, Mann, JJ, & Arngo, V 2012, 'Hippocampal angiogenesis and progenitor cell proliferation are increased with antidepressant use in major depression', *Biological Psychiatry,* vol. 72, no. 7, pp. 562–71.

Boreham, CAG & Riddoch, CJ 2003, 'Physical activity and health across the lifespan', in J McKenna & C Riddoch (ed.), *Perspectives on health and exercise,* Palgrave Macmillan, UK. pp. 11–30.

Brown JC, Huedo-Medina TB, Pescatello LS, Ryan SM, Pescatello SM, Moker E, LaCroix JM, Ferrer RA, Johnson BT 2012, 'The efficacy of exercise in reducing depressive symptoms among cancer survivors: a meta-analysis', *Plos One,* vol. 7, no. 1, e30955.

Chalder, M, Wiles, NJ, Campbell, J, Hollinghurst, SP, Haase, AM, Taylor, AH, Fox, KR, Costelloe, C, Searle, A, Baxter, H, Winder, R, Wright, C, Turner, KM, Calnan, M, Lawlor, DA, Peters, TJ, Sharp, DJ, Montgomery, AA, & Lewis, G 2012, 'Facilitated physical activity as a treatment for depressed adults: Randomised controlled trial', *BMJ,* vol. 344, e2758.

Chen, MJ 2013, 'The neurobiology of depression and physical exercise', in E Panteleimon (ed.), *Routledge handbook of physical activity and mental health,* Routledge, New York, NY. pp. 169–183.

Cooney, GM, Dwan, K, Greig, CA, Lawlor, DA, Rimer, J, Waugh, FR, McMurdo, M, & Mead, GE 2013, 'Exercise for depression', *Cochrane Database of Systematic Reviews,* no. 9, CD004366.

Craft, LL, 2005, 'Exercise and clinical depression: Examining two psychological mechanisms', *Psychology of Sport and Exercise,* vol. 6, no. 2, pp. 151–71.

Craft, LL, 2013, 'Potential psychological mechanisms underlying the exercise and depression relationship', in P Ekkekakis (ed.), *Routledge handbook of physical activity and mental health,* Routledge, New York. pp. 161–183.

Danielsson, L, Noras, AM, Waern, M, & Carlsson, J 2013, 'Exercise in the treatment of major depression: A systematic review grading the quality of evidence', *Physiotherapy Theory and Practice,* vol. 29, no. 8, pp. 573–85.

De Moor, MH, Boomsma, DI, Stubbe, JH, Willemsen, G, & de Geus, EJ 2008, 'Testing causality in the association between regular exercise and symptoms of anxiety and depression', *Archives of General Psychiatry,* vol. 65, no. 8, pp. 897–905.

Ekkekakis, P (eds) 2013a, *Routledge handbook of physical activity and mental health,* Routledge, Oxford, UK.

Ekkekakis, P 2013b, 'Physical activity as a mental health intervention in the era of managed care: A rationale', in P Ekkekakis (ed.), *Routledge handbook of physical activity and mental health,* Routledge, New York. pp. 1–32.

Ekkekakis, P 2015, 'Honey, I shrunk the pooled SMD! Guide to critical appraisal of systematic reviews and meta-analyses using the Cochrane review on exercise for depression as example', *Mental Health and Physical Activity*, vol. 8, pp. 21–36.

Ekkekakis, P, Parfitt, G, & Petruzzello, SJ 2011, 'The pleasure and displeasure people feel when they exercise at different intensities: Decennial update and progress towards a tripartite rationale for exercise intensity prescription', *Sports Medicine*, vol. 41, no. 8, pp. 641–71.

Erickson, K, Voss, MW, Prakash, RS, Basak, C, Szabo, A, Chaddock, L, Kim, JS, Heo, S, Alves, H, White, SM, Wojcicki, TR, Mailey, E, Vieira, VJ, Martin, SA, Pence, BD, Woods, JA, McAuley, E, & Kramer, AF 2011, 'Exercise training increases size of hippocampus and improves memory', *Proceedings of the National Academy of Sciences of the United States of America*, vol. 108, no. 7, pp. 3017–22.

Esmail, N 2009, *Waiting your turn: Hospital waiting lists in Canada, 2009 report*, Fraser Institute, viewed on 10 March 2016, www.fraserinstitute.org/sites/default/files/WaitingYourTurn_2009.pdf.

Faulkner, G & Biddle, SJH 2001, 'Exercise as therapy: It's just not psychology!' *Journal of Sports Sciences*, vol. 19, no. 6, pp. 433–44

Faulkner, G, Hefferon, K, & Mutrie, N 2015, 'Putting positive psychology into motion through physical activity', in S Joseph (2nd ed.), *Putting psychology in practice: Promoting human flourishing in work, health, education, and everyday life*, John Wiley & Sons, Inc, Hoboken, NJ. pp. 207–22.

Faulkner, GE, Trinh, L, & Arbour-Nicitopoulos, KP 2015, 'Physical activity and mental health', in PRE Crocker (3rd ed.), *Sport and exercise psychology: A Canadian perspective*, Pearson Education Canada, Toronto, ON. pp. 341–70.

Ferrari, AJ, Charlson, FJ, Norman, RE, Patten, SB, Freedman, G, Murray, CJ, Vos, T, & Whiteford, HA 2013, 'Burden of depressive disorders by country, sex, age, and year: Findings from the global burden of disease study 2010', *PLos Medicine*, vol. 10, no. 11, e1001547.

Greenberg, PE, Foumier, AA, Sisitsky, T, Pike, CT, & Kessler, RC 2015, 'The economic burden of adults with major depressive disorder in the United States (2005 and 2010)', *Journal of Clinical Psychiatry*, vol. 75, no. 2, pp. 155–62.

Greist, JH, Klein, MH, Eischens, RR, Faris, J, Gurman, AS, & Morgan, WP 1979 'Running as treatment for depression', *Comprehensive Psychiatry*, vol. 20, no. 1, pp. 41–54.

Health and Social Care Information Centre 2014, *Psychological therapies: Annual report on the use of improving access to psychological therapies services: England, 2012 13*, viewed on 10 March 2016, www.hscic.gov.uk/catalogue/PUB13339/psyc-ther-ann-rep-2012-13.pdf.

Hill, AB 1965, 'The environment and disease: Association or causation?', *Proceedings of the Royal Society of Medicine*, vol. 58, no. 5, pp. 295–300.

Hill, AS, Sahay, A, & Hen, R 2015, 'Increasing adult hippocampal neurogenesis is sufficient to reduce anxiety and depression-like behaviors', *Neuropsychopharmacology*, vol. 40, no. 10, pp. 2368–78.

Josefsson, T, Lindwall, M, & Archer, T 2014, 'Physical exercise intervention in depressive disorders: Meta-analysis and systematic review', *Scandinavian Journal of Medicine & Science in Sports*, vol. 24, no. 2, pp. 259–72.

Kessler, RC & Bromet, EJ 2013, 'The epidemiology of depression across cultures', *Annual Review of Public Health*, vol. 34, pp. 119–38.

Krogh, J, Speyer, H, Nørgaard, HC, Moltke, A, & Nordentoft, M 2014. 'Can exercise increase fitness and reduce weight in patients with schizophrenia and depression?', *Frontiers in Psychiatry*, vol. 5, no. 89, pp. 1–6.

Lucas, M, Mekary, R, Pan, A, Mirzaei, F, O'Reilly, EJ, Willett, WC, Koenen, K, Okereke, OI, & Ascherio, A 2011, 'Relation between clinical depression risk and physical activity and time spent watching television among older women: A 10-year prospective follow-up study', *American Journal of Epidemiology*, vol. 174, no. 9, pp. 1017–27.

Mahar, I, Bambico, FR, Mechawar, N, & Nobrega, JN 2014, 'Stress, serotonin, and hippocampal neurogenesis in relation to depression and antidepressant effects', *Neuroscience and Biobehavioral Reviews*, vol. 38, pp. 173–92.

Maio, M, Sabiston, CM, & O'Loughlin, JL 2015, 'Moderate-intensity physical activity moderates the relationship between life events and depressive symptoms in emerging adults', *Journal of Exercise, Movement, and Sport*, vol. 47, no. 1.

Malhi, GS, Bassett, D, Boyce, P, Bryant, R, Fitzgerald, PB, Fritz, K, Hopwood, M, Lyndon, B, Mulder, R, Murray, G, Porter, R, & Singh, AB 2015, 'Royal Australian and New Zealand College of Psychiatrists clinical practice guidelines for mood disorders', *Australian and New Zealand Journal of Psychiatry*, vol. 49, no. 12, pp. 1087–206.

Mammen, G & Faulkner, G 2013, 'Physical activity and the prevention of depression: A systematic review of prospective studies', *American Journal of Preventive Medicine*, vol. 45, no. 5, pp. 649–57.

McCann, IL & Holmes, DS 1984, 'Influence of aerobic exercise on depression', *Journal of Personality and Social Psychology*, vol. 46, no. 5, pp. 1142–7.

Meeusen, R & De Meirleir, K 1995, 'Exercise and brain neurotransmission', *Sports Medicine*, vol. 20, no. 3, pp. pp. 160–88.

Meeusen, R, Thorré, K, Chaouloff, F, Sarre, S, De Meirleir, K, Ebinger, G, & Michotte, Y 1996, 'Effects of tryptophan and/or acute running on extracellular 5-HT and 5 HIAA levels in the hippocampus of food-deprived rats', *Brain Research*, vol. 740, no. 12, pp. 245–52.

Melancon, MO, Lorrain, D, & Dionne, IJ 2012, 'Exercise increases tryptophan availability to the brain in older men age 57–70 years', *Medicine and Science in Sports and Exercise*, vol. 44, no. 5, pp. 881–7.

Millington, B 2012, 'Use it or lose it: Ageing and the politics of brain training', *Leisure Studies*, vol. 31, no. 4, pp. 429–46.

Ministry of Health (2015) *Eating and Activity Guidelines for New Zealand Adults*. New Zealand Government, Wellington.

National Collaborating Centre for Mental Health and National Institute for Health and Clinical Excellence 2010, 'Depression: The treatment and management of depression in adults', British Psychological Society and Royal College of Psychiatrists, Leicester and London, UK.

Nutt, DJ 2008, 'Relationship of neurotransmitters to the symptoms of major depressive disorder', *The Journal of Clinical Psychiatry*, vol. 69, Suppl E1, pp. 4–7.

Nybo, L, Nielsen, B, Blomstrand, E, Moller, K, & Secher, N 2003, 'Neurohumoral responses during prolonged exercise in humans', *Journal of Applied Physiology*, vol. 95, no. 3, pp. 1125–31.

Nyström, MB, Neely, G, Hassmén, P, & Carlbring, P 2015, 'Treating major depression with physical activity: A systematic overview with recommendations', *Cognitive Behavioral Therapy*, vol. 44, no. 4, pp. 341–52.

Pajonk, FG, Wobrock, T, Gruber, O, Scherk, H, Berner, D, Kaiz, I, Kierer, A, Müller, S, Oest, M, Meyer, T, Backens, M, Schneider-Axmann, T, Thornton, AE, Honer, WG, & Falkai, P 2010, 'Hippocampal plasticity in response to exercise in schizophrenia', *Archives of General Psychiatry*, vol. 67, no. 2, pp. 133–43.

Ravindran, AV, Lam, RW, Filteau, MJ, Lespérance, F, Kennedy, SH, Parikh, SV, Patten, SB, & Canadian Network for Mood and Anxiety Treatments (CANMAT) 2009 'Canadian Network for Mood and Anxiety Treatments (CANMAT) Clinical guidelines for the management of major depressive disorder in adults. V. Complementary and alternative medicine treatments', *Journal of Affective Disorders*, vol. 117, Suppl 1, pp. S54–64.

Rosenbaum, S, Tiedemann, A, Sherrington, C, Curtis, J, & Ward, PB 2014, 'Physical activity interventions for people with mental illness: A systematic review and meta analysis', *Journal of Clinical Psychiatry*, vol. 75, no. 9, pp. 964–74.

Sahay, A & Hen, R 2007, 'Adult hippocampal neurogenesis in depression', *Nature Neuroscience*, vol. 10, pp. 1110–5.

Sharma, T, Guski, L, Freund, N, & Gøtzsche, PC 2016, 'Suicidality and aggression during antidepressant treatment: Systematic review and meta-analyses based on clinical study reports', *BMJ*, vol. 352, p. i65.

Silveira, H, Moraes, H, Oliveira, N, Coutinho, ESF, Laks, J, & Deslandes, A 2013 'Physical exercise and clinically depressed patients: A systematic review and meta-analysis', *Neuropsychobiology*, vol. 67, no. 2, pp. 61–8.

Spence, JC, McGannon, KR, & Poon, P 2005, 'The effect of exercise on global self esteem: A quantitative review', *Journal of Sport and Exercise Psychology,* vol. 27, no. 3, pp. 311–34.

Stanton, R & Reaburn, P 2014, 'Exercise and the treatment of depression: A review of the exercise program variables', *Journal of Science and Medicine in Sport*, vol. 17, no. 2, pp. 177–82.

Stubbs, B, Vancampfort, D, Rosenbaum, S, Ward, PB, Richards, J, Soundy, A, Veronese, N, Solmi, M, & Schuch, FB 2016, 'Dropout from exercise randomized controlled trials among people with depression: A meta-analysis and meta regression', *Journal of Affective Disorders*, vol. 190, pp. 457–66.

United States Department of Health and Human Services (US DHHS) 1999, *Mental health: A report of the surgeon general*, U.S. Department of Health and Human Services, Substance Abuse and Mental Health Services Administration, Center for Mental Health Services, National Institutes of Health, National Institute of Mental Health, Rockville, MD.

Ward, MC, White, DT, & Druss, BG 2015, 'A meta-review of lifestyle interventions for cardiovascular risk factors in the general medical population: Lessons for individuals with serious mental illness', *Journal of Clinical Psychiatry*, vol. 76, no. 4, pp. e477–86.

Westerhof, GJ & Keyes, CLM 2010, 'Mental illness and mental health: The two continua model across the lifespan', *Journal of Adult Development*, vol. 17, no. 2 pp. 110–119.

Wilson, WM & Marsden, CA 1996, 'In vivo measurement of extracellular serotonin in the ventral hippocampus during treadmill running', *Behavioural Pharmacology*, vol. 7, no. 1, pp. 101–4.

Work Group On Major Depressive Disorder 2010, *Practice guideline for major depressive disorder in adults*, American Psychiatric Association, Arlington, VA, USA.

World Health Organization (WHO) 2001, *Strengthening mental health promotion*, World Health Organization (Fact sheet no. 220), Geneva, Switzerland.

World Health Organization (WHO) 2012, *Depression: A global crisis*, viewed on 9 March 2016, www.who.int/mental_health/management/depression/wfmh_paper_d epression_wmhd_2012.pdf.

13

NEIGHBOURHOOD ACCESSIBILITY AND ACTIVE TRAVEL

Hugh Barton, Michael Horswell and Paul Millar

Introduction

Neighbourhoods are the flavour of the times, advocated by politicians and campaigners as means of combating environmental and social ills. But there is some equivocation over the degree to which locality still matters. While residents generally feel that they live in a neighbourhood, albeit ill-defined (Minnery *et al.*, 2009), some commentators have long anticipated the imminent death of neighbourhoods in the face of high mobility and the telecommunications revolution (Webber, 1964; Dennis, 1968) and consider our persistence in alluding to them largely nostalgic (Giddens, 1990). The rapid decline of many neighbourhood facilities over the past generation gives some credence to this view: in the UK, local food stores, post offices, banks, clubs, pubs, cottage hospitals and filling stations have vanished from many areas. Despite recent reversal of some of these trends (Competition Commission, 2008), the European Environment Agency reports that people are generally living less local lives, relying on larger, more distant facilities, normally accessed by car, especially in the peripheral areas of towns and cities where lower density, use-segregated, car-based patterns of development ('urban sprawl') predominate (EEA, 2009a). These trends come with an environmental and health cost—including high use of energy resources and land, additional greenhouse emissions, unhealthy air and noise pollution, increases in allergic reactions and lifestyle-related diseases including cardiovascular disorders linked to obesity, physical inactivity or stress (EEA, 2009a, 2009b).

While causal relationships in complex urban systems are notoriously difficult to disentangle (Giles-Corti *et al.*, 2007; Dempsey, 2008; Brownson *et al.*, 2009), official policies have reacted to these concerns, seeking to counteract the trends. The revival of neighbourhoods is held up as a necessary part of a sustainable future (European Commission, 1990; DETR, 1998; Social Exclusion Unit, 2000). The UK government has adopted a localism agenda advocating 'neighbourhood plans', and charitable trusts promoting health have further reinforced this move (CLG, 2010; CRESR, 2010). The benefits of neighbourhood renaissance would, it is held, be increased accessibility to key services for all (reducing social exclusion), better physical and mental health (Corburn, 2005; Rao *et al.*, 2011) and reduced carbon emissions. Concern over climate change has been the key driver since the early 1990s, but recently the issue of obesity—linked to both higher mortality and health inequalities—has given added impetus

(NICE, 2008). Strategies to combat obesity highlight the importance of active travel as a means of increasing levels of physical activity, especially in lower socio-economic groups who typically get much of their exercise through incidental physical activity (Frank *et al.*, 2006; Feng *et al.*, 2009; McDonald *et al.*, 2011). Active travel to nearby facilities also has potential for positive impact on social networks, with benefits to self-reported mental well-being (Calve Blanco, 2010). The revival of neighbourhoods would thus, it is believed, combat the problems of isolation, inactivity and poor facility access which contribute to health inequalities.

While the potential benefits are clear, the practicalities of achieving re-localization are more problematic. The UK government has pursued planning policies of higher residential densities and the concentration of new housing on brownfield sites, as means of urban regeneration, with the intention of achieving the critical mass of population needed to support local services. These policies, though, do not of themselves necessarily deliver neighbourhood revival, as studies in London have shown (Williams, 2000; Barton *et al.*, 2010b). A complementary approach is that of accessibility criteria. The Department for Transport requires the level of access to public transport to be assessed within local transport plans. Many local authorities use the distance of 800 m as an indication of walkable distance to local shopping centres, following the lead of the Greater London Authority (Llewelyn Davies, 1998). Other guides recommend standards for a wide range of local facilities (e.g. Barton *et al.*, 2010a). The quality of the empirical evidence for these standards is varied, often more hunch than firm knowledge. This paper hopes to illuminate the reality of active travel across England, its extent and local variety.

Previous studies of active travel and neighbourhood accessibility

Clearly the policy of neighbourhood revival rests on the critical assumption that long-term trends of decline can be reversed. Can developers, planners and designers, through reshaping the physical environment, alter user behaviour? In academic (as opposed to policy) discourse, this is a contested matter. As a part of the SOLUTIONS research programme, we undertook a systematic review of the literature on active travel and local facilities, very recently updated (Millar and Barton, 2011). Studies have found complex links among neighbourhood characteristics, activity and travel behaviour (Forsyth *et al.*, 2008, 2009). Some studies suggest that land use patterns, particularly in terms of density and land use mix, have only a marginal impact on travel choice (Boarnet and Sarmiento, 1998) and have inconsistent association with health because of social variations (McDonald *et al.*, 2011). Nevertheless, there is a growing consensus that residents in more walkable neighbourhoods (with traditional or neo-traditional form) do undertake more active travel compared with those in modern cul-de-sac layouts (Saelens *et al.*, 2003; Handy, 2005; Frank *et al.*, 2006).

Many of the studies try to tease out the relative importance of social and environmental characteristics in determining behaviour through multiple regression. Necessarily, they select specific indicators thought to be significant. In terms of the environment, common variables are residential density, mixed use, traditional and 'modern' layouts. The conclusions drawn have limited resonance because of the focus on one or two facets only and the lack of a rounded view of place (Barton and Hills, 2005). More detailed attempts to characterize the environment have attempted to itemize each aspect and assess it separately. However, reducing the number of factors studied inevitably tends to reduce the representation of complexity in the real world (Handy, 2005).

Lee and Moudon (2008) investigated the relationship between levels of physical activity and demographic, attitudinal and neighbourhood design variables. They found that the most significant determinant of physical activity in a locality was the existence of neighbourhood facilities (a local centre, convenience store and post office). Winter and Farthing (1997) highlight the degree to which behaviour varies depending on the nature of the facility. When present within a given estate, supermarkets, secondary schools and newsagents, for example, are used by most people in preference to more distant options. By contrast, local dentists, churches and leisure facilities are used by a small minority of people on the estate. The propensity to walk to facilities also varies hugely, with almost all users walking to local play spaces and parks, but few to supermarkets. Winter and Farthing's study is a helpful UK precursor to the current research but is limited by relying on a narrow subset of localities, imprecision on distances and no analysis of urban form issues such as location, density and shape.

There remains, therefore, a surprising dearth of evidence on exactly how people behave in accessing local facilities, and the factors that might explain that behaviour. We lack adequate knowledge about how far people travel to get to different facilities, what mode they use, how far they choose to walk, how that varies between social groups and how it varies between different places. More broadly, we do not really know to what extent people are still using local facilities, and therefore whether the demise of the neighbourhood is reality or myth. There is also uncertainty about the degree to which variations in behaviour are accounted for by self-selection—households selecting locations to suit their modal preferences. Policy-makers are necessarily relying on relatively untested assumptions about the efficacy of neighbourhood planning in shifting user behaviour and tackling the big issues of climate change, obesity and inequality.

Research design

The study is about neighbourhood accessibility and active travel to local facilities. The focus is on English suburban and exurban areas which account on some estimates for 85 per cent of the population (Echenique *et al.*, 2010). In this context, *local* is not defined by set distance threshold (as in some of the studies above) but in terms of function: the non-work facilities that might well be judged as important to daily life, rather than the occasional trip, thus, for example, convenience retail outlets, but not durable goods outlets. Some of those facilities are essential for some or all households (schools and food shops); others are discretionary (pubs, parks and playgrounds). We make an explicit assumption that good accessibility to local facilities, especially by active means, is desirable for health, social inclusion and environmental sustainability reasons. Neighbourhoods in this context are not defined as fixed, bounded units, but as catchment areas for local facilities (Barton, 2000).

The main aim of this paper is to reveal the current pattern of use of local facilities in outer urban areas so as to inform policy-makers and policy-analysts. The research identifies:

- the degree to which local facilities are used
- how far users travel to access them
- what mode of transport they choose
- how far people walk to access facilities
- how this behaviour varies between social groups and
- how it varies between different places.

A second aim is to throw light on the question of whether, through public policy and neighbourhood planning, accessibility could be improved, social inclusion and physical activity promoted and neighbourhoods revived. This is a huge question, involving an understanding of the determinants of residents and market behaviour and of state and community powers to influence that behaviour. The evidence presented here contributes to the data and understanding of this complex issue.

However, it is important at the outset to have a clear view of the complex relationship of independent and dependent variables. The logic model (Figure 13.1) sets out the relationship between the various factors that influence user behaviour. It draws on ecological theories that view behaviour as a result of the interaction of personal, social, cultural and environmental factors. Four sets of factors are distinguished: the population characteristics; the type, scale and location of the facilities; the nature of the place (or neighbourhood); and cultural/attitudinal characteristics of the people. The research is distinctive in exploring all of these factors.

A postal household survey, piloted in Bristol, was carried out in 2007 in 12 localities in four English city regions, London, Newcastle, Cambridge and Bristol. The questionnaire asked for information about destinations and trips in relation to all food outlets, other local services, schools and leisure activities. Based on a physical survey, the questions specified as many facilities as possible by name to ease subsequent spatial analysis. Five thousand, nine hundred and fifty-nine questionnaires were sent out in the 12 neighbourhoods, and 1,619 received, an average response rate of 27.2 per cent, with at least 100 from each place.

Responses were captured in SPSS. Dwellings and facilities were located to post code centres on Geographical Information systems (GIS), and actual trip distances estimated using

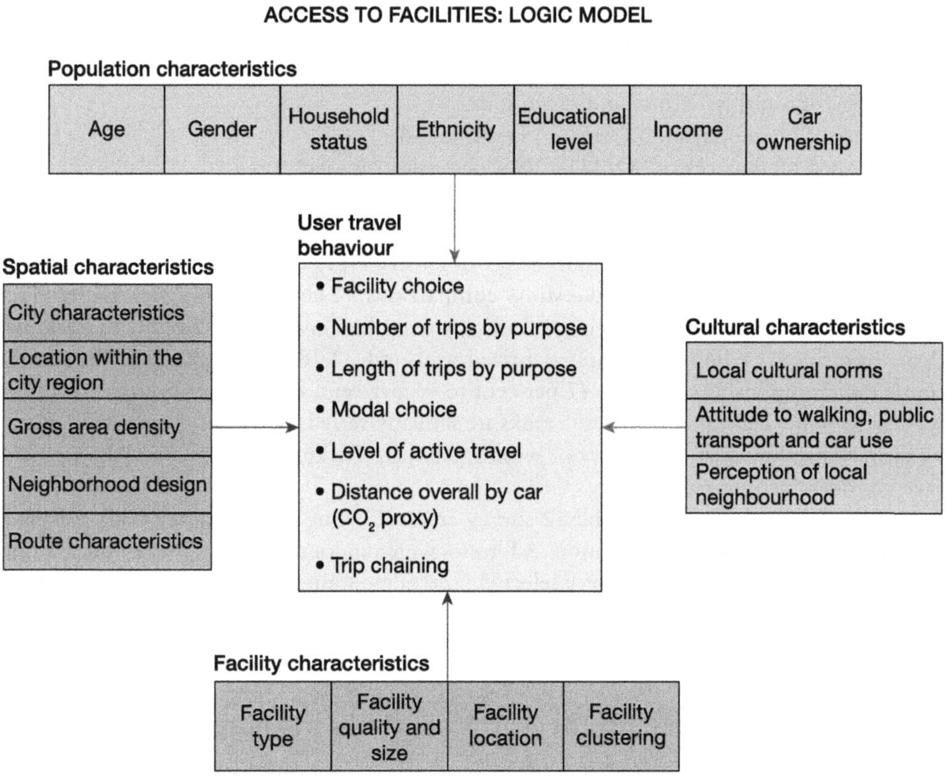

ACCESS TO FACILITIES: LOGIC MODEL

Figure 13.1 Access to local facilities—logic model

the Ordnance Survey Meridian (OSM) dataset. In the vast majority of cases, the facilities used were successfully identified in advance—with the significant exception of leisure destinations. Generally, estimated distances were accurate to within about 100 m. However, in some areas, unknown errors may have occurred due to poor respondent identification of unlisted facilities, and the absence of some purely pedestrian links from the OSM networks. The results enabled the calculation of two important indicators: the overall level of active travel for the relevant purposes (as an indicator of healthy physical activity) and the total distance travelled by car (as a crude proxy for fossil fuel use and transport carbon emissions).

A comparison by trip purpose of our results with those of the National Travel Survey (NTS; DfT, 2005) give grounds for confidence in the quality of our sampling method and assumptions. There is good frequency comparability for education, shopping and leisure trips. Our survey did not include any work-related trips and only a minority of personal business and social entertainment trips, so overall the SOLUTIONS findings relate to 46 per cent of total trips as identified by the NTS—a substantial proportion.

Besides revealing the patterns of facility use and related travel behaviour by social group and place, the questionnaire included attitudinal and perception questions (using a Likert scale), supplemented by focus group discussions in each locality allowing some insight into the theories of behaviour in urban areas (Koger and Winter, 2010) by comparing stated attitudes and actual behaviour.

The case study areas

Twelve case study areas were selected based on the following three criteria:

- a range of social structures and conditions;
- variety of neighbourhood form and location and
- expressed preferences of SOLUTIONS local authority partners.

The 12 localities represent a reasonable cross section of suburban and commuter localities. Table 13.1 distinguishes four locational categories, three types of local urban form and levels of gross density, permitting interesting comparisons. The table specifies population characteristics in terms of income, home and car ownership, and the 2004 Index of Multiple Deprivation rank (1 being the most deprived area and 32,482 being the least deprived). Home ownership levels vary from 47 per cent to 96 per cent, car ownership varies from 57 per cent to 96 per cent, and deprivation ranks are similarly varied. While some neighbourhoods are characterized by relative poverty or wealth (compare Barking and Bradley Stoke), others have considerable internal diversity.

Figure 13.2 illustrates one of the 12 survey areas, showing the location of facilities and the extent of questionnaire distribution. Addresses were randomly selected by computer from council lists. The map identifies every selected postcode—some postcodes representing more than one respondent. Distances were measured along streets and footpaths. Further details about the survey areas are available on www.suburbansolutions.ac.uk.

Overall results: The general pattern by trip purpose

The results of the survey are presented first in an aggregate form, revealing broad patterns from all 12 study areas and their respondents. Disaggregated results then follow.

Table 13.1 Location, names and characteristics of the case study areas

City	Neighbourhood	Location	Reference	Density[a]	Form[b]	Average income (£)	Home ownership (%)	No. of non-car households (%)	Most usual number of cars per household	Deprivation rank
Bristol	Bradley Stoke	Recent outer suburb	Brist—new	Medium	Use-segregated pods	39,000	82	4	2	30,457–31,951
Bristol	Filton Avenue	Older suburb	Brist—old	Low–medium	Traditional/linear	30,000	59	29	2	2,776–26,674
Bristol	Thornbury	Satellite town	Brist—satellite	Low	Neighbourhood cell	37,000	83	13	2	13,499–32,404
Cambridge	Bar Hill	Satellite town	Cam—satellite	Low	Neighbourhood cell	33,000	88	10	1	27,652–31,095
Cambridge	Cherry Hinton	Mixed urban edge	Cam—edge 1	Medium	Neighbourhood cell	32,000	66	20	1	12,397–31,072
Cambridge	Trumpington	Mixed urban edge	Cam—edge 2	Low	Neighbourhood cell	37,000	62	25	1	21,023–21,674
London	Barking	Older suburb	Lond—old 1	High	Traditional/linear	28,000	57	43	1	2,204–10,535
London	Broxbourne	Recent outer suburb	Lond—new	Low	Use-segregated pods	45,000	83	13	2	12,541–26,864
London	Harrow	Older suburb	Lond—old 2	Medium	Traditional/linear	41,000	66	28	2	7,487–28,356
Newcastle	Backworth and Shiremoor	Mixed urban edge	Newc—edge	Low	Use-segregated pods	28,000	47	11	1	4,348–15,826
Newcastle	Cramlington	Satellite town	Newc—satellite	Low–medium	Use-segregated pods	36,000	74	13	2	4,924–30,928
Newcastle	Great Park	Recent outer suburb	Newc—new	Low–medium	Use-segregated pods	43,000	96	16	2	12,331–31,794

Notes:

[a]Density is based on the surveyed census output area (population between 250 and 375 normally), quite tightly drawn around the housing areas. The density ranges are as follows: low = 17–22 ppha; low–medium = 31–35 ppha; medium = 42–51 ppha; high = 71 ppha.

[b]Form is a broad indication only. None of the localities has a simple structure. Areas dominated by 'pods' have hierarchical road systems and cul-de-sac layouts; 'cell' neighbourhoods are relatively distinct and compact; 'linear' areas are part of the urban continuum, with shops along main roads.

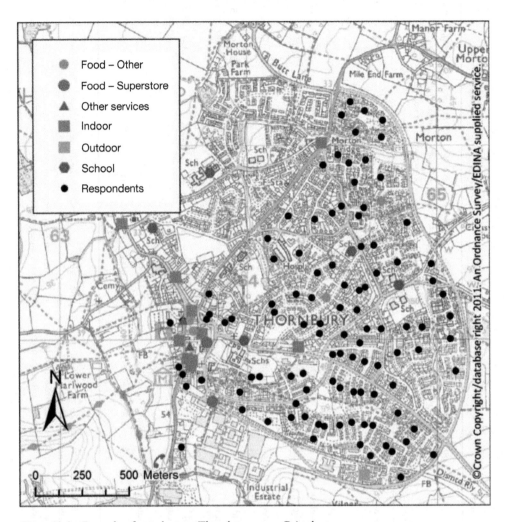

Figure 13.2 Example of a study area, Thornbury—near Bristol

The total number and frequency of trips to different destinations are shown in Figure 13.3. They clearly show the importance of the superstore as a trip generator. Well over 90 per cent of respondents make regular trips to the superstore, with the average frequency being twice a week. Focus group discussions in all the study areas highlighted the significance of superstores for planned or unplanned social contact. The frequency of trips for outdoor and indoor recreation is similar, but only 25 per cent of the respondent households undertake trips for outdoor recreation and 50 per cent for indoor recreation, representing comparably low levels of participation, especially for outdoor recreation which includes parks, playgrounds and walking for pleasure as well as organized sports.

Trips to newsagents and other food stores occur weekly on average. Trips to other facilities cluster around an average frequency of once a fortnight. All these facilities are visited by a substantial majority of households, for example, post offices around 80 per cent and other food shops 85 per cent.

Figure 13.4 shows the range of trip length by trip purpose. The threshold distances of 800 and 1,600 m have been chosen not only because they have a simple resonance (half mile

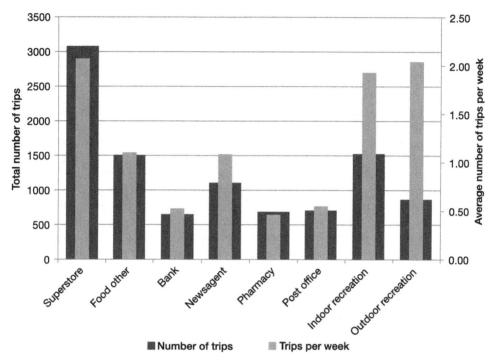

Figure 13.3 The total trips and average number of trips per week by users of each type of facility

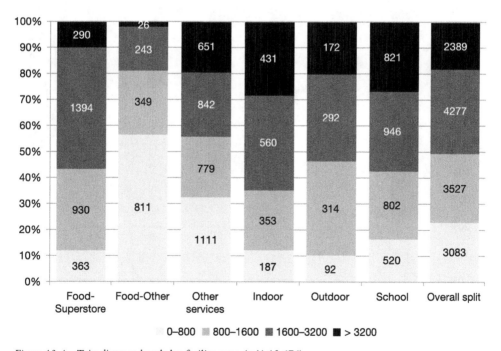

Figure 13.4 Trip distance bands by facility type (*n* ¼ 13,676)

and one mile) but also because they have significance in terms of modal choice (see later). At 800 m about two-thirds of trips, and at 1,600 m about one-third of trips, are by active means. The median distance to most facilities is between 1,600 m and 2,000 m (for all trips it is just over 1,700 m), beyond walking distance for the majority of respondents. Superstores are the least local: only 43 per cent dwellings within the 1,600 m threshold. The exception to the rule is the 'other food' category: used relatively frequently, a median distance of 1,000 m and over 80 per cent within 1,600 m, suggesting general availability and use within the walkable neighbourhood catchment.

The distance people travel to access local facilities—often in excess of 1,600 m (1 mile)—may be due to the absence of facilities or the exercise of consumer choice. The research provides good data to discriminate between these options, finding variations between trip purposes. Almost all households (96%) did 'most' of their food shopping in superstores. Nine of the 12 localities have a nearby superstore, and in all but one instance the closest superstore is also the dominant one—sometimes capturing almost all trade. The one exception was where a new, closer store had not (yet?) managed to supplant traditional loyalties to an older, more distant store. People also normally choose the closest 'other food' stores. In neighbourhoods where there are not many close by, the number of households making 'other food' trips is low.

By contrast, users of indoor and outdoor leisure facilities are more discriminating, often choosing more distant options, reflecting their specialist nature or attractiveness and people being willing and able to access them.

Overall, active travel (walking and cycling) accounts for just under 50 per cent of total trips—as does personal motorized transport (cars, vans, motorbikes and taxis), with public transport relatively unimportant (Figure 13.5). Travel to superstores is dominated by personal

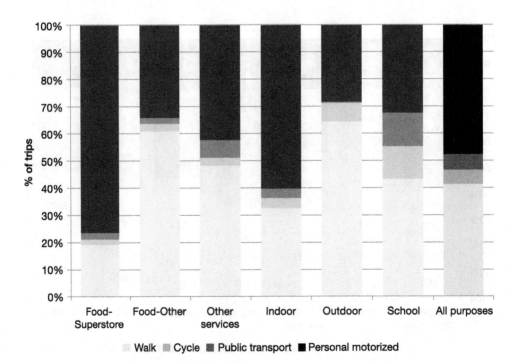

Figure 13.5 Modal split to different facility types.

Note: Statistical significance is high at 0.00; Cramer's *V* is 0.223 and w2 is 1,210

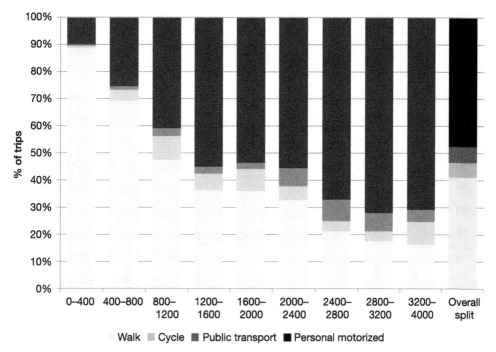

Figure 13.6 Modal choice by distance for all trips.

Note: Statistical significance is high at 0.00; Cramer's *V* is 0.322 and w2 is 2,515

motorized transport—with over three quarters of trips. By comparison, travel to 'other food' shops and to outdoor recreation facilities is predominantly by active means.

The proportion of active travel to superstores decays very fast with distance, with the 50 per cent threshold around 500 m. For school and outdoor recreation trips, however, the 50 per cent threshold is around 2,500 m. Other trips—'other food', services and indoor recreation/leisure—are in-between and all similar in profile, with the 50 per cent threshold around 1,200 m.

Figure 13.6 amalgamates all trip purposes and shows a clear relationship between distance and modal choice. At distances shorter than 400 m, 90 per cent of trips are by active travel, falling to 50 per cent at 1,200 m (about a 15-min walk), and less than a third of trips at 1,600 m. The proportion of trips made using public transport is consistently small but increases with distance.

Figure 13.7 generalizes from the travel distance decay data. It takes active travel proportion by distance and evens out the curve through regression. The three purposes illustrated have been selected, because they illustrate contrasting behaviour patterns. The non-superstore food curve is similar to the 'other services' curve and the average of all trips. It shows a quite rapid decline in the active traveller proportion down to a 50 per cent mark at 1,250 m, then a gradual levelling so that the 25 per cent mark is at 3,250 m, before a decline to zero at 5,000 m. This pattern supports Lee and Moudon's (2008) notion that there are two main kinds of active travellers—those willing to walk only a very modest distance and those willing to walk much further—the sedentary and the active types.

However, the superstore curve suggests that, for this purpose, we are almost all in the sedentary camp, while the minority who participate in outdoor recreation (rather similar to

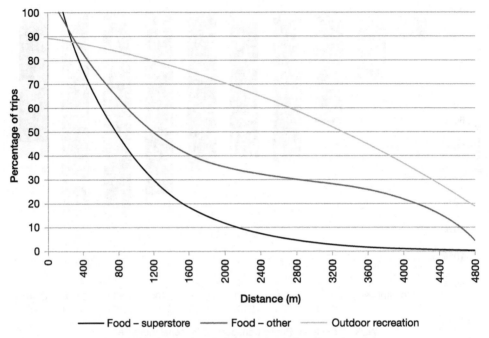

Figure 13.7 Regression lines of active travel distance decay for selected trip purposes

the school trips) fall into the active travel category. It is very clear that different types of destination lead to different travel behaviours. It can be argued that there are three archetypical patterns of travel behaviour to facilities.

The question arises as to what this evidence shows about the nature of neighbourhoods in the twenty-first century. The messages are mixed. Households travel outside the locality for many purposes that might be considered 'local'. The mean travel distance for all purposes was 2,400 m, the median 1,700 m and—with the exception of 'other food shops'—the majority of trips for each purpose was over 1,600 m (1 mile). Recreational trips are often much longer. If 1,600 m is taken as a 'walkable' threshold, then localities do not generally provide the 'local' services people use.

However, local food shops, if present, are well frequented, often by foot; and the *closest* superstore (while often beyond 1,500 m) is used by a substantial majority in preference to others, and visited like a corner shop, twice a week on average. It is apparent that superstore accessibility is generally more important than brand loyalty (or perhaps helps define it). Focus groups (self-selected from the respondents) also emphasized that they considered that they belonged to a neighbourhood or local community and stressed the significance of the superstore in their social contacts. Thus, the neighbourhood, in the catchment sense defined earlier, is not dead but more dispersed than the conventional image, with tentacles stretching out and entangled with the town around, part of the urban continuum. What is striking is the degree to which people in outer suburban areas do still walk. Contrary to popular myth, not everyone relies on the car, even for access to the superstore. Some people (schoolchildren and recreationally active people) walk significantly beyond the 'local', and many are willing to walk 2 km or more to 'local' neighbourhood facilities. The question arises as to whether the habit of active travel applies to particular social groups more than others.

Analysis of demographic variables

This section gives an overview of how modal choice relates to key demographic variables. The literature review showed there has been little research differentiating between groups who may be systematically advantaged or disadvantaged by the pattern of facility availability. An exception is the distinction made by some researchers between sedentary and active groups, discussed above. Table 13.2 shows some key demographic variables that might help explain behavioural differences. The measures here relate to statistical significance and consistency or strength of relationship, not to the size of the relationship. Note the very high significance of age, income and car ownership, but low significance of gender.

It is apparent from Figure 13.8 that age is not a critical determinant of the general pattern of modal choice, despite the consistency of the relationship. The 50–64 group use cars most, while the oldest group (75) use cars least. While the over 75s walk more, the distances are

Table 13.2 Demographic variables in relation to modal choice, in strength order

Variable	Cramer's V	Significance	Effect size
Age	0.203	$p < 0.000$	Medium
Income	0.184	$p < 0.000$	Small
Car ownership	0.096	$p < 0.000$	Small
Ethnicity	0.034	$p < 0.001$	Small
Educational level	0.030	$p < 0.003$	Small
Tenure	0.021	$p < 0.065$	Small
Gender		$p < 0.323$	None

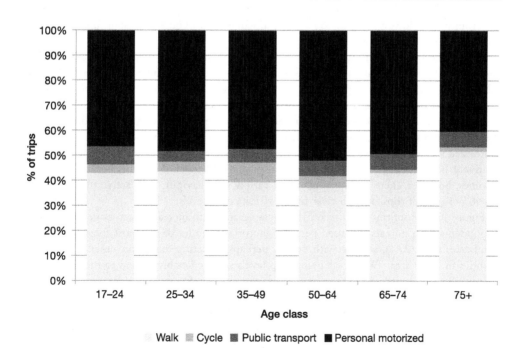

Figure 13.8 Modal choice across all trips by age class

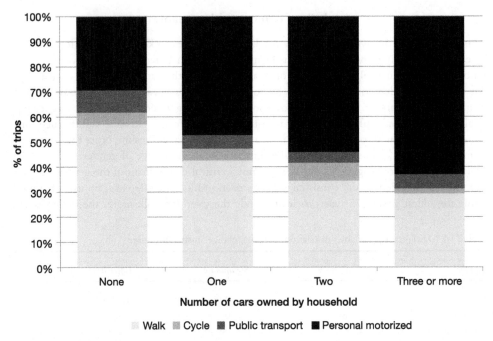

Figure 13.9 Modal choice across all trips by household income band

shorter than other groups. There are interesting variations in the use of the minor modes: the 50–64 age group cycle more than the two youngest and the two oldest groups. Public transport exhibits a different pattern, with the 17–24 age group relying on it more than all the other age groups; use is lowest in the 25–34 age group while levels of public transport use are similar across the three older age groupings.

Modal choice is surprisingly similar in relation to some key social variables. Gender choices are almost identical. Household size (in terms of number of adults) is also not a factor. Educational attainment and ethnicity show a slightly stronger relationship, but the impact is likely masked by more important issues of income and car ownership.

Low income appears a key determinant of travel for some households (Figure 13.9). When the annual household income is less than £20,000, more than half of trips are by non-motorized means; when less than £10,000, over two-thirds are non-motorized, and there is relatively heavy dependence on public transport. For households with medium to high incomes, however, there is surprisingly little variety of behaviour, with active travel around 40–46 per cent of trips, and no clear trend with income levels.

Figure 13.10 confirms that car availability associates with increasing car usage. However, respondents with no cars still used personal motorized modes of transport for a significant number of trips (29%), sharing with others, perhaps reflecting the inconvenience of many facilities in outer areas. While car ownership levels are predictably related to income, there are multiple car owners even at the lowest incomes, and car-free households in every income group up to £60,000.

In summary, it is important to note that the analysis here is limited to only one aspect of local travel—modal choice. In that regard the most important determinant is car owner-ship. However, non-car owners are more reliant on car use than might be expected. At low-income levels, active travel is more common, while at medium and high income

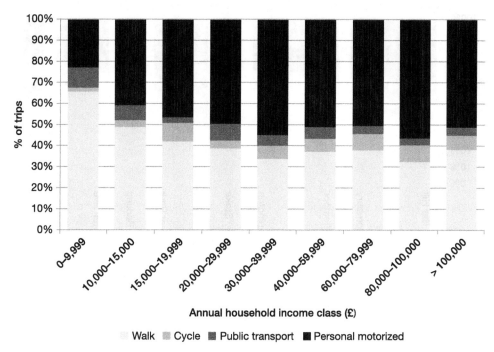

Figure 13.10 Modal choice across all trips by car ownership levels

levels there is little variation in modal choice. Age is a factor, with middle-aged respondents more car dependent, young and old more reliant on walking and public transport, but the variations are modest. However, all the preceding analysis relates to data aggregated across all study areas, whereas substantial differences were in fact found between the study areas.

Findings disaggregated by study area

Aggregating data loses important local detail. The 12 neighbourhoods have different spatial characteristics, and the analysis shows huge variations between them. The proportion of active walking/cycling trips varies by over 200 per cent, ranging from 29 per cent to 64 per cent of total trips. Public transport varies from 1 per cent to 18 per cent. Car use varies from 32 per cent to 79 per cent. It is immediately apparent, therefore, that places and communities vary to a degree which makes generalizations based on average figures potentially very misleading for any particular locality.

Figure 13.11 shows that the new suburbs and commuter settlements are generally more car dependent than the mixed urban edge areas and the older suburbs. There are three localities with very high car use: Broxbourne, Bradley Stoke and Cramlington. While appearing different from each other (unplanned suburban sprawl, planned urban extension and planned new town), they all share a modern car-based cul-de-sac layout with segregated land uses. By comparison, three localities have high levels of active travel and modest car use: Cherry Hinton, Trumpington and Filton Avenue. The first two are peripheral neighbourhoods of Cambridge with mixed-age development and broadly cell-type layouts, while the third is a mid-twentieth century area with a traditional linear pattern. Three other suburbs have

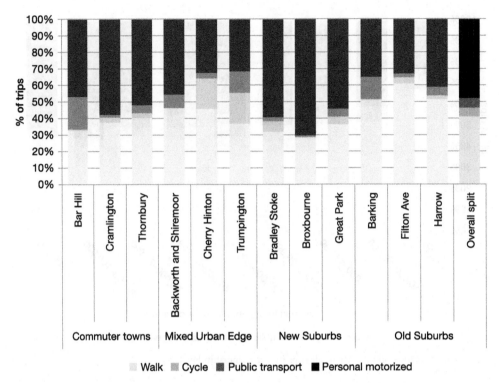

Figure 13.11 Modal split in case study areas, by locational type.

Note: Statistical significance is high at 0.00; Cramer's *V* is 0.241 and w2 is 1,408

above average public transport use: Barking, Harrow and Bar Hill. The first two benefit from the quality of services (including public transport) in London, but the third is very different: a commuter exurb with good bus connection to a commercially dominant Cambridge centre. The remaining study areas of Backworth and Great Park fill intermediate positions.

The modal breakdown reflects the diversity of local area factors: the accessibility of facilities that people use; the qualities of the routes available (e.g. are they perceived as safe and convenient for active travel); the socio-economic characteristics of the population; the local culture and behavioural norms. The variations above can for the most part be explained by their spatial and social characteristics combined with qualitative insights from focus groups of respondents held in each area. In evaluating the results, the *number* of trips is significant as well as the mode. In this respect, all of the neighbourhoods have generally comparable trip numbers per household except for Bar Hill, which had very substantially fewer. The main reasons for this are the high multi-purpose use of one major superstore within the exurb and an unexplained paucity of recreational trips.

Figure 13.12 shows the average trip distance by city and case study areas and shows the average distance (km) travelled by car per respondent per week in each case study area—for all facility types. The solid line indicates the sample average trip distance, and the dashed line the sample median trip distance. In this analysis, the study areas are grouped by city region, to test the theory that behaviour is locally culturally/environmentally influenced.

The variation in average trip distance is a proxy measure of the convenience of local facilities. By and large, as noted earlier, people use the closest available facility—apart from

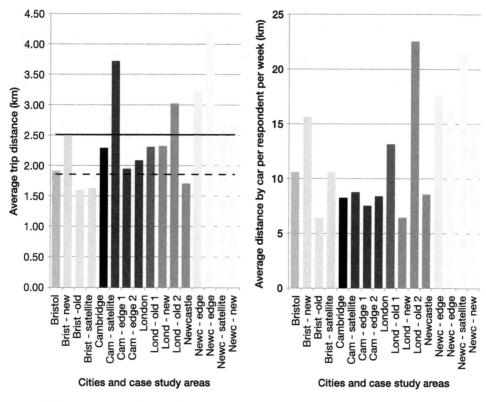

Figure 13.12 Average trip distance for the cities and case study areas, and total distance travelled by car for cities and case study areas

recreational facilities. Areas with higher car dependency generally have higher average trip distance, but this is not a universal rule. Cambridge, which has the highest proportion of active travel, is not associated with the shortest average trip distances. Bristol has the shortest average trip distance, yet has relatively high car dependency.

The total distance travelled by car is a crude proxy for the level of carbon emissions associated with the journeys recorded in the survey. The Newcastle localities stand out for the unfortunate combination of long average distance to facilities and long distances travelled by car. The latter characteristic is shared with the two areas with highest car modal share: Broxbourne and Bradley Stoke.

From the preceding evidence, it is clear that places and communities vary widely. Nevertheless, there are some shared patterns of behaviour, in terms of the propensity to walk and cycle, that suggest the existence of common cultural attitudes in particular cities. For example, behaviour is similar in Trumpington and Cherry Hinton, both 'mixed urban edge' suburbs of Cambridge. In Harrow and Barking, both older London suburbs, the distances people are prepared to walk are surprisingly similar, despite the different social and spatial character. The three survey areas in Bristol city region show broadly similar trip walking distance patterns despite locational, form and social differences. Yet Bradley Stoke is very car dependent, while Filton Avenue has high levels of walking. The variation in modal choice can be explained by geography: the availability of facilities and the permeability of the route network.

The significance of the distinctive cultural/geographical characteristics of each city is illustrated in Figure 13.13. Bristol and Cambridge show very different patterns of behaviour

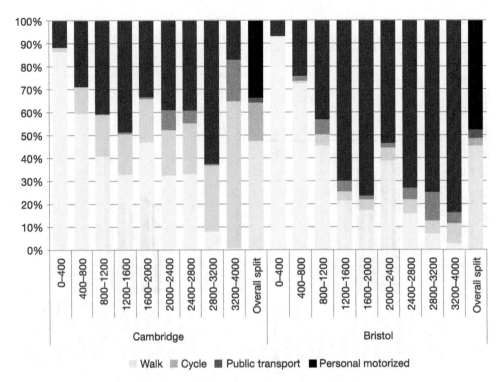

Figure 13.13 Modal choice to all facilities for Bristol and Cambridge

across all trip purposes. This appears to be due to geographical and cultural factors: Cambridge is largely flat with a tradition of cycling; Bristol is in places hilly, with no such tradition. Cambridge is immediately identifiable as a less car dependent city than Bristol—37 per cent as opposed to 52 per cent—and has high use of cycling—15 per cent overall. In Cambridge, walking and cycling together add up to 63 per cent. Even for superstore access active travel— at almost 40 per cent—is surprisingly high and belies the normal image of almost total car dependency. The majority (over 80%) of trips to other food stores and to schools are made on foot or by bicycle.

Attitudes to travel

The question arises as to whether the variations in behaviour between Bristol and Cambridge, which appear to represent cultural differences, reflect respondents' self-confessed attitudes. The questionnaire concentrated on attitudes to walking and cycling. Exercise was cited as an important reason for active travel by nearly 80 per cent of respondents overall and environmental reasons by just over 65 per cent. Across all reasons, Cambridge was consistently 15–25 per cent higher than Bristol and the other cities.

However, stated attitudes were often not reflected in behaviour. Respondents were asked about barriers to walking. The deterrents most often cited were high traffic levels and unsafe streets. Areas with the lowest levels of walking cited no more deterrence factors than the average. Areas citing most concerns about feeling unsafe and where the neighbourhood was not considered attractive were paradoxically among the more active. While overall a substantial majority (76%) felt their neighbourhood was attractive, the figure for the older suburbs fell to less than half, with the London residents in particular finding their locality unattractive. By contrast, over 90 per cent of the residents in the new suburbs thought their locality attractive. This may be partly accounted for by social differences. The new suburbs have very low levels of deprivation, while the older suburbs have socially mixed (in the case of Barking, poorer) populations. However, it is by no means as simple as that. Newcastle respondents, for example, are socially diverse in two of the three areas but rate them as being more attractive than the other cities rate theirs. Perceptions of neighbourhood attractiveness are not, on this evidence, determinants of levels of active travel.

Spatial character, density and active travel

The variation between places is clearly often related to their spatial character. Here, we can only give one angle on the issues involved. Residential density has been highlighted by the literature as an important factor influencing facility accessibility and active travel (ECOTEC, 1993; Handy, 1993; Frank and Pivo, 1995; Hess *et al.*, 1999). But within the relatively limited density range represented by the SOLUTIONS sample—neither inner urban nor rural in character—there is no consistent relationship between density and modal choice. This is true whether we use the densities of the relevant wards and parishes (which often include some industrial, open or rural zones) or more tightly drawn areas.

Figure 13.14 relates the gross population density (ppha) based on wards/parishes to the percentage of active travel trips in each neighbourhood. The density ranges from 17 to 71 ppha.

From detailed analysis of the evidence, it is apparent that some communities with similar social characteristics and similar neighbourhood densities exhibit completely different patterns of behaviour. Diversity is the rule. This is not to argue that density is unimportant when looking across the whole range, but that within the suburban context other aspects of urban

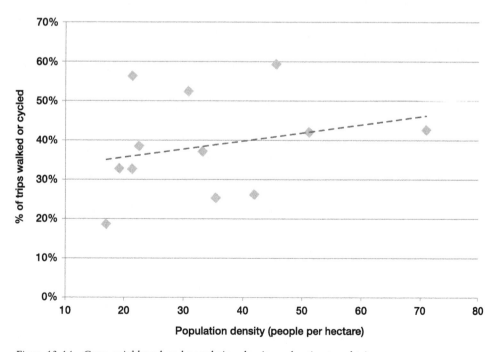

Figure 13.14 Gross neighbourhood population density and active travel trips

form, such as location, networks and use patterns, are much more significant. These other factors are touched on below.

Qualitative comparison of neighbourhoods

This discussion draws together the many strands of analysis above into more integrated pictures of active travel in the 12 neighbourhoods. It is evident that the unique social and spatial characteristics of area cannot be reduced to one or two convenient variables which explain differing behaviours. The analysis here builds on the four key determinants in the logic model—social, attitudinal, spatial and facilities—to differentiate between neighbourhoods and warn against the use of simplistic statistical averaging when planning for active travel in suburbs.

Cherry Hinton and Trumpington stand out as exemplary (by UK suburban standards) in both the proportions of walking/cycling trips to local facilities, and the median distance people are prepared to walk. The positive cultural attitude to active travel in Cambridge, especially to cycling, is clearly distinct from other areas. These distinctive Cambridge attitudes are not easily explained by student car-lessness as few of our respondents were students. The spatial character of the city plays an important part: it is small enough for most of the city to be within cycling distance, it is flat, and planning policy has promoted walking and cycling while constraining car use through capacity constraint and parking policy. Cherry Hinton and Trumpington both benefit from local superstores, within walking distance of many residents, and—in contrast to the findings of Lee and Moudon (2008)—high levels of active travel (50% in the case of one superstore). Both areas have reasonable, though not optimal, permeability and the characteristics of a neighbourhood cell.

Filton Avenue, Harrow South and West Barking also have above average levels of active travel, in spite of being perceived as relatively unattractive. All are older suburbs embedded in their cities, with through bus routes. They are socially distinct: Barking is the poorest and most deprived area, Harrow is socially diverse, with affluent enclaves, and Filton lies between them. They have more car-free households (28–43%) than other areas. Despite having the highest population density in the study, Barking is poorly served by local facilities, with dying retail parades reflecting poverty and a declining population. Distances to effective facilities are therefore long, forcing heavy reliance on long walking trips or bus for those without cars. Nevertheless, car use is higher than the Cambridge suburbs or Filton, and similar to Harrow. Harrow has more and closer facilities, easier to walk to. But neither Barking nor Harrow is optimally permeable by comparison with Filton Avenue's traditional grid structure. The facilities in Filton lie along a spine bus route. All housing is within walking distance, and catchment population has been increased by higher density redevelopment.

The common factor which the three areas share is location: a fair level of integration within the urban area, so that a wide range of facilities is not too distant. However, they contrast in local accessibility. Households without a car are well served in Filton, poorly served in Barking, signifying social exclusion of vulnerable groups, compounding issues of health inequity.

At the other end of the active travel range, in order of car dependence, are Broxbourne, Cramlington, Bradley Stoke, Backworth and Bar Hill. Bar Hill (a Cambridge exurb) is an anomaly for Cambridge in having a low walking/cycling rate. Despite relative affluence and high car ownership, it has also far fewer trips than anywhere else, and an apparent aversion to recreational activities. Backworth's population is similar to Filton Avenue's, with quite high levels of deprivation and a high proportion of social housing, yet car ownership is the second highest out of the 12. Backworth's built form is sporadic, dissected, with permeability reduced by cul-de-sac enclaves and weak provision of local facilities. Despite its social similarity to Filton, its travel behaviour is very different, illustrating how the place impacts on travel choices.

Broxbourne, an area of incremental sprawl, and Cramlington, a planned settlement, are socially varied and lie beyond the city edge. Bradley Stoke is a more recently planned owner-occupied urban extension typical of many outer estates, with no deprivation. All three share design assumptions of full motorization, with pod-based layouts that reduce permeability, compromise walkability and weaken the viability of local facilities. All three study areas have district or town centres nearby but sufficiently distant requiring most trips to be by car.

Taking the two extreme cases, Cherry Hinton and Broxbourne, both are mid-/late-twentieth century suburbs, both have similar deprivation profiles, both have similar gross densities, yet the availability of accessible facilities and the pattern of active travel are completely different. Cherry Hinton's residents travel actively over three times as far and three times the proportion of trips as Broxbourne's (three out of five compared with one out of four). This is due to their cultural/attitudinal differences, their contrasting locational patterns (integrated/dispersed) and long standing planning priorities.

Conclusions

At the general level, the data presented here support some of the findings of earlier researchers. In particular, it shows the critical influence of distance on modal choice—and therefore, if we wish to promote physical activity and reduce car dependence, facilities must be available within walkable distance. What this study adds is more detailed UK evidence about the way in which local facilities are used, the distance people are prepared to walk to them and the degree to which suburbs vary in terms of facilitating active travel to local facilities. We present the findings with some confidence, despite the possibility of respondent bias, given the high levels of significance, consistency with the NTS, and wide range of local behaviour.

The study highlights the fact that many English suburbs are not very walkable at all, but that where there *are* local facilities, people use them. The sheer diversity of local suburban behaviour is striking. The research demonstrates the significance of place and of travel culture.

This diversity suggests that aggregate analysis—i.e. averaging behaviour across many places and communities, looking for statistically valid generalizations and explanations—can be problematic, giving a false impression of universal truth, and in any particular case could be very misleading. There *are* significant shared patterns, but the exceptions are many and complex. Our belief, on the basis of this research, is that it is important to view each place and community holistically and cluster them when similarities occur.

The logic model (Figure 13.1), while presented at the start to orientate the reader, was in fact devised as a result of the research (a post hoc rationalization!) as we became aware of the interacting influences more fully. It is useful in that it distinguishes and emphasizes cultural factors and well as social characteristics, facility provision as well as a rounded view of urban form and design. In this paper, we have not delved deep into each of these determinants, but striven to give an overview. Further research is needed to study a wider range of neighbourhoods, for example in the inner city; to investigate route and facility characteristics fully; to do longitudinal studies on the 12 neighbourhoods and to tie in health/well-being and social capital data.

In terms of practice, it is salutary to note that the suburbs created in the last 20 or 30 years exhibit high levels of car dependence and low levels of active travel, while some of the older or more mixed-age neighbourhoods are less car dependent and have high levels of active travel. There is a hiatus between the expressed purpose of policy—promoting neighbourhood vitality, social inclusion, healthy lifestyles and reduced carbon emissions—and the reality of the development and planning decisions that have shaped suburban places. The divergence in behaviour evident between neighbourhoods derives more from spatial and cultural factor than from population variation. The research suggests that higher residential density—often held up as vital to sustainability—is not the key spatial issue. Neighbourhood location, form, integration (into the town/city), permeability and service catchment viability are all important. The research also highlights the critical significance of cultural attitudes to bike use and to what is a walkable distance; also across most places studied two loose groups are apparent, the more sedentary and the more active. Cultural variation would of course be much *more* marked if we were to compare Dutch and English populations.

There are some patterns of travel behaviour—in terms of thresholds of pedestrian accessibility—which are relatively widespread in the sample neighbourhoods and could provide starting points for policy discussion. One crude threshold is the one kilometre 'standard': local shops and services within this distance are likely to generate a majority of walking trips. However, as local variation is so high, local debate, surveys, spatial analysis and market research are required to define viable principles, relevant to the local community. It is to be devoutly wished that the new UK agenda of 'localism' encourages this sensitivity. The question is: will local communities see planning for active travel—with the concomitant benefits—as their priority?

This chapter has been adapted from: Hugh Barton, Michael Horswell & Paul Millar (2012) Neighbourhood Accessibility and Active Travel, *Planning Practice & Research*, 27:2, 177–201.

References

Barton, H. (2000) *Sustainable Communities: The Potential for Eco-Neighbourhoods* (London: Earthscan).

Barton, H. & Hills, S. (2005) *Sustainability of Land Use and Transport In Outer Areas: WP12: Neighbourhood Accessibility & Social Inclusion Literature Review and Pilot Study*. Available at www.suburbansolutions. ac.uk/DocumentManager/secure0/06B_Neighbourhood%20accessibility%20and%20social% 20inclusion%20(paper).pdf (accessed 13 April 2010).

Barton, H., Grant, M., & Guise, R. (2010a) *Shaping Neighbourhoods—For Local Health and Global Sustainability* (London: Routledge).

Barton, H., Louis, R., & Grant, M. (2010b) Reshaping suburbs—Chapter 7, in: *The Final Report of the SOLUTIONS Project (The Sustainability of Land Use and Transport in Outer Neighbourhoods)*. Available at www.suburbansolutions.ac.uk (accessed 21 February 2012).

Boarnet, M. & Sarmiento, S. (1998) Can land use policy really affect travel behaviour? A study of the link between non-work travel and land use characteristics, *Urban Studies*, 35(7), pp. 1155–1169.

Brownson, R., Hoehner, C., Day, K., Forsyth, A., & Sallis, J. (2009) Measuring the built environment for physical activity, *American Journal of Preventive Medicine*, 36(4), pp. S99–S123.

Calve Blanco, T. (2010) The significance of access to local neighbourhood facilities for social interaction and mental well-being, Draft PhD, University of the West of England.

Centre for Regional Economic and Social Research (CRESR) (2010) *The New Deal for Communities Evaluation: Final report*. Vol. 7 (Sheffield and London: Communities and Local Government Publications, HMSO).

Communities and Local Government (CLG) (2010) *Decentralisation and the Localism Bill: An Essential Guide* (CLG). Available at www.communities.gov.uk/documents/localgovernment/pdf/1793908. pdf (accessed 2 February 2011).

Competition Commission (2008) *The Supply of Groceries in the UK, Market Investigation, Appendix 5.1: Trends in the Number of Convenience and Specialist Grocery Stores* (London: Competition Commission).

Corburn, J. (2005) Urban planning and health disparities: Implications for research and practice, *Planning Practice and Research*, 20(2), pp. 11–126.

Dempsey, N. (2008) Quality of the built environment in urban neighbourhoods, *Planning Practice and Research*, 23(2), pp. 249–264.

Dennis, N. (1968) The popularity of the neighbourhood community idea, in: R. Pahl (Ed.) *Readings in Urban Sociology* (Oxford: Pergamon Press).

Department for Transport (DfT) (2005) *Focus on Personal Travel—2005 Edition—Including the Report of the National Travel Survey 2002/2003* (London: DfT, HMSO).

DETR (1998) *Planning for Sustainable Development: Towards Better Practice* (London: HMSO).

Echenique, M., *et al.* (2010) *Conclusions of the SOLUTIONS Research Project*. Available at www.suburban solutions.ac.uk (accessed 21 February 2012).

ECOTEC (1993) *Reducing Transport Emissions Through Planning* (London: Department of the Environment, HMSO).

EEA (2009a) *About the Urban Environment*. European Environment Agency website. Available at www. eea.europa.eu/themes/urban (accessed 7 June 2009).

EEA (2009b) *Ensuring Quality of Life in European Cities and Towns*. European Environment Report 5/2009 (Luxembourg: Office of Official Publications of the European Communities).

European Commission (1990) *Green Paper on the Urban Environment* (Luxemburg: Office for Official Publications of the European Communities).

Feng, J., Glass, T., Curriero, F., Stewart, W., & Schwartz, B. (2009) The built environment and obesity: A systematic review of the epidemiologic evidence, *Health and Place*, 16, p. 175.

Forsyth, A., Hearst, M., Oakes J., & Schmitz K. (2008) Design and destinations: Factors influencing walking and total physical activity, *Urban Studies*, 45, pp. 1973–1996.

Forsyth, A., Oakes, J., & Schmitz, B. (2009) The built environment, walking, and physical activity: Is the environment more important to some people than others? *Transportation Research Part D: Transport and Environment*, 14(1), pp. 42–49.

Frank, L. & Pivo, G. (1995) Impacts of mixed use and density on utilisation of three modes of travel: Single occupant vehicle, transit and walking, *Transportation Research Record*, 1466, pp. 44–52.

Frank, L., Sallis, J., Conway, T., Chapman, J., Saelens B., & Bachman. W. (2006) Multiple pathways from land use to health: Walkability associations with active transportation, Body Mass Index, and air quality, *Journal of the American Planning Association*, 72(1), pp. 75–89.

Giddens, A. (1990) *The Consequences of Modernity* (Oxford: Polity Press).

Giles-Corti, B., Knuiman, M., Timperio, A., Van Neil, K., Pikora, T., Bull, F., Shilton, T., & Bulsara, M. (2007) Evaluation of the implementation of a state government community design policy aimed at increasing local walking: Design issues and baseline results from RESIDE, Perth Western Australia, *Preventive Medicine*, 46(1), pp. 46–54.

Handy, S. (1993) Regional versus local accessibility: Neo-traditional development and its implications for non- work travel, *Built Environment*, 18, pp. 253–267.

Handy, S. (2005) *Does the Built Environment Influence Physical Activity: Examining the Evidence* (Washington, DC: Transportation Research Board).

Hess, P., Moudon, A., Snyder, M., & Stanilov, K. (1999) Site design and pedestrian travel, *Transportation Research Record*, 1674(1), pp. 9–19.

Koger, S. & Winter, D. (2010) *The Psychology of Environmental Problems* (New York: Psychology Press).

Lee, C. & Moudon, A. (2008) Neighbourhood design and physical activity, *Building Research and Information*, 36(5), pp. 95–411.

Llewelyn Davies (1998) *Sustainable Residential Quality—New Approaches to Urban Living* (London: LPAC).

McDonald, K., Oakes, J., & Forsyth, A. (2011) Effect of street connectivity and density on adult BMI: Results from the Twin Cities Walking Study, *Journal of Epidemiology and Community Health*, Published Online First: 17 January, DOI:10.1136/jech.2010.122556.

Millar, P. & Barton, H. (2011) Active travel and neighbourhood accessibility: A systematic review, Draft paper, University of the West of England. Available at www.uwe.ac.uk/research/who.

Minnery, J., Knight, J., Byrne, J., & Spencer, J. (2009) Bounding neighbourhoods, how do residents do it?, *Planning Practice and Research*, 24(4), pp. 471–493.

NICE (2008) *Promoting and Creating Built and Natural Environments that Encourage and Support Physical Activity*, National Institute of Health and Clinical Excellence (NICE) Public Health guidance 8 (London: NICE).

Rao, M., Barten, F., Blackshaw, N., Lapitan, J., Galea, G., Jacoby, E., Samarth, A., & Buckley, E. (2011) Urban planning, development and non-communicable diseases, *Planning Practice and Research*, 26(4), pp. 373–391.

Saelens, B., Sallis, J., & Frank, L. (2003) Environmental correlates of walking and cycling: Findings from the transportation, urban design, and planning literatures, *Annals of Behavioral Medicine*, 25(2), pp. 80–91.

Social Exclusion Unit (2000) *National Strategy for Neighbourhood Renewal* (London: SEU).

Webber, M. (1964) The urban place and non place urban realm, in: M. Webber *et al.* (Eds.) *Explorations into Urban Structure*, pp. 79–153 (Philadelphia: UPP).

Williams, K. (2000) Does intensifying cities make them more sustainable? in: K. Williams, E. Burton, and M. Jenks (Eds.) *Achieving Sustainable Urban Form* (London: E&FN Spon).

Winter, J. & Farthing, S. (1997) Coordinating facility provision and new housing development: Impact on car and local facility use, in: S. Farthing (Ed.) *Evaluating Local Environmental Policy*, pp. 159–179 (Aldershot: Avebury).

14

THE ENVIRONMENT, PHYSICAL ACTIVITY, RECREATION AND THE OUTDOORS

Barbara Humberstone, Heather Prince and Lois Mansfield

Introduction

The 'outdoors' and the natural environment are significant and arguably, in physical activity research, under-acknowledged spaces/places and ideological contexts in which physical activity recreation and learning take place. These diverse spaces and places co-construct formal, non-formal and informal education and learning arenas with a variety of young and older people and with a variety of aims. Over the last two decades there has been increased interest in the study of outdoor activities which include the study of outdoor education, outdoor recreation, leisure and sport, particularly from social, cultural, educational and environmental perspectives (Humberstone, Prince and Henderson, 2016).

During this time, analyses of physical activities outdoors have benefited from a multiplicity of standpoints. Different schools of socio-cultural analysis have identified outdoor activities as: risk/adventure (Lyng, 1990; McNamee, 2007); alternative sport (Thorpe & Rinehart, 2010); extreme sport (Rinehart & Sydnor, 2003); lifestyle sport (Wheaton, 2004); action sport (Thorpe, 2014); or for socio-environmental analyses, as nature-based sport/sport in nature (Humberstone, 1998; Vanreusel, 1995). The physical and recreational activities considered from these standpoints include activities that generally depend upon the natural environment (landscapes and/or seascapes) and participant's engagement with the elements such as surfing, kayaking, climbing, walking and so forth. These physical activities in nature are the vehicles through which much programmed outdoor learning and outdoor education takes place.[1]

Further, according to much research, being in the natural environment and taking part in outdoor activities have considerable health and wellbeing benefits (Robertson, Lawrence & Heath, 2015; Finlay et al., 2015). In exploring the outdoors as therapeutic media Carpenter and Harper (2016) critique the socio-ecological frameworks drawn upon for ignoring the natural environment. They highlight the mental, physical, social and spiritual benefits of community and environmental contexts for individual and community wellbeing, but fail to recognise the needs and values appended by those that live and work there who may draw a livelihood from the environment in other ways.

The 'outdoors' is thus not only media for learning and promoting human wellbeing, but also an ideological space where individuals either alone or in groups engage actively or passively with the environment or their countryside. For as Crouch (1998: p. 11) maintains,

> Countryside is not only 'outward' as intense ideological practice, or as 'gaze', but also part of enjoying something else, . . . where particular traditions of land availability and regulations (state, commercial) make possible 'being around', being together , taking part in activities, . . . In the doing aspects of 'environment', of countryside, mix with ways of being in space.

This chapter draws attention to theory, policy and practice of the outdoors, the environment and physical activities. It starts with briefly locating policy and practice within tensions highlighted through eco-feminist thoughts, it then points to research that considers the ways in which policy is pertinent in managing these conflicts. The importance of education in promoting sustainable physical activities out of doors is considered in light of current educational policies. Finally, the chapter considers the conflicting demands of key stakeholders or communities of people with different interests in physical activity and the land whilst considering land management.

Policy and practice in relation to the environment and the outdoors can be better understood through attention to theoretical underpinnings and discourses. In this chapter, particular attention is drawn to eco-feminist thought since the contradictions and complexities uncovered through some eco-feminist lenses shine a spotlight onto current fractures between policy and practice in the outdoors. For, as Dobson (2003: p. 83) intimates, social justice and environmental sustainability 'are not always compatible objectives'. There are contradictions and tensions between bounded ideologies; between social justice perspectives, which are human centred, and deep green perspectives, which centre the non-human world. Much eco-feminist thought attempts to break down these boundaries stressing the vital webs of connections between humans and non-human, emphasising how the social, environmental and spiritual interrelate (Humberstone, 2011). It is amongst the few frameworks that has emphasised the powerful interconnection and interdependence between human and more than human which also takes seriously the impact of inequalities through sex, gender, race and so forth. Outdoor physical activities and outdoor learning are systems through which these webs of connections can be experienced and potentially through which inequalities might be challenged.[2] These perspectives, whilst highlighting the fractures and complexities associated with people's interaction with the non-human world, speak little of the actual effects of outdoor physical activity 'consumption' on the degradation of the environment. Nor how this might be addressed and the significance of education in envisioning and enabling greater awareness of and action towards a more sustainable human engagement in physical activities in the outdoors.

In this chapter, we suggest an optimum way to promote a greater understanding of sustainable use of the natural environment is through formal and informal education. Outdoor and environmental education can not only provide opportunities to learn about the environment and webs of connections, but also can foster understanding of health and wellbeing for human and non-human and their interrelations, promoting praxis for eco-feminist thought.

The chapter begins by examining policy, practice and the place of physical activity within outdoor and environmental education in the formal curriculum and the tension arising between attainment setting in the examined curricula and the need to promote a more active and healthy lifestyle. Demands created by introducing people to physical activities outdoors, for outdoor recreation and education, and generated by those who use these landscapes and waterscapes for other purposes are frequently conflictual. The final section locates these tensions in the development of policies that underpin current use of outdoor environments and the key stakeholders and communities involved.

Outdoor and environmental education in the UK: Formal curricular policy and practice

This section examines the place of physical activity within outdoor and environmental education in the formal curriculum and the tension that arises between attainment and reported measures in English, mathematics and science and the need for more active, fit and healthy citizens.

Educational policy in the UK and beyond challenges the balance between political and social ideologies and the individual assertion of identity through leisure (Erickson, 2011). It tends towards a more positivist epistemological framework than a phenomenological approach of gathering evidence (Church & Ravenscroft, 2011) and is influenced by neoliberalist ideologies aligned with the broader value of the environment to other users. There is government recognition of the decline in the number of young people engaging with their environment in physically active ways and the impact that this has on physical and mental wellbeing. However, there is a lack of an overarching strategy (Hayes, 2016) and thus, results in a reductive model to formal curricular provision for every child.

UK educational policy is politically driven and although geographically separate and distinct (from decentralised government departments in England, Wales, Scotland and Northern Ireland and their respective curricula) it shares outcome, performativity and accountability agenda. Standardised tests to measure cognitive attainment have become the norm in formal education (Gorard, Selwyn & Rees, 2002) that have marginalised and devalued less quantifiable learning (Waite, 2015).

In Scotland 'outdoor learning[3] is explicitly positioned to deliver "experience and outcomes" from all eight curricular areas' (Christie et al., 2014), and Education Scotland[4] provides policy and practical guidance to support teachers in embedding it in the curriculum (Education Scotland, 2013; Christie, Higgins & Nicol, 2016). The Curriculum for Excellence places emphasis on young people developing as 'successful learners', 'confident individuals', 'responsible citizens' and 'effective contributors' – the four capacities, and although health, wellbeing and physical activity are not overtly specified in these, they are implicit throughout. In the Curriculum for Wales, and the English national curriculum, adventurous activities (outdoor and adventurous activities in England) are part of the physical education curriculum at Key Stages 2 and 3.[5] Key values in terms of outdoor provision are teaching and learning in the natural environment and through residentials (Curriculum for Wales, 2013), and both emphasise physical activity. In England, an holistic and cross-curricular approach has not been adopted within the formal curriculum (Prince & Exeter, 2015) and outdoor adventurous activities (OAA) have an emphasis on teaching and learning a technical skill. In contrast, in Northern Ireland, the curriculum does not contain physical outdoor activities although there is an emphasis on play in the early years, and on personal development and mutual understanding at Key Stages 1 and 2.

Although the formal physical education curricula might not comprise outdoor education outcomes, particularly the development of self-constructs and meta-skills to encourage lifelong or transferable learning, they do stipulate a range of physical activity, health, fitness and wellbeing outcomes. In many schools, head teachers have introduced initiatives for encouraging or even levering physical activity amongst their pupils such as pre-study physical activity or a weekly school mile run (Gorely et al., 2009) and involve outdoor activities in residential experiences (Kendall & Rodger, 2015), visits or after school clubs. A recent study on out of school activities in primary schools showed that sports and physical activities and after school clubs were positively associated with increased attainment at 11 years (end of Key Stage 2 National Curriculum tests) and also social, emotional and behavioural outcomes. Amongst economically disadvantaged children, out of school activities were the only organised activity positively linked to these outcomes and this has implications for policy makers and practitioners (Chanfreau et al., 2016).

Although physical activity through outdoor education is widely acknowledged to be positive, schools often struggle to implement any kind of meaningful provision due to lack of teacher competence or confidence, cost, perceived issues of health and safety and time, as well as the competing pressures for performativity in core curriculum areas. Some schools, usually with qualified staff, are able to make provision for outdoor activities such as climbing, mountain walking, sailing, kayaking and/or canoeing, often in the context of journeys or expeditions. Those schools without expertise or access to resources and facilities are now encouraging teachers to use local environments including playgrounds, parks and woodlands for environmental education that can be linked to the science or geography curricula, or to fieldwork in secondary education, and although these learning opportunities might not necessarily provide aerobic exercise, they do promote aspects of physical activity. It is hoped that increased funding for the National Citizen Service for 15–17 year olds will enable all young people to take part in adventurous activities and a residential experience (Department for Education (DfE), 2016) as this is the current government's manifesto commitment.

Environmental education is rarely defined as a subject within formal curricula in the UK, but it is encapsulated within outdoor learning, learning for sustainability (LfS) and education for sustainable development, for example. The Scottish Government is committed to an entitlement for all learners to LfS and for every practitioner, school and education leader to demonstrate LfS in their practice following the recommendations in their report (2012). In England, there has been disappointment amongst environmentalists that the most recent iteration of the national curriculum in 2014 makes no reference to sustainable development at any part or any stage of learning, although climate change is reinstated as part of the geography curriculum at KS3 (WWF, 2013).

The Welsh Government is moving towards a new curriculum for implementation by 2018, 'A curriculum for Wales – a curriculum for life' (Welsh Government, 2015) that includes four 'purposes' of which 'ethical informed citizens' and 'healthy confident individuals' are two. Within these, 'show their commitment to a sustainable planet' and 'take part in physical activity' are listed respectively as objectives for pupils to reach, albeit currently in separate lists. Education for Sustainable Development does feature in the Northern Ireland Curriculum Primary and at KS3 (CCEA, 2007) with an emphasis on appreciating and understanding the environment, caring, maintaining and respecting it, and understanding the effect of actions and the need for responsibility.

It can be seen that environmental education is not a focus in any of these curricula although it may become so through (learning for) sustainability education. In terms of policy it lacks a theoretical framework and support, rendering it 'largely ineffective' (Scott & Reid, 1998: p. 222). A recent review of environmental and sustainability education policy research (Aikens, McKenzie & Vaughter, 2016) suggests that there are not only competing paradigms and identities but also that this educational content often exists where there are 'multiple policy discourses competing for primacy' (2016: p. 348).

Given this curriculum paralysis in the subject area, many schools have embedded environmental education through their own bespoke approaches or projects such as Forest School (Knight, 2015) or (wildlife) gardening (Ohly et al., 2016) and through initiatives with organisations such as the Council for Learning Outside the Classroom (CLOtC), Learning through Landscapes (LTL) and Open Air Laboratories (OPAL).

> Despite the lack of an overarching government strategy, public bodies, environmental charities and sector-led organisations are developing new ways of engaging children of all ages with the outdoor world and, in so doing, broadening and deepening their education and skills.
>
> *Hayes, 2016: p. 18*

A shift towards less prescribed curriculum content has allowed schools more autonomy to choose the ways in which they can enable children to engage in learning outdoors tailored to the needs of their learners, location and opportunity supported by a recent government White Paper, *Educational Excellence Everywhere* (DfE, 2016). Furthermore, physical activity is integrated through being and learning outdoors, whether it is predominantly focused on outdoor or environmental education or in many cases, a combination of the two.

Learning in the outdoors in natural environments has been shown to have personal, social, developmental, educational and health outcomes in both formal and non-formal settings (Dillon & Dickie, 2012; Rickinson et al., 2004; Fiennes et al., 2015). In terms of the enhancement of physical activity in schools, research has shown the benefits in relation to the development of motor skills (Scholz & Krombholz, 2007) including through play (Fjørtoft, 2004) and increased levels and engagement in physical activity more widely (Lovell, 2009).

The intersectionality in critical policy theory and methodology (Aikens et al., 2016) to encourage a more physical active nation was a driver for the UK government's latest sporting strategy (HM Government, 2015). In this there is a commitment to a widening of the interpretation of engagement in physical activity including the introduction of a new measure of 'active lives' by the end of 2016. The 'Getting Active Outdoors' report (Gordon, Chester & Denton, 2015) identified that being outdoors is itself the most important factor to the majority of outdoor users and where physical activity is driven by emotional purposes and revolves around exploring and learning. It would seem that this holistic and integrated engagement in the outdoor environment, bringing outdoor and education policy communities together, is beginning to be reflected in both formal education practice and broader political policy in the UK. This is to be welcomed in terms of enhancing the scope of physical activity, widening access and inclusivity.

However, this can only increase demands on land and water. This dilemma is clearly evident in other countries. For example Aall et al. (2011) highlight the issues of increased use and over use of the environment through some outdoor activities in Norway that require the use of more manufactured equipment. In raising this problem, they argue the need for policies that can encourage more sustainable outdoor activities' practices that require fewer manufactured goods and promote a greater awareness of active care for the environment. In a study of land/water use in Wales, Church and Ravenscroft (2011) raise the issue of conflict arising between the key stakeholders around access and use of land and waterways for kayak participants. They suggest that policy for managing sustainable access of physical activities in nature requires policy-makers to better understand the life-worlds of the all those engaged in the politics of access to water to provide potential solutions to the debate.

The next section locates these debates in the development of policies that underpin current use of the environment and draws attention to key stakeholders involved.

Appreciating the outdoor canvas

Physical activity in the outdoors, such as walking, canoeing or climbing, necessarily places demands on the access to, and management of, land and water. Whilst there is increasingly developed policy of how the public can engage with the outdoors as a learning environment, the demands of outdoor activities through the various forms of recreation, leisure and education and those who are using these landscapes for other purposes are sometimes contradictory. Government policy has mainly focused on the designation of National Parks (National Parks & Access to the Countryside 1949) and Areas of Outstanding Natural Beauty with recreation remits (Countryside Act 1968), reduction of impact (House of Commons, 1995) and the enactment of very specific access legislation (Countryside & Rights of Way Act 2000). The outdoor sector continues to demand increased right of access, most notably on water, and there is no joint policy position, strategy or organisation which creates this type of formal consensus; the process is left to individual bodies to work at a local level.

Furthermore, outdoor environments comprise places where many stakeholders have a vested interest in the resource base, whether tangible or intangible in character (for example, Church & Ravenscroft, 2011). Their objectives, attitudes and behaviour vary, which creates cognitive conflict and dissonance influencing the relationship between recreationalists, those that live and work there and those who seek to conserve or preserve it. The challenge is deepened by political and social ideologies that can support or undermine the relationships between different stakeholders. In this section, it is argued that the relationship between outdoor recreationists taking part in physical activity and other environmental stakeholders is rooted in historical materialism, supported by changing land use contexts, land ownership, property rights, government and governance.

Changing land use contexts: Political ideologies at work

Traditionally, in Western society, the outdoor environment has been used to provide for society's physiological needs of food, timber for construction, mineral wealth for industrial processes and/or a potable water supply – 'primary land uses'. Initially, this was achieved through feudalism prioritising subsistence: Land was owned by the monarch, bestowed to his barons and managed by serfdom. In the UK, piecemeal private enclosure of open commons and waste (1300 to 1700) was followed by legislated enclosure (1760 to 1890), as the mode of production shifted to a capitalist system (Overton, 1996). This was underpinned by technological change, agricultural and industrial revolution, food surplus creating financial profit and a changed active social status from serfdom to a mainly landless proletariat.

The result of Enclosure limited people's access to the outdoors unless it was to work either as an owner occupier or a tenant. This mass privatisation of the UK countryside ran parallel to immigration into urban areas by the landless as the Industrial Revolution unfolded. In 1815 90 per cent of populace lived and worked in the countryside, by 1870 two thirds were urbanised; most in squalid, cramped, unhealthy conditions. Simultaneously the nature conservation movement began to evolve intent initially on preserving birds (Sea Birds Preservation Act 1869) and then wider countryside from the 'ravages' of technological change and urban sprawl, encapsulated by the formation of the Commons Preservation Society in 1865 (now the Open Spaces Society) (Evans, 1992). These developments were the impetus to encourage people to return the countryside, not to work there, but to appreciate and enjoy clean air, landscape beauty and healthy physically active pastimes such as walking and later cycling. It led to the emergence of 'secondary land use'; that is, outdoor recreational physical activities and nature conservation, predicated on the existence of the products of primary land use.

Outdoor recreation as a pastime accelerated in popularity throughout the early twentieth century supported by the advent of bicycles, then cars, development of 'Wakes Weeks' and eventually the five-day working week (Bunce, 1994). Post War designation of National Parks in 1949, with their twin aims of recreation and conservation of iconic landscapes whilst supporting agricultural land use, aided opportunities for people to return to the countryside. Thus, the environment was still productivist at its core, supported by political process through the Town & Country Planning Act 1947 and the Agriculture Act 1947, although with recognition of the loss of our environment (Carson, 1962; Shoard, 1980). This continued into the 1980s, only being challenged institutionally on the world stage with regard to food overproduction, surpluses and protectionist food production policies of the European Union (Mansfield, 2011). However, now policy and decision makers are more interested in the 'additionality' land uses can bring through their activities, manifested by more directed financial support for rural development and environmental management. Termed ecosystem goods and services, these represent the entire panoply of phenomena created by human activity outside and how they can benefit society (Table 14.1). As a consequence, our environment is now truly multifunctional of which outdoor recreational physical activities and food are but two parts of the greater objective (Figure 14.1), all be they underpinned by a range of historical, political and social ideologies.

Land ownership and outside physical activity: A clash of political and social ideologies

Probably the biggest clash of ideologies comes from land owning classes and access to land by the landless proletariat with its roots in the political history of land ownership in the UK

Table 14.1 Characteristics of ecosystem services

Ecosystem Service	Characteristics and Examples
Provisioning services	Products obtained directly from functioning ecosystems which provide human needs such as nutrition, shelter and safety. E.g. food, timber
Regulating services	Benefits created through the regulation of ecosystem services and are particularly important in terms of issues such as climate change and natural disasters. E.g. flood management, carbon sequestration
Cultural services	Non-material benefits that we can acquire through spiritual enrichment, cognitive development, educational values, sense of place, social relations, recreation and so on. These are experienced by people most often and help raise public awareness and support for protecting ecosystems. E.g. outdoor education and recreation, health and well being, sense of place
Supporting services	Those necessary for the production of all other ecosystem services, probably the most complex to understand as their value is indirect. E.g. soil and water management

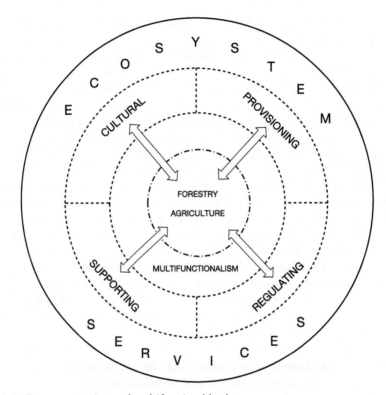

Figure 14.1 Ecosystem services and multifunctional land use

(Shoard, 1987). This has limited physical activity in open spaces where other land use objectives operate with no real heedance to physical activity and recreation. There are three central issues: misinterpretation of common land, damage to livelihoods and land ownership constructs. Large tracts of land had the Right of Common upon it, confirmed by the Statute of Merton in 1235.[6] Common land is not, as the name suggests, common to all. Instead, in England and Wales, common land might be owned by one person, but access to, and use of, the land is bestowed on others. Legally, a common is recognised as land that has rights attached to it, whereby: 'A person may take some part of the produce of, or property in, the soil owned by another' (Aitchison & Gadsden, 1992: p. 168).

The right can include grazing rights (typical of upland areas), dead wood collection from the ground (estover), peat extraction (turbary), fishing (piscary) or pig grazing (pannage), as well as other rights such as bracken or gorse gathering, or mineral exploitation (Aitchison et al., 2000). It did not, until 2000, give people the right to walk where they like (see below) other than on historic highways[7] or Rights of Way derived from custom and practice through common law.

In the early 1930s less than 1 per cent of open moorland was accessible to the public as the land owning gentry did not want the 'masses' wandering on their land citing crop and fishery damage, and disturbance of deer and grouse as the main economic reasons. As a result, there began a long power struggle between rural landowners and the public to win back their rights to walk these areas again. Shoard (1999) gives a passionate account of the battles to secure greater access, culminating in the famous mass trespass of Kinder Scout in England's Peak District in 1932. Nevertheless it was only with the enactment of the National Parks and Access to the Countryside Bill 1949 and the later Countryside (Scotland) Bill 1967 that the first steps were taken to secure access (*not* ownership) to these areas. The issue was only finally resolved with the Land Reform (Scotland) Act 2003 and the Countryside and Rights of Way Act (CROW) 2000 whereby open access is limited to open land above the last wall up a hillside. In England, for example, this means the public now have access to 865 thousand hectares for quiet enjoyment, to walk, cycle or ride horses.

Unfortunately, the enactment of these two pieces of legislation has only served to re-enforce the previous concerns of landowners and managers who perceive lack of recognition of their livelihoods (McVittie et al., 2005) with careless behaviour of the public. Thus, the Country Code was set up in the 1950s and updated in 2012 as the CROW Act rolled out; a code that resonates with the 'Leave No Trace' principles of North America.

From the historical evolution of this struggle have emerged three land ownership constructs which influence outdoor recreation's relationship with the broader environmental milieu: private, public and community. The importance of these forms of historical materialism cannot be underestimated, but are often ignored, as they place physical and cultural limits on accepted behaviour and opportunities for physical activity. Private ownership is sometimes referred to as the paternalistic countryside, whereby a few landowners shape the development of the outdoor landscape (Marsden, 1998). In England, Wales and Scotland over 80 per cent of rural land is privately owned by individuals, family trusts or corporations. The largest 100 landowners control about 2m ha (8.2%) of the land, many in Scotland. The majority of national parks are in private ownership, for example, over 8 per cent of the Peak District is owned by water companies and private charitable organisations such as the National Trust that owns c.2 per cent. Private landowners are at liberty to pursue their own agendas contrary or integrated with the needs of outdoor recreation and leisure but they are able to plan for the long term with regard to natural resource management and have to abide by laws and jurisdiction. Today, some land owners encourage physical activity through additional facilities, such as forestry companies providing mountain biking trails, whereas others, often sole owners, discourage it actively through deliberate neglect of path (trail) egress and access.

A particular private land ownership worthy of mention is that of water supply. The UK water industry has moved from private to public and back to private during the same time period as the explosion in demand for outdoor recreational physical activity has occurred. This shift has been underpinned by neoliberalisation, the commodification and commercialisation of common property resources[8] via privatisation forming market environmentalism, whereby natural resources are regulated to provide economic and environmental needs. Whilst there are many proponents and detractors of market environmentalism (Bakker, 2005), the reality is that land previously publicly owned by the state is now in private hands. As a result land owners eliminate anything which may detract from their core aims or increase costs to themselves, for example footpath erosion deposits soil into water courses.

In contrast, public ownership refers to land owned by the state, which occupies about 20 per cent of land in Great Britain. Governance employs synoptic or incremental planning systems, regulations and controls devised by the state through statute and policy implementation. The largest public land owner is the Forestry Commission, owning about 1.06m ha, along with the Ministry of Defence (260,000 ha) and the state controlled Scottish Natural Heritage (34,000ha), Natural Resources Wales (126,000 ha) and Natural England (63,000 ha). Little of the national parks is in public ownership which substantially reduces choice of physical activity. However, the Brecon Beacons is an exception with 16 per cent publicly owned. This is in direct contrast to National Parks elsewhere in the world. Because the land is acquired with tax payers' money, access is therefore obligatory unless without due cause, as long as it does not interfere with commercial operations, such as timber harvesting. The only exceptions are nature reserves with limited access due to wildlife disturbance or situations where there is demonstrable danger to the public. The challenge with publicly owned land is to manage within a consistent policy framework over long time scales; quangos[9] are often at the mercy of the politicians reacting to public and constituents concerns. Emotive issues such as the escape of wild boar, or the browsing behaviour of deer in the south east are classic examples which negatively affect those simply out for a walk or jog (ECOS, 2014).

Land owned by communities are very much governance systems driven by approaches to planning and controlled through some representation mechanism that allows a community to influence their operation or use and to enjoy the benefits arising. Probably the most well-known of these in the UK is the community buy out of the Island of Eigg, Inner Hebrides in 1997.

Ownership versus property rights: Social ideologies

Where there is no clear understanding of property rights and if no one is policing access, use and/or management, each user will take what they need regardless of its deleterious effect on another user. In other words, for those who think they are simply out for a walk or a ride on their bike, their actions can have a negative effect on someone else's property rights. The classic outdoor example of this is the use of a Right of Way. Whilst the public have the legal right to use the route, they may inadvertently, through use, cause biophysical deterioration.[10]

Property rights refer to 'authorised actions pertaining to a resource' and are created via *de jure* (the law) or *de facto* (what actually happens in practice due to cultural norms) of which land is only one, but the main type of property. Some resources change from public to private ownership, thus creating a transfer of property rights, as in the water supply discussed above. As the switch occurs, private owners are faced with the dilemma of how to protect their property from other users used to public access of these resources.

Furthermore, different stakeholders (such as an owner or authorised entrant, like a walker) can have different combinations of property rights. As a result individuals or organisations are said to have *bundles of property rights* (Quinn et al., 2010) and this makes management of the outdoors complex. One could be dealing with a landowner, different stakeholders with different rights for the same resource, as well as a resource having multiple uses or users, all of which have evolved over long time periods, in some cases hundreds of years, which requires collaboration to solve particular resource challenges.

Government and governance: A move to co-management

The third strand of the relationship between outdoor recreation and leisure with the wider environment is the way in which resource use is governed. Governance through co-management relies on groups of people working together to be able to benefit in the way each group wishes without affecting other groups negatively. This provides an ideal environment for outdoor users usually at odds with each other to compromise and benefit for their own interests. With respect to the environment the driving political ideology was, and remains, mainly a system of centralised organisations which maintain power and control using a synoptic planning approach (Figure 14.2). A range of Government agencies have a cursory overview in relation to physical activity outside. The overall effect is to provide control by Government and quango 'experts' to instigate the change they believe to be the correct one

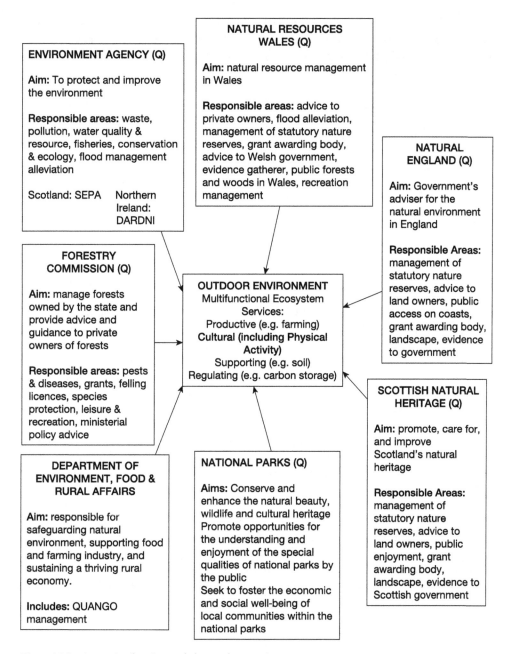

Figure 14.2 Synoptic planning and the outdoor environment

in a simple and straightforward manner in line with their primary function. Developments for the benefit of physical activity are therefore limited focused on those Government agencies owning or controlling land through active provision of infrastructure (car parks, rights of way, land access, cycling routes) and for all, passive tolerance of those seeking physical activity affecting their resource base. Perhaps the most direct manifestation of a more active engagement comes through the recent work of Natural England who are beginning to explore the arguably related health and wellbeing agenda via their 'Learning in Natural Environments and Outdoors for All' initiative along with the report series 'Outdoors for All: Fair access to a good quality natural environment' (http://publications.naturalengland.org.uk/category/6502695238107136 Accessed: 08/11/16).

Added to this is a broader shift towards a more governance-based outlook, sometimes referred to as co-management (Carlsson & Berkes, 2005) such as a stakeholder partnership whereby every organisation or individual with a vested interest is involved in decision making. An outdoor example is how access rights to land are upheld and managed on the ground in Scotland through the Land Reform (Scotland) Act 2003. Local Authorities and National Park Authorities (known as *access authorities*) have a duty to uphold the right of access, develop plans for a system of core paths[11] and ensure the formation of a stakeholder led local access forum. One attempt to do this has been explored by the Cairngorms National Park and their Access Strategy (CNPA, 2007).

Conclusion

In this chapter, we have drawn attention to some of the complex and conflicting issues and interests around policy and policy making as they relate to the aspects of physical activity associated with outdoor education and recreational physical activities. We have emphasised the webs of connections between human and more-than-human and the inherent conflicts between human groups and between human and non-human interests. Figure 14.2 identified these interlinking webs highlighting that the practice of physical activity in nature is not undertaken in isolation, but rather takes place within particular outdoor environments that are shaped and influenced by many years of changing legislation fuelled by shifting social and political ideologies and changing land usage. More recently emerging from changes in legislation, policy and decision-making are more moderate co-management styles. We have also emphasised that recreational physical activities in nature and physical activities outside of school are only a small part of the whole picture. We traced government policy on school curriculum. And have shown how physical activity outdoors in various guises is made available and accessible through aspects of schools' programmes, thus providing a holistic approach to the provision of outdoor activities through outdoor and environmental education adopted by many schools. Embodied in the physical practice through much of outdoor and environmental education is the notion of sustainability and lifelong learning which embeds in young people something of the interconnections between human and non-human health and wellbeing. Nevertheless, who has access to natural environments for recreational physical activities, how land and seascapes can equitably and sustainably be utilised and how an environmental ethic can become embedded into people's psyche are issues that still remain under-researched.

Notes

1   See Humberstone, Prince & Henderson (2016), part 2 Formal education in outdoor studies (p. 79–150) and part 3 Non-formal education and training in/for/about outdoor studies (p. 151–268).
2   See Humberstone, Prince & Henderson (2016), part 5 Social and environmental justice and outdoor studies (p. 333–418).
3   There has been a shift from 'Outdoor Education' to 'Outdoor Learning' in many contexts but the terms are used interchangeably here (see Christie, Higgins & Nicol, 2016: p. 115).
4   Education Scotland is the Scottish Government's education support agency: www.educationscotland.gov.uk.
5   Key Stage 2 (KS2), 7–11 years; Key Stage 3 (KS3); 11–14 years.

6 Right of Common continues to the present day, re-affirmed by the Commons Registration Act 1965 and the Commons Act 2006.

7 Highway – Land that is a highway means the public have the right to pass and re-pass along it. Any other form of use is considered trespass in law. Currently there are 190,000km of RoW in England and Wales.

8 Common Property Resources – Rivalrous (they can be diminished) and non excludable (we cannot stop people taking advantage of them) resources which on use can deteriorate. This relates directly to Hardin's 'tragedy of the commons' (Concept Box 4), something which exercises many resource managers. Examples are water bodies and RoW.

9 QUANGO – A quasi-autonomous non-governmental organisation which has devolved power from the UK government, including non-departmental public bodies, non-ministerial departments and executive agencies; an example of which is the Forestry Commission.

10 Biophysical deterioration – Damage to the physical and ecological character of a resource. In the case of a footpath this is usually observed in order of occurrence: vegetation trampling; vegetation loss; exposure of bare soil and soil erosion.

11 Core path – A system of paths identified by the access authority sufficient for the purpose of giving the public access throughout their authority area.

References

Aall, C., Grimstad Klepp, I., Brudvik Engeset, A., Skuland, S.E. & Støa, E. (2011). Leisure and sustainable development in Norway: Part of the solution and the problem, *Leisure Studies, 30*(4), 453–476.

Aikens, K., McKenzie, M. & Vaughter, P. (2016). Environmental and sustainability education policy research: A systematic review of methodological and thematic trends. *Environmental Education Research, 22*(3), 333–359. DOI: 10.1080/13504622.2015.1135418.

Aitchison, J., Crowther, K., Ashby, M. & Redgrave, L. (2000). *The Common Lands of England: A Biological Survey*. Aberystwyth: University of Aberystwyth.

Aitchison, J. & Gadsden, G. (1992). 'Common land', in Howarth, W. and Rodgers, C.P., *Agriculture, Conservation and Land Use – Law and Policy Issues for Rural Areas*. Cardiff: University Press of Wales.

Bakker, K. (2005). Neoliberalising nature? Market environmentalism in water supply in England and Wales. *Annals of the Association of American Geographers, 95*(3), 531–555.

Bunce, M. (1994). *The Countryside Ideal Anglo-American Images of Landscape*. Oxford: Routledge.

Cairngorms National Park Authority (CNPA) (2007). *Enjoying the Cairngorms, Cairngorms National Park Outdoor Access Strategy 2007–2012*. CNPA: Grantown on Spey.

Carlsson, L. & Berkes, F. (2005). Co-management: Concepts and methodological implications. *Journal of Environmental Management, 75*, 65–76.

Carpenter, C. & Harper, N. (2016). Health and wellbeing benefits of activities in the outdoors. In B. Humberstone, H. Prince & K.A. Henderson (Eds.). *Routledge International Handbook of Outdoor Studies*, pp. 59–68. Oxford: Routledge.

Carson, R. (1962). *Silent Spring*. New York: Houghton Mifflin.

CCEA (2007). Northern Ireland Curriculum. Retrieved August 30, 2017 from: http://ccea.org.uk/curriculum.

Chanfreau, J., Tanner E., Callanan, M., Laing, K., Skipp, A. & Todd, L. (2016). *Out of School Activities During Primary School and KS2 Attainment*. London: University College London, Institute of Education, Centre for Longitudinal Studies.

Christie, B., Beames, S., Higgins, P., Nicol, R. & Ross, H. (2014). Outdoor learning provision in Scotland. *Scottish Educational Review, 46*(1), 48–64.

Christie, B., Higgins, P. & Nicol, R. (2016). Curricular outdoor learning in Scotland. In B. Humberstone, H. Prince & K.A. Henderson (Eds.). *Routledge International Handbook of Outdoor Studies,* pp.113–120. Oxford: Routledge.

Church, A. & Ravenscroft, N. (2011). Politics, research and the natural environment: The lifeworlds of water-based sport and recreation in Wales. *Leisure Studies, 30*(4), 387–405.

Crouch, D. (1998). Countryside at leisure, *Leisure Studies Association Newsletter,* No 50.

Curriculum for Wales (2013). Physical Education in the national curriculum for Wales. Retrieved August 30, 2017 from: http://learning.gov.wales/docs/learningwales/publications/130425-physical-education-inthe-national-curriculum-en.pdf.

Department for Education (DfE). (2016). *Educational Excellence Everywhere*. U.K. Government White Paper. Retrieved August 30, 2017 from: www.gov.uk/government/publications/educational-excellence-everywhere.

Dillon, J. & Dickie, I. (2012). *Learning in the Natural Environment: Review of Social and Economic Benefits and Barriers*. Natural England Commissioned Reports. London: King's College London.

Dobson, A. (2003). Social justice and environmental sustainability: Ne'er the twain shall meet? In J. Agyeman, R.D. Bullard & B. Evans. *Just Sustainabilities: Development in an Unequal World*, pp. 83–98. London: Earthscan.

ECOS. (2014). A Review of Conservation Vol. 35(34/4). Retrieved August 30, 2017 from: www.banc.org.uk.

Education Scotland (2013). *Experience and Outcome Guides for Outdoor Learning*. Glasgow: Education Scotland.

Erickson, B. (2011). Recreational activism: Politics, nature and the rise of neoliberalism. *Leisure Studies*, *30*(4), 477–494.

Evans, D. (1992). *A History of Nature Conservation in Britain*. London: Routledge.

Fiennes, C., Oliver, E., Dickson, K., Escobar, D., Roman, A. & Oliver, S. (2015). *The Existing Evidence-Base about the Effectiveness of Outdoor Learning*. London: Institute for Outdoor Learning, Blagrave Trust, UCL & Giving Evidence Report.

Finlay, J., Franke, T., McKay, H. & Sims-Gould, J. (2015). Therapeutic landscapes and wellbeing in laterlife: Impacts of blue and green spaces for older adults. *Health & Place*, 34, 97–106. DOI: 10.1016/j.healthplace.2015.05.001.

Fjørtoft, I. (2004). Landscape as playscape: The effects of natural environments on children's play and motor development. *Children, Youth and Environments*, *14*(2), 21–44.

Gorard, S., Selwyn, N. & Rees, G. (2002). Privileging the visible: A critique of the National Learning Targets. *British Educational Research Journal*, *28*(3), 309–325.

Gordon, K., Chester, M. & Denton, A. (2015). *Getting Active in the Outdoors: A study of Demography, Motivation, Participation and Provision in Outdoor Sport and Recreation in England*. London: Sport England and Outdoor Industries Association. Retrieved from: www.sportengland.org/media/3275/outdoors-participation-report-v2-lr-spreads.pdf.

Gorely, T., Nevill, M.E., Morris, J.G., Stensel, D.J. & Nevill, A. (2009). Effect of a school-based intervention to promote healthy lifestyles in 7–11 year old children. *International Journal of Behavioral Nutrition and Physical Activity*, *6*(5). DOI: 10.1186/1479-5868-6-5.

Hayes, D. (2016). Special report, policy outdoor learning. *Children and Young People Now*, 10–23 May 2016, 17–25.

House of Commons (1995). *The Environmental Impact of Leisure Activities. Fourth Report: Report, Together with the Proceedings of the Committee Relating to the Report. Volume 1*. Great Britain: Environment Select Committee of Parliament.

Humberstone, B. (1998). Re-creation and connections in and with nature: Synthesizing eco-logical and feminist discourses and praxis? *International Review for the Sociology of Sport*, *3*(4), 381–392.

Humberstone, B. (2011). Embodiment and social and environmental action in nature-based sport: Spiritual Spaces, Special Issue – Leisure and the politics of the environment. *Journal of Leisure Studies*, *30*(4), 495–512.

Humberstone, B., Prince, H. & Henderson, K. (eds.) (2016). *Routledge International Handbook of Outdoor Studies*. Oxford: Routledge.

HM Government (2015). *Sporting Future: A New Strategy for an Active Nation*. London: Cabinet Office.

Kendall, S. & Rodger, J. (2015). *Paul Hamlyn Foundation. Evaluation of Learning Away. Final Report*. Leeds: York Consulting.

Knight, S. (2015). Forest School in the United Kingdom. In B. Humberstone, H. Prince & K.A. Henderson (Eds.). *Routledge International Handbook of Outdoor Studies*, pp. 244–250. Oxford: Routledge.

Lovell, R. (2009). *An Evaluation of Physical Activity at Forest School*. Edinburgh: School of Clinical Sciences and Community Health, University of Edinburgh.

Lyng, S. (1990). Edgework: A social psychological analysis of voluntary risk taking. *American Journal of Sociology*, *35*(1), 851–886.

Mansfield, L. (2011). *Upland Agriculture & the Environment*. Bowness-on-Windermere: Badger Press.

Marsden, T. (1998). 'Theoretical approaches to rural restructuring: Economic Perspectives', Ch.2 in Ilbery, B.W., *The Geography of Rural Change*. London: Longman.

McNamee, M. (Ed.). (2007). *Philosophy, Risk and Adventure Sports*. Oxford: Routledge.

McVittie, A., Moran, D., Smyth, K. & Hall, C. (2005). *Measuring Public Preferences for the Uplands. Final Report*. Hackthorpe, Cumbria: International Centre for the Uplands.

Ohly, H., Gentry, S., Wigglesworth, R., Bethel, A., Lovell, R. & Garside, R. (2016). A systematic review of the health and well-being impacts of school gardening: Synthesis of quantitative and qualitative evidence. *BMC Public Health, 16*(1), 1–36.

Overton, M (1996) *Agricultural Revolution in England: The Transformation of the Agrarian Economy 1500-1850*. Cambridge, UK: Cambridge University Press.

Prince, H. & Exeter, D. (2015). Formal curricular initiatives and evaluation in the UK. In B. Humberstone, H. Prince & K.A. Henderson (Eds.). *Routledge International Handbook of Outdoor Studies*, pp.141–150. Oxford: Routledge.

Quinn, C.H., Fraser, E.D.G., Hubacek, K. & Reed, M.S. (2010). Property Rights in UK uplands and the implications for policy and management. *Ecological Economics, 69*(6), 1355–1363.

Rickinson, M., Dillon, J., Teamey, K., Morris, M., Choi, M.Y., Sanders, D. & Benefield, P. (2004). *A Review of Research on Outdoor Learning*. London: National Foundation for Educational Research and King's College London.

Rinehart, R. & Sydnor, S. (Eds.). (2003). *To the Extreme: Alternative Sports, Inside and Out*. Albany, NY: State University of New York Press.

Robertson, M. Lawrence, R. & Heath, G. (Eds.) (2015). *Experiencing the Outdoors: Enhancing Strategies for Wellbeing*. Holland: Sense Publishers.

Scholz, U. & Krombholz, H. (2007). A study of the physical performance ability of children from wood kindergartens and from regular kindergartens. *Motorik, 1*, 17–22.

Scott, W. & Reid, A. (1998). The revisioning of environmental education: A critical analysis of recent policy shifts in England and Wales. *Educational Review, 50*(3), 213–223. DOI:10.1080/0013191980500301.

Scottish Government. (2012). *Learning for Sustainability. Report of the One Planet Schools' Ministerial Advisory Group*. Edinburgh: Scottish Government.

Shoard, M. (1980). *Theft of the Countryside*. London: Temple Smith.

Shoard, M. (1987) *This Land is Our Land: Struggle for Britain's Countryside*. London: Paladin Books.

Shoard, M. (1999). *A Right to Roam*. Oxford: Oxford University Press.

Thorpe, H. & Rinehart, R. (2010). Alternative sport and affect: Non-representational theory examined. *Sport in Society, 13*(7/8), 1268–1291.

Thorpe, H. (2014). *Transnational Mobilities in Action Sport Cultures*. London: Palgrave Macmillan.

Vanreusel, B. (1995). From Bambi to Rambo: Towards a socio-ecological approach to the pursuit of outdoor sports. In O. Weiss & W. Schulz (Eds.). *Sport in Space and Time*, pp. 273–282. Vienna: Vienna University Press.

Waite, S. (2015). Supporting early learning outdoors in the UK. In B. Humberstone, H. Prince & K.A. Henderson (Eds.). *Routledge International Handbook of Outdoor Studies*, pp.103–112. Oxford: Routledge.

Welsh Government (2015). *Qualified for life: A Curriculum for Wales – A Curriculum for Life*. Retrieved August 30, 2017 from: http://gov.wales/docs/dcells/publications/151021-a-curriculum-for-wales-a-curriculum-for-life-en.pdf .

Wheaton, B. (Ed.). (2004). *Understanding Lifestyle Sports, Consumption, Identity and Difference*. London: Routledge.

WWF. (2013). *New Curriculum Contains Climate Change, but Not Sustainability*. Retrieved from: www.wwf.org.uk/wwf_articles.cfm?unewsid=6741.

15

SPORT POLICY

Pippa Chapman

Introduction

Sport and physical activity can be conceived as being one and the same thing, or can be seen as two very separate areas of policy and practice. The two are not necessarily mutually exclusive and while there are specific examples of the two overlapping, they also occupy different policy spaces and often seek to achieve completely different objectives. This chapter explores sport policy contexts and how sport sometimes overlaps with physical activity policy and at other times is conceived as something quite separate. This chapter draws predominantly on examples from British sport policy but despite this focus on the UK, elements of the central policymaking decisions and programmes that are in place in the UK, along with the justification for the UK government's policy approach, could be applied to other similar nations. The sport policy landscape incorporates domestic stakeholders including governments, sports councils, national governing bodies of sport (NGBs), Olympic and Paralympic committees and delivery partners such as local authorities and sports clubs. There is also an international dimension to the sport policy landscape that involves international federations and other international bodies such as the International Olympic Committee (IOC) and the World Anti-Doping Agency (WADA).

Mapping sport and physical activity policy

Houlihan (1991: 5) asserts that public policy is "concerned with the actions and positions of the state" and "is the product of a pattern of decisions". Governments' positions relating to sport policy and the decisions they make tend to focus around two key components: elite sport and mass participation. The relative importance of these two central policy concerns may fluctuate depending on the political leadership, the availability of public money to invest and the wider national and international climate.

In the UK, the government's interest and involvement in sport began in the 1960s and since then successive governments have included sport in their policies and the prominence of sport as a concern for government has grown over time, particularly in the past 20 years. Early policies for sport focused on mass participation and the British government endorsed the Council of Europe's "Sport for All" campaign. The programme was delivered through the newly established Sports Council and aimed to achieve increased participation at all levels of sport through raising awareness of "the value of sport to the mass of the people" (Coghlan, 1990: 69). In 1982, the Sports Council published *Sport in the Community: The Next Ten Years*, which focused on the quality of provision for sport, targeting specific age groups and linking participation in sport to health benefits (Houlihan and White, 2002). In 1995, the Conservative government led by John Major published *Sport: Raising the Game*, which moved the sport policy focus from mass participation to young people's sport, especially sport in schools, and elite sport.

The participation policy agenda re-emerged following the election of the Labour government and their sport policy document *A Sporting Future for All* in 2000. This policy included a focus on the potential for sport to contribute to achieving social outcomes, in particular tackling social exclusion. This notion was reinforced by the Labour government's next sport policy paper, *Game Plan*, which was a joint publication between the DCMS and the Prime Minister's Strategy Unit. One example from Game Plan of the government's thinking at this time for using sport to support social outcomes is "[u]sing sport to promote social inclusion can also help to build social capital through developing personal skills and enlarging individuals' social networks" (DCMS/Strategy Unit, 2002: 60). Green (2004: 374) described an "explicit emphasis being placed upon the symbiotic, and overtly instrumental, relationship between sport (and increased physical activity, in general), education and health policy" in the *Game Plan* policy. Participation in sport continued to be a concern for the government from the early part of the 21st century as the successful bid for hosting the London 2012 Olympic and Paralympic Games began to dominate policymaking and, along with the hosting of the Games and the fortune of the British athletes, plans for achieving a sport and physical activity legacy from the Games emerged. The legacy of London 2012 will be discussed in greater detail later in this chapter.

In 2015, the Minister for Sport in the UK, Tracey Crouch, declared that a new national sports strategy was needed and a public consultation was opened guided by a publication from DCMS. In this document, the new government's ideas around the cross-cutting nature of sport and the delineation of responsibility for various health and social concerns that might relate to sport within the UK government were explicit. Senior ministers with responsibilities including sport, culture, public health, transport and the environment all introduced sections of the public consultation and proposed questions relating to the role of sport and physical activity. In this consultation document, the UK government declared its conception of sport and physical activity as separate policy areas, albeit all under the auspices of a sport policy consultation, and noted the separate challenges and objectives but with a recognition that they need to work together.

Later in 2015 and following the consultation period, the government published *Sporting Future: A New Strategy for an Active Nation*. There were two key changes in this strategy compared with the government's previous sport policies. Firstly, a move from focusing on simply sport to sport *and* physical activity and, secondly, a set of outcomes that are sought through sport. In the past 20 years while physical activity has been a feature of sport policies, especially when there has been any reference to healthy lifestyles, the focus has been on sport with funding being channelled in to national governing bodies of sport (NGBs) and often underpinned by a notion that participation in sport means competitive sport. In the new strategy there is an acknowledgement of the contribution of more traditional forms of sport but the thinking moves beyond this and incorporates dance, walking, utility cycling (for example, cycling to commute to work) and outdoor recreation. These types of activity are seen as particularly important when it comes to involving those sections of the population who are, or are at risk of being, inactive, including older people, girls and women, disabled people and those in lower socio-economic groups.

The five central outcomes in the new strategy are: physical wellbeing; mental wellbeing; individual development; social and community development; and economic development (DCMS, 2015). The strategy is centred on the principle of sport and physical activity as vehicles for achieving these outcomes. The importance of these outcomes is described in the document thus: "this new strategy for sport and physical activity moves beyond merely looking at how many people take part. It will consider what people get from participating and what more can be done to make a physically active life truly transformative" (HM Government, 2015b: 10).

As the British government's aims around sport change, so too have its ideas around how these policies can be implemented and the aims achieved, and it has stated its openness to broadening the range of funding recipients and partnerships. This may include organisations that have not previously been part of the sport landscape, in particular building relationships with the health sector and increasing involvement with third sector organisations that may have similar aims in terms of personal, health and social development. A key challenge for implementing the policy is measuring the achievement of the outcomes, including isolating the contribution of sport or physical activity, while in the past participation in sport has been measured by numbers alone. The changes to sport policy that are presented in the strategy could be perceived as an opportunity for the sport sector to contribute more to health and social outcomes but the government's openness to diversification of partners for implementing the strategy could be seen as a threat to the traditional sport structures.

One consideration when examining sport policy and physical activity policy is to determine similarities and differences between the two policy areas. A key difference between the two may be the motivation or intended outcome of a policy. Physical activity policy is likely to focus on achieving a health outcomes through increasing levels of physical activity and drawing attention to the health benefits of being active. Sport policy may include health benefits but will often have a wider concern in terms of sport achieving specific outcomes and the pursuit of excellence in sport. Overlaps may exist in these motivations and may also exist in the nature of activity. For example, swimming might be seen as a useful way of being more active to achieve health benefits but swimming is also a sport in the sense that people train for and compete within the sport.

In order to determine what organisations they recognise and work with, Sport England, which is responsible for programmes and distribution of public monies to support participation in sport in England, uses the Council of Europe Sports Charter's definition of sport. This definition describes sport thus: "all forms of physical activity which, through casual or organised participation, aim at expressing or improving physical fitness and mental wellbeing, forming social relationships or obtaining results in competition at all levels" (Council of Europe, 1992). In this definition, sport is recognised as being a form of physical activity and while sport by its very nature always involves being active, not all types of physical activity can be classified as sport because they do not have the same aims and may lack the competitive element included in this definition. To say that sport is merely a subset of physical activity may be particularly challenged by those organisations and individuals working at the elite end of sport: while those engaged in the pursuit of excellence are indeed physically active, the notion of physical activity is unlikely to be part of their consciousness as they focus on intense, targeted training in their sport in order to achieve at the highest level. This suggests that a way of delineating sport from physical activity is to identify the context in which it is being used, as well as the policy objective.

The relationship between sport and physical activity can be seen as sport being a subset of physical activity. An alternative would be to see them as overlapping policy communities. Houlihan (1991) stated that policy communities may overlap due to challenge for control of a certain issue or acceptance that an issue concerns more than one policy community. Marsh and Rhodes (1992) noted that one of the key characteristics of a policy community is limited membership: only those organisations or individuals with specific concern for the policy area will be a member of a given policy community but they might be a member of more than one community. In the case of a physical activity policy community, the membership would include organisations with a health and physical activity interest, for example organisations focused on specific populations such as older people, school-age children or people with disabilities or specific illnesses, leisure providers such as gym brands or local authorities and could include NGBs as they have a remit with regards to participation in sport and recreation. A sport policy community would also include NGBs but would then have a separate membership including Olympic and Paralympic committees, organisations that provide funding and/or services for elite athletes such as sports institutes or sports councils and other providers of sport such as clubs and universities.

The overlap between sport and physical activity policy communities could lead to unintended benefits (or challenges) to each of the specific policy areas due to the phenomenon of policytaking. Policytaking is a change to policy that occurs as a by-product of efforts within another policy area and is distinct from policymaking, which is a specific action within a given policy area to achieve a specific outcome for that area (Dery, 1999). For example, a policy to increase physical activity for health reasons with a specific focus on cycling could result in more people discovering an enjoyment and aptitude for cycling as a sport and progressing to take up cycling at a competitive level, which could result in talent being identified, thus supporting sport policy around talent identification and development. The emergence of talent would not be of concern for the physical activity policy community as their intended outcome is more people realising the health benefits of cycling but would be highly valued by the sport policy community.

A sport policy community might have overlaps with other areas of public policy as well as physical activity. Houlihan (1991) cited examples whereby a sport policy community might overlap with other policy communities including the issue of football hooliganism being of concern to sport, foreign policy and law and order policy communities. Sport could overlap with the policy community for international relations due to the international nature of elite sport, hosting of major events, governance and anti-doping. A potential challenge for a sport policy community is how well it can exert influence and defend its position to ensure that its role is understood and appreciated by policymakers. As noted above, the British government's new sport strategy presents such as challenge as the government has indicated its willingness to look outside of the traditional sport sector to other organisations providing sport and physical activity opportunities that might fulfil the government's aims around personal, health and social outcomes.

Sport policy contexts

As noted earlier in this chapter, political leadership, funding and the wider political context can influence the prevalence of sport policy and its relationship with other policy areas, including physical activity. This section will explore key factors that might impact upon sport policy and physical activity policy at a national and international level.

International contexts

Sport policy around the world is multi-faceted and constitutes elements including mass participation in sport, sport for development, elite sport, hosting of major events, combatting corruption, anti-doping and governance and, as noted in the introduction, there are multiple stakeholders in the sport policy landscape at both the domestic and international levels. The Council of Europe's "Sport for All" campaign in 1966 was, as Coghlan (1990) stated, the first time a group of nations had agreed specific action to promote physical activity and sport. Over time, governments have become more interested in sport and have therefore developed explicit policies to achieve their visions for the development of sport including specific priorities and often allocation of public monies to support their policies. With specific reference to elite sport, there has been considerable policy convergence between countries, especially more economically development countries (Houlihan, 2009; Houlihan and Zheng, 2013; De Bosscher et al., 2008), and increased government spending and centralised programmes for supporting elite athletes have been key features of these policies. It should be noted that, for the most part, government intervention for elite sport systems tend to focus on Olympic and Paralympic disciplines rather than professionalised sports such as rugby and football as these sports have sufficient income through commercial partnerships and broadcasting deals to fund their elite programmes without government support so their lack of need of financial support means they are generally not so connected to government interest at the elite level.

A further convergence at the international level is the growth in the number of countries bidding for the biggest sports events. Emerging economies such as India (hosted the Commonwealth Games in 2010), Brazil (hosted the FIFA World Cup in 2014 and the Olympic Games in 2016) and South Africa (hosted the FIFA World Cup in 2010) are now more involved and there is a stronger interest from wealthy nations in the Middle East (Qatar will host the 2022 FIFA World Cup and Doha was a candidate city for the 2020 Olympic Games). However, Bloyce and Smith (2010) noted that bidding for hosting the Olympic Games has become less fierce with increasing concerns around cost and uncertainty around the return for the host city and country. Indeed there have been high profile withdrawals from the bidding process for the 2020 Olympic Games (Rome) and 2022 Winter Olympic Games (Oslo) due to economic concerns and a lack of public and political support respectively (Guardian, 2014). So the diversity of countries involved in the processes of bidding and hosting has expanded but there may be fewer countries overall for each bid.

In addition to policy convergence between countries, supra-national organisations have also acknowledged the importance of sport: for example, the United Nations (UN) has incorporated sport and play in to the Convention of the Rights of the Child and Convention on the Rights of Persons with Disabilities. Furthermore, the UN has formed a close relationship with the International Olympic Committee (IOC): the IOC is a permanent observer of the United Nations and worked with the United Nations Office for Sport Development and Peace until the office's closure in 2017.

The International Olympic Committee (IOC), whilst fundamentally responsible for the Olympic Games and all of the organisations, international federations and national committees and sports organisations that fall within its influence, also has a keen interest in international development. In a report to the United Nations in 2015, the IOC advocated for contribution of sport and physical activity to the achievement of the Millennium Development Goals and the post-2015 development agenda (IOC, 2015). It should be noted that in this report, the IOC discussed sport and physical activity together in general terms but also separated them to reflect on specific elements of the development agenda. For example, with specific reference to healthy living, physical activity was described as a way to improve and maintain health and avoid specific conditions such as cardiovascular disease while sport was described as "a valuable informational and educational platform for health and development messages" (IOC, 2015: 4).

Sport for development means the use of sport to achieve specific personal or community-focused outcomes in order to improve people's lives. As noted above, the British government has taken this approach in the past in terms of tackling social issues such as crime and this notion has re-emerged more recently in relation to sport and physical activity as a vehicle to achieve personal health and social outcomes. In both practice and research, sport for development is particularly prevalent in the context of international development and there has been a marked increase in this area of sport policy in recent years. Kay (2011: 281) described a reason why this increased prevalence has occurred: "[t]he growth of sports-based initiatives within international development work reflects the perceived compatibility of sport with the wider international development agenda". Sport for development in the international context usually involves governments or non-government organisations (NGOs) in wealthy nations initiating programmes and giving financial support to less wealthy nations in order to address specific issues. As Kay (2011) noted, this practice by wealthy nations is founded on their own countries' beliefs about the benefits of sport, for example beliefs about sport improving education and promoting health, so sport is used to carry educational messages and encourage healthy lifestyles including raising awareness of specific issues such as HIV and AIDS.

National contexts

As noted above, there are common elements of sport policy between different nations in terms of what that nation's government is seeking to achieve but there may be differences in the reasons for a government prioritising sport and physical activity. Bloyce and Smith (2010) identified governments' recognition of the social significance of sport as a driver for the development of government involvement in sport. Collins (2011) highlighted the significance of sport with regards to national pride as a driver of government interest in and policies for sport in New Zealand while Thibault (2012) identified health concerns are being at the heart of Canadian policies for sport and physical activity. Grix and Houlihan (2014: 576) stated that elite sport "can be utilised by governments in the pursuit of both domestic and international policy objectives" and Grix and Carmichael (2012) identified three specific reasons for government investment in elite sport: to improve their international image, to reinforce a sense of national identity and to encourage the general population to participate in sport, which will be explored later in the chapter with specific reference to London 2012. UK Sport, the British government's elite sport agency, has an objective to "inspire the next generation through school and community sport" (UK Sport, 2015: 7), which involves athletes that are part of the organisation's World Class Programme visiting schools and communities to share their experiences of being an elite athlete and encourage young people to get involved in sport, thus linking the realm of elite sport back to the wider participation agenda. This relates to Grix and Carmichael's (2012) comments about the use of sports people as role models for the wider population which, despite its widespread rhetorical use, is not founded in robust evidence.

In addition to identifying reasons for a government having policies relating to sport and physical activity, the mechanisms employed for implementing these policies can also be examined. Houlihan (2009) used the term governmentalisation to explain the increased government interest in elite sport but it could be applied to sport policy more widely. Governmentalisation is "the development of a state apparatus for the delivery and management of services that were previously the primary or sole responsibility of organisations of civil society" (Houlihan, 2009: 55). The nature of these "apparatus" may be closely linked to constitutional arrangements or existing government organisations and these structures will reflect the nuances of specific countries' governments.

In the UK devolution has a strong influence over the organisational arrangements for funding and implementing sport and physical activity policies. The home country sports councils, Sport England, Sport Wales, **sport**scotland and Sport Northern Ireland hold responsibility for the development of community sport and increasing sport participation. They are responsible for distributing and monitoring the use of public funds that are used to support NGBs, develop facilities and implement initiatives to increase participation. As well as the sports councils and NGBs, organisations have emerged that focus on the sports activities of specific populations including the Youth Sport Trust, which was founded in 1995 and focuses on physical education and sport for young people, Women in Sport (previously known as the Women's Sport Foundation and later the Women's Sport and Fitness Foundation), which focuses on the experiences of women including their participation levels, and Sporting Equals, which seeks to promote participation in sport amongst the black and minority ethnic population. The complexity of the organisational arrangements for delivering mass participation sport in the UK may seem problematic but the four sports councils respond to their devolved governments' priorities; thus it could be argued that their initiatives are more relevant and it is more feasible for them to work with other devolved policies and services such as health and social care.

Connecting elite sport with physical activity through major event legacies

As noted above, the interest in bidding to major events continues to be very competitive. The hosting of major events has become an increasingly important focus for academic research in recent years including studies on the economic impact of hosting, policy processes and the notion of legacy, which is now one of the pillars of the Olympic Games following a change to the Olympic Charter in 2007 (Girginov and Hills, 2009). London's bid for the 2012 Olympic and Paralympic Games included legacy elements relating to urban regeneration and participation in sport and physical activity.

Case study: London 2012 and physical activity legacy

Sport policy in the UK in the past decade has been heavily influenced by London's successful bid to host the 2012 Olympic and Paralympic Games. After London won the bid in 2005, British sport policy was shaped around parts of the bid in order to achieve a legacy from the hosting of the Games. A key part of hosting the Games was the construction projects required that included building new housing, which was used as the athletes' village during the Games, and new sports stadia including an aquatics centre, velodrome and central stadium used for the opening and closing ceremonies and the athletics. There was also a significant increase in the amount of public money allocated to UK Sport in order to support the preparation of the British teams for the Games to ensure the British team was represented in all sports and won as many medals as possible. A further legacy that the government sought was to increase the number of people regularly participating in sport and being more active across the country. Masterman (2013) cited the London bid's focus on participation, particularly amongst young people, as being one of the key factors that led to the bid being successful.

In 2008, DCMS produced two key documents focusing on sport policy. *Before, During and After: Making the Most of the 2012 Games* focused on the Games very specifically and incorporated five key promises: making the UK a world-leading sporting nation, transforming the heart of East London, inspiring a generation of young people, making the Olympic Park a blueprint for sustainable living, demonstrating the UK is a creative, inclusive and welcoming place to live in, visit and for business (DCMS, 2008a).

These promises were all linked to the London 2012 bid and the UK government's aspirations for hosting the Games and the legacy it sought to achieve from the Games. This detailed document included allocation of duties at national and regional levels, a timeline of specific events and milestones and case studies of existing or planned programmes of activity. DCMS stated an aspiration under promise one for "more people of all ages playing more sport and being more physically active than event before" (DCMS, 2008a: 20). In this document the government described the difference between sport and physical activity: "Physical activity is more than just sport. It includes 'everyday' forms of exercise, such as walking, recreational cycling and dancing. Sport means activities that are often more vigorous and undertaken competitively" (DCMS, 2008a: 22). This shows that the government saw a marked difference between the two terms but valued both for delivering health benefits and saw increasing participation in both as achievable through the hosting of the Games.

Playing to Win: A New Era for Sport, the other document published by DCMS in 2008, focused on sport participation and excellence and set out a ten-year vision for developing sport. It included the notion of increased participation as a legacy from hosting London 2012 and asserted this with some confidence: "An important legacy from the 2012 Games *will be* increased levels of physical activity throughout the country" (DCMS, 2008b: 18 – emphasis added). It is important to note here that the term "physical activity", and not "sport participation", was used and in this section it was stated that DCMS's drive for more people playing sport must sit alongside other government departments' work to increase physical activity including the Department of Health and the Department for Transport. Again, this demonstrates the government's awareness of the differences between physical activity and sport and also gives some description of the membership of the overlapping policy communities.

The aspiration to increase participation in sport and physical activity amongst the general public as a result of hosting the Games and the British team being successful is known as the demonstration effect or the inspiration effect (Weed et al., 2015; Grix and Carmichael, 2012). Despite no evidence to support the assertion, increasing sport participation was a key element of the government's justification for spending billions of pounds of public money on hosting the Games. This notion was central to government rhetoric on the Games including being part of policy documents, as noted above, and in the more general public discourse around the Games. The Labour government stated an aim of getting 2 million more people active in England by the time London hosted the Games (DCMS, 2008a; 2008b). The Coalition government abandoned this specific target when it came to power in 2010 but the new government retained the same aspiration around using the Games to inspire people to be more active, especially young people (DCMS, 2010).

As noted by Weed et al. (2015), London 2012 was the first host of the Olympic Games to proactively seek increased participation in sport as an outcome of hosting the Games but the UK was not alone in stating a connection between the hosting and increasing participation, and they cited examples from Australia and New Zealand where similar assertions have been made. Weed et al. (2015) conducted a systematic review of evidence seeking to understand the potential of a demonstration effect whereby the general public are encouraged to participate in sport as a result of seeing their nation's elite sports people succeed. The review of the evidence found no support for the demonstration effect in terms of encouraging someone to begin participating in sport, however the study found that there is evidence that shows that there can be an impact on increasing the frequency of participation amongst those already participating and on re-establishing participation amongst those who have lapsed.

While Weed et al.'s study focused on the specific notion of participation as a legacy of hosting, Grix and Carmichael (2012) examined how governments use participation as a more general justification for investing in elite sport. A key finding of their study was the prevalence, and indeed the "privileging" (Grix and Carmichael, 2012: 86), of the idea of a "virtuous cycle" of sport. This refers to a notion that elite success encourages people to participate in sport, which results in improved health and a widening of the potential talent pool, which in turn leads to more success at the elite level and so the cycle begins again.

Since London 2012, the government and Mayor of London's office have produced annual reports examining the progress of the legacy of London 2012. The reports bring together information under five key headings: Sport and Healthy Living, Regeneration of East London, Economic Growth, Bringing Communities Together and the Legacy from the Paralympics. The Sport and Healthy Living sections of these reports focus on elements such as allocation of monies from specific Sport England funds, including participation and facilities development, hosting of events and government partnerships and the publication of strategies. In response to the legacy aim of encouraging more people to be active, one of the elements that is reported on is the number of people participating in sport on a regular basis as captures by APS. The 2013 report showed that 15.3 million people aged 16 years and over in England were participating in sport once per week; this figure rose to 15.6 million in the 2014 report then fell to 15.5 million in the 2015 report (HM Government/Mayor of London, 2013; 2014; 2015a). The notion of a participation legacy continued to be part of political rhetoric and public discourse for some time after the conclusion of the Games in 2012 and these figures would suggest that the participation legacy did not manifest, an issue that was repeatedly noted by the media, resulting in headlines such as "Golden promises of London 2012's legacy turn out to be idle boasts" (*Guardian*, 2015). The Conservative government's new *Sporting Future* strategy moves away from discussion of participation legacy and London 2012 is mentioned only briefly in the document with reference to events and volunteers, although the "inspiration" effect remains part of the rhetoric in support of hosting events, broadcasting and investing in elite success.

Conclusions and implications

It is clear that sport and physical activity policies overlap, sometimes intentionally and at other times more coincidentally, with one policy area benefitting from something quite separate. Where the overlaps are intentional, this is usually due to mutual or complementary motivations or intended outcomes. Sport and physical activity policy decisions come from what a government wants to achieve and how they believe it is best to achieve those aims. This chapter has shown that for the most part British sport policy in the past decade has been dedicated to encouraging participation in sport and physical activity either directly through funding Sport England and the NGBs or indirectly through funding elite athletes and the hosting of major sports events in an attempt to inspire people to participate. The current climate, however, is one of support for both sport and physical activity and the British government's new sport strategy has explicitly and intentionally coupled sport and physical activity and asserted that there is a role for both to play in achieving a set of personal, health and social outcomes whether an individual's aspirations are to participate in a traditional sport setting or in physical activity for enjoyment or utility.

As the government's attention has moved more to health and wellbeing, and without London 2012 as a driver for sports policy in the UK, there could be a loss of the platform for sport, and Olympic/Paralympic NGBs in particular, in terms of accessing government funding and influencing the direction of government policy. The new strategy indicates the potential for more partnership with organisations outside of the traditional sport structure in order to achieve the government's aims, which could contribute to a dilution of the power of the sport sector. Indeed, it is possible that smaller NGBs with fewer staff and a smaller participation base may find it challenging to prove their worth in terms of being in a position to fulfil any of the government's planned outcomes for sport and physical activity and therefore may be hit by severe funding cuts that could threaten their survival. Meanwhile, organisations that have previously been on the periphery of the sport sector as they are more aligned with physical activity, or even organisations that have not been involved in the sector at all, might find that they benefit hugely through their ability to respond to the aims of the strategy.

For those NGBs that do continue to receive funding from the British government, there are many challenges including developing partnerships with new organisations, establishing new offers to attempt to achieve the government's aims and finding a way of measuring the impact of their work for achieving the five outcomes outlined in the strategy. These challenges will occur in addition to the existing remit of these organisations of continuing to encourage people to participate in their sport. So there remains a degree of uncertainty in how the government's strategy will be delivered and how organisations will measure their efforts against the five outcomes. While this uncertainty may be problematic, it also opens the door for new partnerships and innovation in the sector that has been somewhat lacking in the past decade.

From a research perspective, the changes in the sector brought about by the new strategy may present interesting opportunities across the spectrum of academic interest in sport and physical activity including examining whether sport and physical activity can achieve the outcomes stated in the strategy, the impact on the sport sector from a policy perspective and the development of new partnerships with the health sector.

References

Bloyce, D., and Smith, A. (eds) (2010). *Sport Policy and Development: An Introduction.* London: Routledge.

Coghlan, J. F. (1990) *Sport and British Politics Since 1960,* Basingstoke, UK: Falmer Press

Collins, S. (2011) 'Sports development and adult participation in New Zealand' in B. Houlihan, & M. Green (eds.) *Routledge Handbook of Sports Development,* Abingdon: Routledge, pp. 231–242

Council of Europe (1992) European Sports Charter https://wcd.coe.int/ViewDoc.jsp?Ref=Rec(92)1 3&Sector=secCM&Language=lanEnglish&Ver=rev&BackColorInternet=9999CC&BackColorIntr anet=FFBB55&BackColorLogged=FFAC75 (accessed 31/10/2015)

De Bosscher, V., Bingham, J., Shibli, S., van Bottenburg, M. and De Knop, P. (2008) *The Global Sporting Arms Race: An International Comparative Study on Sport Policy Factors Leading to International Sporting Success,* Oxford: Meyer and Meyer Sport

DCMS/Strategy Unit (2002) *Game Plan: A Strategy for Delivering Government's Sport and Physical Activity Objectives,* London Cabinet Office

DCMS (2008a) *Before, During and After: Making the Most of the London 2012 Games,* London: DCMS

DCMS (2008b) *Playing to Win: A New Era for Sport,* London: DCMS

DCMS (2010) *Plans for the Legacy from the 2012 Olympic and Paralympic Games,* London: DCMS

DCMS (2015) *A New Strategy for Sport: Consultation Paper,* London: DCMS

Dery, D. (1999) 'Policy by the way: When policy is incidental to making other policies', *Journal of Public Policy,* 18(2), pp. 163–176

Girginov, V. and Hills, L. (2009) 'The political process of constructing a sustainable London Olympics sports development legacy', *International Journal of Sport Policy and Politics,* 1(2), pp. 161–181

Green, M. (2004) 'Changing policy priorities for sport in England: The emergence of elite sport development as a key policy concern', *Leisure Studies,* 23(4), pp. 365–385

Grix, J., and F. Carmichael. 2012. 'Why do governments invest in elite sport? A polemic.' *International Journal of Sport Policy and Politics,* 4(1), pp. 73–90.

Grix, J. & Houlihan, B. (2014) 'Sports mega-events as part of a nation's soft power strategy: The cases of Germany (2006) and the UK (2012). *The British Journal of Politics and International Relations,* 16(4), pp. 572–596.

Guardian (2014) 'Oslo withdrawal from Winter Olympics bidding is missed opportunity – IOC', Available online: www.theguardian.com/sport/2014/oct/02/oslo-withdrawal-winter-olympics-2022-ioc (accessed 31/10/2015)

Guardian (2015) 'Golden promises of London 2012's legacy turn out to be idle boasts', Available online: www.theguardian.com/uk-news/blog/2015/mar/25/olympic-legacy-london-2012-idle-boasts (accessed 31/10/2015)

HM Government/Mayor of London (2013) *Inspired by 2012: The Legacy from the London 2012 Olympic and Paralympic Games. A Joint UK Government and Mayor of London Report*, London: Cabinet Office

HM Government/Mayor of London (2014) *Inspired by 2012: The Legacy from the London 2012 Olympic and Paralympic Games. Second Annual Report – Summer 2014. A Joint UK Government and Mayor of London Report*, London: Cabinet Office

HM Government/Mayor of London (2015a) *Inspired by 2012: The Legacy from the London 2012 Olympic and Paralympic Games. Third Annual Report – Summer 2015. A Joint UK Government and Mayor of London Report*, London: Cabinet Office

HM Government (2015b) *Sporting Future: A New Strategy for an Active Nation*, London: Cabinet Office

Houlihan, B. (1991) *The Government and Politics of Sport*, London: Routledge

Houlihan, B. (2009) 'Mechanisms of international influence on domestic elite sport policy', *International Journal of Sport Policy*, 1(1), p. 51–69

Houlihan, B., & White, A. (2002). *The Politics of Sports Development: Development of Sport or Development through Sport*. London: Routledge.

Houlihan, B. and Zheng, J. (2013) 'The Olympics and elite sport policy: Where will it all end?', *The International Journal of the History of Sport*, 30(4), pp. 338–355

International Olympic Committee (IOC) (2015) 'The Contribution of Sport to the Sustainable Development Goals and the post-2015 Development Agenda', Available online: www.olympic.org/documents/olympism_in_action/sport_contribution_to_post_2015_agenda-eng-feb.pdf (accessed 31/10/2015)

Kay, T. (2011) 'Sport and International development. Introduction: The unproven remedy' in B. Houlihan, & M. Green (eds.) *Routledge Handbook of Sports Development*, Abingdon: Routledge, pp. 281–284

Marsh, D. and Rhodes, R. A. W. (1992) 'Policy communities and issue networks: Beyond typology', in D. Marsh and R. A. W. Rhodes (eds.) *Policy Networks in British Government*, Oxford: Clarendon Press

Masterman, G. (2013). Preparing and winning the London bid. In V. Girginov (Ed.), *The Handbook of the London 2012 Olympic and Paralympic Games. Volume One: Making the Games*, Abingdon: Routledge, pp. 29–42.

Thibault, L. (2012) 'Sports development and adult sport participation in Canada' in B. Houlihan, & M. Green (eds.) *Routledge Handbook of Sports Development*, Abingdon: Routledge, pp. 243–252

UK Sport (2015) 'The United Kingdom Sports Council Grant-in-Aid and Lottery Distribution Fund Report and Accounts for the year ended 31 March 2015', Available online: www.uksport.gov.uk/~/media/files/annual-reports/2014_15_annual_report.pdf?la=en (accessed 31/10/2015)

Weed, M., Coren, E., Fiore, J., Wellard, I., Chatziefstathiou, Mansfield, L. and Dowse, S. (2015) 'The Olympic Games and raising sport participation: A systematic review of evidence and an interrogation of policy for a demonstration effect', *European Sport Management Quarterly*, 15(2), pp. 195–225

16

YOUNG PEOPLE, PHYSICAL ACTIVITY AND 'ACTIVE PLAY' PROMOTION IN CANADA

Stephanie Alexander

Introduction

In Canada, as in the United States and in a growing number of European and African countries (Ebbeling et al., 2002, Onywera et al., 2013, Tremblay et al., 2014), there has been a surge of interest in measuring, evaluating and taking action on physical inactivity and obesity in the population, particularly among children and youth (PHAC, 2010, WHO, 2004, WHO, 2010b, WHO, 2012, Kohl et al., 2012, Piggin and Bairner, 2014, WHO, 2010a). Much of the literature on physical activity amongst children and youth focuses on preventing obesity by determining the most important factors influencing physical activity. Indeed, many studies have examined behavioural (i.e., individual) factors or family-based (i.e., contextual) factors, while others have examined the social and physical environment factors that shape physical activity behaviours and others the pharmacological interventions directly addressing child obesity (Ebbeling et al., 2002).

Sallis et al. (2000) published a seminal review of studies addressing a large range of potential correlates of physical activity for children and adolescents aged 3 to 18 years. The authors evaluated 108 studies for variables related to physical activity, and despite the inconsistent associations of variables with physical activity for youth and adolescents, they found that physical activity for both groups was shaped by access to recreational facilities and programmes (Sallis et al., 2000). In their review, they emphasise the need for better physical environment supports for physical activity promotion, and recommend addressing the modifiable variables for physical activity through education and family programmes, and also through changes to environments and policies (p. 972). Developing on the argument that the physical environment significantly influences children's physical activity, Davison and Lawson (2006) conducted a review of literature on the physical environment specifically. They similarly found that publicly available recreation facilities and transportation infrastructures (i.e., sidewalks, controlled intersections, public transportation) were positively related to children's participation in physical activity (Davison and Lawson, 2006). Given the numerous influences on child and youth physical activity, Sallis et al. (2006) proposed the development of multilevel interventions based on an ecological approach to target the many areas that shape physical activity (i.e., individual, social and physical environment, policies), and they specifically suggest that four domains of active living should be addressed: recreation, transportation, occupation and household activities (Sallis et al., 2006). Most recently, the growing concerns about a so-called *global* childhood obesity epidemic prompted the WHO (2010a) to develop a set of *Global Recommendations on Physical Activity for Health,* which include a section specifically recommending appropriate levels of physical activity for children and youth, globally.

The numerous health risks linked to childhood obesity, the significant research on factors shaping childhood physical activity, as well as the growing discussions about the *global* obesity epidemic have all provided the fuel behind the "anti-obesity" campaigns developed in Canada. In particular the organisations *Active Health Kids Canada* and *ParticipACTION* take an ecological approach in their work evaluating and promoting the factors most affecting children's physical activity in Canada. They widely promote recommendations for child and youth physical activity, attempt to mobilise government and non-government organisations for changes to the social and physical environments and aim to influence family and peers, schools and communities for increasing physical activity opportunities (Tremblay et al., 2015). Within this work, an increasing number of their campaigns have focused on the promotion of "active play" and outdoor leisure as a way to increase children's levels of physical activity (Active Healthy Kids Canada, 2012, Grove, 2012, ParticipACTION, 2012).

While the promotion of physical activity and active play within these interventions is clearly aimed to improve the health and lives of children in Canada, this chapter aims to identify possible unintended consequences of such interventions. Taking this work as its starting point, the chapter raises a series of questions about child and youth focused physical activity promotion strategies in Canada. Specifically, the hope is to make visible some of the political and social influences shaping the seemingly neutral and objective public health and physical activity interventions aimed at children. In order to engage the contemporary physical activity promotion trend for Canadian children, this chapter first traces a brief history of physical activity promotion in Canada, and discusses the emergence of "active play" as a central activity within health promotion strategies. The chapter then outlines three modes of thought, or assumptions, inherent in Canadian physical activity promotion. I discuss the practices involved in the promotion of active play and show how messages about health and play shape children's knowledge and behaviours through a series of bio-pedagogical practices (Wright and Harwood, 2009), and furthermore, how these practices shape contemporary Canadian childhood.

Physical activity promotion to Canadian children

The singular most recognisable name in physical activity promotion in Canada is undoubtedly that of ParticipACTION (Lamb Drover, 2014). Coming to life in 1971 amid a new momentum to promote sports and athletics in Canada, ParticipACTION has come to be known as the primary public face of Canadian physical activity promotion. Receiving significant funding from the Canadian government, for 30 years ParticipACTION mobilised physical fitness in the Canadian population through a series of highly circulated and popular national social marketing campaigns (for a history of ParticipACTION, see Lamb Drover, 2014; for examples of ParticipACTIONS's early campaigns, see their *Archive Project,* ParticipACTION, 2015h).

One effect of the widely disseminated campaigns produced by ParticipACTION in the 1970s, were nascent discussions about a national physical inactivity crisis in Canada. While still small in scope in the 1970s compared with the contemporary narrative of an "obesity epidemic" and related inactivity and sedentary behavior, ParticipACTION campaigns in the

1970s focused primarily on mobilising Canadian adults into engaging in more physical activity through what Lamb Drover (2014, p. 292) has called a "performance of citizenship through physical fitness". The first iterations focused primarily on adults, but later campaigns addressed children and youth and were ubiquitous on Canadian television and radio in the 1970s and 1980s. This had the effect of creating of ParticipACTION a brand name that was synonymous with a Canadian-variety of physical fitness (Lamb Drover, 2014). In 2001 ParticipACTION was shut down due to government budget cuts to the programme; the core funds were cut back so far that ParticipACTION preferred to cease operations than try to run its programme on significantly fewer funds (Edwards, 2004). Furthermore, due to changing media and television environment, some suggest that another reason for its decline in 2001 was that ParticipACTION had not "move(d) quickly enough with the times" and had as a result "lost its edge" (Lagarde, 2004, p. S20).

In 2007 ParticipACTION was re-launched by the newly elected Canadian government, this time with funds both from the federal government (e.g., Public Health Agency of Canada and Sport Canada), and with new private sector funds (e.g., among others, Coca-Cola Canada, who provided $10 million in support over ten years) (ParticipACTION, 2015c).[1] With the revival of ParticipACTION in 2007, and Canada generally being caught up in the momentum around the so-called childhood obesity "epidemic",[2] it is unsurprising that the organisation was mandated to focus its preventive efforts primarily on children and youth (Bauman et al., 2009, Craig et al., 2009).

Drawing on research conducted by the Canadian Fitness Lifestyle Research Institute (CFLRI, 2015) ParticipACTION began the production of a new set of interventions geared towards children and youth between the ages of 5 and 18. The interventions emphasised the need for children and youth to engage in scientifically determined amounts of physical activity per day (i.e., at least 30 minutes), and to be active as much as possible (CSEP, 2011). However, particular to this new iteration of ParticipACTION was the need for the televised and web-based media campaigns to address and engage a new target audience: children. One of the central means by which this was done was by focusing on children's leisure activities. Indeed, research on which ParticipACTION relied underscored that children's leisure time was an area rife for physical activity intervention and as such the campaigns began to link children's play with physical activity interventions (CFLRI and ParticipACTION, 2011). One of the current and more popular ParticipACTION campaigns adopting this approach is entitled "Bring Back Play!". The campaign, which has been aired primarily on television and online, draws on generalised nostalgia about the past to convince Canadians that children's play had all but disappeared, and that collective efforts should be made to bring back play (i.e., physically active play) for children (ParticipACTION, 2012, ParticipACTION, 2015g).

Up until July 2015, one of ParticipACTION's long-standing partners was Active Healthy Kids Canada (hereafter, AHKC). AHKC was a not-for profit organisation established in 1994 to promote physical activity specifically to children and youth through the provision of "expertise and direction to policy makers and the public on how to increase, and effectively allocate resources and attention toward physical activity", expertise which was based largely on research and surveillance data from various regional and national surveys addressing children and youth (Colley et al., 2012, p. 321). Between 2005 and 2014 the AHKC produced yearly *Report Cards on Physical Activity for Children and Youth* (Active Healthy Kids Canada, 2013) which broadly assessed and reported on the state of physical activity among Canadian children and youth (Active Healthy Kids Canada, 2014). The evidence base for the *Report Cards* was compiled from various sources of literature and government and non-governmental organisations in order to develop and evaluate indicators for physical activity, related to different facets of children's lives (Colley et al., 2012, p. 321, ParticipACTION, 2015a, Tremblay et al., 2015). The indicators are developed, refined and evaluated through consensus by a group of experts in physical activity research, to assess how children in Canada are doing and to evaluate the country's physical activity opportunities for children and youth (Active Healthy Kids Canada, 2014). Chief Scientific Officer of AHCK, Dr. Mark Tremblay, writes that the

> report cards represent a synthesis of the best available evidence across a series of indicators related to individual behaviors (overall physical activity, organized sport participation, active transportation, active play, sedentary behavior), sources of influence (family and peers, schools, and the built environment), and strategies and investments (government and nongovernment), and then interpreted by a national expert consensus panel which results in the assigning of a "grade".
>
> *Tremblay et al., 2015, p. 297*

The annual *Report Cards* thus present the physical activity evaluations using an academic letter grade approach (i.e., A, B, C, D, F) (Colley et al., 2012, p. 321), and the results from each *Report Card* are designed as a knowledge translation instrument, used to shape programs, and create better policies, and serve as an "advocacy mechanism to drive social action by stimulating debate, motivating policy, practice, and behavior modification and inspiring change in Canada" (Tremblay et al., 2014, p. S113, Active Healthy Kids Canada, 2014).

It was in 2008, not long after ParticipACTION had been reinstated to address children's physical inactivity, that the notion of "active play" entered the vocabulary of the AHKC *Report Cards* (Active Healthy Kids Canada, 2008). As a result a new indicator was created to effectively distinguish between different types of children's leisure – "active" and "inactive". Merged into the concept of "active play", children's physically active leisure was for the first time included as one of the central health indicators in the AHKC *Report Card*, to be measured, evaluated and finally promoted as another important form of physical activity (Alexander et al., 2014a). Subsequent AHKC *Report Cards* were produced to emphasise the concern that children were not playing actively enough, bearing titles such as: "It's time to unplug our kids" (Active Healthy Kids Canada, 2008) and "Is active play extinct?" (Active Healthy Kids Canada, 2012).

In 2014 the development of the *Report Cards* was taken over by ParticipACTION, and the 2015 *Report Card* was for the first time produced and promoted by ParticipACTION. Still focused on reshaping children's leisure activities, the 2015 *Report Card* turned its focus to the risks of keeping children indoors to play: "The Biggest Risk is Keeping Kids Indoors" (ParticipACTION, 2015b), and the most recent media campaign based on the 2015 Report Card bears the slogan "Get Out of the Way and Let Them Play" (ParticipACTION, 2015d). As such, in the mid-2000s both ParticipACTION and AHKC, in their attempts to promote children's physical activity, turned to children's leisure activities as a means of doing so; children's play and children's leisure time thus became the new target of governmental efforts to turn the tides of childhood obesity.

The most recent development of the *Report Cards* is their global expansion through the newly established *Active Healthy Kids Global Alliance* between 15 countries,[3] and which has recently grown to 39 countries (Tremblay et al., 2014). ParticipACTION is continuing to work with AHKC's former strategic research partner, Healthy Active Living and Obesity

Research Group (HALO) to work on the *Active Healthy Kids Global Alliance* (Tremblay et al., 2014). Their aim is to:

> expand our work as a global community of childhood PA researchers and advocates to learn from one another and challenge conventional within country solutions with international cross-fertilization of ideas and approaches. This may be facilitated by the creation of a global federation or network of active healthy kids organizations or research or advocacy groups.
>
> *Tremblay et al., 2014, p. S122*

With the *Report Card* results from the countries in the Global Alliance, a "global matrix" of indicators has been developed that are common to all countries in the alliance, but each country grades the indicators independently. According to Tremblay et al. (2014), the Global Matrix "not only assesses global variation in indicators related to PA, but also serves as a tool to motivate change, facilitate advocacy, and cross-fertilize efforts aimed at empowering *the movement to get kids moving* around the world" (p. S113–S114). The expansion of the "global matrix" of grades for children's physical activity is to be released in 2016 (Tremblay et al., 2014).

Having set out a brief history of the development of Canadian physical activity interventions for children, the chapter now explores several key themes emerging from my doctoral research (2009–2013) (Alexander, 2014), which included the discursive analysis of texts promoting physical activity to Canadian children, and from more recent examinations of campaigns conducted by the two central physical activity organisations in Canada: ParticipACTION and the former Active Healthy Kids Canada.

The themes presented illustrate the biopedagogies at work in the promotion of physical activity for children in Canada. The concept of biopedagogies, theorised by scholars in the field of critical obesity research (Harwood, 2009, Jette et al., 2014) draws on Michel Foucault's idea of biopower (Foucault, 2008, Foucault, 2003, Foucault, 1980).[4] The concept of biopedagogies brings the notion of biopower together with that of pedagogy – to form a "pedagogy of bios" (Harwood, 2009, p. 15). Burrows (2009) writes that the state, as represented by government programmes and interventions, operates through biopedagogical practices, which include "a diffuse set of technologies to govern the actions of families, but also constitute families' understanding of themselves as viable, good and healthful" (p. 127). Campaigns such as those produced by ParticipACTION and AHKC are exemplary of such biopedagogical practices, as they create normalising mechanisms outlining appropriate practices for health regulation (e.g., weight) as well as the appropriate means of achieving given norms (e.g., physical activity levels, forms of active play) (Rail and Lafrance, 2009). As such, children and their families are indeed "'taught', via biopedagogies, to be 'healthy' (and good) citizens" (Harwood, 2009, p. 17). These approaches are useful for casting light on, and problematising, the promotion of physical activity and active play to children.

Dominant assumptions underlying physical activity promotion to children in Canada

Presented below are three dominant assumptions that underlie and inform many physical activity campaigns produced by Canadian physical activity organisations, such as those outlined above. The three assumptions are entitled: "Playing should be productive", "Play and pleasure are equated with physical activity" and "Playing actively: A part of Canadian national identity". As these themes represent assumptions that are often implicit, they are infrequently brought to the surface and questions for their legitimacy or their potentially negative effects are typically not addressed. As such, highlighting themes this way serves to shed light on our modes of thinking about children and physical activity, which is pertinent, as reflecting on these may ultimately inform future action.

Playing should be productive

A central assumption within the physical activity promotion campaigns can be summed up in a statement made by ParticipACTION (2012), that "active play may be fun, but it's certainly not frivolous" (ParticipACTION, 2012). In this frequently cited statement, active playing is accepted as fun, but it must also have a purpose: the physical health and fitness of Canadian children. This is a sentiment that can be seen in both AHKC and ParticipACTION campaigns, that physically active ways of playing are valued precisely because of this productive potential. One example of how playing is rendered productive for children comes in the form of the ParticipACTION worksheets published as part of their "Think Again" campaign. These worksheets encourage children to record their favourite (physically active) activities, and to calculate how they are improving each week. They suggest to children:

> Pick an activity that you love or try a new one. Don't forget to track how much time you spend doing your activity each week. See if you can beat your weekly total. Now turn off the TV and all your electronic toys and get ready, get set, PLAY!
>
> *2015i, p. 2*

The worksheets also suggest that children and parents should assign a grade to children's activities based on how many minutes they have been playing actively:

> Have your kids track their daily physical activity. At the end of the week, see how many days they've hit 60 minutes per day. Use the handy chart to assign a weekly mark. Get ready, set, go! . . . Post one for each child in the house and see who can have the most fun getting an A.
>
> *2015i, p. 2*

In this way, ParticipACTION's campaigns, which reach children and families via workbooks, but also through television ads and the internet, are an important means through which the values of playing actively are instilled in children's lives. It also illustrates how play and children's pleasure is instrumentalised to productively promote healthy, disciplined youth and adults. However, by advancing play as a form of physical activity and by asking children to record, evaluate and reform their leisure time to be more active, children's play activities may inadvertently be transformed into a form of work (i.e., activity to be graded). Indeed, by drawing a parallel between the competition and evaluation of academic work and children's self-governing of their play activities, children's play becomes linked with competition and academic achievement. Under these circumstances, active play as a governed and evaluated activity appears to relate very little to the spontaneous pleasure, fun and enjoyment which children are being encouraged to gain from their leisure time.

Yet the motivation behind these campaigns is more than just for the production of healthy children and adults. Beneath the enthusiastic active play promotion within physical activity programmes, is the promised impact on obesity reduction, and the implications that this may have for the country's economic situation. As suggested by Canadian public health organisations, there are significant fears about the social and economic consequences linked to the growth of childhood obesity (PHAC, 2010). These consequences reinforce the importance of promoting active play as a critical component of Canadian society, and a direct link is made between children's play and the social and economic prosperity of the country. Behind the assumption that play promotes children's health lies another important value: active play, viewed as a way to combat obesity, becomes critical to the future growth of Canadian society. Playing (as a form of physical activity) thus becomes productive for the country: healthy citizens, young and old, are not a drain on the health care system.

The promotion of physical activity to children by organisations such as ParticipACTION has flourished within a neo-liberal governmental rationality. For instance, Lemke (2001) writes that a central characteristic of neo-liberal rationalities is that they developed techniques for regulating the behaviour of individuals without being responsible for them; neo-liberal strategies made individuals responsible for their own lives (Lemke, 2001, Foucault, 2008). This neoliberal economic configuration has also come to shape modern public health approaches, in which individuals, and increasingly children, are encouraged to "assume responsibility for insuring, monitoring, and acting upon their own health statuses" (Nadesan, 2008, p. 108). This is relevant for understanding how families and children are being incited to monitor and manage their health-related and leisure activities, and importantly, for how it shapes obesity preventive interventions. Viewing the interventions around children's active play as existing within current neo-liberal forms of governing prompts us to question *who* is being made responsible for children's "appropriate", "healthy" or "normal" forms of leisure, and how children's play is becoming economically relevant in the context of obesity prevention.

Play and pleasure is equated with physical activity

In their essay on pleasure and public health Coveney and Bunton (2003) argue that the topic of pleasure has been absent from much public health research and practice, likely because pleasure is viewed as too frivolous to become integrated into serious health research (Coveney and Bunton, 2003). The authors argue that while the experiences of pleasure or pleasure-seeking activities are characterised by freedom and spontaneity, within the realms of public health research and intervention they are also considered irrational, unhealthy and risky and thus surrounded by regulation, management and control (Coveney and Bunton, 2003). While this is certainly true for much public health that addresses adult populations, pleasure and fun is *not* evacuated from Canadian physical activity campaigns aimed at children. Rather, the notion of pleasure has been especially salient in the promotion of children's physical activity, in which it has also been reframed within public health discussions.

In much of the physical activity literature, playing and the pleasure derived from it have been constructed as a proxy for physical activity. For instance, in their 2014 "Bring Back Play!" campaign, ParticipACTION (2012) writes:

> With only 5% of kids meeting the Canadian Physical Activity Guidelines of 60 minutes of physical activity EVERY day, play might be one of the easiest, most affordable and fun ways for our kids to get moving – if we all make the effort to Bring Back Play.

As such, campaigns for children's physical activity draw on the notions of pleasure or fun as tropes for physical activity, frequently invoked to promote physical activities and sports.

ParticipACTION's "Think Again" campaign similarly suggests numerous "Active Ways To Play!" (ParticipACTION, 2015i). Within the campaign they imply that being active and having fun coexist for all children, suggesting: "Hey kids, this is your free time, and your only job is to make it active and to have fun!" (p. 3). In this case, free time is prescribed to be "active and fun", but it is also conceived of as a child's "job". This not only links play and pleasure to physical activity, but also invokes work and obligation as an essential component of a child's free time.

The physical activity messages discussed also imply that fun and pleasure are the qualities that all children experience when being physically active, and as a consequence, the pleasure attributed to playing is *assumed* to be a necessary experience of physical activity for children. However, by prescribing play as a type of physical activity these messages also underscore the primary function that these organisations attribute to leisure and play: a physical health practice. Indeed, since pleasure and fun are already firmly integrated in the promotion of physical activity to children, these affective notions themselves become instrumentalised. Pleasure (as defined by public health through active play) becomes a prescribed experience for children engaging in physical activity.

What is paradoxical in this is that through the promotion of play as an activity engaged in for a productive health end, playing itself and the associated pleasures may lose some of its playful, fun and spontaneous quality (Frohlich et al., 2012). This can be seen in a recent study in which children between the ages of 7 and 11 photographed and discussed their ideas about playing (Alexander et al., 2014b). Several children in the study suggested that when their play activities were too scheduled, structured or were too goal oriented (e.g., lessons or sports teams), the activity sometimes felt more like a duty or an obligation than play (Alexander et al., 2014b). One way that such interventions and campaigns targeting children can be understood is as a form of biopolitics *through* leisure. Children are encouraged to enjoy and gain pleasure from disciplining their activities and playing more actively, and there is a push to have children take the lead when it comes to initiating the right kinds of leisure activities, and engaging in the right kinds of physically active play. As such, while the public health discourse on children's play is evidently not "pleasure averse", pleasure and play, it appears, become instrumental for promoting and disciplining children's physical activities, though this may, as a consequence, reshape the experiences of play for children.

Playing actively: A part of Canadian national identity

Among the campaigns and documents recently produced by ParticipACTION and AHKC, there has been a return to the idea that physical activity is a significant component and symbol of Canadian national identity. As Lamb Drover (2014) has suggested, ParticipACTION, in its first iteration as a physical activity promoter in the 1970s explicitly drew on and helped construct a Canadian physical activity identity. Citing a 1981 ParticipACTION booklet that explicitly promotes the mandate of "not just getting individuals fit, but of building a fit nation" (Lamb Drover, 2014, p. 297), Lamb Drover (2014, p. 297) suggests that this national marketing strategy instigated the Canadian population to "perform their patriotism through physical activity.

When ParticipACTION resurfaced with their new mandate in 2007, the organisation again labelled itself "Canada's premier physical activity brand" (ParticipACTON, 2015) and again promoted physical activity on the basis of a national Canadian identity, and this time aiming the messaging at both children and adults. This has expressed itself especially in

ParticipACTION's recent policy statement entitled: "Healthy, Prosperous, United: An active Canada is a better Canada" (ParticipACTION, 2015e). The policy statement suggests:

> From our local playgrounds to our inspiring high-performance athletes, sport and physical activity are vital to the cultural fabric of our nation.
>
> *p. 2*

Similarly, their 2015 "Impact Report" (ParticipACTION, 2015f) draws on Canada's national sport – hockey – and on the assumed unifying capacity that "our team's" overtime win has for children and adults alike:

> Physical activity, playground to podium, unites our country in ways almost nothing but an overtime goal can. 2015 is the *Year of Sport* in Canada, celebrating the power of sport and physical activity to enhance the lives of all Canadians.
>
> *ParticipACTION, 2015*

National identity has also been invoked to promote particular ways of playing and engaging in sport, which the organisation defines as particularly Canadian. As part of ParticipACTION's "Bring Back Play!" campaign, ideas are proposed for bringing back Canadian winter play. Families are urged to play actively outdoors, even when it is cold, as this is part of what it is to be Canadian:

> Let's warm up to winter and embrace what being Canadian is all about. Help us Bring Back Winter Play by getting outside for at least 60 minutes of active fun each day. Invite your friends and family to join by sharing #WinterPlay.
>
> *ParticipACTION, 2013*

Lastly, in a trenchant example of how play and physical activity are linked to national identity in Canada, the growing momentum around active play promotion has been taken up by the sports, home and hardware company called Canadian Tire (Canadian Tire, 2015). The company makes a direct link between children, health and national prosperity, first through the company's motto: "Strong kids = Strong Families = Strong Nation",[5] but then more explicitly in their popular 2013 advertisement. In this advertisement, Canadian Tire explicitly draws on the momentum around active play promotion, creating their own slogan "We all play for Canada" Anthem (Canadian Tire, 2013b). The following text is part of their first 2013 advertisement, for which the company won a series of awards (Canadian Tire, 2013a). The text is read over orchestral music that builds in momentum during the 1-minute advertisement. The opening light-hearted piano music accompanies archival footage of children playing outdoors; the non-specified past is indicated by sepia colours and 1970s fashions. However, the mood changes with the words "but have you noticed . . . play doesn't come out to play as much anymore". The video darkens as it shows a dilapidated basketball court, abandoned swings and contemporary children at home playing video games and watching TV. With the rallying call to "bring back play", the music shifts to become anthem-like, gains in intensity and comes to a crescendo as the video shows children sports equipment, the National Hockey League's Stanley Cup and children (all wearing the Canadian Tire logo) playing soccer and baseball, playing in the backyard, at a park and swimming pool. The last scene shows three children running up a hill together carrying a large Canadian flag. As they fade into the horizon, the last words are spoken: "We all play for Canada".

Through seasons that changed and smiles that didn't, no company has shared this nation's passion for play like *Canadian Tire*. But have you noticed? . . . Play doesn't come out to play as much anymore. As a company that cares deeply about families knowing half our kids aren't active matters . . . for a country without strong children cannot stay strong. So Canadian Tire is rallying this country's most influential partners to *bring back play* . . . And with it, all the confidence, creativity and strength that serves to remind: **We all play for Canada.**

Canadian Tire, 2013b, my emphasis

Playing sports outdoors, more than physical activity alone, has thus become a symbol of being *truly* Canadian; a citizen who displays a physical hardiness and outdoorsy character, by playing actively outside no matter the weather. The aim appears to be to unite Canadians in a collective effort to engage all children in this kind of active play, for the sake of children's health, but fundamentally, for the sake of Canada as a "nation". While the explicit aim is to promote the health of children and improve the health status of Canadians as a whole, at least one important question arises from this: what does so strongly linking physically active play and Canadian identity and nationalism mean for those individuals who do not – or cannot – "play this way" for Canada?

Conclusion

The aim of this chapter was to make visible some of the assumptions that shape what appear to be neutral and objective physical activity interventions for children and how these also shape contemporary Canadian childhoods. For instance, Ian Hacking's writings about "making up people" (Hacking, 2002) describe the way certain kinds of humans (e.g., those who are suicidal) and human acts (e.g., suicide) emerge at particular historical moments alongside the very categories that are created to describe them, and this through various statistical analyses and scientific research. Drawing on Hacking's work allows us understand how the social and economic fears linked to childhood obesity that have emerged over the course of the last three decades have led to the creation of new categories for childhood health, and new ways of acting (i.e., playing) as a child. What is now called (and often vilified as) "screen play" (i.e., TV, Computer, Electronic games, etc.) and sedentary leisure (distinguished from "active" leisure) are terms that came into being in public health discourse only as the growing fears of childhood obesity became tied to the expansion of electronic media and technologies for children. The appearance of these new concepts has provided the space for the creation of a new kind of behaviour for children – active play – as a category of its own; part of an identifiable and newly measurable activity within the repertoire of children's activities.

Thinking of physical activity interventions as being part of a broader discourse on childhood, physical activity and health (Foucault, 1972) means also thinking of them as being part of the organising principles that guide social practices in a given place and time, which also function to form the objects of which they speak (Markula and Pringle, 2006). The discourses around physical activity, childhood and play shape the possibilities for what can be acted upon (i.e., obesity, play, elements of childhood), and thus the kinds of childhoods that are accepted and promoted. Indeed, emerging alongside the newly defined categories and concepts around children's play (i.e., active play, sedentary play) is also a new kind of *child subject*: the child who is happily physically active, an outdoor playing child; one who is fit and not overweight (according to growth/weight charts); one who enjoys monitoring, adjusting and engaging in the healthy and active leisure activities; and one who can easily recognise and easily embodies the notion of "active play".

Furthermore, public health and physical activity organisations play a central role in the instrumentalisation of social practices more generally and shape the way the realms of the social (including practices related to pleasure and play) become integrated into health matters. One concern with this, highlighted by Meyer and Schwartz (2000), is that when social issues are increasingly viewed exclusively through a public health lens – and in which action is justified only in the name of health – this may narrow the scope of how the "social" is understood. Promoting children's play primarily within a productive health optic does indeed narrow the scope of what children's play can mean (i.e., it becomes relevant only for health and development) and thus also what can be included within its scope (i.e., play as active, healthy). This is a process Meyer and Schwartz (2000, p. 1189) have called the "public healthification" of the social. With regard to the issues raised in this chapter, a process of "public healthification" appears to underlie the development of interventions addressing children's health and play. As such, one implication for future physical health practice is the need to re-consider the way notions such as "play", "pleasure" and "fun" are being taken up and used to promote children's physical activity. Furthermore, it would require asking: does the possible benefit (e.g., more active play, possibly less obesity) outweigh the possible unintended consequences (e.g., play related to mainly as goal-oriented, health-related, a duty)?

Areas for future research

The assumptions presented in this chapter prompt several other important themes for future research and practice. First, one important consideration involves the unintended consequences of the kinds of childhoods being produced through such interventions. For instance, given this work, it will be relevant to examine the kinds of childhoods that are being relegated or side-lined (or even stigmatised) through the dominant promotion of the "actively playing child". Related to this is an examination of children's leisure activities themselves, particularly those that are deemed less active, labelled "sedentary", and therefore also unhealthy. For instance, it will be important to examine the possible effects (other than reduction in obesity) that a decrease in "sedentary play" activities may have. That is, to consider how a decrease in the calm and restful play that children do alone, quietly, and sometimes "inactively" (e.g., puzzles, art, reading, computer or watching a movie) might reshape the way children relate to their daily activities, their free time and to their friends and families.

Notes

1 The implications of the public-private partnerships on the direction of these programmes are clearly of critical importance, however, due to limited space cannot be discussed in the context of this chapter.

2 In 2006, the Canadian House of Commons Standing Committee on Health initiated an extensive study on childhood obesity in Canada, the findings in 2007 suggesting the need to focus government action on childhood obesity prevention (Parliament of Canada, 2007).

3 The 15 countries included in the 2014 Global Alliance: Australia, Canada, Colombia, England, Finland, Ghana, Ireland, Kenya, Mexico, Mozambique, New Zealand, Nigeria, Scotland, South Africa, United States (Tremblay et al., 2014). By 2016 there were already a total of 39 countries registered (see map: www.activehealthykids.org/registered-countries/).

4 Foucault described biopower as 18th century efforts on the part of a state to solidify itself through the regulation and disciplining of the lives and health of the population through various "technologies of power" (i.e., statistical surveys, demography, medical institutions). The knowledge collected

about the population resulted in the establishment of norms for desirable and healthy behaviour against which the population was evaluated and measured (Foucault, 1980; Foucault, 2003).

5 Website and advertisement produced by Canadian Tire, entitled: "We all play for Canada / Nous jouons tous pour le Canada" Anthem (Canadian Tire, 2013b) (see: www.youtube.com/watch?v=qmfgsQSoJW4).

References

Active Healthy Kids Canada. 2008. The Active Healthy Kids Canada Report Card on Physical Activity for Children and Youth. Toronto, Canada: Active Healthy Kids Canada.

Active Healthy Kids Canada. 2012. Is Active Play Extinct? Report Card on Physical Activity for Children and Youth. Toronto, Canada: Active Healthy Kids Canada.

Active Healthy Kids Canada. 2013. *About Us: Who We Are* [Online]. Toronto, Ontario. Available: www.activehealthykids.ca/AboutUs.aspx [Accessed March 2013].

Active Healthy Kids Canada. 2014. Global Summit of Physical Activity for Children: Conference Proceedings. Global Summit of Physical Activity for Children, May 19–22 2014 Toronto.

Alexander, S. A. 2014. *"All work and no play . . . ?": A critical investigation of an emerging public health discourse on children's play*. PhD, Université de Montréal.

Alexander, S. A., Frohlich, K. L. & Fusco, C. 2014a. "Active play may be lots of fun . . . but it's certainly not frivolous": The emergence of active play as a health practice in Canadian public health. *Sociology of Health & Illness,* 36, 1188–1204.

Alexander, S. A., Frohlich, K. L. & Fusco, C. 2014b. Problematizing 'Play for Health' Discourses Through Children's Photo-elicited Narratives. *Qualitative Health Research,* 24, 1329–1341.

Bauman, A., Cavill, N. & Brawley, L. 2009. ParticipACTION: The Future Challenges for Physical Activity Promotion in Canada. *International Journal of Behavioral Nutrition and Physical Activity,* 6, 1–4.

Burrows, L. 2009. Pedagogizing Families through Obesity Discourse In: Wright, J. & Harwood, V. (eds.) *Biopolitics and the 'Obesity Epidemic': Governing Bodies.* New York: Routledge.

Canadian Tire. 2013a. *Awards and Recognitions* [Online]. Toronto, Canada: Canadian Tire. Available: http://corp.canadiantire.ca/EN/AboutUs/Pages/AwardsRecognition.aspx - 2013 [Accessed October 2015].

Canadian Tire. 2013b. *We All Play for Canada* [Online]. Toronto: Candian Tire.

Canadian Tire. 2015. *Canadian Tire* [Online]. Available: www.canadiantire.ca/en.html.

CFLRI. 2015. *Canadian Fitness Lifestyle Research Institute,* [Online]. Available: www.cflri.ca [Accessed October 2015].

CFLRI & ParticipACTION. 2011. The Influence of After-School Programs on Children's Physical Activity Levels. *In:* Canadian Fitness Lifestyle Research Institute (ed.) *The Research File.* Ottawa, Canada.

Colley, R. C., Brownrigg, M. & Tremblay, M. S. 2012. A Model of Knowledge Translation in Health: The Active Healthy Kids Canada Report Card on Physical Activity for Children and Youth. *Health Promotion Practice,* 13, 320–330.

Coveney, J. & Bunton, R. 2003. In Pursuit of the Study of Pleasure: Implications for Health Research and Practice. *Health: An Interdisciplinary Journal for the Social Study of Health, Illness and Medicine,* 7, 161–179.

Craig, C. L., Bauman, A., Gauvin, L., Robertson, J. & Murumets, K. 2009. ParticipACTION: A Mass Media Campaign Targeting Parents of Inactive Children; Knowledge, Saliency, and Trialing Behaviours. *International Journal of Behavioral Nutrition and Physical Activity,* 6, 1–7.

CSEP. 2011. Canadian Physical Activity Guidelines: For Children 5–11 Years. Canadian Society for Exercise Physiology.

Davison, K. K. & Lawson, C. T. 2006. Do Attributes in the Physical Environment Influence Children's Physical Activity? A Review of the Literature. *International Journal of Behavioral Nutrition and Physical Activity,* 3.

Ebbeling, C. B., Pawlak, D. B. & Ludwig, D. S. 2002. Childhood Obesity: Public-Health Crisis, Common Sense Cure. *The Lancet,* 360, 473–482.

Edwards, P. 2004. No Country Mouse Thirty Years of Effective Marketing and Health Communications. *Canadian Journal of Public Health / Revue Canadienne de Santé Publique,* 95, S6–S13.

Foucault, M. 1972. *The Archaeology of Knowledge,* London: Routledge.

Foucault, M. 1980. The Politics of Health in the Eighteenth Century. *In:* Gordon, C. (ed.) *Power/ Knowledge: Selected Interviews and Other Writings 1972–1977.* New York: Pantheon Books.

Foucault, M. 2003. *"Society Must Be Defended": Lectures at the Collège de France, 1975–1976.* New York: Picador.

Foucault, M. 2008. *The Birth of Biopolitics: Lectures at the Collège de France 1978–1979.* New York: Palgrave Macmillan.

Frohlich, K. L., Alexander, S. A. & Fusco, C. 2012. All Work and No Play? The Nascent Discourse on Play in Health Research. *Social Theory & Health, 11*(2), 1–18. doi:10.1057/sth.2012.18.

Grove, J. 2012. Bringing Back Play: ParticipACTION's Kelly Murumets. *Active For Life Magazine.*

Hacking, I. 2002. Making Up People. *Historical Ontology.* Cambridge, Massachusetts: Harvard University Press.

Harwood, V. 2009. Theorizing Biopedagogies. *In:* Wright, J. & Harwood, V. (eds.) *Biopolitics and the 'Obesity Epidemic': Governing Bodies.* New York: Routledge.

Jette, S., Bhagat, K. & Andrews, D. L. 2014. Governing the Child-Citizen: 'Let's Move!' as National Biopedagogy. *Sport, Education and Society,* DOI: 10.1080/13573322.2014.993961.

Kohl, H. W. R., Craig, C. L., Lambert, E. V., Inoue, S., Ramadan Alkandari, J., Leetongin, G. & Kahlmeier, S. 2012. The Pandemic of Physical Inactivity: Global Action for Public Health. *The Lancet,* 380, 294–305.

Lagarde, F. 2004. The Mouse Under the Microscope: Keys to ParticipACTION's Success. *Canadian Journal of Public Health,* 95, S20–S24.

Lamb Drover, V. 2014. ParticipACTION, Healthism, and the Crafting of a Social Memory (1971–1999). *Journal of the Canadian Historical Association,* 25, 277–306.

Lemke, T. 2001. 'The Birth of Bio-politics': Michel Foucault's Lecture at the Collège de France on Neo-Liberal Governmentality. *Economy and Society,* 30, 190–207.

Markula, P. & Pringle, R. 2006. *Foucault, Sport and Exercise: Power, Knowledge and Transforming the Self.* New York: Routledge.

Meyer, I. H. & Schwartz, S. 2000. Social Issues as Public Health: Promise and Peril. *American Journal of Public Health,* 90, 1189–1191.

Nadesan, M. 2008. *Governmentality, Biopower, and Everyday Life.* New York: Routledge.

Onywera, V. O., Héroux, M., Jáuregui Ulloa, E., Adamo, K. B., Taylor, J. L., Janssen, I. & Tremblay, M. S. 2013. Adiposity and Physical Activity among Children in Countries at Different Stages of the Physical Activity Transition: Canada, Mexico and Kenya. *African Journal for Physical, Health Education, Recreation and Dance,* 19, 132–142.

Parliament of Canada. 2007. *Healthy Weights for Healthy Kids. Report of the Standing Committee on Health.* Canada: Canadian Parliament.

ParticipACTION. 2012. *Bring Back Play!* [Online]. Available: www.participaction.com/get-moving/ bring-back-play/ [Accessed July 2012].

ParticipACTION. 2013. *Bring Back Winter Play!* [Online]. Toronto, Canada: ParticipACTION. Available: www.participaction.com/get-moving/bring-back-winter-play/ [Accessed October 2015].

ParticipACTION. 2015a. *Archived Report Cards* [Online]. Toronto, Canada. Available: www.participac- tion.com/report-card-2015/about-the-participaction-report-card/archived-report-card/ [Accessed September 2015].

ParticipACTION 2015b. The Biggest Risk Is Keeping Kids Indoors. The 2015 ParticipACTION Report Card on Physical Activity for Children and Youth. Toronto: ParticipACTION.

ParticipACTION. 2015c. *Coca-Cola's Involvement* [Online]. Toronto, Canada: ParticipACTION. Available: www.participaction.com/teen-challenge/coca-colas-involvement/ and www.participac- tion.com/teen-challenge/frequently-asked-questions [Accessed October 2015].

ParticipACTION. 2015d. *Get Out of Their Way and Let Them Play* [Online]. Toronto, Canada: ParticipACTION. Available: www.participaction.com/wp-content/uploads/2015/03/2015- Report-Card-Tips-Sheet-EN-FINAL.pdf.

ParticipACTION 2015e. Healthy, Prosperous, United: An Active Canada is a Better Canada: National Policy Considerations. Toronto: ParticipACTION.

ParticipACTION 2015f. Impact Report 2015: Plays of the Year — Our Latest Achievements as Champions of Physical Activity and Sport Participation in Canada. Toronto: ParticipACTION.

ParticipACTION. 2015g. *Our Campaigns* [Online]. Available: www.participaction.com/about/our- campaigns/ [Accessed October 2015].

ParticipACTION. 2015h. *The ParticipACTION Archive Project* [Online]. Regina, Canada: Saskatchewan Council for Archives and Archivists & ParticipACTION. Available: http://scaa.sk.ca/gallery/participaction/english/home.html [Accessed October 2015].

ParticipACTION. 2015i. *Think Your Kids Are Active Enough After School? THINK AGAIN* [Online]. Toronto, Canada: ParticipACTION. Available: www.participaction.com/pdf/par_schoolsout_englishforwebsite.pdf [Accessed October 2015].

ParticipACTON. 2015. *Our Vision* [Online]. Toronto, Canada: ParticipACTON. Available: www.participaction.com/about/our-vision/ [Accessed October 2015].

PHAC. 2010. Curbing Childhood Obesity: A Federal, Provincial and Territorial Framework for Action to Promote Healthy Weights. Ottawa: Public Health Agency of Canada.

Piggin, J. & Bairner, A. 2014. The Global Physical Inactivity Pandemic: An Analysis of Knowledge Production. *Sport, Education and Society*. DOI: 10.1080/13573322.2014.882301.

Rail, G. & Lafrance, M. 2009. Confessions of the Flesh and Biopedagogies: Discursive Constructions of Obesity on Nip/Tuck. *Medical Humanities*, 35, 76–79.

Sallis, J. F., Cervero, R. B., Ascher, W., Henderson, K. A., Kraft, M. K. & Kerr, J. 2006. An Ecological Approach to Creating Active Living Communities. *Annual Review of Public Health*, 27, 297–322.

Sallis, J. F., Prochaska, J. J. & Taylor, W. C. 2000. A Review of Correlates of Physical Activity of Children and Adolescents. *Medicine and Science in Sports and Exercise*, 32, 963–975.

Tremblay, M. S., Gonzalez, S. A., Katzmarzyk, P. T., Onywera, V. O., Reilly, J. J. & Tomkinson, G. 2015. Physical Activity Report Cards: Active Healthy Kids Global Alliance and the Lancet Physical Activity Observatory. *Journal of Physical Activity and Health*, 12, 297–298.

Tremblay, M. S., Gray, C. E., Akinroye, K., Harrington, D. M., Katzmarzyk, P. T., Lambert, E. V., Liukkonen, J., Maddison, R., Ocansey, R. T., Onywera, V. O., Prista, A., Reilly, J. J., Rodriguez Martinez, M. D. P., Sarmiento Duenas, O. L., Standage, M. & Tomkinson, G. 2014. Physical Activity of Children: A Global Matrix of Grades Comparing 15 Countries. *Journal of Physical Activity and Health*, 11, S113–S125.

WHO. 2004. *Obesity: Preventing and Managing the Global Epidemic*. Geneva, Switzerland: World Health Organization.

WHO. 2010a. *Global Recommendations on Physical Activity for Health*. Geneva, Switzerland: World Health Organization Press.

WHO. 2010b. *Population-Based Prevention Strategies for Childhood Obesity: Report of the WHO Forum and Technical Meeting*. Geneva: World Health Organization.

WHO. 2012. *Population-Based Approaches to Childhood Obesity Prevention*. Geneva, Switzerland: World Health Organization.

Wright, J. & Harwood, V. 2009. *Biopolitics and the 'Obesity Epidemic': Governing Bodies*. New York: Routledge.

17

EDUCATION, PHYSICAL EDUCATION AND PHYSICAL ACTIVITY PROMOTION

Andy Smith, Ken Green and Miranda Thurston

Introduction

The promotion of physical activity (PA) is a significant priority of much national, international and global policy in public health (Department of Health, 2011; Public Health England [PHE], 2014; World Health Organization [WHO], 2010) and related policy sectors, including education and sport (DCMS, 2015; Sport England, 2016). Indeed, education is frequently identified as an important policy context for the enhancement of PA through subjects such as physical education (PE) and as part of whole school approaches to health and wellbeing (e.g. PHE, 2015). This policy emphasis reflects a widely accepted view that schools not only provide universal access over a sustained period to children and youth regardless of family background; they are also believed to have the potential to deliver numerous education, social and health outcomes (Eccles and Roeser, 2011; PHE, 2015). Over the past decade or more, policy makers in most high-income countries have been urging schools to embrace an expanding and increasingly diverse public health agenda alongside their core educational goals (Rossi et al., 2016). This has reinforced the emphasis placed on PA promotion as *the* solution for improving the current and future health and wellbeing of children and youth. Thus, schools and teachers (especially PE teachers) are increasingly likely to be held accountable for a range of health outcomes relating to physical health (e.g. overweight and obesity and, by extension, cardio-metabolic health), mental illness (e.g. depression, anxiety and self-harm) and mental wellbeing (psychosocial health) which are the target of much contemporary public health policy.

The central object of this chapter is to examine: (i) the policy rationale for viewing education generally, and schools in particular, as an appropriate setting for PA promotion; (ii) the apparent role PE – which has long been viewed as the specific setting within which PA *should* be promoted – is expected to have in fostering lifelong participation in PA and sport; and (iii) the limits of education in promoting PA given the significance of wider social inequalities in families and the wider societies of which they are a part.

Education as a setting for physical activity

Education is commonly regarded as an important site of socialization, which refers to the processes through which people acquire or are 'taught' (either directly or indirectly, explicitly or implicitly, intentionally or unintentionally) and internalize the values, beliefs, expectations, knowledge, skills, habits and practices prevalent in their groups and societies. This is most straightforwardly seen through *physical* education, which involves the socialization of young people into sporting and PA cultures (including sport) and the knowledge and skills that sustain them. Socialization in sport and PA in schools can occur through many processes: single subjects involving active participation like PE; through other curricula which give access to knowledge about PA (e.g. science); cross-curricular subjects (e.g. Personal, Social and Health Education) where knowledge of PA in the context of broader lifestyles might be promoted; and in other activities as part of an alleged whole school approach to PA (such as extra-curricular activities, including the use of break-times for free or structured play).

The promotion of PA in school (via PE) is not new and some of the earliest justifications for school-based PA related to physical health (cardiometabolic, prevention of overweight and obesity, improving bone and muscle strength) and the prevention of future health problems. The international guidelines developed by the WHO (2010) reflect this focus, recommending that between the ages of 5–17 years of age, children should accumulate 60 minutes a day of moderate to vigorous activity (MVPA). In England, concern about increases in childhood and youth overweight and obesity is discussed in the context of the proportion of young people not meeting these recommendations. The rationale for focusing on PA has been given further impetus by research on sedentary behaviour (SB) (defined as any waking behaviour characterized by an energy expenditure ≤1.5 METs while in a sitting or reclining position), which has been identified as an independent risk factor for cardiometabolic health (Tremblay et al., 2012). Canada, for example, has published '24 hour movement guidelines' for children and youth aged 5–17 years, which incorporate the WHO PA recommendations alongside guidance on SB (no more than two hours per day) and sleep (Tremblay et al., 2016) – in recognition of the fact that children and young people can accumulate both large amounts of MVPA *and* sedentary behaviour within 24 hours (Ekelund et al., 2006), including at school.

In recent years, however, PA has been increasingly associated with a range of health outcomes beyond physical health, including improved mental health and wellbeing and, relatedly, cognition and academic achievement. However, evidence of the benefits of PA to the mental health of children and young people (e.g. Biddle and Asare, 2011; Brown et al., 2013), and to cognition and academic achievement (Hillman et al., 2017), is mixed. For example, in their review of reviews, Biddle and Asare (2011) noted that PA promotion may be beneficial for reducing depression and anxiety, and improving self-esteem (at least in the short-term) and cognitive functioning (including academic performance). However, these associations were identified as being usually small, inconsistent, and derived from mainly cross-sectional studies regarded as involving low quality intervention designs.

Notwithstanding the lack of rigorous scientific evidence for the assumed role PA is expected to make in this regard, the benefits of PA continue to be used by policy makers to argue that schools provide an optimum setting for addressing an expanding array of outcomes on the assumption that healthier pupils are more likely to be effective learners (e.g. PHE, 2014, 2015). In the next section we examine what might reasonably and realistically be expected of PE teachers in terms of socializing children and youth into PA (via sport, among other things) and the significance of PE for developing in young people an habitual and lifelong participation in PA.

Physical education as a setting for physical activity promotion

It is commonly assumed that PE can have a positive effect on PA among young people, not only by educating them about the well-documented benefits of PA, but also by making PA a habitual part of their lives. Regarding what might be termed a 'PE effect' on PA, it is widely believed, in and beyond the PE 'profession' itself, that school PE *is* or, at the very least, *can* (even *should*) be a crucial socializing vehicle for enhancing youngsters' engagement with PA, physically active recreation (typically, but not exclusively, in the form of sport) in their leisure and, in the longer run, over the life-course (see Vanreusel and Scheerder, 2016).

At first glance, this all seems perfectly reasonable. After all, PE teachers tend to have a captive audience at least once each week (during school time), for a decade or more, at a formative phase of young people's lives when their predispositions (or habitus) towards PA is most impressionable (Haycock and Smith, 2014, 2016; Stuij, 2015). There remains however a dearth of evidence demonstrating a 'PE effect'. Indeed, the precise nature of the relationship between PE and socialization into PA (and sport) is seldom explored other than in implicit, speculative and discursive ways that take for granted the positive socializing effects of PE on young people's engagement with physically active recreation in the short, medium and longer terms. So what might the potential socializing effects of PE on youths' current and future involvement in PA at the elementary and secondary school levels be?

PE during the elementary years and childhood

Elementary school PE is a secondary socialization process that continues *alongside* ongoing parental (primary) socialization. It is, however, questionable whether elementary PE can influence PA or sport participation, or whether what actually occurs amounts to a 'selection effect' wherein those youngsters who already possess the necessary attributes for successful engagement with PA are the ones who engage most with PE. For Parry, the answer is relatively clear: youngsters' prior participation in sport (and, by extension, PA) is likely to be more significant for PE, even at the elementary stage, than *vice-versa*. Parry's (2013) use of the 1970 British Cohort Study revealed an absence of school PE effects on elementary children's sports participation *beyond* school. He concluded, however, that it is likely that childhood sports participation affects their perceived ability and enjoyment and this, in turn, can lead to enthusiastic engagement with elementary PE. On this view, not only does enjoyment of sport beyond school increase the likelihood that children will seek out further opportunities for PA in the form of sport *inside* school, but as we shall examine later, the influence of family context is likely to be the primary driver of inequalities in participation and experience of PA inside school.

At elementary school, children are more-or-less guaranteed opportunities to engage in PA and sport weekly, which means that PE has the potential to, if not generate interest in PA and sport, then, at the very least, reinforce the emergent sporting habits of some youngsters. In very many countries, this is thought to be achieved through the content of early elementary PE curricula, which revolve around encouraging children to enjoy a variety of physical activities and games. In recent decades, PE curricula at both the elementary and secondary school levels have broadened to incorporate activities beyond the confines of conventional sports. Contemporary PE curricula tend to incorporate not only competitive game-contests (i.e., conventional sports including football, hockey, basketball and badminton) but also less competitive, less organized, recreational versions of these sports, as well as more recreationally oriented physical activities and exercise (aerobics, cycling, skateboarding, health and fitness gyms, surfing, cheerleading, dance, parkour and so forth) variously referred to as 'lifestyle', 'lifetime' and adventure sports and activities (see Gilchrist and Wheaton, 2016). Despite this broadening and diversification of much PE curricula, there appears limited potential for a primary or elementary 'PE effect' on PA promotion. This is most likely to be attributable to the 'traditional' model of delivering PE in elementary schools in the UK (Blair and Capel, 2011) and worldwide (Tsangaridou, 2012) whereby a so-called 'generalist' classroom teacher is responsible for teaching all curriculum subjects to the class, including PE. Limited experience of PA (as well as sporting capital) among generalist teachers, together with negative memories of school PE, are often exacerbated by limited preparation for teaching PE during initial teacher education (Elliot et al, 2013; Morgan and Hansen, 2008). The upshot is that 'A significant number of [elementary] school teachers have low levels of confidence, do not possess the skills and knowledge to deliver appropriate PE instruction, have limited content knowledge and do not feel competent teaching PE' (Tsangaridou, 2012: 281).

More recently, however, as part of the trend towards the marketization of education in countries such as England (e.g. Evans and Davies, 2010, 2014; Smith, 2015), Australia and New Zealand (Williams and Macdonald, 2015), economic and political imperatives articulated in policy have resulted in the increasing use of outsourcing of activity to (often) private providers such as sports coaches to deliver elements of PA promotion via curricular and extra-curricular PE. Sports coaches have become popular in part because they offer a relatively cheap and enthusiastic specialist alternative to generalist elementary teachers who are perceived to have a number of sporting shortcomings (see Jones and Green, 2015; Smith, 2015). Whether or not a shift away from delivery of elementary PE by generalist classroom teachers towards greater use of sports coaches constitutes a 'good' or 'bad' thing – in terms of encouraging PA – is a moot point. Coaches may well shift the content of PE lessons back towards the sports and games they favour (Smith, 2015), but it is possible that their expertise and apparent enthusiasm may enhance some pupils' competence, enjoyment and engagement with PA via sport.

Physical education during the secondary years and the onset of youth

Whatever the effect of elementary PE on the formation of predispositions towards PA, childhood serves as a form of anticipatory socialization during which emergent activity habits and portfolios can be rehearsed before the secondary school years and youth life-stage where drop-off and drop-out from PA and sport increase. By the time they arrive at secondary school, very many children have already begun to adopt the leisure practices that will come to form the core of their youth and, eventually, adult leisure lifestyles (Roberts, 1999, 2016). If such PA and sporting foundations are not built by this stage, and sustained throughout youth, it is unlikely that individuals will play sport regularly into and then throughout adulthood (Roberts, 2016; Roberts and Brodie, 1992).

Although habitus formation is most impressionable during childhood, deep-seated predispositions can and do change, typically as a consequence of significant events and/or repeated exposure to particular experiences (Haycock and Smith, 2014, 2016; Stuij, 2015). According to Feinstein, Bynner and Duckworth (2007: 307), there can be '"turning points" [in people's habitus] where the predicted route changes direction in response to new sources of influence'. Transitioning from elementary to secondary school is potentially one such turning point. As Symonds (2015) observes, youngsters are rarely faced with such a powerful set of personal and social changes than those which are experienced during the transition from elementary to secondary school, and during adolescence in particular. When youngsters' lives begin to unfreeze and re-form, PE teachers may help initiate, reinforce or even reverse past developmental trends. During the early secondary years, youngsters' lifestyles remain relatively fluid, and their participation in PA and sport still bears the imprint of their childhood habits and engagement. Thus, youngsters remain – in principle, at least – available for recruitment to and retention in (or, for that matter, alienation from) PA during the early years of secondary schooling. This is not simply due to the fact that they are obliged to take part in PE whether they like it or not. Rather, it is because many children are positively predisposed towards PA (including sport) as they make the transition from primary to secondary school (Dismore and Bailey, 2010; Haycock and Smith, 2011, 2014). Many arrive in secondary schools still on an upward trend in motivation towards, and participation in, PA and sport. As they make the transition from elementary to secondary school, youngsters are entering the period in which sport participation (in and out of school) is approaching its peak, prior (i.e. roughly between ages 12–14) to a long, steady decline as the early years of youth (i.e. the mid-teenage years) are more typically a time for cutting-down, rather than building-up, repertoires for engagement in PA and sport (Haycock and Smith, 2016; Roberts, 2016).

Where youngsters have or develop significant reservations about school PE these tend to revolve around a perceived shift from fun, enjoyment and recreational participation in primary PE to a more serious, skills-based focus on sport, in its competitive guise, at secondary school (Dismore and Bailey, 2010). The competitive sporting environment that greets them in secondary school PE – and that largely passes for education in PA – is likely to impact upon youngsters' enjoyment of, and attachments to, PA and sport by emphasizing performance and encouraging peer comparisons of ability (Evans and Davies, 2010; Parry, 2013). Youngsters transitioning from primary to secondary schooling may not only be under-prepared for PE in secondary schools, but those not yet committed to physically active recreation *per se* may well feel alienated by such a performative culture (Dismore and Bailey, 2010; Evans and Davies, 2010). Rather than sustaining primary-aged youngsters' involvement, secondary PE provision may exacerbate already widening inequalities in PA and sport participation that have roots outside school (Evans and Davies, 2010; Parry, 2013). If PE in this form erodes or undermines young people's feelings of competence, involvement and enjoyment as well as identity, then it contributes to young people's disengagement from PA and sport.

If engagement in PE (especially in the secondary years) is to play any part in involving and retaining young people in PA and sport, as well as recruiting those already marginalized or alienated, the content, form, delivery and context of PE require careful consideration. This has been examined in detail elsewhere (e.g. Green, 2014), though it is worth noting that whatever the consequences for the levels of PA during PE lessons, there is no substantial evidence that increasing the *amount* of school PE impacts significantly on youngsters' dispositions towards engaging in PA beyond school, or into adult life. The content and style of PE curricular delivery do appear important, however, for, as we noted earlier, where multi-activity PE programmes have the potential to contribute to the promotion of PA via a 'PE effect' is in providing youngsters with a broad base of skills and interests. The recipe for lifelong participation in PA and sport involves, among other things, the construction of rich, diverse 'wide sporting repertoires' (Roberts and Brodie, 1992) to which PE curricula might contribute through the provision of a portfolio of sports and physical activities. Some of these will endure while others will be replaced, supplemented or even dropped as their lives unfold; not least because the particular forms of activity in which young people find pleasurable excitement often develop and/or change as they grow older (Roberts and Brodie, 1992). Finally, engagement in PE might positively influence experiences of PA by providing more choice of activities which are non-threatening, recreational and self-directed and which enable young people to make their own decisions, based on their personal needs, in an environment where they become motivated towards engaging in PA because they wish to repeat satisfying experiences (Green, 2014; Smith et al., 2009).

Physical activity, inequality and the limits of education

To adequately understand the potential role PE may have in the promotion of PA and sport participation requires us to recognize the significance of global educational policy contexts and activities, as well as the importance of broader social inequalities which beset the lives of children, young people and their families. As Ball (2012, 2013) has noted, educational policy in many countries is increasingly defined by a concern with economic competitiveness and a correlative downgrading in the emphasis placed on the social purposes of education. This, he argues, is clearly expressed in the development of a global context of education policy making (as part of broader public service reform), the global convergence of education systems and increased commodification and marketization of education (e.g. Ball, 2012, 2013). These developments are currently expressed in 'a *generic global policy ensemble* that rests on a set of basic and common policy technologies . . . the market, management and performativity' (Ball, 2013: 46; emphasis in original) which have significant direct and indirect impacts on the practices of schools. In a prevailing neo-liberal policy climate which emphasizes *inter alia* the importance of highly prescriptive systems of accountability and inspection, competition and standards, choice and voice and target-hitting, teachers are thus increasingly 'caught between the imperatives of prescription and the disciplines of performance. Their practice is both "steered" *and* "rowed"' (Ball, 2013: 173; original emphasis).

PE teachers, and others responsible for the promotion of PA in education, are not immune to the effects of these neo-liberal trends and are constrained by their mutual independence with others, and by the prescriptions of policy (including curricula), to think and act in a variety of (often contradictory) ways. In England and Wales, teachers and schools are expected to promote PA – via PE and other subjects – for a variety of education, health and social outcomes, but they are required to do so in an already heavily congested curriculum which often prioritizes core subjects (e.g. mathematics, science) and skills such as literacy and numeracy. The existence of subject hierarchies (Ball et al., 2012) in which PE is frequently ranked lower than other so-called 'important' subjects often means that more time, money and attention is devoted to teaching and performance in those subjects. Consequently, opportunities for children and young people to engage in PA can be marginalized (particularly in the elementary and later secondary years), and time spent being sedentary increases, as teachers manage the constraints on them to deliver PE alongside 'academic' subjects which are the focus of particular attention during inspections, in league tables and by parents (Ball, 2012, 2013). The enactment of education policy by teachers (especially PE teachers) and how this is shaped significantly by the context of schooling is thus central to understanding the potential for PA promotion (and other policy goals) in contemporary education (Ball et al., 2012).

Despite the significance of education policy and practice for PA promotion, as Bernstein (1970) famously noted, policy which is based on the assumption that education can and does compensate for wider social inequalities is at best hugely misguided, and at worst based on a series of heavily value-laden and deficit-type views of children, their families and the reality of their circumstances. While the process of education and schooling *may* help to alleviate some of the effects of social inequality and disadvantage experienced by pupils, this is *only possible within certain limits* relative to the social and economic circumstances in which schools are located and which characterize the lives of their pupils (Bernstein, 1970). Policy expectations that education will help overcome the corrosive effects of inequality and their impact on the propensity for young people to engage in (more) PA are clearly wide of the mark. They also detract attention from the very significant deep-seated social inequalities which are more likely to be expressed and reinforced in schools than be narrowed by them (Evans and Davies, 2010; Smith and Haycock, 2016). As Hartas (2014: 48) has noted, the 'home lives of children are unequal and this inequality is translated into educational inequality, a part of larger systemic patterns of inequality that persist across generations', including in relation to the propensity for children and young people to engage in PA during and away from school, and in later life. In relation to PA, the roots of these inequalities can often be traced back to differences in primary socialization which occur from birth and which tend to give rise to differences in childhood predispositions for PA and degrees of sporting capital. While malleable, unequal dispositions towards PA (or not) are rooted in childhood – an especially formative phase of life when tastes, habits, predispositions and personalities are developing – and find expression in present-day PE.

Research findings suggest these early dispositions towards or away from sport appear to be transmitted during childhood, primarily through families (see Birchwood et al., 2008; Haycock and Smith, 2014, 2016; Quarmby and Dagkas, 2010; Wheeler, 2014). Some parents (especially those from the middle classes) are more likely to intentionally engage in the 'concerted cultivation' of their children's PA and sporting habits (Smith and Haycock, 2016; Wheeler, 2014). Others (lower-working-class parents, for example) have a tendency to leave PA and sports socialization to chance and/or to the education system. Whether parents are pro-active and strategic, or reactive and ambivalent, about their children's sporting experiences and capital, early childhood experiences tend to result in youngsters developing particular orientations to PA and sport *per se* prior to or, at the very least, alongside the early elementary school years. Consequently, even at ages 5 to 6, children arrive at elementary schools embodying different levels and forms of experience and abilities (i.e. sporting capital) alongside differential orientations towards PA and sport (i.e. sporting habitus) (Evans and Davies, 2010; Haycock and Smith, 2014; Wheeler, 2014). It would be implausible to suggest that the effectiveness of attempts to promote PA and sport in education settings were somehow immune from these broader trends.

Conclusion

In this chapter we have been centrally concerned with examining the policy rationale for viewing education (especially schools) as an appropriate setting for the promotion of PA, and the apparent role of – as well as the limits of relying upon – PE in fostering lifelong participation in PA and sport in contexts of social inequality. It has been suggested that engaging in PE may help promote PA among young people in schools, and may strengthen their sporting predispositions and biographies which are structured by, and structuring of, their broader social relations and habituses. The relationships developed between young people and their teachers, peers and significant others in education settings have been shown to help shape participation in, and experiences of, PA during and after school. These experiences, however, are to a large extent shaped by the particular diet of sports and physical activities provided by teachers (and increasingly coaches, especially in primary schools), by the contextual dimensions of schools (e.g. sporting traditions, availability of facilities and resources and the 'kinds' of pupils who attend them), and by the many complex features of increasingly marketized and commercialized approaches promoted by neo-liberal inspired policy decisions.

We have also argued, however, that the degree to which the content, organization and delivery of curricula promotes PA often depends on the predispositions, habits and experiences that are, to a large degree, acquired and reproduced outside of education in childhood and family contexts characterized by varying degrees of social inequality. In this regard, it might be argued that the promotion of PA through PE is most likely to be effective within what Birchwood et al. (2008) refer to as the minimum–maximum range to which young people are already predisposed by virtue of their socialization into, or away from, PA and sport in the family. In other words, where PE might make a difference to the promotion of PA and sport seems likely to be restricted, for the most part, to those youngsters already predisposed towards doing so. Indeed, any assumed relationship may, in fact, be spurious. If the findings of Birchwood et al. (2008) are anything to go by, family socialization appears a far better bet than PE (and education generally) as a major 'cause' of an immediate and enduring propensity to engage in PA and sport among young people. In short, we may simply have to accept that there are strong, relatively determining constraints on involvement in PA and sport through school-based PE that simply lie outside the scope of formal (physical) education programmes or curricula and are deep-seated features of social inequality (Evans and Davies, 2010). At the very least, we should recognize that participation in, and experiences of, education are 'affected by these inequalities in a whole variety of complex ways' (Ball, 2013: 214) which seriously questions the continued propensity for policy makers to 'position education as a key means of addressing them' (Ball, 2013: 214).

References

Ball, S. (2012). *Global education inc.: New policy networks and the neoliberal imaginary*. London: Routledge.

Ball, S. (2013). *The education debate* (2nd ed). Bristol: Policy Press.

Ball, S., Maguire, M. & Braun, A. (2012). *How schools do policy: Policy enactments in secondary schools*. London: Routledge.

Bernstein, B. (1970). *A critique of the concept of 'compensatory education'*. In: D. Rubinstein and C. Stoneman (Eds.) *Education for Democracy*. London: Penguin.

Biddle, S. & Asare, M. (2011). Physical activity and mental health in children and adolescents: A review of reviews. *British Journal of Sports Medicine, 45*, 886–895.

Birchwood, D., Roberts, K. & Pollock, G. (2008). Explaining differences in sport participation rates among young adults: Evidence from the South Caucasus. *European Physical Education Review, 14*(3), 283–298.

Blair, R. & Capel, S. (2011). Primary physical education, coaches and continuing professional development. *Sport, Education and Society, 16*(4), 485–505.

Brown, H., et al. (2013). Physical activity interventions and depression in children and adolescents. *Sports Medicine, 43*, 195–206.

DCMS (2015). *Sporting future*. London: DCMS.

Department of Health (2011). *Start active, stay active: A report on physical activity for health from the four home countries' Chief Medical Officers*. London: Department of Health.

Dismore, H. & Bailey, R. (2010) 'It's been a bit of a rocky start': Attitudes toward physical education following transition. *Physical Education and Sport Pedagogy, 15*(2), 175–191.

Eccles, J. & Roeser, R. (2011). Schools as developmental contexts during adolescence. *Journal of Research on Adolescence, 21*(1), 225–241.

Ekelund, U., Brage, S., Froberg, K., Harro, M., Anderssen S. A., Sardinha, L. B. et al. (2006). TV viewing and physical activity are independently associated with metabolic risk in children: The European Youth Heart Study. *PLoS Med, 3*(12), e488. DOI: 10. 1371/journal.pmed.0030488. PMID:17194189.

Elliot, D.E., Atencio, M., Campbell, T. & Jess, M. (2013). From PE experiences to PE teaching practices? Insights from Scottish primary teachers' experiences of PE, teacher education, school entry and professional development. *Sport, Education and Society, 18*(6), 749–766.

Evans, J. & Davies, B. (2010). Family, class and embodiment: Why school physical education makes so little difference to post-school participation patterns in physical activity. *International Journal of Qualitative Studies in Education, 23*(7), 765–784.

Evans, J. & Davies, B. (2014). Physical Education PLC: Neoliberalism, curriculum and governance. New directions for PESP research. *Sport, Education and Society, 19*(7), 869–884.

Feinstein, L., Bynner, J. & Duckworth, K. (2007). Young people's leisure contexts and their relation to adult outcomes. *Journal of Youth Studies, 9*(3), 305–327.

Gilchrist, P. & Wheaton, B. (2016). Lifestyle and adventure sports among youth. In: K. Green and A. Smith (Eds.) *The Routledge Handbook of Youth Sport*. London: Routledge.

Green, K. (2014). Mission impossible? Reflections on the relationship between physical education, youth sport and lifelong participation. *Sport, Education and Society, 19*(4), 357–375.

Hartas, D. (2014). *Parenting, family policy and children's well-being in an unequal society*. Basingstoke: Palgrave Macmillan.

Haycock, D. & Smith, A. (2014). A family affair? Exploring the influence of childhood sports socialisation on young adults' leisure-sport careers in north-west England. *Leisure Studies*, 33(3), 285–304.

Haycock, D. & Smith, A., 2016. Youth, sport and leisure careers. In: K. Green and A. Smith (Eds.) *The Routledge Handbook of Youth Sport*. London: Routledge.

Hillman, D., Erickson K. & Hatfield, B. (2017). Run for your life! Childhood physical activity effects on brain and cognition. *Kinesiology Review*, 6(1), 12–21.

Jones, L. & Green, K. (2015). Who teaches primary physical education? Change and transformation through the eyes of subject leaders. *Sport, Education and Society*, DOI: 10.1080/13573322.2015.1061987.

Morgan, P.J. & Hansen, V. (2008). The relationship between PE biographies and PE teaching practices of classroom teachers. *Sport, Education and Society*, 13(4), 373–391.

Parry, W. (2013). *Experiences of physical activity at age 10 in the British Cohort Study*. London: Centre for Longitudinal Studies, Institute of Education.

Public Health England (PHE) (2014). *Everybody active, every day. An evidence-based approach to physical activity*. London: Public Health England.

Public Health England (PHE) (2015). *Promoting children and young people's emotional health and wellbeing: A whole school and college approach*. London: Public Health England.

Quarmby, T. & Dagkas, S. (2010). Children's engagement in leisure time physical activity: Exploring family structure as a determinant. *Leisure Studies*, 29(1), 53–66.

Roberts, K. (1999). *Leisure in contemporary society*. Wallingford: CABI Publishing.

Roberts, K. (2016). Youth leisure as the context for youth sport. In: K. Green and A. Smith (Eds.) *The Routledge Handbook of Youth Sport*. London: Routledge.

Roberts, K. & Brodie, D. (1992). *Inner-city sport: Who plays, and what are the benefits?* Culemborg: Giordano Bruno.

Rossi, T., Pavey, A., Macdonald D. & McCuiag, L. (2016). Teachers as health workers: Patterns and imperatives of Australian teachers' work. *British Educational Research Journal*, 42(2), 258–276.

Smith, A. (2015). Primary school physical education and sports coaches: Evidence from a study of School Sport Partnerships in north-west England. *Sport, Education and Society*, 20(7), 872–888.

Smith, A. & Haycock, D. (2016). Families, youth and extra-curricular activity: Implications for physical education and school sport. In: S. Dagkas and L. Burrows (Eds.) *Families, Young People, Physical Activity and Health*. London: Routledge.

Smith, A., Green, K. & Thurston, M. (2009). 'Activity choice' and physical education in England and Wales. *Sport, Education and Society*, 14(2), 203–222.

Sport England (2016). *Towards an active nation*. London: Sport England.

Stuij, M. (2015). Habitus and social class: A case study on socialisation into sports and exercise. *Sport, Education and Society*, 20(6), 780–798.

Symonds, J. (2015). *Understanding school transition. What happens to children and how to help them*. London: Routledge.

Tremblay, M. & the Sedentary Behaviour Research Network. (2012). Letter to the Editor: Standardized use of the terms "sedentary" and "sedentary behaviours". *Applied Physiology, Nutrition and Metabolism*, 37, 540–542.

Tremblay, M., Carson, V. & Chaput, J-P. (2016). Introduction to the Canadian 24-hour movement guidelines for children and youth: An integration of physical activity, sedentary behaviour, and sleep. *Applied Physiology, Nutrition and Metabolism*, 41, iii–iv.

Tsangaridou, N. (2012). Educating primary teachers to teach physical education. *European Physical Education Review*, 18(3), 275–286.

Vanreusel, B. & Scheerder, J. (2016). Tracking and youth sport: The quest for lifelong adherence to sport and physical activity. In: K. Green and A. Smith (Eds.) *The Routledge Handbook of Youth Sport*. London: Routledge.

Wheeler, S. (2014). Organised activities, educational activities and family activities: How do they feature in the middle-class family's weekend? *Leisure Studies*, 33(2), 215–232.

Williams, B. & Macdonald, D. (2015). Explaining outsourcing in health, sport and physical education. *Sport, Education and Society*, 20(1), 57–72.

World Health Organization (WHO) (2010). *Global recommendations on physical activity for health*. Geneva: WHO.

PART II

Practices

THEME D INTRODUCTION
People, places and physical activity

The fourth theme in the Handbook focuses on the people who take part in physical activity and the places and spaces where they participate. The chapters on age, gender and disability examine selected aspects of the stratified character of societies and discuss the ways that difference and diversity are both reinforced and challenged in policy making and practice in the physical activity sector. Of vital importance to the discussions in these chapters is the idea that opportunities for and access to physical activity are characterised by wider social inequalities which shape patterns of engagement in and experiences of physical activity. The chapters on families, workplaces, schools and prisons recognise that physical activity takes place in different contexts and spaces. These chapters illustrate that people's physically active identities are spatialised and shaped by their everyday relations in different and diverse contexts; something that needs to be recognised in physical activity policy making, promotion and practice.

Cassandra Phoenix and Emmanuelle Tulle highlight that physical activity and inactivity are key policy concerns in relation to an ageing population. The authors argue that the prevailing medicalisation of ageing has led to physical activity policy focused almost exclusively on managing the ageing process and assuring good health. Physical activity is prescribed and regulated for older people in policy and recommended guidelines which also serve to homogenise the ageing process, and reduce physical activity to a medical treatment intervention. Phoenix and Tulle propose that physical activity policy for older people needs to recognise the different needs and preferences of older people to ensure that taking part becomes a pleasurable experience rather than a prescriptive one.

Philippa Velija and Louise Mansfield explore UK and international policy responses to the underrepresentation of girls and women in physical activity. They outline the long and complex history of exclusion of girls and women from physical activity and show that in many countries of the world, participation rates for girls and women are still lower than for boys and men. The chapter identifies and discusses both UK and worldwide policy and practice responses aimed at increasing physical activity for women and girls. The chapter illustrates that both legislation and advocacy has been successful in creating opportunities for girls and women in physical activity. It is also emphasised that national and international physical activity policy making and enactment for girls and women is important in addressing gender discrepancies in participation. The authors conclude though that the local and diverse needs of girls and women must become a part of policy making to ensure its relevance and impact.

Toni Williams and Brett Smith critically examine policy and practice in terms of physical activity for people living with disabilities. Despite legislation assuring the rights of disabled people in accessing health and wellbeing services, they remain a largely inactive population. Williams and Smith detail the personal, social and environmental barriers still facing those with disabilities in seeking to take part in physical activity. The chapter then focuses on the significance of healthcare professionals (HCPs) in promoting and supporting physical activity for people with disabilities. The central issue is the contradiction that healthcare professionals are best placed to encourage and engage disabled people in physical activity but their knowledge and understanding of opportunities for and access to appropriate programmes emphasising physical activity for health and behaviour change is limited. Healthcare professionals focus on more immediate rehabilitation than increasing physical activity levels in the long-term. The chapter proposes an emphasis on ensuring inclusive policy recommendations through the development of better training for HCPs within the healthcare system to ensure a comprehensive understanding of the health benefits of physical activity and more effective promotion of life-long physical activity for those living with disabilities.

John Day examines the ways that family relationships impact on people's physical activity habits. For Day, whilst families have been found to be pivotal in understanding health and wellbeing, family dynamics have been somewhat overlooked in physical activity policy and practice. Household composition, socio-economic status and parental role are identified in this chapter as significant in shaping types and levels of engagement in physical activity. Day's analysis suggests that families are more motivated by the wellbeing benefits of physical activity than the health ones. A policy focus on physical activity and quality of life, then, would be a significant development. Moreover, furthering an understanding of ways in which parenting can embrace an active lifestyle would make a contribution to developing tailored policy recommendations for families.

Continuing with the idea of active living and wellbeing, the next chapter by David McGillivray discusses workplace physical activity policy and practice. Documenting a shift from recreational and social workplace programmes to more explicit health and wellbeing ones, McGillivray examines the regulatory role of physical activity in work contexts. The chapter argues that whatever the precise rationale for workplace physical activity programmes they are centrally focused on producing fitter, more productive and happier workers. For McGillivray, there is little evidence that physical activity policy and promotion in the workplace improves health and wellbeing. Workplace policy agendas tend to provide physical activity interventions that may suit some but not all and they tend to ignore diverse needs and the complexities in the way work 'fits' into people's daily lives. The chapter concludes that there is scope for a more holistic approach to policy and practice which includes the workplace as one community setting amongst many for taking part in physical activity.

Jordan Smith, David Lubans and Rodney Lyn's chapter returns to the issue of school-based physical activity, examined by Smith et al., in Theme C of the Handbook. This chapter focuses on the USA context and examines the potential of multi-component physical activity interventions for improving health and education outcomes. For the authors, realising the potential of schools to increase physical activity needs to involve effective policy and practice in relation to physical education lessons, physical activity before, during and after school, the involvement of staff and the role of family and communities. Approaches which develop integrated strategies for understanding school-based contexts, expert delivery of physical activity programmes and partnerships between teachers, families and communities are suggested in this chapter as vitally important for effective policy and practice for physical activity in schools.

The last chapter in this theme is by Mark Norman and discusses penal policy and physical activity and the complexities of promoting and delivering physical activity in prisons. The chapter identifies various types of physical activity delivered for different reasons in prison systems. Prisoners can be involved in punitive physical labour, regulated outdoor recreation and leisure-type physical pursuits. The degree to which different physical activities are included in prisons is interconnected with differences in prison types, the overarching system of prisoner control and diversity in the prison population. For Norman, difference and diversity in prisons is rarely considered in the promotion and opportunities for physical activity and should be further explored in developing the potential of physical activity to improve the health and wellbeing of those incarcerated in penal institutions.

18

PHYSICAL ACTIVITY AND AGEING

Cassandra Phoenix and Emmanuelle Tulle

Introduction

Over the past decade, research at the intersection of the ageing body and physical activity has been slowly shifting from an almost exclusive focus on the health benefits of physical activity in older age (e.g. Chodzko-Zajko et al. 2009) to a broader comprehension of physical activity as a cultural practice and personal endeavour in older age. Debates and discussions surrounding the intersection of ageing and physical activity are taking place across numerous disciplines including health sciences, social gerontology, sociology of sport, and geography to name but a few and subsequently, the literature incorporates a divergent range of approaches, theoretical positions and methodologies. While still dominated by positivist epistemologies, more critically informed, interpretive research examining the experiences of physical activity in older adults has emerged in recent years (see Tulle 2008a, Eman 2012, Tulle and Phoenix 2015). As Phoenix and Grant (2009) note, these other ways of knowing can offer rich insight into the organisation and dynamics of physical activity in context, along with the diversity of meanings that older people give to their involvement.

Within this body of work, scholars have examined a range of topics including the influence of (spousal) relationships on physical activity behaviours (Dionigi et al. 2012, Barnett et al. 2013), the enjoyment of competition (Dionigi 2006, Tulle 2008a, Berlin and Klenosky 2014), the value of social networks facilitated by exercise settings (Bidone et al. 2009, Capalb et al. 2014), the influence of cultural beliefs (D'Alonzo and Sharma 2010, Jette and Vertinsky, 2011, Ceria-Ulep et al. 2011) and gender (Liechty et al. 2014, Humberstone and Cutler-Riddick, 2015) on experiences of physical activity; the impact of physical and social environments (Aronson and Oman, 2004; Chaudhury et al. 2012) including residential care settings (Kluge et al. 2012) and the changing dynamics of long-term involvement in sport and exercise (Heuser 2005, Griffin and Phoenix 2014, Evans and Sleap 2015).

This work illuminates how the ageing body is a key site for "acting out" physical activity policies and practices. It also highlights how older adults' experiences of physical activity can be diverse, shaped by a variety of socio-economic factors and lifestyle choices that cannot be separated from the wider context and culture within which they take place (Gullette 2004). In this chapter we provide an overview of key issues that demonstrate the ways in which physical activity and inactivity have come to be recognised as core concerns in relation to growing older. We then draw attention to three strands of research within this domain, which we believe have much to offer our understanding of the paradoxes and tensions regarding physical activity policy and promotion that arise in the context of older age. Finally, we offer a number of future directions that researchers committed to focusing a critical spotlight on physical activity policies and practice may wish to pursue.

Aged embodiment

Ageing has traditionally been framed by biomedical knowledge, which has encouraged an understanding of growing older primarily in terms of corporeality as bodily manifestations (Tulle-Winton 2000). The implications of this have encompassed not only biological, but also cultural processes in that ageing has typically been perceived as a medical and social "problem" with images of older people and the meaning of ageing itself being conflated with ill health, frailty, disability, disengagement and dependency on the health care system (Blaikie 1999). Such a scenario has allowed our relationship in Western society with the ageing process to be dominated by the *narrative of decline* (Gullette 1997), a narrative that portrays "a tragedy of accumulating deficits, diminishing reserves, and deteriorating attractiveness and strength: nothing more than denouement" (Randall and McKim 2008, p. 4). The prevalence of this narrative has damaging implications for the ageing body because it presents ageing as a process of passively *getting* rather than actively *growing* old, and as a body at risk. This seemingly legitimises the increased levels of control that the ageing body is subjected to via welfare and health professionals. Such social control can become internalised, enabling self-surveillance to become an important mechanism for perpetuating this narrative. It also further facilitates the management and movement of ageing bodies out of public spaces including the labour market and visual media (Tulle 2008a, p. 3). Indeed, as Tulle rightly reminds us, "older bodies are subjected to forms of professional control and surveillance, whether at home or in institutions, justified and legitimated by their declining properties". For her, these forms of domination are imposed on ageing bodies by broader structures and narratives that encompass socially contingent expectations of age appropriate behaviour. They also restrict the scope in which aged embodiment can be imagined. By embodiment we mean the complex interplay of cultural, social and personal norms which frame not only how people manage and present their bodies and themselves but also how they are perceived. Precisely how physical activity, by giving primacy to a different kind of physicality, enables people to become embodied in ways which challenge the narrative of decline and give way to more imaginative ways of being is worthy of investigation.

For Gilleard and Higgs (2000, 2013, see also Jones and Higgs 2010), the practices of choice and consumption can provide opportunities for protecting identity and retaining a sense of agency alongside an ageing, changing body. Ageing, they assert, is not what it once was, to the extent that:

> old age as a distinct social category has collapsed while ageing itself has lost much of its former coherence. Age as 'old age' has been replaced by the feared social imaginary of a 'fourth age' . . . while the ageing 'process' has become caught up in the puzzling cultural complexity that is the 'third age'.
>
> *2013, p. vii*

Emerging from this blend of fear, hope and confusion, a number of scholars have noted a new kind of ageing appearing, characterised by "the expansion of more promising possibilities of self-construction" in later life (Gergen and Gergen 2000, p. 282). This "new" model of ageing has been conceptualised in various ways, including, but not limited to, successful ageing, positive ageing, productive ageing, healthy ageing and ageing well (Phoenix and Sparkes 2009, Andrews 2009, Boudiny 2013).

Linked to these conceptualisations has been the notion of *active ageing* – a term that rapidly permeated into cultural consciousness during the early 2000s through policy and practice discourse about the ageing population and the welfare of older people, particularly in the United Kingdom (see Stenner et al. 2010). While certainly not *the* single defining feature of active ageing, being physically active in one's older age undoubtedly constitutes a core element. Stenner et al. (2010, p. 467) describe active ageing as "a broad and internally complex notion that plays a key role in a global strategy for the management of ageing populations". For them, an important component in its internal complexity is its intertwining of political/ ethical (normative) and scientific (descriptive/explanatory) concerns. In relation to health, these authors argue that active ageing policy urges individual citizens and families to make "personal efforts to adopt positive personal health practices at all stages of life" (World Health Organization, 2002, p.17). Indeed, the role that active ageing policy plays in reinforcing neoliberal ideologies of health is a common criticism (see Clarke and Warren 2007, Holstein and Minkler 2007), along with its oppression of marginalised and disadvantaged elders (see Ranzijn 2010) and reinforcement of anti-ageing discourse (Cardona 2008). Yet Stenner et al. (2010, p. 2) also remind us that it is not the domain of health and social policy alone at work here. Rather, health and physical activity *researchers* contribute by providing data on what such positive personal health practices might entail, while *businesses and politicians* collaborate to fund the research and supportive environments that appear to make "the healthy choices the easy choices" .

"Declining to decline" through physical activity

It is against this contextual backdrop that an interest has emerged in recent years regarding the ways in which physical activity can be utilised as a key resource in older age for embodied resistance to the dominant narrative of decline. For example, research focusing on veteran elite runners (e.g. Tulle 2007, 2008a) and older natural bodybuilders (e.g. Phoenix and Smith, 2011) suggests that sports participation in later life may reflect and can even instigate social change, by increasing embodied agency and widening the range of culturally available ageing identities beyond that of unitary, universal and inevitable decline. These studies show how participation in sport and physical activity in later life has the potential to generate *counterstories* through which social actors might develop these "resistant" identities as they age.

Understanding how resistance to the notion of inevitable decline in older age might be enacted through sport and physical activity is important. Not least because exercise is commonly positioned as a key weapon in the fight against disease and, by extension, the ageing process. This has been accentuated, argues Tulle (2008b) by the attentions of the discipline of human kinesiology / sport sciences, wherein researchers have become concerned with the impact of increasing age on performance, the potential impact of exercise on ageing processes, and the role played by exercise on illness prevention and life extension. In doing so, she argues, sport science (and by association sport and exercise) is a powerful constituent of the anti-ageing project (Vincent 2006), and as such "may perhaps be actively involved in the increased medicalisation of ageing by reconstructing the ageing body as malleable, open to intervention" (Tulle 2008b, pp. 341–342). The danger in such a construction is that it becomes geared towards the elimination of ageing as process and burden. In doing so, it reinforces the social construction of ageing as associated with decline, a problem to map out and solve via science. It also gives professionals leave to delve more deeply into older people's lives, a feature of what is arguably a natural extension of the anxieties about physical activity: the concern with sedentary behaviour.

Sedentary behaviour: A vital politics in older age

Also relevant for physical activity policy and practice in older age is the somewhat new problem of late modern affluent societies that has been identified: inactivity or, more precisely, sedentary behaviour. Of note here this is more than a fanciful question of nomenclature – using the term "sedentary behaviour" brings inactivity into the realm of disease. The apparent discovery, by Owen et al. (2010a), of physiological changes as a result of prolonged sitting is the justification to make it a health risk in its own right, which overlaps with, and is also additional to, the lack of physical activity. Thus one could be engaging in sport several times a week but sitting for long periods of time, and the physiological benefits of these bouts of physical activity would not compensate for the deleterious effects of being inactive, a type of behaviour which has been described as the "Active Couch Potato" (Owen et al. 2010a, p. 108). This process of specification and naming is in a semantic space with the sedentarisation of Western lives explanation, according to which technological improvements and labour-saving devices have transformed our working lives and our leisure time (Owen et al. 2010b). It is the negative aspect of these transformations which is highlighted – that we no longer need to expend the levels of energy that our forebears would have done in more physically demanding occupations and in the absence of motorised transport, and this has made us lazy, to the detriment of our health. This is of course a very broad and somewhat inaccurate generalisation of past habits.

Elsewhere Tulle (2014) conducted an analysis of sedentariness in early medical treatises and showed that the languor, which we associate with late 20th century lifestyles, had a long history among the affluent and powerful classes of the 18th and 19th centuries. For physicians such as Tissot and one hundred years later Yorke-Davies, sedentary behaviour was a problem of the intellectual, of the writer and of anyone who did not have to do physical labour to earn a living, and its nefarious health consequences were already visible: weight gain, heart disease, unwelcome expansion of the waistband and general listlessness (Tulle 2014)! What distinguishes the 18th century sedentarian from his contemporary counterpart lies not in physiology, but in the way the problem is framed and in the target population.

Unlike in the classical and the Victorian periods, the contemporary sedentary person is old, often female and US African American (Baruth et al. 2013, Nies et al. 2013). This person watches too much television. In a systematic review of articles on sedentary behaviour Rhodes et al. (2012) are well aware that the range of "activities" that people are doing when they are not in motion is broad, yet it is screen viewing which attracts the most attention and commentary and from which older people should, it seems, be weaned. Similarly, contemporary physical activity policy recommendations require people to deploy greater asceticism, which, allied with the singling out of screen viewing time as the bad component of sedentary behaviour, betrays a moral concern that people, irrespective of age, should conduct their lives in appropriate ways (see for instance Hamilton et al. 2008, Kikuchi et al. 2013, Paterick 2013). This is problematic for a number of reasons.

First, commonly used interventions aimed at addressing sedentary behaviour include the use of strategies to support behaviour change, such as telephone-based physical activity advice delivered by either a professional or a peer mentor (Castro et al. 2011) or internet-based exercise programmes and the adoption of wearable technologies (e.g. accelerometers) designed to prompt people to move (Dobbins et al. 2013, Kerr et al. 2013). The totality of people's lives, more precisely how people use their spare time, here and now, is now under scrutiny.

Second, despite relying on the sedentarisation explanation to understand the increase in inactivity, the target of intervention is the individual although not a passive one, but through the transformation of his or her dispositions (to sit down and watch TV), a wholly complicit one. Individuals have to recognise that their past dispositions to sit are inherently pathological. Third the war metaphor fuels the sense of panic, reinforced by moral overtones targeted at both individual patients but also professionals, the inference here being that health care practitioners are not doing their job properly and that patients lack the wherewithal to make appropriate decisions. The historical, political, economic or discursive context within which lives are led is largely absent and how these lives are evaluated is carried out almost exclusively in terms of health outcomes, overshadowing other realms of experience such as the hidden pleasures that people, including older people, might derive from their activities, sedentary or otherwise. Nevertheless the implications of this concern with sedentariness can be conceptualised as a vital politics (Rose 2007) in older age.

Absent pleasures

Being active in older age has been almost entirely overshadowed by health initiatives (with health outcome measures) and the slightly more elusive anti-ageing narratives alluded to above. To that end, a particularly noteworthy strand of inquiry, which has much to offer critical scholarship on physical activity policy and practice, coheres around the embodied pleasures of physicality in later life. This area of analytical interest reflects and extends an increasing interest in affect, emotion and, in some instances, the use of phenomenological approaches to understand physical cultural practices (see Pringle 2009, Thorpe and Rinehart 2010, Wellard 2012, Throsby 2013, Allen-Collinson and Leledaki 2015, Allen-Collinson and Owton, 2015).

Although still in its infancy, the small amount of research that examines the pleasures of physicality in relation to the ageing body has illustrated how encountering pleasure with and through the moving, ageing body goes some way to challenging foreclosing assumptions about what the ageing body can and should do, produce and represent. For example, informed by a carnal sociology Nettleton (2013, 2015) argues that attention to the visceral basis of meaning gives insight into why older fell runners continue to participate in this intense, transformative activity in later life. Such an approach, she asserts, highlights the often profound, existential reasons for sustained participation that go beyond health pronouncements and the notion of a responsible citizen. Indeed, Nettleton explains how the imperative to run and experience a passion inherent (and to a certain extent exclusive) to the fell running community ensures that many older adults continue running, often against recommendations from health professionals that they should "slow down" and engage in activity less risky to the older body.

Differing ideas around the benefits and risks of exertion is a theme also discussed by Jette and Vertinsky (2015). Conscious that health care policies and lifestyle prescriptions often lack sensitivity to social location, cultural nuance, and the power relations that they (re)produce, these authors turned their attention to traditional Chinese understandings of health geographies of the body (that differ vastly from those in Western society) to examine how varying body ontologies lead to a divergence in bodily practices that are conducted in the name of health. Drawing from in-depth interview data with Chinese origin women aged 65 and over and now living in Canada, Jette and Vertinsky argued that these women undertook their physical activity practices in pursuit of happiness and life balance. This was characterised by their practice of Tai Chi as "playing Tai Chi" and a counter to neoliberal notions of personal responsibility for health based upon a Western calculus of risk (p. 115).

Pleasure, however, is not a singular, uni-dimensional concept, but can be experienced as different types in, with and through the ageing body. Furthermore, it can be encountered across various temporalities and spaces, in some instances beyond where and when the activity was undertaken. These were the findings of research conducted by Phoenix and Orr (2014), which employed in-depth interviews and photo elicitation techniques to understand the impact of physical activity on older adults' perceptions and experiences of (self-)ageing (see Orr and Phoenix, 2015). Their analyses revealed four different types of pleasure, which were used to construct a typology of pleasure in later life. For example, Phoenix and Orr (2014) noted how pleasure could be *sensual* by coming into being through the senses (i.e. the smell of a freshly mown pitch, the touch of water against one's body as it moves in the swimming pool). It could also be encountered through the process of *documenting* one's activities (i.e. times, routes, descriptive accounts) or by *immersing* oneself in the moment of that activity (i.e. meditative state often accomplished in yoga). For some of the participants, pleasure was not induced through the act of physicality itself, but via the sense of routine and *habit* it brought to the rhythm of their daily life.

Concluding comments and implications for physical activity policy

In this chapter, we have presented a small but significant selection of key issues that hold relevance for how the ageing body intersects with physical activity policy and practice. Until relatively recently, biomedical perspectives and positivist methodologies dominated our knowledge of the ageing body and its physicality. These have often reduced the experiences and meanings of physical activity practices in older age almost exclusively to health pronouncements and contributed to a broader social "war on old age" (see Vincent 2007, p. 941). Critical scholarship focusing upon active embodiment in later life has highlighted how physical activity in later life is also political. To that end, we have alluded to the ways in which physical activity – through its alignment with the broader concept of "active ageing" – can be understood as a complex notion that plays a key role in the management of ageing. We have also shown how the physically active ageing body can act as a site of resistance to the identity-damaging narrative of decline, although in some circumstances, such resistance is so fierce that it reinforces the war *on ageing* per se, rather than a war on the socially situated, largely negative meanings surrounding it. Through a critically informed discussion of sedentary behaviour, we also illuminate how in recent years, sitting still has rapidly and indeed purposefully been positioned as a lifestyle choice, characterised by excessive screen time particularly in the form of television viewing. The act of sitting is deemed as being immoral and irresponsible – irrespective of how the time sitting might be used. Indeed people might be *actively* sitting, engaged in reminiscing, resting, reading or doing crosswords or even socialising with friends and family. Finally, we exemplified how emerging research into the pleasures of physical activity offers new ways of relating to the ageing body that are currently excluded not only from narratives of ageing, but physical activity policy and practice too.

In terms of implications for physical activity policy and practice, we contend that prescriptive guidelines frequently projected through policy discourse in relation to later life physical activity are often disconnected from the everyday experiences of those that it aims to serve. Specifically, like other age groups, older adults are rarely cognisant of prescriptive figures concerning frequency, intensity, time and type of activity. Nor does the justification of "disease prevention", often touted by health policy, tend to form the singular or even primary motivation for older adults' affinity toward being physically active in later life (Tulle 2008a). Rather, adults come to, leave, return to and remain physically active throughout their ageing process for a number of reasons including: the status of their relationships with significant others (caring, cared for, supportive, discouraging); their ability to see themselves as, or embrace the identity of, someone who exercises; and the various pleasures that they experience from being physically active across different times and spaces. Accordingly, the drivers for physical activity initiatives should not simply be the transformation of the old body from a body of decline to an active, fit, almost ageless body, but one concerned with enriching the whole lives of older people.

That said, instigating such initiatives requires a commitment to sustainable and sustaining levels of funding, which with the erosion of local authority budgets and the de-legitimisation of the welfare state is currently under considerable pressure. Indeed, the paucity of such provision is consistent with a form of government strongly inflected by neoliberal ideology (Dardot and Laval 2010), which prioritises prescription within a marketised model of provision. That noted, shifting the emphasis within physical activity programmes to a focus on experiential and affectual encounters rather than instrumental gains might offer one relatively cost-effective, yet promising step forward. This is particularly so given the work highlighting the importance of emphasising affect (as opposed to health education messages alone) for maintaining motivation towards exercise behaviours (see Segar and Richardson 2014, Taylor and Pescatello 2016), coupled with the relative absence of affect within health policy discourse. Shifting away from the demonising of sitting in older age and incorporating the affectual and experiential aspects of movement might contribute to more productive and appealing recommendations for later life physical activity policy and practice in the future.

References

Allen-Collinson, J. and Leledaki, A., 2015. Sensing the outdoors: A visual and haptic phenomenology of outdoor exercise embodiment. *Leisure Studies*. ISSN: 0261–4367.

Allen-Collinson, J. and Owton, H., 2015. Intense embodiment: Senses of heat in women's running and boxing. *Body & Society*. ISSN: 1357–034x.

Andrews, M., 2009. The narrative complexity of successful aging. *International Journal of Sociology and Social Policy* (Special issue on Theorising Aging Studies) 29(1–2), 73–83.

Aronson, R. E. and Oman, R. F., 2004. Views on exercise and physical activity among rural-dwelling senior citizens. *Journal of Rural Health*, 20(1), 76–79.

Barnett, I., Guell, C. and Ogilvie, D., 2013. How do couples influence each other's physical activity behaviours in retirement? An exploratory qualitative study. *BMC Public Health*, 13, 1197.

Baruth, M., Sharpe, P. A., Hutto, B., Wilcox., S. and Warren, T. Y., 2013. Patterns of sedentary behavior in overweight and obese women. *Ethnicity & Disease,* 23(3), 336–342.

Berlin, K. L. and Klenosky, D. B., 2014. Let me play, not exercise! *Journal of Leisure Research*, 46(2), 127–152.

Bidone, M., Goodwin, D. L. and Drinkwater, D. T., 2009. Older women's experiences of a fitness program: The importance of social networks. *Journal of Applied Sport Psychology*, 21, S86–S101.

Blaikie, A., 1999. *Ageing and popular culture*. Cambridge, UK: Cambridge University Press.

Boudiny, K., 2013. 'Active ageing': From empty rhetoric to effective policy tool. *Ageing & Society*, 33(6), 1077–1098.

Capalb, D. J., O'Halloran, P. and Liamputtong, P., 2014. Why older people engage in physical activity: An exploratory study of participants in a community-based walking program. *Australian Journal of Primary Health*, 20(1), 74–78.

Cardona, B., 2008. 'Healthy ageing' policies and anti-ageing ideologies and practices: On the exercise of responsibility. *Medical Health Care and Philosophy*, 11, 475–483.

Castro, C. M., Pruitt, L.A., Buman, M. P. and King, A. C., 2011. Physical activity program delivery by professionals versus volunteers: The TEAM randomized trial. *Health Psychology,* 30(3), 285–294.

Ceria-Ulep, C. D., Serafica, R. C. and Tse, A., 2011. Filipino older adults' beliefs about exercise activity. *Nursing Forum,* 46(4), 240–250.

Chaudhury, H., Mahmood, A., Michael, Y. L., Campo, M. and Hay, K., 2012. The influence of neighborhood residential density, physical and social environments on older adults' physical activity: An exploratory study in two metropolitan areas. *Journal of Aging Studies,* 26(1), 35–43.

Chodzko-Zajko, W., Schwingel, A. and Park, C. H., 2009. Successful aging: The role of physicalactivity. *American Journal of Lifestyle Medicine,* 3(1), 20–28.

Clarke, A. and Warren, L., 2007. Hopes, fears and expectations about the future: What do older people's stories tell us about active ageing? *Ageing & Society,* 27, 465–488.

D'Alonzo, K. T. and Sharma, M. 2010. The influence of marianismo beliefs on physical activity in midlife immigrant Latinas: A photovoice study. *Qualitative Research in Sport and Exercise,* 2(2), 229–249.

Dardot, P. and Laval, C., 2010. *La nouvelle raison du monde: Essai sur la société néoliberale.* Paris: Editions La Découverte.

Dionigi, R., 2006. Competitive sport as leisure in later life: Negotiations, discourse and aging. *Leisure Sciences,* 28(2), 181–196.

Dionigi, R., Fraser-Thomas, J. and Logan, J., 2012. The nature of family influences on sport participation in masters athletes. *Annals of Leisure Research,* 15(4), 366–388.

Dobbins, C., Fergus, P., Stratton, G., Rosenberg, M. and Merabti, M., 2013. Monitoring and reducing sedentary behavior in the elderly with the aid of human digital memories. *Telemedicine Journal and E-Health: The Official Journal of the American Telemedicine Association,* 19(3), 173–185.

Eman, J., 2012. The role of sports in making sense of the process of growing old. *Journal of Aging Studies,* 26(4), 467–475.

Evans, A. B. and Sleap, M., 2015. Older adults' lifelong embodied experiences of leisure time aquatic physical activity in the United Kingdom. *Leisure Studies,* 34(3), 335–353.

Gergen, K. J. and Gergen, M. M., 2000. The new aging: Self construction and social values. In R. W. Schaie and J. Hendricks, eds. *The evolution of the aging self: The societal impact of the aging process.* New York: Springer. 281–306.

Gilleard, C. and Higgs, P., 2000. *Cultures of ageing, self, citizen and the body.* Harlow: Prentice Hall.

Gilleard, C. and Higgs, P., 2013. *Ageing, corporeality and embodiment.* London: Anthem Press.

Griffin, M. and Phoenix, C., 2014. Learning to run from narrative foreclosure: One woman's story of ageing and physical activity. *Journal of Aging & Physical Activity,* 22, 393–404.

Gullette, M. M., 1997. *Declining to decline: Cultural combat and the politics of the midlife.* Charlottesville, VA: University of Virginia Press.

Gullette, M. M., 2004. *Aged by culture.* Chicago, IL: The University of Chicago Press.

Hamilton M, T., Healy G, M., Dunstan, D.W., Zderic, T. W. and Owen, N., 2008. Too little exercise and too much sitting: Inactivity physiology and the need for new recommendations on sedentary behavior. *Current Cardiovascular Risk Reports,* 2(4), 292–298.

Heuser, L., 2005. We're not too old to play sports: The career of women lawn bowlers. *Leisure Studies,* 24(1), 45–60.

Holstein, MB. and Minkler, M. (2007) Critical gerontology: Reflections for the 21st century. In: Bernard M, Scharf T (eds) *Critical perspectives on ageing societies.* Bristol: Policy Press. 13–26.

Humberstone, B. and Cutler-Riddick, C., 2015. Older women, embodiment and yoga practice. *Ageing & Society,* 35(6), 1221–1241.

Jette, S. and Vertinsky, P., 2011. Exercise is medicine: Understanding the exercise beliefs and practices of older Chinese women immigrants in British Columbia, Canada. *Journal of Aging Studies,* 25(3), 272–284.

Jette, S., and Vertinsky, P., 2015. The contingencies of exercise science in a globalizing world: Ageing Chinese Canadian and their play and pleasure in exercise. In E. Tulle and C. Phoenix, eds. *Physical activity in sport and later life: Critical perspectives.* London: Palgrave Macmillan. 113–123.

Jones, I. R. and Higgs, P. F., 2010. The natural, the normal and the normative: Contested terrains in ageing and old age. *Social Science & Medicine,* 71, 1513–1519.

Kerr, J., Marshall, S. J., Godbole, S., Chen, J., Legge, A., Doherty., A. R., et al. 2013. Using the SenseCam to improve classifications of sedentary behavior in free-living settings. *American Journal of Preventive Medicine,* 44(3), 290–296.

Kikuchi, H., Inoue, S., Sugiyama, T., Owen, N., Oka, K. and Shimomitsu, T., 2013. Correlates of prolonged television viewing time in older Japanese men and women. *BMC Public Health*, 13, 213.

Kluge, M. A., Tang, A., Glick, L., LeCompte, M. and Willis, B., 2012. Let's keep moving: A dance movement class for older women recently relocated to a continuing care retirement community. *Arts & Health: An International Journal for Research, Policy and Practice*, 4(1), 4–15.

Liechty, T., Dahlstrom. L., Sveinson K. and Rossow-Kimball, B., 2014. Canadian men's perceptions of leisure time physical activity and the ageing body. *Qualitative Research in Sport, Exercise & Health*, 6(1), 20–44.

Nettleton, S., 2013. Cementing relations within a sporting field: Fell running in the English Lake District and the acquisition of existential capital. *Cultural Sociology*, 7(2), 196–210.

Nettleton, S., 2015. Fell running in later life: Irresponsible intoxication or existential capital? In E. Tulle and C. Phoenix, eds. *Physical activity and sport in later life: Critical perspectives*. Basingstoke, UK: Palgrave. 124–136.

Nies, M. A., Troutman-Jordan, M., Branche, D., Moore-Harrison, T. and Hohensee, C., 2013. Physical activity preferences for low-income sedentary urban African American older adults. *Journal of Gerontological Nursing*, 39(6), 20–29.

Orr, N. and Phoenix, C., 2015. Photographing physical activity: Using visual methods to 'grasp at' the sensual experiences of the ageing body. *Qualitative Research*, 15(4), 454–472.

Owen, N., Healy, G. N., Matthews, C. E. and Dunstan, D. W., 2010a. Too much sitting: The population-health science of sedentary behavior. *Exercise and Sport Sciences Review*, 38(3), 105–116.

Owen, N., Sparling, P. B., Healy, G. N., Dunstan, D. W. and Matthews, C. E., 2010b. Sedentary behavior: Emerging evidence for a new health risk. *Mayo Clinic Proceedings*, 85(12), 1138–1141.

Paterick, T. E., 2013. The corpulent and sedentary society: Epitome of a healthcare crisis. *The Journal of Medical Practice Management*, 29(1), 32–34.

Phoenix, C. and Grant, B., 2009. Expanding the agenda for research on the physically active aging body. *Journal of Aging and Physical Activity*, 17(3), 362–381.

Phoenix, C. and Orr, N., 2014. Pleasure: A forgotten dimension of ageing and physical activity. *Social Science and Medicine*, 115, 94–102.

Phoenix, C., and Smith, B., 2011. Telling a (good?) counterstory of aging: Natural bodybuilding meets the narrative of decline. *The Journals of Gerontology, Series B*, 66(5), 628–639.

Phoenix, C. and Sparkes, A. C., 2009. Being Fred: Big stories, small stories and the accomplishment of a positive ageing identity. *Qualitative Research*, 9(2), 83–99.

Pringle, R., 2009. Defamiliarizing heavy-contact sports: A critical examination of rugby, discipline and pleasure. *Sociology of Sport Journal*, 26, 211–234.

Randall, W. L. and McKim, A. E., 2008. *Reading our lives: The poetics of growing old*. New York, NY: Oxford University Press.

Ranzijn, R., 2010. Active ageing – Another way to oppress marginalized and disadvantaged elders? *Journal of Health Psychology*, 15(5), 716–723.

Rhodes, R., Mark, R. and Temmel, C., 2012. Adult sedentary behavior: A systematic review. *American Journal of Preventive Medicine*, 42(3), e3–28.

Rose, N., 2007. *The politics of life itself: Biomedicine, power, and subjectivities in the 21st Century*. Princeton: Princeton University Press.

Segar, M. L. and Richardson, C. R., 2014. Prescribing pleasure and meaning: Cultivating walking motivation and maintenance. *American Journal of Preventative Medicine*, 47(6), 838–841.

Stenner, P., McFarquhar, T. and Bowling, A., 2010. Older people and 'active ageing': Subjective aspects of ageing actively. *Journal of Health Psychology*, 16(3), 467–477.

Taylor, B. A. and Pescatello, L. S., 2016. For the love of it: Affective experiences that may increase physical activity participation among older adults. *Social Science & Medicine*, 161, 61–63.

Thorpe, H. and Rinehart, R., 2010. Alternative sport and affect: Non-representational theory examined. *Sport in Society*, 13(7–8), 1268–1291.

Throsby, K., 2013. "If I go in like a cranky sea lion, I come out like a smiling dolphin": Marathon swimming and the unexpected pleasures of being a body in water. *Feminist Review*, 103, 5–22.

Tulle, E., 2007. Running to run: Embodiment, structure and agency amongst veteran elite runners. *Sociology*, 41(2), 329–346.

Tulle, E., 2008a. *Ageing, the body and social change: Running in later life*. Basingstoke, UK: Palgrave Macmillan.

Tulle, E., 2008b. Acting your age? Sports science and the ageing body. *Journal of Aging Studies,* 22(4), 291–294.

Tulle, E., 2014. Are you sitting comfortably? Think again. *Discover Society,* Issue 11, www.discoversociety.org/2014/08/05/are-you-sitting-comfortably-think-again/ [accessed online 1/10/15].

Tulle, E. and Phoenix, C., eds., 2015. *Physical activity and sport in later life: Critical approaches.* Basingstoke: Palgrave Macmillan.

Tulle-Winton, E., 2000. Old bodies. In P. Hancock, B. Hughes, E. Jagger, K. Paterson, R. Russell, E. Tulle-Winton and M. Tyler, eds. *The body, culture and society: An introduction.* Buckingham, UK: Open University Press. 64–84.

Vincent, J., 2006. Ageing contested: Anti-ageing science and the cultural construction of old age. *Sociology,* 40(4), 681–698.

Vincent, J., 2007. Science and imagery in the 'war on old age'. *Ageing and Society,* 27(6), 941–961.

Wellard, I., 2012. Body-reflexive pleasures: Exploring bodily experiences within the context of sport and physical activity. *Sport, Education and Society,* 17(1), 21–33.

World Health Organization, 2002. Active ageing policy framework. Online document. Available from: www.who.int/ageing/publications/active/en/index.html [accessed 1/03/13].

19

GIRLS, WOMEN AND PHYSICAL ACTIVITY

Philippa Velija and Louise Mansfield

Introduction

Worldwide participation rates for physical activity tend to be lower for women and girls compared to boys and men. Typically, physical activity is taken to mean any bodily movement, produced by the contraction of skeletal muscle that increases energy expenditure (World Health Organization, 2017). There are too many types of physical activity to list individually, all taking place in diverse contexts including communities, education and workplaces. Patterns of participation in physical activity are most often measured by the frequency, time and intensity of the activities themselves and the pattern is certainly characterised by gendered differences in many countries of the world. Whilst there are large differences between countries, Hallal et al. (2012) explain that of the 105 countries of the world there is data for, the proportion of young people not achieving 60 min per day of physical activity is around 80 per cent in 56 of those countries in boys, and 95 per cent of the 105 countries for girls. The gender disparities in participation rates continue as people get older and women take part less often in physical activity than men. Data from the World Health Organization (WHO) illustrates that in high income countries, 26 per cent of men and 35 per cent of women are insufficiently active. Whilst evidence indicates that the gap between men and women's participation has decreased over time, prevailing gender differences reflect the relative exclusion of women and girls from taking part in physical pursuits (Green et al., 2015). A history of exclusion has resulted from opposition to the involvement of women and girls in physical activities that have been variously argued to be damaging to their bodies and minds, and unattractive and counter to dominant ideas about femininity. International, national and local policies focusing on increasing physical activity for women and girls have developed in response to the under-representation of females in physical activity. Overall such policy responses have emphasised two broad agendas: (1) women's rights in relation to equitable access to and opportunities for physical activity, and (2) women's welfare in terms of promoting health and fitness. This chapter examines policy development on physical activity for girls and women in selected countries around the world. It begins with a brief historical overview of the exclusionary ideologies and practices that have left a legacy of under-representation of women and girls in physical activity. A discussion of UK policy and practice aimed at increasing levels of physical activity amongst girls and women is presented. The chapter examines a number of global policy approaches to female involvement in physical activity. It concludes with a comment about the impact of formal policy agendas on rates of participation and experiences of women and girls in physical activity.

A gendered history of participation and physical activity

The gendered history of physical activity has been well documented. This history of exclusion is multifaceted, but one enduring issue is the impact of medical discourses in the 19th century which defined girls and women's bodies as weak, fragile and in need of protection to preserve fertility. The common belief was that females were less suited to vigorous exercise because it would cause physical and mental illness particularly connected to risk of damage to child bearing capacities (Vertinsky, 1990). These medical discourses, supported in varying degrees by the predominantly male medical profession, underpinned the relative exclusion of females from physical activity although there were class differences in access and opportunity. The notion of free time for women's leisure was determined in part by class divisions, and sports such as golf and tennis and sports such as climbing, sailing were accessible by upper middle class women for whom participation was a sign of social status (Hargreaves, 1994).

The emergence of modern sport and its governance reflects a history of maleness and masculinity in opportunities for, access to and control over participation in physical activity in a range of contexts. The following sections are structured around two key opportunities for physical activity that illustrate gendered practices of exclusion and the policy context for increasing participation by girls and women: schooling, education and physical education, and leisure time physical activity.

Females, schooling and education through the physical

Being involved in physical activity at a young age can lead to the development of sporting habits and physically active lifestyles (Green, 2010). Physical education was significant in presenting challenges to early 19th century images of female frailty and exclusion from physical activity by pioneering therapeutic exercise and sport (Atkinson, 1973). Girls' access to physical education and the types of physical activity that were provided through the curriculum was again largely dependent on social class. Whilst girls' public schools encouraged games, such as cricket and hockey, publicly funded schools followed more callisthenic-related activities based on the Swedish traditions (Kirk, 2002). Today in the UK most young people are involved in physical activity through school which provides the context for a formal physical education curriculum as well as extracurricular opportunities for physical activity. Yet a gender gap in participation in physical activity is reflected in UK physical education with data consistently highlighting that girls tend to be less physically active both in and out of school settings (Green, 2010). This is despite the introduction of the 1992 National Curriculum in England and Wales for all children in state schools (schools which are funded by the UK government with no charge to attend) which was posited as a way for the curriculum to meet the needs of all pupils. The national curriculum is compulsory for all pupils and was partially designed to be inclusive, yet to some extent the gendered nature of the NCPE contributes to negative experiences for girls and does not inspire lifelong participation. Critical perspectives express concern about the gendered character of the NCPE. Such concerns are three-fold and consider issues connected to: (1) the emphasis on games, (2) the optional nature of dance and (3) the place and status of outdoor education. The continued dominance of games over other forms of physical activity has implications for gender equity for two reasons. First, the content of games in PE has been most persistently associated with sex differentiated provision and the delivery of these activities has been closely associated with gendered patterns of participation (Penney, 2002). Games can be delivered in ways that challenge gender stereotypes. Wider education policy connected to teacher training has a role to play in engaging student teachers in dialogue that challenges current thinking about what games should be available to male and female pupils, whether desegregated provision is appropriate and the relative merits of mixed-sex physical education. However, Penney (2002) argues that current policy concerning teacher training and established teaching practices restrict opportunities for student teachers to develop critical readings of any aspect of the national curriculum. Gender differences prevail in the teaching of games through segregated teaching and ideological views about the physical (in)capabilities of girls in sport which are reinforced though education policy and the training of PE teachers. Boys continue to play football, rugby and cricket whilst girls participate in netball, hockey and rounders (Hargreaves, 1994). The marginalisation of other activities through the NCPE includes a rejection of compulsory dance for girls and boys. Whilst teaching dance can embrace progressive attitudes to gender and dance, being allowed to exclude dance teaching restricts the likelihood of girls and boys experiencing dance at all, avoids dancing together in mixed sex groups and therefore reduces opportunities for learning human movement skills collaboratively. Where dance is taught in schools it invariably becomes positioned as a female appropriate activity (Waddington et al., 1998). Like dance, outdoor education tends to be marginalised in the curriculum as it is an optional activity. The potential for outdoor activities to support inclusive physical activity that challenges gender stereotypes through adventurous physical pursuits for both boys and girls and approaches to collaborative across genders are lost when outdoor activities are not on the agenda for curriculum-based physical education (Humberstone, 2012). Within the NCPE there arguably needs to be more consideration for the inclusion of broader forms of physical activity that might support, encourage or motivate girls to stay active.

Outside of the UK specific education policy aimed at rebalancing gender inequity has been made which has had implications for sport. The most notable example is that of the USA Title IX 1972 of the Education Amendments Act. The legalisation ruled that any institution receiving federal funding is not permitted to exclude participants on the basis of sex, and that funds should be equally distributed. The impact of the legalisation is evidenced in the rise in women competing in college sport. According to the NCAA Gender Equity Report (2004–2010) there has been a 14 per cent increase in the proportion of female student athletes in Division I, a 21 per cent increase for women in Division II and a 14 per cent increase for women in Division III. Increased participation of females does not necessarily mean gender equality has been achieved. USA College sport remains a site for discrimination and sexualisation of female athletes (Nelson and Rowe, 1994) and women are underrepresented in leadership positions (Morrison, 1993). Although the participation of women in USA Colleges remains considerably lower than men's, the legislation has increased participation and enables legal challenges to state funded institutions who do not comply (Carpenter, 1993). A recent suggestion in the UK that reflects this legislative approach to gender equality in sport and physical activity is to utilise the UK Public Sector Equality Duty Act to enforce equity of spending in physical education (DCMS, 2014).

Some policy-led initiatives for increasing physical activity have employed school-community partnership approaches in developing strategies for promoting and engaging girls and women in physical activity. Many of these represent a response to growing evidence illustrating that females are deterred from engaging in physical education because of lack of choice, overly competitive games, lack of confidence, poor body image, and that many girls do not value being good at PE because of a focus on academic studies. A recent study *Changing the Game for Girls*, by the UK's Women and Sport Fitness and Foundation (WSFF, 2015) found that 51 per cent of girls were put off physical activity by negative experiences of physical education. An evidence-based strategy *Changing the Game for Girls: In Action* (WSFF, 2015) was developed in response to the finding and supported a two-year pilot programme, launched to include a network of 25 schools involved in adapting existing provision to deliver supportive environments. A range of initiatives were employed including; involving teachers, developing a primary transition toolkit, bringing in local role models, supporting the girls to have a voice in shaping provision and supporting the school to make use of a number of local partnerships. These initiatives were supported by addressing more complex issues about how physical activities were advertised and how images of sporty pupils, which discourage participation, could be changed. The project reflects a multifaceted approach and recognises that one policy solution will not meet the needs of diverse groups of girls and women seeking to be involved in physical activity.

Gendered leisure and physical activity

The gendered patterns of participation in physical activity in education settings are mirrored in leisure time physical activity participation. Across all ages girls' and women's participation is lower than for boys and men (Green, 2010). Historically, as outlined earlier in the chapter, medical discourses and restriction on females based on beliefs about heteronormative femininity and suitable activity restricted women's access to physically active forms of leisure. Policy development and decision making about leisure time activity from the mid-to-late 20th century in the UK offer an important consideration in understanding more contemporary gender differences in physical activity. In the UK, for example, a policy agenda of 'Sport for All' was connected to political movements around gender equity and the 'Women and Sport' campaign was part of the UK Sports Council strategy that specifically supported girls and women's participation (Deem and Gilroy, 1998). Policies at this time focused on recreation, access to physical activity and improving facilities to increase participation (Green, 2006). The UK Sports Council had a number of targets to increase participation that emphasised physical activity for all and not the few, but these initiatives have remained limited in fully recognising the barriers to girls and women's participation, as well the diversity of girls and women's needs (Hargreaves, 1994). More recent policy-driven attempts seek to avoid a one-size-fits-all approach to the promotion and practice of girls and women's physical activity and have recognised the importance of local knowledge and understanding and tailored programmes of delivery. For example, in a recent project funded by Sport England 'I Will if you Will' was delivered by Bury Council in partnership with private and public sector groups and local clubs. The project aimed to change the sporting habits of local girls and women by providing a range of different activities in different spaces, at different times and supporting childcare and facility development. The project has included updating the sporting infrastructure and facilities, and offered local clubs and private gyms a grant to support those working directly with women and girls. The activities offered are diverse and cover both traditional sports such as netball, but also include Belrobics, Ballroom dancing and Mum Fitness classes. The target is to increase participation and expects to achieve 45,000 girls and women participating. These targets are not just about getting girls and women to participate once, but consider sustainability by retaining participants and a target of 10,000 is set to ensure girls and women continue to be physically active. The 'I Will if you Will' approach addresses three interrelated processes by which the barriers to female participation might be addressed: listening to what women want and providing it, developing facilities to make them user friendly for women and being sustainable by offering low or no cost projects that local sports and physical activity providers can support. Similar approaches to understanding the complexities of participation and the need to tailor programmes to the participants and to the skills, expertise and resources of organisations, are gaining momentum through Sport England's priorities for engaging inactive people (Mansfield et al., 2015). The realisation that an innovative and tailored policy and evidence-led approach is needed to understand the diversity of girls and women physical activity needs as well as considering partners in the local area to deliver projects that engage girls and women in physical activity. Going beyond one-time activity participation and examining ways to sustain physical activity levels throughout the life course is emerging as a central tenet in current UK policy on physical activity for girls and women, as it is in other countries world-wide.

Contemporary physical activity policy for girls and women in the UK: The Women and Sport 2014–2015 Report

Whilst women's and girls' physical activity has been influenced by legislation indirectly concerned with such participation, contemporary government is increasingly concerned with policy agendas directly linked to physical activity opportunities and barriers. Reflecting both the rights and welfare agenda, such policy focuses on ensuring equality of access and opportunity for the health and wellbeing of women and girls. The UK Women and Sport 2014–2015 Report is one example. Implemented through the UK's Department for Digital, Culture, Media and Sport (DCMS) select committee, the report is a vehicle for making recommendations to support future policy developments and funding decisions; in this case about women in sport where sport is thought of broadly and includes a range of physical activities beyond competitive games (Velija and Mansfield, 2017). Drawing on evidence from oral testimonies of key stakeholders the report makes recommendations about attracting new female participants, inspiring women and the role of National Governing Bodies of Sport. Some of the well-known and historic barriers that females face in their sporting engagement are emphasised. Issues identified include the limited range of sports on offer, poor experiences of physical education (PE) and narrow options for after school sport, a lack of suitable and available facilities and inequitable access to such facilities. The report draws out a comprehensive list of key recommendations, some of which have been alluded to in this chapter including: measuring children's levels of physical activity, raising the quality of PE training, encouraging diverse provision of sport and physical activity in education settings, forging stronger connections for girls between schools and clubs, ensuring equitable spending on boys and girls sport programmes in school, allying sport facility development with public health, encouraging community-use of school facilities, engaging communities (particularly diverse groups of girls and women) in decision making and funded provision of sport and physical activity for females. The report emphasises that the media constructs discriminatory messages about female sport, unlikely to be inspirational to the current generation of potential female participants. The issues relate to inequitable media coverage of women's sports compared to men's and the associated reduced opportunities for and scale of sponsorship deals for women. Recommendations for resolving such issues include: an emphasis on ethical journalism that focuses on positive aspects of women's performances and avoids reducing reporting to commentary on appearance, raising the profile of women's sport via increased coverage, the promotion of good practice examples of women's sports which have successful media attention. Highlighting the role of National Governing Bodies (NGBs) of sport in raising participation for women and girls, the report concludes that NGBs remain the central organising agents for both mass participation and elite performance in sport in the UK. NGBs in the UK are responsible for strategic planning and managing their sport in terms of administration, coaching and playing from grassroots to international level (Trimble et al., 2010). The report emphasises the importance for good governance in NGBs including the need for funding to be linked to the achievement of set targets for female participation. Notwithstanding the important role of NGBs, the report makes a case for other delivery partners to support participation. USGirls, for example, is cited as a successful model created to increase and sustain young females' participation in disadvantaged communities and based on the StreetGames approach of delivering to young women at the right time, for the right price, in the right place and in the right style (Hills et al., 2013). Over 30,000 young women have engaged in sporting activities through UsGirls projects which highlight the significance of working 'with' and 'for' girls and women as well as the importance of designing and delivering programmes tailored to the needs of local communities. In concluding, The Women and Sport Report 2014–2015 provides four key policy-related priorities for future developments in women's sport and physical activity which represent a commitment to increasing participation: (1) to continue to encourage greater participation in sport for girls and women using most up to date research insight and designing activities that appeal to female participants, (2) to continue to ensure women are represented at all levels in sporting bodies, (3) to upskill NGB's personnel in marketing their sport to commercial investors and (4) to work with media to increase their commitment to raising the profile of women's game. The political significance of the report is in the high profile, government-centred status given to the issue of women's sport and physical activity but the impact of this on practice remains to be seen (Velija and Mansfield, 2017).

Contemporary physical activity policy for girls and women in international contexts

The politicisation of and policy agenda for physical activity for women and girls has been variously influenced by feminist advances and the rights and welfare politics of western governments. However, a formalised international development agenda for gender equity in physical activity has been emerging since the late 20th century. The International Working Group on Women and Sport (IWG) formed in 1994 recognised the inequitable support, funding and opportunities for girls and women globally. The women who formed IWG were already active in leadership positions in national sporting structures and came together to share their national strategies and to discuss an international platform for women and sport (Hargreaves, 2000). From this came the Brighton Declaration on Women and Sport, a strategy that outlines principles for supporting girls and women through access to facilities, school and junior sport, women's mass participation, high performance sport, leadership in sport, education, training and development, sport research and international co-operation (Hargreaves, 2000). Four years later at the 2nd World Conference on Women and Sport, in Windhoek Namibia the principles were reaffirmed and global issues such as women's and girls' health and wellbeing, and the role of sport and physical activity in addressing broader health inequalities were emphasised. More recently the IWG conference was held in Helsinki in 2014 and brought together people from 100 countries and called for a *Lead the Change, be the Change* programme. A 20 year report on the IWG work thus far illustrates a focus on new objectives and priorities moving forward including: addressing child care provision, supporting retired female athletes, ensuring sport is free from sexual harassment and bullying and emphasising female leadership in referring, coaching and decision making (Fasting et al.,

2014). The IWG has been instrumental in the wider gender and development movement, but some criticisms remain over whose female voices are represented in policy and decision making, and how these may marginalise some groups. More recently Pike and Matthews (2014) have questioned whether there has been a coherent global movement for women and sport that represents a diverse range of women across a multitude of sport and physical activity contexts, because these organisations have predominantly consisted of White Western women.

One of the most recent impacts on supporting girls and women around the globe in physical activity is the Sport for Development and Peace (SDP) Movement. Whilst in 2008 only 30 of the 264 projects identified by the international platform on Sport and Development were targeted towards girls or women (Saavedra, 2008), the inception of the Millennium Development Goals (MDG) and Sustainable Development Goals (SDG) led to increasing numbers of SDP projects using sport and physical activity to empower girls and women. These include projects that focus on local issues such as poverty, levels of literacy, sexual violence, human trafficking, disease, drugs and alcohol, knowledge of rights and impacts of war (Saavedra, 2009). Created by the UN, the MDG (2000) provide a target driven approach to addressing poverty, disease and exclusion as well as education, environmental sustainability and gender equity. Sport is highlighted as mechanism to realise the MDG (Rhind et al., 2011). Through the MDG, sport became a vehicle for meeting wider social outcomes and further legitimatised the growth of sport for development projects (Coalter, 2008). In 2016 the MDG were further developed into 17 Sustainable Development Goals (SDG) which also explicitly focus on gender equality and empowerment of all women and girls. Adopted by the world leaders at a UN summit on 1 January 2016, the aim of SDG #5 is to end all forms of discrimination, eliminate violence against women and girls, recognise unpaid work and domestic work, enable women to work and have leadership opportunities in political and public life, access to economic resources and to support the development of gender quality and empowerment through sound policies. Sport is once again identified as a tool for achieving these goals and is widely promoted through the United Nations office on Sport for Development and Peace. These agendas have all contributed to the sport for development programmes and two examples are discussed below the *Go Sisters* project in Zambia (Kay et al., 2015) and the GOAL programme that started in India (Hayhurst et al., forthcoming).

'Go Sisters' Zambia: Girls, sport, empowerment and HIV/AIDS

The Go Sisters programme was launched in 2002 by the EduSport Foundation in Lusaka, Zambia. EduSport was founded in 1999 as a Non-Governmental Organisation (NGO) to 'empower underserved communities through their active participation in sport' (Hayhurst et al., 2011). Girls are involved in leadership roles in all EduSport programmes and Go Sisters was one of the first programmes to be developed to help girls and young people to pursue equality (Kay et al., 2015). Go Sisters is a peer-mentoring programme that aims to achieve its goal through promoting sport, with the main aim to 'provide extra-family social, supportive, networks, a safe social space and reduce social isolation of females' (Coalter, 2007:83). The activities also take place in public spaces and therefore are visible and provide positive female role models in the community. As well as supporting education for girls the programme is part of Kicking Aids Out and therefore educates on HIV/AIDS issues through games. Go Sisters is often discussed as an example of a sustainable SDP programme and is specifically mentioned in the MDG as an example of how sport can help achieve gender equity and empowerment. In 2008 the purpose of Go Sisters became aligned with the MDG #3 'promoting gender equity and empowerment of girls and women'. As part of the funding for Go Sisters EduSport were increasingly required to adopt monitoring and evaluation procedures, and as such a partnership between staff at Brunel University London and Go Sisters developed (Kay et al., 2015). The approach adopted by the research team at Brunel was developed to avoid some of the positivistic traditions in M&E work that limits local knowledge and experience and to reduce the negative association with this form of external monitoring. The partnership approach also focused on embedding building the research capacity of those delivering Go Sisters to develop a sustainable approach to monitoring and evaluation. This partnership demonstrates the importance of working with groups and not on them to develop methods of data collection that are relevant and authentic so that they can support the development to enhance the delivery of existing programmes. The benefit of this partnership work is evidenced in Museke et al.'s review of the programme (2015) in which it is argued that the project: (1) has enabled girls to feel empowered to make decisions in their own lives and (2) has improved knowledge and understanding about HIV/AIDS. The research partnership also allowed for a more critical dialogue about the program design, delivery and evaluation supporting the notions of addressing cultural and local specificity for research quality in SDP settings.

The 'GOAL' Project, India: Girls, sport and life skills

Another example of a girls physical activity and empowerment project is GOAL, a programme run by the NAZ foundation (India) Trust. Supported by the Standard Chartered Bank as part of their corporate social responsibility to invest in local communities. The GOAL programme uses netball as a medium to engage young women aged 13–19 with the aim of delivering a programme of sport education and life skills in Delhi's poor communities. The programme has now expanded to China, Nigeria, Zambia and Jordan (Hayhurst et al., forthcoming). Topics covered in the educational modules included communication, health and hygiene, human rights and financial literacy, and there is a standardised curriculum designed by Standard Chartered in collaboration with population council (Hayhurst et al., forthcoming). This curriculum can be adapted to local contexts, but as Hayhurst et al. (forthcoming) note, examples are not provided and the curriculum and training is limited in supporting a localised approach. Kay's (2011) initial evaluation of the GOAL programme outlines the way in which the project was successful in fostering individual empowerment, both physically but also in relation to self-esteem. In particular, GOAL provided a space for girls to discuss issues and develop confidence to communicate their concerns and ask questions pertaining to their health. She also notes how the girls had an impact on those around them, and they were able to disseminate knowledge about health and wellbeing to mothers and sisters, acting as female agents of change in their local communities (Kay, 2011). Nevertheless, since Kay's (2011) evaluation and the growth of the programme Hayhurst et al. (forthcoming) discuss some of the issues around GOAL and applying a postcolonial feminist international relations theory critique some elements of programmes. In particular, there are concerns about the role of corporate social responsibility funding which align such programmes to the global economy of entrepreneurism at the expense of empowering women through a focus on local contexts.

The two programmes discussed are examples of plus sport programmes where sport is used as a tool to support a number of non-sport outcomes associated with education, health and wellbeing (Wilson, 2012). Nevertheless, they aim to empower girls through physical activity and have become a significant part of international development programmes. The focus of these programmes has been predominantly for girls and delivered in local contexts. This means they are not necessarily embedded in national policies to support girls' and women's physical activity, nor do they necessarily represent government policies. They are, however, closely aligned to the MDG and SDG and they attract funding on this basis. It should be noted that the use of sport and physical activity programmes to 'do good' can be overstated, and the sustainability of the projects is not always outlined (Coalter, 2008, Kay et al., 2015, Wilson, 2012). Understanding the impact of such projects is challenging as evaluation is complex. Collaborative approaches to monitoring and evaluation that involve local people and understand global and local contexts is one way to support the development of effective girls' programmes of physical activity at a local level in international contexts (Kay et al., 2015).

Conclusion

It is widely recognised that girls and women are less physically active than boys and men. Issues that have prevented girls and women from being physical activity include the dominance of (gendered) medical discourses, lack of facilities and opportunities, cost of participation, lack of time, stereotypes that emphasise girls and boys should have different interests and practical issues around travel and the safety of girls and women. These are complex and intersecting issues that serve to constrain female participation in physical activity. Recognition of the issues that affect female participation has resulted in the development of both local and global policy agendas and decision making that aim to increase participation in physical activity. Both direct legislation and advocacy have been employed in the development of widening participation opportunities for female physical activity. High level national and international policy, demanding and promoting physical activity for women and girls, is important in setting agendas and ensuring programming and promotion directly targets female participation. Yet such policy making needs to be developed with an understanding of the local and diverse needs of girls and women for whom policy is being set. Only then does policy become enacted with and for those girls and women for whom it is intended (Mansfield et al., 2017).

References

Atkinson, P. 1973. "Fitness, Feminism and Schooling" in S. Delamont and L. Duffin, eds., *The Nineteenth-Century Woman: Her Cultural World*. London, UK: Croom Helm.

Carpenter, L.J. 1993. "Letters home: My wife with Title IX.". In G. Cohen, ed., *Women in Sport. Issues and Controversies*. Newbury Park, CA: SAGE, pp. 79–94.

Coalter, F. 2008. *A Wider Social Role for Sport: Who's Keeping Score?* Oxon, UK: Routledge.

DCMS 2014. *Women and Sport: First Report of Session 2014–15*. London, UK: House of Commons.

Deem, R. & Gilroy, S. 1998. "Physical Activity, Life-long Learning and Empowerment — Situating Sport in Women's Leisure." *Sport, Education and Society* 3 (1): 89–104.

Fasting, K., Svela Sand, T., Pike, E. & Matthews, J. 2014. "From Brighton to Helsinki: Women and Sport Progress Report 1994–2014," Publication of the Finish Sports Confederation. http://iwggti. org/common_up/iwgnew/files//Brighton_Plus_Helsinki_2014_Declaration.pdf [Accessed 28th March 2017]

Green, K. 2010. *Key Themes in Youth Sport*. London: Routledge.

Green, K., Thurston, M., Vaage, O. & Mordal Moen, K. 2015. "Girls, young women and sport in Norway: A case of sporting convergence amid favourable socio-economic circumstances." *International Journal of Sport Policy and Politics* 7 (4): 531–550.

Green, M. 2006. "From 'Sport for All' to Not About 'Sport' at All?: Interrogating Sport Policy interventions in the United Kingdom." *European Sport Management Quarterly* 6 (3): 217–238.

Hallal, P. C., Anderson, L., Bull, F., Guthold, R., Haskell, W. & Ekelund, U. 2012. "Global Physical Activity levels: Surveillance progress, pitfalls and prospects." *The Lancet,* 380 (9838): 247–257.

Hargreaves, J. 1994. *Sporting Females: Critical Issues in the History and Sociology of Women's Sport*. London, UK: Routledge.

Hargreaves, J. 2000. *Heroines of Sport: The Politics of Difference and Identity*. London Routledge.

Hayhurst, L., MacNeil, M. & Frisby, W. 2011. "A postcolonial feminist approach to gender, development and EduSport", in Houlihan and Green, eds., *Routledge Handbook of Sports Development*. Oxon, UK: Routledge. 353–367.

Hayhurst, L.M.C., Sundstrom, L., & Waldman, D. (Forthcoming). "Postcolonial Feminist International Relations Theory and Sport for Development" in J. Cauldwell, L. Mansfield, B. Wheaton and J. Watson, eds., *The Handbook of Feminisms in Sport, Leisure and Physical Education*. London: Palgrave.

Hills, L., Maitland, A. & Croston, A. 2013. "Us Girls: Engaging Young Women from Disadvantaged Communities in Sport an Independent Evaluation by Brunel University on behalf of StreetGames." July 2013. London: Brunel University.

Humberstone, B. 2012. "Bringing Outdoor Education into the Physical Education Agenda: Gender Identities and Social Change." *Quest* 47 (2): 144–157.

Kay, T. 2011. "Development through sport? Sport in support of female empowerment in Delhi, India" in B. Houlihan and M. Green, eds., *Routledge Handbook of Sports Development*. Oxon, UK: Routledge. 308–323.

Kay, T., Mansfield, L. & Jeanes, R. 2015. "Researching with Go Sisters, Zambia: Reciprocal learning in sport for development" in L. Hayhurst, T. Kay and M. Chawansky, eds., *Beyond Sport for Development and Peace: Transnational Perspective on Theory, Policy and Practice*. London: Routledge. 214–244.

Kirk, D. 2002. "Physical education: a gendered history" in D. Penney, *Gender and Physical Education: Contemporary Issues and Future Directions*. London: Routledge.

Mansfield, L., Anokye, N., Fox-Rushby, J. & Kay, T. 2015. "The Health and Sport Engagement (HASE) Intervention and Evaluation Project: Protocol for the Design, Outcome, Process and Economic Evaluation of a Complex Community Sport Intervention to Increase Levels of Physical Activity." *BMJ Open* 5 (10): p.e009276.

Morrison, L. 1993. "The AIAW: Governance by women for women" in G.L. Cohen, ed., *Women in Sport: Issues and Controversies*. London: SAGE. 59–69.

Museke, S., Namukanga, A. & Palmer-Felgate, S. 2015. "Reflection on Researching with Go Sisters, Zambia: Reciprocal Learning in Sport for Development" in L. Hayhurst, T. Kay and M. Chawansky, eds., *Beyond Sport for Development and Peace: Transnational Perspective on Theory, Policy and Practice*. London: Routledge. 230–237.

Nelson, M.B. & Rowe, C. 1994. *The Stronger Women Get, the More Men Love Football: Sexism and the American Culture of Sports*. New York: Harcourt Brace.

Penney, D. (ed.) 2002. *Gender and Physical Education: Contemporary Issues and Future Directions*. London: Routledge.

Pike, E. & Matthews, J. 2014. "A Post-Colonial Critique of the International Movements for Women and Sexuality in Sport" in J. Hargreaves and E. Anderson, eds., *Routledge Handbook of Sport, Gender and Sexuality*. London, UK: Routledge.

Rhind, D., Brackenridge, C., Kay, T. and Owusu-Sekyere, F. 2011 "Child Protection and SDP: The Post-MDG Agenda for Policy, Practice and Research" in L. Hayhurst, T. Kay & M. Chawansky, eds., *Beyond Sport for Development and Peace: Transnational Perspective on Theory, Policy and Practice*. London: Routledge.

Saavedra, M. 2008. "Chapter 5: Dilemmas and Opportunities in Gender and Sport-in-Development" in R. Levermore, A Beacon, *Sport and International Development*. Basingstoke, UK: Palgrave Macmillan.

Trimble, L., Buraimo, C., Grecic, D. & Minten, S. 2010. *Sport in the UK*. Exeter, UK: Learning Matters.

Velija, P. with Mansfield, L. 2017. "The UK House of Commons Women and Sport Repot 2014–2015 Policy, Evidence and Impact" in L. Mansfield, J. Caudwell, B. Wheaton & R. Watson, eds., *Handbook of Feminisms in Sport, Leisure and Physical Education*. UK Basingstoke: Palgrave Macmillan.

Vertinsky, P. 1990. *The Eternally Wounded Woman: Women, Doctors and Exercise in the Late Nineteenth Century*. Illinois, USA: University of Illinois Press.

Waddington, I., Malcolm, D. & Cobb, J. 1998. "Gender Stereotyping and Physical Education." *European Physical Education Review* 4 (1):34–36.

Wilson. B. 2012. *Sport and Peace: A Sociological Perspective*. Canada: Oxford University Press.

Women's Sport and Fitness Foundation (WSFF) 2015. Changing the Game for Girls: A Toolkit to Help Teachers Get More Girls Involved in PE and School Sport www.womeninsport.org/wp-content/uploads/2015/04/Changing-the-Game-for-Girls-Teachers-Toolkit.pdf [Accessed 11th November 2016].

World Health Organization (WHO), 2017. Health topics: Physical activity. Online document. Available from: http://www.who.int/topics/physical_activity/en/ [accessed 8/09/17].

20

DISABILITY AND PHYSICAL ACTIVITY

Toni Williams and Brett Smith

Introduction

Disabled people have the rights, by law, to access services in all areas of citizenship including attaining the highest standards of health, and participation in sport and leisure activities. Despite these rights, disabled people lead insufficiently active lifestyles, which negatively impacts upon their health, well-being and quality of life. Thus, health promotion through physical activity (PA) is a significant and timely issue for disabled populations. In this chapter, first we explore how disability is explained and understood, and the consequences this has on shaping medical practices and public health programmes for disabled people. We then explore the relationship between disability, health and leisure time physical activity (LTPA). Here, we offer a contextual example in spinal cord injured populations of the barriers to a physically activity lifestyle and the dilemmas encountered by the healthcare professionals (HCPs) tasked with promoting PA. Lastly, we offer some implications for future policy and practice, and a critical approach to PA promotion, to effectively support disabled people to be physically active for life.

Understanding disability and health

There are a variety of models and theories which aim to define disability with often contrasting perspectives and profoundly different implications for the lives of disabled people. Therefore in the first instance, it is imperative to critically examine how disability is explained and understood. As Smith and Bundon (*in-press*) describe, having a grasp on how disability is explained and understood is vital for individuals working with disabled people in any context. This is because the definition of disability is fundamental in shaping medical practices and public health programmes – including PA – and how research with disabled people is carried out (McDermott & Turk, 2011).

Medical model of disability

Historically, the medical model (sometimes referred to as the individual model of disability) was the dominant model for understanding disability. Through this model, disability was defined as the inability to perform a task considered "normal" for any person due to impairment (Thomas, 2007). Therefore in the medical model, disability is described as "caused" by parts of the body that do not work "properly" (Smith & Perrier, 2015). Despite this dominant medical discourse traditionally shaping how people understand disability, the medical model has been profoundly criticised. One problem with the medical model is that by defining disability based on biological assumptions of normality, the role of wider social-cultural, physical and political forces that construct "normal" are overlooked and unchallenged (Brittain, 2004; Meekosha & Shuttleworth, 2009). Another criticism of the medical model is that it depicts disability as a personal physical tragedy or a psychological trauma that should be *overcome* (Brittain, 2004). Furthermore, the medical model locates the "problem" of disability within the individual (Goodley, 2013; Smith & Bundon, *in-press*). By locating the cause of disabled people's problems squarely within them and their impairments, disabled people become solely responsible for their own health (Brittain, 2004; Smith & Perrier, 2015). Accordingly, any societal factors that contribute to the experience of disability and the consequences to health – such as access to PA opportunities – are overlooked by the medical model.

Social model of disability

To address the limitations of the medical model, a social model of disability was proposed that shone light on the social and cultural meaning of disability. The social model rejects the causal link between impairment and disability and instead asserts that disability results from the social restrictions (or barriers) imposed upon people with impairment. Thus, improvements to the lives of disabled people require the removal of oppressive disablist social barriers and the development of social policies and practices that facilitate total societal inclusion and citizenship (Thomas, 2007). A key strength of the social model was its impressive political power. It was at the heart of the disabled people's movement in the UK and influenced anti-discrimination legislation through the Disability Discrimination Act 1995 (Lutz & Bowers, 2005; Shakespeare, 2014). Consequently, disabled people, by law, should have equal access and total inclusion within society including attaining the highest standard of health, and participation in leisure and sport activities.[1]

Many important achievements have been accomplished under the social model of disability. For example, under anti-discrimination law all sports clubs and leisure providers are legally obligated to make reasonable adjustments to their services to ensure everyone has access (EFDS, 2013). However, the social model has also faced intense criticism. One critique of the social model is that a focus on barrier removal is impractical as it is not possible to change the natural environment to positively impact all disabled people (Shakespeare, 2014). For instance, wheelchair users can be restricted assessing areas of remote wilderness or climbing rocky mountains (Smith & Perrier, 2015). Furthermore the social model has been critiqued for creating a dualism by separating impairment from disability (Thomas, 2007). By setting aside impairment and focusing on social barriers, the reality of dysfunction, illness and bodily pain is ultimately excluded from understandings of disability (Martin, 2013). Moreover, the importance of impairment, people's lived experience of disability, and how the body can be a social source of disablism is overlooked (Hughes & Paterson, 1997; Shakespeare, 2014). For instance, by providing ramped access to a sport or leisure facility social barriers – and in theory disability and disablism – are removed (Smith & Perrier, 2015). Yet these transformations alone do not address the underlying disablist values and institutional structures within society (Brittain, 2004). Society can still restrict sport and leisure participation of people with impairments through disablist attitudes, comments and behaviours.

Conceptual models of disability

Accordingly, neither the medical model nor social model reflects the multifaceted nature of disability (Lutz & Bowers, 2005). Given all this, conceptual models of disability have been developed that contend disabled people live lives shaped by impairment *and* the effects of disabling and discriminatory cultural, social and environmental conditions that impede their function, everyday activities and/or social participation (Emerson et al., 2012; World Health Organization, 2015). These conceptual models importantly expand our understanding of the physical and social experiences of disability in relation to PA policy and practice. One such conceptual model developed to encompass the complexity of disability was the social *relational* model (Thomas, 2007). Importantly, this model encompasses and extends disablism by recognising that people can experience many forms of social oppression (i.e. structural disablism and psycho-emotional disablism) that emerge not from within the individual but from relationships with structures and people (Smith & Bundon, *in-press*). For example, psycho-emotional disablism may involve being stared at by staff and other members in the gym or having jokes made about an impairment during a sports game. These various forms of social oppression are more clearly recognised by the Equality Act 2010, which replaced the Disability Discrimination Act 1995. The Equality Act strengthens previous laws in important ways by helping to tackle harassment or discrimination arising from disability (Government Equalities Office, 2010). Hence, the social relational model can provide a platform to analyse the social relations within health, leisure and sporting environments that construct, institutionalise and perform disability (Smith & Perrier, 2015).

Disability, health and physical activity

The discriminatory cultural, social and environmental conditions that construct disability pose numerous challenges to the life-long health and well-being of disabled people. As Emerson et al. (2012) explain, "[g]iven that all disabled people (by definition) have a health condition or impairment, it is necessarily true that disabled people (as a group) will have poorer health that non-disabled people" (p.254). Disabled people experience poorer health for numerous reasons. These include reduced access to timely and effective healthcare, exposure to social determinants of poorer health and a predisposition to secondary health conditions or impairments (Emerson et al., 2012). For example, following a spinal cord injury (SCI) people are faced with an immediate loss of function, reduced mobility and are at risk of developing a plethora of secondary health conditions (Canning & Hicks, 2014; Gorgey, 2014). These secondary health conditions associated with SCI include pressure ulcers, urinary tract infections, chronic pain, obesity, respiratory dysfunction and cardiovascular disorders (Chen et al., 2011; Canning & Hicks, 2014). Additionally these secondary health conditions can present as risk factors for poor mental health, increased disability and a decrease in quality of life and life expectancy (Krause & Saunders, 2011; Canning & Hicks, 2014).

To improve and maintain health and well-being, it is important to include into one's habits a physically active lifestyle. This is because PA has been identified as a means to alleviate or prevent many of the health and well-being complications associated with disability. For example, PA has been shown to reduce levels of perceived musculoskeletal and neuropathic pain (Norrbrink, et al., 2012), decrease the risk factors of cardiovascular disease and type 2 diabetes (Buchholz et al., 2009) and lead to greater functional capacity such as ease of transfer thereby improving quality of life (Martin Ginis et al., 2012). Furthermore, being physically active can improve well-being through reducing depression and facilitating experiences that promote psychological growth (Martin Ginis et al., 2012; Tomasone et al., 2013; Day, 2013). Despite the array of health and well-being benefits to be gained from regular PA, most disabled people live insufficiently active lifestyles. In SCI populations for instance, an estimated 50 per cent are completely sedentary (Martin Ginis et al., 2010a). The human cost of physical inactivity is vast as individuals unnecessarily endure acute and chronic secondary health conditions preventable through exercise (Gorgey, 2014). This link between primary impairments and secondary health conditions is additionally mediated by social processes (Emerson et al., 2012) such as access to PA opportunities. Therefore, health promotion through PA, including the factors that promote and constrain a physically activity lifestyle, is a significant and timely issue. Important in this process of promotion are the people (i.e. who) that are deemed credible to convey PA messages and the contexts (i.e. where) in which this might effectively occur. We shall now explore these factors for people with SCI in the context of general LTPA. Here, LTPA is defined as an activity people chose to partake in their spare time such as exercising in the gym, playing recreational sport or general wheeling (Martin Ginis et al., 2010a; Smith, 2013).

Barriers to a physically active lifestyle

In line with the social relational model of disability, people with SCI face a multitude of personal, environmental and social barriers that prevent them from leading a physically active lifestyle. Despite improvements to health and well-being from being physically active, people with SCI report personal barriers such as poor health and well-being as a barrier to participating in sport and exercise (Williams et al., 2014). Issues such as loss of bodily control, pain, depression, lack of self-confidence and feelings of social exclusion all contribute to a lack of LTPA (Levins et al., 2004; Stephens et al., 2012). Furthermore, a disruption to people's body-self relationship, and a loss of an able-bodied identity also restrict LTPA (Williams et al., 2014). In addition, even with anti-discriminatory acts protecting the rights of disable people to engage in sporting and leisure opportunities, aspects of the material, geographical and social environment substantially impact engagement in LTPA. In terms of the material and geographical environment, a lack of both personal and communal resources, inadequate finances and a lack of accessible facilities prevent people from being physically active (Kehn & Kroll, 2009; Stephens et al., 2012; Smith, 2013). The importance of relationships in restricting activities – as outlined in the social relational model – is further evidenced in SCI populations as a perceived lack of social support is another social environmental barrier to LTPA (Williams et al., 2014).

A further significant barrier for people with SCI to lead a physically activity lifestyle concerns knowledge on LTPA (Williams et al., 2014). As with other physical disabilities (Saebu, 2010; Martin Ginis et al., 2012; Mulligan et al., 2012), a lack of knowledge about where and how to exercise is a significant constraint to LTPA participation. To find knowledge and information regarding PA, people with SCI turn to their healthcare professionals (HCPs). This is because HCPs are trusted and valued as credible messengers of PA information (Letts et al., 2011; Smith et al., 2015). In addition, rehabilitation in SCI centres has been identified as a key context of the start of lifelong health and well-being through PA promotion (Letts et al., 2011; Smith et al., 2015). Moreover, within formal rehabilitation and the community, it is the physiotherapists (or physical therapists) which have also been identified as the healthcare professional (HCP) best placed to convey PA messages (Morris & Williams, 2009; Walkeden & Walker, 2015). For example, their role as "promotors, preventers and rehabilitators puts them in an ideal position to influence exercise behaviours in every individual they treat" (McGrane et al., 2015, p.11). Likewise physiotherapists in rehabilitation have a responsibility to provide knowledge and support for disabled people to attain independence and be physically active for their lifelong health and well-being (Mulligan et al., 2011). Yet in spite of physiotherapists being identified as the ideal HCP to promote PA, active PA promotion is not a structured or integral component of physiotherapy practice (Mulligan et al., 2011; Williams et al., 2016).

Dilemmas to promoting physical activity

There are three significant dilemmas faced by physiotherapists and other HCPs in relation to promoting a physically active lifestyle to people with SCI. The first of these is a lack of knowledge translation to enable effective promotion and prescription of PA. For example, physiotherapists lack any formal training and education in sport and exercise (Williams et al., 2016). As Williams et al. (2016) highlighted, physiotherapists in neurological rehabilitation do recognise the value of people with SCI living a physically active lifestyle for physical health, well-being, the prevention of future illness and quality of life. In other words, the physiotherapist understood the importance of LTPA for people with SCI beyond the medical model of disability which typically prioritises physical and functional restoration outcomes. Yet this is *tacit knowledge* acquired through experience of working with people with SCI over time rather than *explicit knowledge* gained from other sources (e.g. policy documents, physiotherapy degree courses, sport and exercise scientists or workshops in rehabilitation centres). Furthermore physiotherapists perceive they do not have the skills required to change health behaviour. Consistent with research in stroke rehabilitation (Morris et al., 2014), physiotherapists in SCI rehabilitation perceived they were unable to change behaviour and motivate those patients who had little interest in PA (Williams et al., 2016). The evidence suggests that knowledge about health promotion through PA is lacking not just in physiotherapists, but also in other HCPs. For example, a survey study of HCPs (mainly doctors) in SCI rehabilitation across four countries (UK, the Netherlands, Belgium and Republic of Ireland) reported inadequate training in health promotion and behaviour strategies which limited their ability to deliver health advice to people with SCI (Wong et al., 2015).

The second dilemma concerns a lack of clarity and support within the healthcare system as to the roles and responsibilities of HCPs in health promotion. According to the World Confederation of Physical Therapy, physiotherapists have been hailed as the health-promotion professionals (WCPT, 2012). Furthermore they claim "physiotherapists use the health promotion approach of participation and empowerment in their treatment of people and groups to improve their lifestyles and health through physical activity" (p.16). Yet it is not just physiotherapists who are tasked with health promotion including PA. In the UK, national policy stipulates that all HCPs have a responsibility to deliver health promotion (NHS Future Forum, 2012). Under the "Making Every Contact Count" policy, every contact made with a patient by any HCP is viewed as an opportunity to deliver brief interventions on health behaviours including PA (Walkeden & Walker, 2015). In spite of this, in the UK and Ireland rehabilitation context, not all physiotherapists considered their role to include health promotion through PA (Williams et al., 2016). Furthermore, echoing research in the UK (Walkeden & Walker, 2015) and other countries such as Sweden and New Zealand (Mulligan et al., 2011), physiotherapists identified multiple barriers to PA promotion within their healthcare system. For example, the physiotherapists in UK and Ireland raised concerns that there was an absence of people embedded within the community to help people with SCI become physically active for life (Williams et al., 2016).

The third dilemma faced by physiotherapists in promoting PA concerns managing their patients' hopes and expectations of physical recovery following a neurological impairment such as SCI. Patients need hope for the future if they are to engage in rehabilitation and learn the required skills to manage their SCI (Soundy et al., 2010; Harvey et al., 2012). Yet on the other hand, physiotherapists need to ensure they foster hopefulness without promoting false hopes of recovery following SCI (Soundy et al., 2013). Thus, managing hopes and expectations is essential if people are to remain physically active for their long-term health and well-being once their functional recovery has reached a plateau (Harvey et al., 2012; Soundy et al., 2013; van Lit & Kayes, 2014). With this in mind, physiotherapists do not promote LTPA opportunities which they perceive foster false hope of recovery. For example, community-based LTPA opportunities such as activity-based rehabilitation (ABR) – which aim to maximise an individual's physiological, functional and neurological potential through intensive exercise – are problematic to physiotherapists. This is because some physiotherapists perceive ABR to focus on non-functional activities, such as gait training and assisted walking, and in turn promote a restitution narrative (Williams et al., 2016).

The restitution narrative in this context refers to a common storyline in SCI that follows the plot "yesterday I was able-bodied, today I'm disabled, but tomorrow I'll be able-bodied again" (Smith & Sparkes, 2005, p.1096). Indeed, the restitution narrative, with its associated *concrete hope* of restoring a former abled-bodied self, is a strong motivator for people with SCI to be physically active (Perrier et al., 2013; Williams et al., 2014; Papathomas et al., 2015). With a focus on overcoming disability, the restitution narrative aligns with the medical model of disability. The dangers with an *exercise is restitution* narrative (see Papathomas et al., 2015) that resonates with the medical model of disability, arise through the possible adverse consequences on health and well-being when the hope for recovery is not fulfilled. Specifically, a pre-occupation with recovery could restrict individuals from partaking in other LTPA opportunities which may be psychologically fulfilling, limit people's ability to envision a range of potential outcomes other than a cure, and inhibit other areas of life such as community integration (Perrier et al., 2013; Williams et al., 2014; Papathomas et al., 2015). However, a lack of understanding regarding LTPA initiatives such as ABR highlights a breakdown in communication between physiotherapists in SCI rehabilitation and community health practitioners in LTPA initiatives such as ABR (Williams et al., 2016). Moreover, in line with the social relational model of disability that highlights the social imposition of restricting activity for people with SCI, not promoting PA through ABR could be viewed as a form of social oppression. In other words, physiotherapists are enacting psycho-emotional disablism (Thomas, 2007) by denying their patients the option to remain physically active through community-based LTPA initiatives such as ABR.

Implications for future physical activity policy and practice

There are a plethora of policies aiming to reduce health inequalities and promote LTPA. Yet as Emerson et al. (2012) warn, all too often they pay little attention to the situation of disabled people. This is because disabled people are rarely featured as a target of health promotion (Kehn & Kroll, 2009; Smith et al., 2015). Moreover, there is no consideration as to whether the benefits of population-level health and LTPA interventions can foster behaviour change equally across different social groups. Therefore there is a real risk that without attention to the specific situation of disabled people they will not benefit from "generic" social policies and will become more socially disadvantaged and oppressed (Thomas, 2007; Emerson et al., 2012). For example, a recent focus of health promotion has specifically targeted the need to reduce *sedentary behaviour* as well as increase LTPA. Sedentary behaviour in this context refers to "sitting time" (Biddle et al., 2015). Research into sedentary behaviour has identified that too much sitting can increase many health outcomes such as cardio-metabolic risk factors, type 2 diabetes and premature mortality (e.g. Dunstan et al., 2012; Biddle et al., 2015). Such is the impact of this research that headlines like "too much sitting kills you" and "sitting is the new smoking" have received widespread media attention (Verschuren et al., 2015). Health promotion messages such as #SittingKills and #SitLessWalkMore feature regularly on social media sites (e.g. Twitter and Facebook) and are uncritically promoted by many health organisations. The issue with such discourses that target "sitting" as the problem is that they are disablist. In other words, in light of the social relational model, these health promotion messages exclude and oppress disabled people (e.g. those with mobility impairments or wheelchair users) who are unable to reduce the amount of time they spend sitting.

Behaviour change interventions aimed at reducing health inequalities and promoting LTPA are likely to more effective if they are tailored to the specific situations (e.g. social and cultural contexts) of disabled people (Emerson et al., 2012). The barriers to LTPA participation and dilemmas faced by HCPs in LTPA promotion identified earlier in this chapter also need to be addressed if disabled people are to be physically active for life. In light of these factors, there are several implications for policy and practice aimed at improving LTPA promotion and reducing the barriers to LTPA for disabled people. These implications include the need to improve knowledge translation, the consideration of PA beyond sport, and the need for support within the healthcare system. Lastly, we will highlight the possible adverse consequences of promoting exercise as medicine.

Knowledge translation

To enable HCPs to promote and prescribe LTPA as a structured and integral component of their practice, effective knowledge translation is needed across the macro, meso and micro fields. Effective knowledge translation requires the combined efforts of national policy makers, healthcare systems, HCPs, academics and community-based expertise (Morris & Williams, 2009; Tomasone et al., 2014; Wong et al., 2015). Starting with knowledge production, at the macro level, PA policy makers need to engage with academics to drive meaningful guidelines on PA for disabled people (Williams et al., 2016). Currently in the UK, the PA guidelines do not include any specific information for people with disabilities (Department of Health, 2011). In the absence of specific guidelines, The National Health Service recommends that wheelchair uses simply try and adapt the general PA guidelines (NHS, 2015). However, comprehensive, realistic and sustainable PA guidelines specifically for people with SCI would address the barrier raised by physiotherapists regarding a lack of knowledge and confidence in PA prescription and promotion (Williams et al., 2016). Therefore evidence-based comprehensive guidelines need to be developed and embedded into UK policies if they are to be received and utilised by HCPs tasked with promoting regular engagement in LTPA (Williams et al., 2016). As part of this, guidelines should include specific details about the types, amounts and intensity of physical activities to achieve health benefits in disabled populations (Martin Ginis et al., 2011).

To translate knowledge produced at the macro level into practice at the meso and micro level, appropriate training needs to be delivered (Williams et al., 2016). Without appropriate guidelines and training, HCPs have insufficient knowledge to promote a physically active lifestyle to disabled people (McGrane et al., 2015; Wong et al., 2015). At the meso level university degree courses should educate HCPs on the importance of LTPA both as a component of their rehabilitation treatment, and promotion of lifelong health and well-being in the community (Williams et al., 2016). HCPs need to understand the relationship between the factors that constrain a physically active lifestyle, and those factors that facilitate engagement in regular sport and exercise (Williams et al., 2014). At the micro level, it is essential that hospitals deliver mandatory training to reinforce HCPs understanding of their role in health promotion (Walkeden & Walker, 2015). Furthermore, to maximise the potential of PA promotion resulting in an increase in PA uptake, HCPs need the skills required to change behaviour. HCPs should additionally be educated in psychosocial factors such as motivational interventions to foster positive health behaviour change (Morris et al., 2014; McGrane et al., 2015). One way to translate knowledge about PA to HCPs "in a way that attracts people, holds their attention, and gets under their skin" (Smith et al., 2015, p.310) is through narrative. Smith et al. (2015) demonstrated that evidence-based stories were effective in disseminating LTPA research knowledge to HCPs in SCI rehabilitation. Moreover, these evidence-based stories can be utilised by HCPs as a resource to share knowledge on PA with people with SCI and move them towards behaviour change.

Support within the healthcare system

In addition to knowledge translation practices, there needs to be support within the healthcare system to facilitate a physically active lifestyle for disabled people. Research from countries such as the UK, Ireland, Sweden and New Zealand highlights an international pattern in HCPs facing barriers to PA promotion that are located with the healthcare system (Mulligan et al., 2011; Williams et al., 2016). The perception from HCPs is that disabled people are unable to access PA opportunities because they do not have the support to do so (e.g. lack of social support, restricted finances and geographical isolation, etc.). In other words, disablism in general needs to be addressed in the operation of the healthcare system and beyond, by providing additional support for disabled people to access PA opportunities available to able-bodied people (Emerson et al., 2012). This support may come from greater alignment between the healthcare system and the various organisations championing the rights of disabled people to be physically active for life. For example, the English Federation of Disability Sport (EFDS) is a national charity in the UK dedicated to engaging disabled people in sport and PA. The "Charter for Change" set out by the EFDS in 2015 calls upon everybody (e.g. those in Government, healthcare, sport, leisure) to support disabled people to be active and promote positive public attitudes towards participation (see www.efds. co.uk/charter). Similarly, the leading disability charity – Disability Rights UK – has set up partnership with Sports England to increase PA participation for disabled people through the "Get Yourself Active" project. One of the aims of this project is to urge healthcare providers to see sport and PA as a legitimate way to improve the health and well-being of disabled people (see www.disabilityrightsuk.org/how-we-can-help/get-yourself-active). Furthermore, HCPs themselves can address the constraints of their healthcare system by educating and advocating that accessing PA is an important component of the health and well-being of disabled people (Mulligan et al., 2011; Williams et al., 2016). Indeed, in line with the social relational model of disability, all HCPs should act as disability allies in addressing common disablist issues for their patients (Roush & Sharby, 2011).

Physical activity is more than sport

The knowledge on PA shared with physiotherapists and other HCPs needs to include the diversity of PA opportunities available to people with disabilities. A key reason for this is that the emphasis of PA in rehabilitation centres can predominantly focus on sport (Williams et al., 2016). This could be problematic for numerous reasons. Firstly, sport can be empowering and promote health and well-being, but if HCPs simply promote this kind of activity, there is the risk of perpetuating the "supercrip" narrative. A supercrip is a disabled athlete that with courage, dedication and hard work proves that the odds can be beaten, the impossible can be accomplished and one can heroically triumph over the "tragedy" of disability (Smith & Sparkes, 2012). The UK's Channel 4 "Freaks of Nature" campaign for the 2012 Paralympics (Silva & Howe, 2012), and more recently the Invictus Games for wounded, injured and sick service personal, are examples of the supercrip narrative in action. The concern with supercrip athletes, as noted by Berger (2008, p.648), "is that these stories of success will foster unrealistic expectations about what people with disabilities can achieve, what they should be able to achieve, if only they tried hard enough". This, in turn, could lead to blaming disabled people who do not wish to, or are unable for bodily, structural or economic reasons, to engage in disability sport (Smith & Sparkes, 2012). Equally, whilst for some people a supercrip narrative might interpellate (i.e. hail) them into disability sport, for others it can push people away from sport (Smith, 2013).

Secondly, a preoccupation with sport may inhibit psychological growth and well-being in other ways (Williams et al., 2014). For example, Kleiber and Hutchinson (1999) caution that "vigorous physical activity (and particularly sport) is at best a temporary palliative to 'the crisis' of physical disability for spinal injured men and at worst an impediment to a more complete personal transformation following the injury experience" (pp.135–136). In other words, the desire for men to be physically active is brought about by cultural ideals which value a hyper-masculine hero narrative following illness and injury. Participating in sport may therefore perpetuate the ideology that men are valuable solely for their strong and able bodies rather than providing any alternative narratives (Williams et al., 2014). This may prevent men with disabilities from expressing masculinity in ways outside of physical power and strength and value other dimensions of the self. This may be particularly so for people within the military who become disabled and are funnelled into sport programmes such as the Paralympics and Invictus Games.

Thirdly, an exclusive focus on sport could discourage an active lifestyle for those who do not like para-sport. For instance, people with SCI often report wanting to do other activities outside of a competitive sports environment, including aerobic exercise, resistance training and general wheeling (Martin Ginis et al., 2010b). A lack of motivation and interest to engage in disability sport can arise from disappointment in wheelchair versions of able-bodied sports and the lack of inclusivity for able-bodied friends (Williams et al., 2014). Furthermore, women with SCI can find it difficult to participate with men in disability sports when they are in the minority (Levins et al., 2004). Thus, a wider range of options to be physically active need to be offered. Community-based LTPA options such as ABR need to be considered by HCPs as a viable opportunity for disabled people to be physically active. The concerns HCPs have with ABR, such as promoting an unrealistic restitution narrative and concrete hope of walking again, arise from their professional ethic to keep their patients safe (Morris et al., 2014). However, these concerns held by HCPs need to be resolved with community based health practitioners to enable disabled people to make informed decisions about engaging in LTPA opportunities. To facilitate this, closer communication and engagement should be implemented at the micro level between HCPs working with disabled people and health practitioners in the community (Williams et al., 2016).

Possible adverse consequences of promoting exercise as medicine

Although it is undisputed that PA provides multiple benefits for people with disabilities, a more critical approach to PA promotion is needed. The potential dangerous consequences of promoting an *exercise is restitution* narrative and the associated "false" hope of recovery have already been highlighted. However, there are other concerns regarding health and PA promotion that HCPs and policymakers need to be aware of. Due to the extensive research on the relationship between PA and health, exercise as a form of medicine is an emerging concept of growing popularity within healthcare, policy and practice (Sallis, 2009). As such, the *exercise is medicine* narrative has therefore been proposed as an ideal story to promote a physically active lifestyle for disabled people (Papathomas et al., 2015). This is because the *exercise is medicine* storyline provides an alternative to restitution whereby participating in LTPA is aimed at improving health and well-being without the promise of cure or recovery.

One concern is that by promoting an *exercise is medicine* narrative a neoliberal health role is also promoted (Smith & Perrier, 2015). Smith and Perrier (2015) comment that the health role in this context "calls on the individual to be a responsible citizen who must personally take care of his or her own health by doing things like exercising regularly" (p.98). This attitude negates any social responsibility and leaves the individual accountable for being physically active. In other words, the *exercise is medicine* narrative aligns with the individualist mentality of the medical model of disability. As emphasised earlier in this chapter, the medical model of disability is problematic for disabled individuals because it neglects the social factors that restrict activity. For instance, people with SCI do take an active role to responsibly take care of their body and health (Smith, 2013). Yet despite developing a sense of body-compassion, and wanting to be physically active, there are still multiple environmental and social barriers that prevent people from participating in PA (Williams et al., 2014). The neoliberal health role therefore risks ignoring societal aspects of being able to participate in PA and consequently overlooks disablism and social oppression (as understood in the social relation model of disability) (Smith & Perrier, 2015). When an individual is motivated to exercise, but cannot because they are unable to access any PA opportunities, this could negatively impact upon their health and well-being (Williams et al., 2014).

Furthermore, HCPs and health practitioners need to be aware that initial PA experiences following physical impairment can actually heighten distress. As Day (2013) warned, PA can highlight the limitations associated with disability and it is only by overcoming these struggles and difficulties that post-traumatic growth can be achieved. As these concerns emphasise, people need to be sensitive to the narratives they promote regarding PA. The *exercise is restitution* narrative and *exercise is medicine* narrative are only two of the multiple typologies associated with LTPA participation which present different possibilities, limitations and dangers for the storyteller (see Perrier et al., 2013; Papathomas et al., 2015). The typologies of narrative allow the storyteller – be it the disabled person or HCP – to critically reflect on the narrative that guides them and the influence it has on their broader lives (Frank, 2013). It is therefore a valuable tool for those HCPs and health practitioners promoting PA and implementing PA interventions, to categorise these narrative typologies and act upon them when necessary. In addition, HCPs and health practitioners need to promote a range of PA narratives as the more narratives available, the greater the chance that people can find one that fits their experiences of PA (Smith, 2013).

Conclusion

In this chapter, we have located the "problem" of physical inactivity for people living with disability within the disablist social and environmental barriers that impede participation in sport and exercise. Thus, we have drawn attention to the inequalities experienced by disabled people in being able to attain the highest standard of health and well-being through engagement in PA. As illustrated in our examples of the research in SCI and LTPA, we have also identified the importance of knowledge about how and where to exercise as a significant constraint to being physically active. Conversely, despite policy stipulating the role of HCPs to deliver health promotion, and HCPs being trusted and valued messengers of PA information, we have highlighted the multiple dilemmas experienced by HCPs in promoting PA. In addition, we have problematised "generic" behaviour change interventions that fail to consider the specific situations of disabled people. In light of all this, we have offered several implications for policy and practice aimed at improving LTPA promotion and reducing the disablist barriers preventing disabled people from engaging in sport and exercise. These implications emphasise the need for effective knowledge translation and the need for support from the healthcare system. We hope that these implications can assist policy makers, HCPs, rehabilitation centres and community-based LTPA initiatives in supporting disabled people to be physically active for life.

Note

1 The human rights of disabled people are further recognised by the United Nations Convention of the Rights of Persons with Disabilities (United Nations, 2006).

References

Berger, R. J. (2008) Disability and the dedicated wheelchair athlete: Beyond the "supercrip" critique. *Journal of Contemporary Ethnography*, 37(6), 647–678.

Biddle, S. J. H., Mutrie, N., & Gorely, T. (2015) *Psychology of physical activity. Determinants, well-being and interventions.* 3rd ed. Oxon: Routledge.

Brittain, I. (2004) Perceptions of disability and their impact upon involvement in sport for people with disabilities at all levels. *Journal of Sport & Social Issues*, 28(4), 429–452.

Buchholz, A. C., Martin Ginis, K. A., Bray, S. R., Craven, B. C., Hicks, A. L., Hayes, K. C., Latimer, A. E., McColl, M. A., Potter, P. J., & Wolfe, D. L. (2009) Greater daily leisure time physical activity is associated with lower chronic disease risk in adults with spinal cord injury. *Applied Physiology, Nutrition, and Metabolism*, 34(4), 640–647.

Canning, K. L., & Hicks, A. L. (2014) Secondary health conditions associated with spinal cord injury. *Critical Reviews in Physical and Rehabilitation Medicine*, 26(3–4), 181–191.

Chen, Y., Cao, Y., Allen, V., & Richards, S. (2011) Weight matters: Physical and psychosocial well-being of persons with spinal cord injury in relation to body mass index. *Archives of Physical Medicine and Rehabilitation*, 92(3), 391–398.

Day, M. C. (2013) The role of initial physical activity experiences in promoting posttraumatic growth in Paralympic athletes with an acquired disability. *Disability and Rehabilitation*, 35(24), 2064–2072.

Department of Health (2011) *UK physical activity guidelines*. www.gov.uk/government/publications/uk-physical-activity-guidelines [accessed 10 October 2015].

Dunstan, D. W., Howard, B., Healy, G. N., & Owen, N. (2012) Too much sitting – A health hazard. *Diabetes Research and Clinical Practice*, 97, 368–376.

EFDS (2013) *English Federation of Disability Sport sports clubs and the Equality Act 2010*. www.efds.co.uk/assets/0000/8224/Fact_sheet_Sports_Clubs__The_Equality_Act_final_Dec2013_x.pdf [accessed 16 March 2016].

Emerson, E., Vick, B., Graham, H., Hatton, C., Llewellyn, G., Madden, R., Rechel, B., & Robertson, J. (2012) Disablement and health. In N. Watson, A. Roulstone, & C. Thomas, eds. *Routledge handbook of disability studies*. London: Routledge. (pp.253–270).

Frank, A. W. (2013) *The wounded storyteller*. 2nd ed. London: University of Chicago Press.

Goodley, D. (2013) Dis/entangling critical disability studies. *Disability & Society*, 28(5), 631–644.

Gorgey, A. S. (2014) Exercise awareness and barriers after spinal cord injury. *World Journal of Orthopedics*, 5(3), 158.

Government Equalities Office (2010) Equality Act 2010: What do I need to know? A quick start guide for private clubs and other associations. www.gov.uk/government/uploads/system/uploads/attachment_data/file/85018/private-clubs.pdf [accessed 01 May 2016].

Harvey, L. A., Adams, R., Chu, J., Batty, J., & Barratt, D. (2012) A comparison of patients' and physiotherapists' expectations about walking post spinal cord injury: A longitudinal cohort study. *Spinal Cord*, 50(7), 548–552.

Hughes, B., & Paterson, K. (1997) The social model of disability and the disappearing body: Toward a sociology of impairment. *Disability and Society*, 12(3), 325–340.

Kehn, M., & Kroll, T. (2009) Staying physically active after spinal cord injury: A qualitative exploration of barriers and facilitators to exercise participation. *BMC Public Health*, 9, 168–178.

Kleiber, D. A., & Hutchinson, S. L. (1999) Heroic masculinity in the recovery from spinal cord injury. In A. Sparkes, & M. Silvennoinen, eds. *Talking bodies: Men's narratives of the body and sport*. Jyvaskyla: SoPhi University of Jyvaskyla. (pp.125–155).

Krause, K. S., & Saunders, L. L. (2011) Health, secondary conditions, and life expectancy after spinal cord injury. *Archives of Physical Medicine and Rehabilitation*, 92(11), 1770–1775.

Letts, L., Martin Ginis, K. A., Faulkner, G., Colquhoun, H., Levac, D., & Gorczynski, P. (2011) Preferred methods and messengers for delivering physical activity information to people with spinal cord injury: A focus group study. *Rehabilitation Psychology*, 56(2), 128–137.

Levins, S. M., Redenbach, D. M., & Dyck, I. (2004) Individual and societal influences on participation in physical activity following spinal cord injury: A qualitative study. *Physical Therapy*, 84(6), 496–509.

Lutz, B. J., & Bowers, B. J. (2005) Disability in everyday life. *Qualitative Health Research*, 15(8), 1037–1054.

Martin, J. J. (2013) Benefits and barriers to physical activity for individuals with disabilities: A social-relational model of disability perspective. *Disability and Rehabilitation*, 35, 2030–2037.

Martin Ginis, K. A., Latimer, A. E., Arbour-Nicitopoulos, K. P., Buchholz, A. C., Bray, S. R., Craven, B. C., Hayes, K. C., Hicks, A. L., McColl, M. A., Potter, P. J., Smith, K., & Wolfe, D. L. (2010a) Leisure time physical activity in a population-based sample of people with spinal cord injury Part I: Demographic and injury-related correlates. *Archives of Physical Medicine and Rehabilitation*, 91(5), 722–728.

Martin Ginis, K. A., Arbour-Nicitopoulos, K. P., Latimer, A. E., Buchholz, A. C., Bray, S. R., Craven, B. C., Hayes, K.C., Hicks, A.L., McColl, M.A., Potter, P.J., Smith, K., & Wolfe, D. L. (2010b) Leisure time physical activity in a population-based sample of people with spinal cord injury part II: Activity types, intensities, and durations. *Archives of Physical Medicine and Rehabilitation*, 91(5), 729–733.

Martin Ginis, K. A., Hicks, A. L., Latimer, A. E., Warbuton, D. E. R., Bourne, C., Ditor, D. S., Goodwin, D. L., Hayes, K. C., McCartney, N., McIlraith, A., Pomerleau, P., Smith, K., Stone, J. A., & Wolfe, D. L. (2011) The development of evidence-informed physical activity guidelines for adults with spinal cord injury. *Spinal Cord*, 49, 1088–1096.

Martin Ginis, K. A., Jörgensen, S., & Stapleton, J. (2012) Exercise and sport for persons with spinal cord injury. *PM&R*, 4(11), 894–900.

McDermott, S., & Turk, M. A. (2011) The myth and reality of disability prevalence: Measuring disability for research and service. *Disability and Health Journal*, 4(1), 1–5.

McGrane, N., Galvin, R., Cusack, T., & Stokes, E. (2015) Addition of motivational interventions to exercise and traditional physiotherapy: A review and meta-analysis. *Physiotherapy*, 101, 1–12.

Meekosha, H., & Shuttleworth, R. (2009) What's so 'critical' about critical disability studies? *Australian Journal of Human Rights*, 15, 47–75.

Morris, J. H., & Williams, B. (2009) Optimising long-term participation in physical activities after stroke: Exploring new ways of working for physiotherapists. *Physiotherapy*, 95(3), 227–233.

Morris, J. H., Oliver, T., Kroll, T., Joice, S., & Williams, B. (2014) From physical and functional to continuity with pre-stroke self and participation in valued activities: A qualitative exploration of stroke survivors', carers' and physiotherapists' perceptions of physical activity after stroke. *Disability and Rehabilitation*, 37(1), 64–77.

Mulligan, H. F., Hale, L. A., Whitehead, L., & Baxter, G. D. (2012) Barriers to physical activity for people with long-term neurological conditions: A review study. *Adapted Physical Activity Quarterly*, 29(3), 243–265.

Mulligan, H., Fjellman-Wiklund, A., Hale, L., Thomas, D., & Hager-Ross, C. (2011) Promoting physical activity for people with neurological disability: Perspectives and experiences of physiotherapists. *Physiotherapy Theory and Practice*, 27(6), 399–401.

NHS (2015) *Fitness advice for wheelchair uses.* Available from: www.nhs.uk/Livewell/Disability/Pages/fitness-for-wheelchair-users.aspx. [accessed 10 October 2015].

NHS Future Forum (2012) *The NHS's role in public health. A report from the NHS Future Forum.* London: Future Forum. Available from: www.gov.uk/government/uploads/system/uploads/attachment_data/file/216423/dh_132114.pdf [Accessed 10 August 2015].

Norrbrink, C., Lindberg, T., Wahman, K., & Bjerkefors, A. (2012) Effects of an exercise programme on musculoskeletal and neuropathic pain after spinal cord injury – Results from a seated double-poling ergometer study. *Spinal Cord*, 50(6), 457–461.

Papathomas, A., Williams, T. L., & Smith, B. (2015) Understanding physical activity participation in spinal cord injured populations: Three narrative types for consideration. *International Journal of Qualitative Studies on Health and Well-being.* DOI: 10.3402/qhw.v10.27295.

Perrier, M-J., Smith, B., & Latimer-Cheung, A. E. (2013) Narrative environments and the capacity of disability narratives to motivate leisure-time physical activity among individuals with spinal cord injury. *Disability and Rehabilitation*, 35(24), 2089–2096.

Roush, S. E., & Sharby, N. (2011) Disability reconsidered the paradox of physical therapy. *Physical Therapy*, 91(12), 1715–1727.

Saebu, M. (2010) Physical disability and physical activity: A review of the literature on correlates and associations. *European Journal of Adapted Physical Activity*, 3(2), 37–55.

Sallis, R. E. (2009) Exercise is medicine and physicians need to prescribe it! *British Journal of Sports Medicine*, 43, 3–4.

Shakespeare, T. (2014) *Disability rights and wrongs revisited.* Oxford: Routledge.

Silva, C.F., & Howe, P.D. (2012) The (in)validity of supercrip representation of Paralympian athletes. *Journal of Sport and Social Issues,* 36(2), 174–194.

Smith, B. (2013) Disability, sport and men's narratives of health: A qualitative study. *Health Psychology*, 32(1), 110–119.

Smith, B., & Bundon, A. (*in-press*). Disability models: Explaining and understanding disability sport. In I. Brittain, ed. *Palgrave handbook of Paralympic studies.* Basingstoke: Palgrave.

Smith, B., & Perrier, M-J. (2015) Disability, sport and impaired bodies: A critical approach. In. R. Schinke & K. R. McGannon, eds. *The psychology of sub-culture in sport and physical activity: Critical perspectives.* London: Psychology Press, Taylor & Francis. (pp.95–106).

Smith, B., & Sparkes, A. C. (2005) Men, sport, spinal cord injury and narratives of hope. *Social Science & Medicine*, 61(5), 1095–1105.

Smith, B., & Sparkes, A. C. (2012) Disability, sport and physical activity. A critical review. In N. Watson, A. Roulstone, & C. Thomas, eds. *Routledge handbook of disability studies.* London: Routledge. (pp.336–347).

Smith, B., Tomasone, J. R., Latimer-Cheung, A. E., & Martin Ginis, K. A. (2015) Narrative as a knowledge translation tool for facilitating impact: Translating physical activity knowledge to disabled people and health professionals. *Health Psychology*, 34(4), 303–313.

Soundy, A., Smith, B., Butler, M., Lowe, C. M., Dawes, H., & Winward, C. H. (2010) A qualitative study in neurological physiotherapy and hope: Beyond physical improvement. *Physiotherapy Theory and Practice*, 26(2), 79–88.

Soundy, A., Smith, B., Dawes, H., Pall, H., Gimbrere, K., & Ramsay, J. (2013) Patients' expressions of hope and illness in three neurological conditions: A meta-ethnography. *Health Psychology Review*, 7(2), 177–201.

Stephens, C., Neil, R., & Smith, P. (2012) The perceived benefits and barriers of sport in spinal cord injured individuals: A qualitative study. *Disability and Rehabilitation*, 34(24), 2061–2070.

Thomas, C. (2007) *Sociologies of disability and illness: Contested ideas in disability studies and medical sociology.* Basingstoke: Palgrave Macmillan.

Tomasone, J. R., Martin Ginis, K. A., Estabrooks, P. A., & Domenicucci, L. (2014) Changing minds, changing lives from the top down: An investigation of the dissemination and adoption of a Canada-wide educational intervention to enhance health care professionals' intentions to prescribe physical activity. *International Journal of Behavioural Medicine*, 22(3), 336–44.

Tomasone, J. R., Wesch, N., Martin Ginis, K. A., & Noreau, L. (2013) Spinal cord injury, physical activity, and quality of life: A systematic review. *Kinesiology Review*, 2(1), 113–129.

United Nations. (2006) *Convention on the Rights of Persons with Disabilities and Optional Protocol.* Available from: www.un.org/disabilities/default.asp?id=150 [accessed 28 July 2014].

van Lit, A., & Kayes, N. (2014) A narrative review of hope after spinal cord injury: Implications for physiotherapy. *New Zealand Journal of Physiotherapy*, 42(1), 33–41.

Verschuren, O., Mead, G., & Visser-Meily, A. (2015) Sedentary behaviour and stroke: Foundational knowledge is crucial. *Translational Stroke Research*, 6(1), 9–12.

Walkeden, S., & Walker, K. M. (2015) Perceptions of physiotherapists about their role in health promotion at an acute hospital: A qualitative study. *Physiotherapy*, 101, 226–231.

WCPT (2012) *Active and healthy: The role of the physiotherapist in physical activity (briefing paper).* Available from: www.google.com/webhp?sourceid=chrome-instant&ion=1&espv=2&ie=UTF-8#q=Active +and+healthy%3A+the+role+of+the+physiotherapist+in+physical+activity [accessed 10 August 2015].

WHO (2015) *International Classification of Functioning, Disability and Health (ICF).* Available from: www.who.int/classifications/icf/en/ [accessed 08 January 2015].

Williams, T. L., Smith, B., & Papathomas, A. (2014) The barriers, benefits and facilitators of leisure time physical activity among people with spinal cord injury: A meta-synthesis of qualitative findings. *Health Psychology Review,* 8, 404–425.

Williams, T.L., Smith, B., & Papathomas, A. (2016) Physical activity promotion for people with spinal cord injury: Physiotherapists' beliefs and actions. *Disability & Rehabilitation.* DOI: 10.1080/09638288. 2016.1242176.

Wong, S., van Middendorp, J., Belci, M., van Nes, I., Roels, E., Smith, É., Hirani, S. P., & Forbes, A. (2015) Knowledge, attitudes and practices of medical staff towards obesity management in patients with spinal cord injuries: An international survey of four western European countries. *Spinal Cord*, 53, 24–31.

21

PHYSICAL ACTIVITY, FAMILIES AND HOUSEHOLDS

John Day

Introduction

Thompson *et al.*'s (2009) finding that all members of a family household are rarely active together and Hart, Herriot, Bishop and Truby's (2003) conclusion that exercise involvement is of low priority within the context of family lifestyle decisions suggest physical activity is not a widespread family practice. Nevertheless, from life course and physical activity promotion perspectives, family relationships are likely to have a profound bearing on people's physical activity habits. Arguably, the sticking point most relevant to family life and policy is how parents identify engaging in physical activity with their children as a childrearing task and not worthwhile physical activity for themselves (Hamilton & White, 2010). This is somewhat at odds with the evidence-based health argument that doing something rather than nothing has significant benefits (Weed, 2016). Much of our knowledge about physical activity within family contexts has been constructed with an explicit intention to raise population levels of physical activity for desirable public health outcomes. Instead of implying that physical activity is something that people 'should' be doing more often, this chapter is written from the position that being active is, for the most part, conducive to human wellbeing (Wellard, 2014). Critically, the social environment of family is more pivotal to both wellbeing and happiness than factors associated with health (Layard, 2011). This is a point consistently overlooked in studies of families informed by the paradigm of physical activity promotion. In reviewing our existing knowledge of the area, the chapter focuses on the key topics of childhood socialisation by parents, the influence of various household compositions and the role played by parents as both physical activity participants and providers. In closing the chapter, the main implications for physical activity policy and practice are outlined.

Families, households and popular approaches in physical activity research

Secularisation, greater acceptance of homosexual relationships, an increase in the number of marriages ending in divorce, more single person households and ever shifting patterns of migration have required us to rethink what we mean by the term *family* in contemporary societies (Chambers, 2012; Cheal, 2002). Since the middle of the twentieth century in the West, there has gradually been a reduced influence from Christian infused modes of thought concerning how adults should go about starting a family (Cheal, 2002). It is no longer expected that couples must be married before they can participate in sexual intercourse, reside with one another or raise children. The subsequent diversification of family units who live together and apart has seen family scholars in social and policy sciences investigate and test the ideas of personal life, kinship, friendship, community and family practices in an effort to sufficiently depict the intimacies of people's valued relationships (Chambers, 2012). Although each of us hold an idea of what a family is, contrasting familial socialisation experiences give rise to differing and sometimes contradictory images of this idea, contradictions and differences that seldom emerge in family studies (Bernardes, 1987). Therefore, as a research concept and primary group in our early biographical experiences, families are simultaneously a familiar and strange point of collective reference. Such a critical awareness of the term 'family' encourages researchers to consider a series of reflexive and methodological issues when conducting family research. Although this is not the place to comprehensively unpack these essential research considerations, readers would be well advised to revisit the thought-provoking exchange between Jon Bernardes (1987, 1988) and Patricia Wilson and Ray Pahl (1988) in *The Sociological Review*. Drawing upon this debate in account of the way family focused physical activity research is currently conducted, it is argued that this body of knowledge would benefit from making more definitive distinctions between the study of households and families. Wilson and Pahl (1988; pp. 236–7) are worth quoting at length about the debilitating mix-up that emanates from failing to establish a differentiation:

> Commentators seem wilfully determined to define households with different compositions as being different family types. The conflation of 'household composition' with 'family type' has become so much part of contemporary conventional wisdom that the terminology now appears in official statistics. Thus, for example, households based solely on dependent children with only one parent present are referred to as 'one-parent families'. The second, absent, parent may or may not be alive but, if the former, the children certainly have two parents in their family, even if they have only one in their household. Once 'family' has been redefined as 'household type' the scope for muddle and confusion is substantially increased.

As discussed later in the chapter, research that claims to examine the effect of 'family structure' on the physical activity of family members because they live together is particularly misleading in this regard. Household refers to living arrangements, whereas family is defined by the intimate relationships of its members (Cheal, 2002). There is often considerable overlap, but the distinction has been crucial since images of isolated, permanent and static living arrangements invoked by the model of the nuclear family became less credible (Cheal, 2002). The study of family intimacies requires gaining an insight into the close associations that family members are involved, and the privileged knowledge that they share amongst, about and trust each other with (Jamieson, 1998).

Though the predominant approach of attempting to establish statistical correlations between parental demographics and child physical activity overlooks the lived experience of the intimacies that epitomise family life, such studies also serve as examples of the pressure on parents to raise healthy children. Moreover, mixed and sometimes conflicting findings from quantitative studies of family influences on physical activity involvement have uncovered a number of trends that underscore the significance of families in shaping the physical activity of its members. Gustafson and Rhodes's (2006) systematic review of parental correlates of child physical activity found results from previous studies of the number of parents in the family, family socio-economic status, ethnicity and the sex of family members to be ambiguous. The only finding to emerge from the review with a relatively strong evidence base was that children with active parents receive more parental support to be active and are generally more active than children with non-active parents. Pugliese and Tinsley's (2007) meta-analysis of the effect of parental behaviours on child and adolescent physical activity also upholds a moderate positive relation between parental support and child physical activity levels. The discrepancy between these two analyses concerns the extent to which, if at all, the modelling of parental behaviours by children mediates the influence of the support provided by active parents. Pugliese and Tinsley's meta-analysis suggests that it is not possible to separate the likelihood that children will replicate the active behaviours of active parents from the simultaneous encouragement provided by active parents for their children to follow their active behaviours. Whereas Gustafson and Rhodes argue that although the modelling of the active behaviours of parents may increase the chances of an active childhood, modelling does not provide children with the opportunity to be active as the transportation and financial resource aspects of parental support can. The complexities of physical activity socialisation are further highlighted by Edwardson and Gorely's (2010) systematic review of parental influence on the types and intensities of children's physical activity, which concluded that adolescent physical activity is more closely related to, and influenced by, fathers' levels of physical activity than mothers'. Moreover, Pugliese and Tinsley acknowledge that active children are also likely to have some degree of influence on their parent's physical activity habits. With regard to physical activity patterns it would thus seem that there is as much going on *within* families, in terms of the power relations of family relationships, as there is *between* family units, such as the opportunities and constraints of contrasting socio-economic resources. However, the dominant and most popular approach to researching the active habits of family members focuses on how parents go about socialising their children, which is informed by the notion that an active childhood significantly increases the likelihood of being regularly active throughout the life course.

Family and the socialisation thesis of lifelong physical activity

Research informed and justified by the active child socialisation thesis of lifelong physical activity participation tends to be confined to families comprised of two parents in a heterosexual relationship residing in the same household as their biological children. Families referred to by Bois, Sarrazin, Brustad, Trouilloud, and Cury (2005; p. 385) and Quarmby and Dagkas (2010; p. 56) as 'intact'. Such a line of thought implies that families falling outside of the heterosexuality and biological parenting of 'intact' family households are unstable and broken in some way (Chambers, 2012). Although the majority of studies therefore narrowly depict family environments as static and singular, the means by which parents influence their children's physical activity habits within this form of household are still multifaceted.

Eriksson, Nordqvist and Rasmussen (2008) contend that the association between child and parent physical activity patterns among early adolescent sons may be mediated by athletic competence. The engagement of sons in sport and vigorous physical activities, who had either two parents that regularly participated in sport or a highly active father, was positively related to their athletic competence. In spite of Eriksson *et al.*'s cross-sectional design, meaning the direction of the relationship between son's athletic competence and the likelihood of their participation in sport and vigorous physical activity is unclear, the study marks out the significance of father-son relationships to the childhood physical activity habits of males. Should assumptions regarding the consequences of childhood physical activity levels for participation across the life course hold any ground, fathers' engagement in physical activity during the childhood of their sons would appear to be of central importance. The influence of fathers upon their male and female children's physical activity patterns was also telling in Bois *et al.*'s (2005) investigation of the interplay between 9 to 11-year-old children's self-perceptions of physical competence, parents' perceptions of their children's physical competence and children's physical activity levels. Congruent with a largely consistent evidence base, it was found that, on the whole, children with higher self-perceptions of physical competence were more likely to be involved in physical activity. Also directly related to children's physical activity levels were fathers' perceptions of their children's physical competence, with higher perceptions of the physical competence of their children increasing the chances of higher levels of physical activity. Bois *et al.* theorise that this direct relationship could be a case of fathers providing their children with more opportunities to be active when holding higher perceptions of their children's physical competence, and fewer opportunities when perceptions are lower. Bois *et al.* also indicate that the values children associate with physical activity may mediate the association between fathers' perceptions of their child's physical competence and children's physical activity levels, as the study did not account for this variable. Although mothers' perceptions of their children's physical ability were not directly correlated with children's physical activity levels, the perceptions they held of their children's physical competence did inform the children's self-perceptions of physical competence. It therefore seems that the influence of mothers and fathers impacts their children's physical activity habits in contrasting ways.

Some studies do not support the belief that more active parents are likely to rear more active children. This raises questions about the philosophical underpinning that allegedly justifies the intense research focus on what parents are, could and 'should' be doing to increase their children's physical activity levels. Findings from Anderssen, Wold and Torsheim's (2006; p. 520–1) longitudinal investigation of the interrelationships between the physical activity practices of children and parents 'did not support the view on physical activity socialization' of a parental influence upon their children's physical activity. Anderssen *et al.* attribute this to the possible bearing that social factors might have, such as parental encouragement and financial resources, which were not included in the study. Like a sizeable proportion of studies concerning the effect of family relationships upon physical activity habits, Anderssen *et al.*'s research is informed by behavioural epidemiology and the frequency of physical activity involvement, as opposed to a deeper understanding of how the intimacies of family relationships inform people's values and attitudes toward physical activity. In this sense, the conventional behavioural epidemiology approach to parental influence upon children's physical activity habits studies what *might* be the behavioural consequences of socialisation, but not the intricacies of the socialisation process. Qualitative research on the experiences and attitudes of parents with intentions of socialising their children into regular physical activity habits also sheds further doubt on the strength of their influence in constructing an active childhood for their children. Hesketh, Hinkley and Campbell's (2012) unstructured focus groups with people who had become parents during the past 12 months and parents with children between 3 and 5 years of age uncovered some of the circumstantial constraints in attempting to maximise the time that their children spent being physically active. Parents with a firstborn child less than a year old were hopeful of minimising the time that their child would spend watching television and successfully encouraging them to be highly active throughout childhood. An optimism not shared by many of those with at least three years' experience of being a parent, some of whom used the television as a babysitter to give them sufficient time to complete household duties. The more experienced parents were aware that such strategies were not ideal, but saw some screen time for children as necessary and effective in balancing their time between caregiving and household chores. Parents from both groups also shared the belief that children are 'naturally' physically active. This perception might have implications for the extent to which parents act upon their intentions to integrate physical activity into the early years of their children's lives. The idea that physical activity is a natural aspect of childhood is also referred to by the parents of children aged 3 to 5 years, who participated in a focus group study undertaken by Dwyer, Higgs, Hardy and Baur (2008). Some parents felt that more or less from birth, children were automatically active, but this 'hard-wired' behaviour was gradually socialised out of their children by an increasingly technological society. According to these parents, the main constraint to their children's physical activity were enticing and largely sedentary technology-based pastimes, such as television viewing and using hand-held screen devices, meaning some parents were of the opinion that they were fighting a losing battle.

For the most part, it appears that parental influence over shaping children's physical activity engagement wanes as both parents and their children age (Alderman, Benham-Deal & Jenkins, 2010). Alderman *et al.*'s (2010) study suggests that the moderate physical activity association between parents and their preschool age children has dwindled away by the time children enter adolescence. Or as Anderssen *et al.* (2006; p. 520) conclude, 'the frequency and the time that adolescents spend on leisure-time physical activity tend to vary somewhat with time, and, parents' own physical activity does not seem to play an important role in those variations'. This is not to say that the way children are socialised into various types of physical activity by parents does not have any impact on how they relate to and value physical activity throughout the lifespan. However, with regard to the level of children's engagement with physical activity, and particularly the patterning of this engagement, the influence of parents' physical activity habits is significant during early childhood but has often worn thin by adolescence. As children age they are generally exposed to wider social influences, such as friends they make at school, and may perceive teachers as alternative or complementary role models to parents (Alderman *et al.*, 2010). Invariably, when building relationships outside of the family unit, children develop interests that may not be shared by parents. Adolescence is an important stage of the life course in this respect, as it is at this age when children begin to establish influential relationships outside of their immediate family environment and make decisions with a greater degree of independence (Cheal, 2002). Along these lines, David Cheal (2002; p. 96) has conceptualised adolescence as a phase of anticipatory socialisation, when children 'seek out experiences which help them to develop attitudes and skills that they believe they will need in later life'. It is therefore to be expected that as children enter adolescence and begin to construct some of their own values and socialisation experiences that parents are likely to have less impact on their children's behaviours. With this in mind, the *quality* of the relationship between parents and their children is likely to be relevant, significant and meaningful to any sustained influence that parents maintain over their children's behaviour from adolescence onwards. Unfortunately, variables symptomatic of the quality of parent-child relationships, such as personal time spent together and communication, have been largely neglected in longitudinal and prospective physical activity research (Lim & Biddle, 2012).

A notable exception to the majority of longitudinal studies of parental influence on adolescent physical activity, which does account for the quality of parent-child relationships, was undertaken by Ornelas, Perreira and Ayala (2007). Using data from the US National Longitudinal Study of Adolescent Health, the authors found family cohesion, parent-child communication and the number of everyday activities that parents and children engaged in together to be significantly and positively related to higher levels of moderate to vigorous physical activity one year later. This points not only towards the power of sway that a meaningful relationship between parent and child can have upon an ageing adolescent's behavioural tendencies, but also how the closeness of parent-child ties can endure over time. A form of closeness likely to be distinguishable from other meaningful but non-familial relationships that emerge during a child's anticipatory socialisation (Cheal, 2002). Variables indicative of the quality of family relationships, such as family cohesion, communication and time spent together, as well as profound and enduring yet fluctuating feelings of closeness fall within the concept of intimacy. Crucial distinctions between studying a group of people because they live together or because they are intimately involved in one another's personal lives on a long-standing basis have yet to be considering in reference to physical activity. Although family-oriented studies of physical activity are yet to fully embrace the concept of intimacy, there has been some recognition of alterations to the composition of households through analyses of the influence of 'family structure' on the activity inclinations of its members. These studies claim to scrutinise the influence of 'family structures' on physical activity habits, but actually investigate the effects of various household compositions on children's physical activity (see Gorely, Atkin, Biddle & Marshall, 2009; Hesketh, Crawford & Salmon, 2006; Quarmby & Dagkas, 2010). In summary, it remains to be seen whether fixed surface-level comparisons *between* the make-up of people's households carry any worthwhile implications for social policy at a time of notable changes to the intimacies of family life (Chambers, 2012).

Physical activity and household structure and composition

Anthony Giddens's (1992) claim that 'pure' egalitarian relationships are now possible following the individualisation and democratisation of intimate interpersonal relationships has been met with considerable doubt (Chambers, 2012). Less refuted is his suggestion that our increasingly democratic relations with kin and friends are inextricably linked to the diversification of households (Chambers, 2012). According to the 2014 UK Labour Force Survey, there were approximately 26.7 million households in the UK, with around 18.6 million of these constituting some form of family household, defined as 'a married, civil partnered or cohabiting couple with or without children, or a lone parent with at least one child who live at the same address' (Office for National Statistics, 2015; p. 1). Within most nation states of the Western world, such as the UK, it is rare for all living generations of the same family to dwell together (Cheal, 2002). In most Western cultures it is expected that children live with and are cared and provided for by their biological parents who inculcate them with the skills and values required to eventually care and provide for themselves, so that they are able to start their own households and families, if they wish. This notion of family life as a perpetual routine, a remnant of the 'family cycle' paradigm dominant in family sociology until the 1980s, has gradually become more of an ideal than a typical experience for most people (Allan & Crow, 2001; Chambers, 2012). Over time, the structure provided by the stability of family relationships, especially between couples involved in a romantic relationship, has become less secure. As noted by Chambers (2012; p. 4),

> Individuals now expect much more from intimate relationships and are much more prepared to get divorced or move on to the next relationship if either party feels trapped or no longer feels fulfilled ... expectations of a life-long conjugal relationship involving having and bringing up children, with wife as homemaker and husband as breadwinner, have gone.

Adjoined to the increased prevalence of divorce in Britain since the early 1970s, when the 1969 Divorce Reform Act took effect, is the detachment of sexual intercourse from marriage (Allan, 1999; Giddens, 1992). Taken collectively, the ramifications for the composition of Western households are far-reaching, with conventional family units more likely to break-up and the increased possibility of newborn children being reared within single-parent households. The consequences for family demographics mean that academics are continuously required to reconsider what is meant by the term 'family' and national household surveys regularly redesigned.

Initial investigations of unconventional but increasingly common family environments reveal significant effects on family members' propensity to be regularly active. Again, as with most family-oriented physical activity literature, the main emphasis is on the activity habits of children, rather than all members of a family or household. Quarmby and Dagkas's (2010) exploratory examination of children's experiences of leisure time physical activity proposes parents' values and beliefs pertaining to physical activity are paramount and frequently reproduced in children's construction of their own values and beliefs towards physical activity. 'Family structure' appeared decisive in shaping the physical activity inclinations and behaviours of children aged between 11 and 14 years, with those from single-parent households more likely to be engaged in more sedentary activities than those children residing with both biological parents. The additional time stress experienced by single parents situated within the constraints of work commitments and being solely responsible for childcare and household duties served to limit the leisure time available to spend time with and provide physical activity opportunities for their children. While household circumstances might be relevant to children's physical activity behaviours, the generational transmission of the value of being more or less active from parents to children is likely to be more pertinent to lifelong physical activity habits and beliefs. Thus, the frequency of children's opportunities to be active seems to be related to the make-up of the household and would appear to either augment or restrain the biographical physical activity views of parents, instilled in and reproduced by their children. Family norms within low-income single-parent households often restrict opportunities for children to be physically active (Quarmby & Dagkas, 2013). Ultimately, limited opportunities to be more active become manifested in household routines and family activities characterised by sedentariness.

Parent-child relationships are commonly presented as a one-way dictatorship from authoritative parents to passive children, as opposed to a two-way negotiation of contested power relations (Edwards & Weller, 2014). Workings of power and influence within non-conventional household situations are better outlined in Ruseski, Humphreys, Hallmann and Breuer's (2011) inquiry into the economics of physical activity within family households. The paper by Ruseski et al. is also of notable value as time spent being active through sport participation is measured for all household members and not solely children, including those who do not have children. Unlike Quarmby and Dagkas, Ruseski et al. did not reduce their study to differences in circumstance between 'intact' and 'non-intact' households. Instead, Ruseski et al. use marital status, the presence or absence of children in the household and household size as the basis for analysis of 'family structure'. From the 1,934 questionnaire responses, including 408 provided by parents on behalf of their 3 to 17 year-old children, it was identified that the presence of children in a household reduces both the possibility of sports participation and the amount of time spent participating for all members of a household. Especially interesting was the trend indicating 'the overall effect of children on time spent by adults in participating in sport is unclear, as the presence of children reduces time spent while active children increase the time adults spend practicing sport' (Ruseski et al., 2011;

p. 65). A spillover of children's physical activity to their parents has also been unearthed in a subsequent study by Berniell, de la Mata and Valdés (2013), with fathers more likely to engage in light physical activity during the implementation of health education initiatives at the elementary schools attended by their children. The evidence points towards an intergenerational interaction of physical activity influences between parents and their children. Whilst those household compositions which include children might reduce the likelihood of physical activity for members of family households, early research shows that as children age, require less care and engage with physical activity at school, familial physical activity influences become intergenerational and more interdependent.

Nonetheless, the vast proportion of research is preoccupied with only the physical activity habits of children. Hesketh *et al.* (2006) analysed data on 2,458 children collated from the 2001 Children's Leisure Activity and 2002/3 Health, Eating and Play surveys in Australia. This paper makes an interesting offering to our knowledge of children's physical activity, by distinguishing between the intensities of activity that children are most inclined to engage in according to their household composition. Low-intensity activity was more prevalent among children from single-parent households and children without siblings. Whereas children with siblings, especially girls, spent more time doing moderate-to-vigorous activities. Sparse mentions of sibling relationships in the existing literature signal that sibship may have a prominent role in childhood physical activity (Ramanathan & Crocker, 2009; Ziviani, Macdonald, Ward, Jenkins & Rodger, 2006). Although in the vast proportion of research, children tend to be referred to as 'boys' and 'girls', rather than being contextualised in their family roles as sons, daughters, brothers and sisters. The study also stresses the significance of the make-up of family households for the physical activity of children, as 'the measures of family composition (number of parents in the home and presence of siblings) were more consistently related to children's physical activity than were the socioeconomic indicators' (Hesketh *et al.*, 2006; p. 36). This reiterates the point that future research would be well informed to examine more closely what happens *within* families in terms of physical activity, to make better sense of the numerous quantitative trends that have been recognised as existing between family households. This is further reinforced by the finding that the cultural background of a family seems to be crucial to children's activity levels in the two-hour period after they have left school for the day (Hesketh, Graham & Waters, 2008).

Physical activity and parents as participants and providers

A greater proportion of contemporary academic discussions position parents as physical activity providers rather than participants, which implicitly prioritises being active during childhood over adulthood. This gradual precedence of one stage of the life course over another is attached to the intensification and expansion of parenting over the last four decades (Faircloth, 2014). Portrayed as having absolute power over the behaviours of their children, parental demographics are often used as independent variables to examine the influence that they have over the activity patterns of children. For example, Zecevic, Tremblay, Lovsin and Michel (2010; p. 7) concluded that 'whereas being an older parent is a negative correlate of children's PA, marital status, language, educational levels, and household income were not'. Overlooked is that all parents were once children, young parents may be in adolescence themselves and that parent-child relationships involve interactive negotiations of power as soon as children begin to communicate. Implicit to the dominant approach to the research then, is the greater degree of importance attached to the physical activity of children over adults and parents, despite a discourse, prevalent in this research area, which champions the value of physical activity involvement at all stages of the life course. Drawing on parents' experiences, this contradiction may extend beyond the literature and be encountered in the struggle to remain active throughout the transition to becoming a parent. The mothers and fathers interviewed by Hamilton and White (2010) all found they had to alter their physical activity behaviours as a consequence of parenthood. For the majority of participants, this alteration comprised of a decreased frequency and intensity of physical activity involvement. Some parents organised their physical activity participation by being active with their children, such as walking the dog together. Whereas other parents managed to arrange time to engage in structured activities without their offspring, which they described as a stress-free luxury. However, a persistent theme in the interviews with parents was the perception that their own physical activity was less important than their children's physical activity. A group of the parents embraced the challenges of parenthood and the balancing act required to be active when this desire clashed with the responsibility to provide and care for their children. A section of the parents also expressed their envy of those who had remained active following entry into parenthood. This resentment was directed at both partners and parents from other families, especially husbands and friends. Combined with the findings from the quantitative studies already discussed, there is sufficient evidence to postulate that once family households become multigenerational and increase in size, a messier negotiation of family life is required for adult members to remain active should they be motivated to do so.

The challenge to remain active once becoming a parent is more complex than the successful negotiation and organisation of family life, and is further convoluted by the gendered identity of what is to be expected of mothers and fathers in contemporary society. According to Lewis and Ridge (2005), entry into motherhood presents an obstacle for the physical activity behaviours of some females and an increased purpose to be active for others. Mothers hold conflicting opinions about whether being regularly active should be part of a 'good' mother's lifestyle (Lewis & Ridge, 2005). The less active mothers interviewed by Lewis and Ridge tended to identify with being active as something that they did not have time for, as their participation would represent a self-centred neglect of their motherly duties. In contrast, more active mothers valued their involvement in physical activity as an essential part of being a responsible mother. These women justified their standpoint through valuing physical activity as a practice which afforded them with a pleasurable break from the routine of being a mother and also supplied them with what they saw as an opportunity to be healthy role models for their children and families. Lewis and Ridge therefore argue that the rationales behind the contrasting choices made by mothers about whether or not to be regularly active are informed by either more egalitarian or more domesticated ideas of motherhood. In line with Giddens's (1992) proposition of a greater balancing between the social status of males and females involved in heterosexual partnerships with one another, Lewis and Ridge conclude that frequent physical activity participation has become more of a legitimate leisure pursuit for many mothers. Whereas less active mothers subscribed to a more traditional, constraining and self-sacrificing doctrine of motherhood by prioritising their children's wellbeing over their own. Lewis and Ridge also assert that active mothers symbolise a new identity of motherhood, which challenges the well-established domestic obligations and restrictions of being a mother while remaining devoted to the overall health and wellbeing of their families.

With regard to mothers' and fathers' strivings to frequently engage in physical activity, another study by Hamilton and White (2012) suggests that parents are more likely to intend to participate if they are supported by their friends and have active friends with comparable parental responsibilities to their own. Additionally, having an active identity not only independently predicted that parents were more likely to intend to be active, but was also related to an increased likelihood of parents following through with their intentions to be active and participating in physical activity. Higher levels of family focused social support, such as help with child care and household tasks, significantly increased the intentions of mothers to involve themselves in regular physical activity, but this was not the case for fathers. To these ends, the quantitative data upon which Hamilton and White base their analysis would appear to offer an insight into how the power relations between spouses involved in heterosexual relationships are played out and impact upon physical activity tendencies. The indication from this data is that fathers need little to no support or approval from their partners to be active, whereas mothers are not able to exercise such freewill and require some level of support from husbands or other family members to be physically active. The work of Hamilton and White (2010, 2012) is symptomatic of a split in the literature that de-contextualises the everyday family circumstances juggled by parents through separating parents' own participation in physical activity from the provision and management of their children's activity habits. Bevan and Reilly (2011) have made reference to the persistent stress experienced by mothers attempting to effectively organise a healthy and active lifestyle for their children and Lewis and Ridge (2005) found that some but not all mothers sacrifice their own physical activity involvement to care for their preschool aged children. Yet there is little research which captures a more holistic perspective of how physical activity features within the broader everyday experience of being a parent within family life.

Macdonald *et al.* (2004) bridge this gap to a certain extent, albeit briefly and indirectly, via an investigation of the physical activity aspects of the family lives of 6- to 9-year-old children. Most of the parents interviewed recalled how they had become less active upon entering parenthood due to increased time constraints and their willingness to give up some of their own physical activity time to allow their children to be as active as possible. Physical activity engagement was therefore seen by parents as a dimension of family lifestyle which required their constant governance. At a time when fathers are reportedly taking on an increased share of childcare responsibilities within Western families, the bargaining between heterosexual couples with regard to the parental governance of the physical activity of families remains unclear. There is also a discord between the existing quantitative and qualitative data in this respect. Quantitative evidence indicates that the influence of fathers is more powerful than that of mothers, which might suggest that children pay greater attention to their fathers in this domain of family life and, if this is the case, fathers may also be the parent most likely to be active and play with their children (Harrington, 2006). Whereas qualitative explorations underline how the role of physical activity provider tends to fall within the remit of a mother's duties. Moreover, fathers barely feature in studies of this sort, with a leaning towards the experiences of mothers and investigations of 'parenting' comprised exclusively of female participants (see Lewis & Ridge, 2005; Hesketh *et al.*, 2012). With this in mind, future research into fathers' experiences of physical activity as both participant and provider would be worthwhile. In terms of provision, Kay (2007) found that fathers regularly involved in organising and supporting their sons' football participation were sometimes troubled by contradictions between emerging expectations of nurturant fatherhood and the role of household provider. Unlike the bulk of the literature concerning physical activity more generally, this research captures a more realistic representation of father-son relationships, which fathers viewed as more of an interdependent friendship than a relationship they controlled. Males are born into father-son relationships not of their choosing, but a mutual interest in a leisure pursuit such as sport is likely to lay the foundations for a friendship of choice that extends beyond the son's childhood. Parental support of children's physical activities of shared interest might therefore provide an additional dimension of intimacy to parent-child relationships and possibly enhance the wellbeing experienced through the parenting of physical activities, which often demand a considerable sacrifice of parents' leisure time.

Implications for physical activity policy and practice

Although the pertinence of engaging in regular physical activity during childhood to lifelong participation is unclear, parental modelling and family socio-economic status are noteworthy correlates. These trends are interesting but any explanation demands an understanding of what goes on within the context of specific families. Often replicated by their children, parental physical activity behaviours have symbolic power and are concomitant with intergenerational transmission and reproduction of parent's physical activity values. Conjoined to this is the issue of developing the type of embodiment essential for lifelong physical activity. This would appear to be a consequence of the interplay between family resources and parental modelling as manifested in children's embodied reproduction of both the social class position and physical activity biographies of their parents (Evans & Davies, 2010). Children who are not socialised into embodied performances characteristic of sustained engagement in physical activity tend to belong to families of lower socio-economic status. Therefore, the lifelong consequences of physical activity involvement during childhood extend beyond the issue of parents' economic resources. It is as a consequence of the intergenerational reproduction of embodiment that 'targeting' children belonging to families of lower socio-economic status by offering opportunities to be active at a reduced cost or free of charge have not been effective (Evans & Davies, 2010). From a family socialisation perspective, these complex sets of relationships indicate that there is greater value for policy to focus upon parents to increase the likelihood of lifelong physical activity participation amongst their children, who are already engaged in some form of physical activity as a compulsory aspect of education.

Parents who are active with their children after being regularly active prior to parenthood are stuck between the health benefits of doing something rather than nothing but are not active in a manner they perceive to be worthwhile for themselves. They generally perceive participation in physical activity with their children as another parenting duty rather than a pursuit they will gain improved health or wellbeing from (Hamilton & White, 2010). Thinking outside of the increased public attention devoted to parents' childrearing practices, the relevance of physical health to people's lives is that it contributes to feelings of happiness and overall life satisfaction (Layard, 2011). Current UK Department of Health (2011) physical activity guidelines claim to adopt a life course perspective, although are more indicative of biological age-specific recommendations for maximal benefits in physical health. The family-oriented physical activity literature reviewed here illustrates that active parents are motivated more by the perceived benefits to individual and family wellbeing than potential improvements in physical health. In this sense, the addition of potential gains in quality of life for family members to physical activity guidelines would be worthwhile. For most, entry into parenthood is associated with a decline in physical activity levels, so to better our understanding of how active parenthood is negotiated a more detailed knowledge of the less common instances of becoming more active through parenthood is required. Ultimately, the majority of our knowledge about physical activity within family life is restricted by researcher adherence to the intensification of childrearing, meaning that the majority of focus is uncritically placed upon how much or little physical activity parents provide for their children. More holistic studies are stifled by confusion between household and family, with single-parent households referred to as single-parent families and then passed off as a legitimate 'family type' or 'family structure'.

References

Alderman, B., Benham-Deal, T. & Jenkins, J. (2010). Change in parental influence on children's physical activity over time. *Journal of Physical Activity and Health, 7,* 60–67.

Allan, G. (1999). Introduction. In G. Allan (Ed.), *The sociology of the family: A reader* (pp. 1–7). Oxford: Blackwell.

Allan, G. & Crow, G. (2001). *Families, households and society.* Basingstoke: Palgrave Macmillan.

Anderssen, N., Wold, B. & Torsheim, T. (2006). Are parental health habits transmitted to their children? An eight year longitudinal study of physical activity in adolescents and their parents. *Journal of Adolescence, 29,* 513–524.

Bernardes, J. (1987). 'Doing things with words': Sociology and 'family policy' debates. *The Sociological Review, 35,* 679–702.

Bernardes, J. (1988). Whose 'family'? A note on 'the changing sociological construct of the family'. *The Sociological Review, 36,* 267–272.

Berniell, L., de la Mata, D. & Valdés, N. (2013). Spillovers of health education at school on parents' physical activity. *Health Economics, 22,* 1004–1020.

Bevan, A. & Reilly, S. (2011). Mothers' efforts to promote healthy nutrition and physical activity for their preschool children. *Journal of Pediatric Nursing, 26,* 395–403.

Bois, J., Sarrazin, P., Brustad, R., Trouilloud, D. & Cury, F. (2005). Elementary schoolchildren's perceived competence and physical activity involvement: The influence of parents' role modelling behaviours and perceptions of their child's competence. *Psychology of Sport and Exercise, 6,* 381–397.

Chambers, D. (2012). *A sociology of family life: Change and diversity in intimate relations.* Cambridge: Polity Press.

Cheal, D. (2002). *Sociology of family life.* Basingstoke: Palgrave Macmillan.

Department of Health (2011). *Start active, stay active: A report on physical activity for health from the four home countries' Chief Medical Officers.* London: Crown Copyright.

Dwyer, G., Higgs, J., Hardy, L. & Baur, L. (2008). What do parents and preschool staff tell us about young children's physical activity: A qualitative study. *International Journal of Behavioral Nutrition and Physical Activity, 5,* 66.

Edwards, R. & Weller, S. (2014). Sibling relationships and the construction of young people's gendered identities over time and in different spaces. *Families, Relationships and Societies, 3,* 185–199.

Edwardson, C. & Gorely, T. (2010). Parental influences on different types and intensities of physical activity in youth: A systematic review. *Psychology of Sport and Exercise, 11,* 522–535.

Eriksson, M., Nordqvist, T. & Rasmussen, F. (2008). Associations between parents' and 12-year-old children's sport and vigorous activity: The role of self-esteem and athletic competence. *Journal of Physical Activity and Health, 5,* 359–373.

Evans, J. & Davies, B. (2010). Family, class and embodiment: Why school physical education makes so little difference to post-school participation patterns in physical activity. *International Journal of Qualitative Studies in Education, 23,* 765–784.

Faircloth, C. (2014). Intensive parenting and the expansion of parenting. In E. Lee, J. Bristow, C. Faircloth & J. Macvarish (Eds.), *Parenting culture studies* (pp. 25–50). Basingstoke: Palgrave Macmillan.

Giddens, A. (1992). *The transformation of intimacy: Sexuality, love and eroticism in modern societies.* Cambridge: Polity Press.

Gorely, T., Atkin, A., Biddle, S. & Marshall, S. (2009). Family circumstance, sedentary behaviour and physical activity in adolescents living in England: project STIL. *International Journal of Behavioral Nutrition and Physical Activity, 6,* 33.

Gustafson, S. & Rhodes, R. (2006). Parental correlates of physical activity in children and early adolescents. *Sports Med, 36,* 79–97.

Hamilton, K. & White, K. (2010). Understanding parental physical activity: Meanings, habits and social role influence. *Psychology of Sport and Exercise, 11,* 275–285.

Hamilton, K. & White, K. (2012). Social influences and the physical activity intentions of parents of young-children families: An extended theory of planned behavior approach. *Journal of Family Issues, 33,* 1351–1372.

Harrington, M. (2006). Sport and leisure as contexts for fathering in Australian families. *Leisure Studies, 25,* 165–183.

Hart, K., Herriot, A., Bishop, J. & Truby, H. (2003). Promoting healthy diet and exercise patterns amongst primary school children: A qualitative investigation of parental perspectives. *Journal of Human Nutrition and Dietetics, 16,* 89–96.

Hesketh, K., Crawford, D. & Salmon, J. (2006). Children's television viewing and objectively measured physical activity: Associations with family circumstance. *International Journal of Behavioral Nutrition and Physical Activity, 3*, 36.

Hesketh, K., Graham, M. & Waters, E. (2008). Children's after-school activity: Associations with weight status and family circumstance. *Pediatric Exercise Science, 20*, 84–94.

Hesketh, K., Hinkley, T. & Campbell, K. (2012). Children's physical activity and screen time: qualitative comparison of views of parents of infants and preschool children. *International Journal of Behavioral Nutrition and Physical Activity, 9*, 152.

Jamieson, L. (1998). *Intimacy: Personal relationships in modern societies*. Cambridge: Polity Press.

Kay, T. (2007). Fathering through sport. *World Leisure Journal, 49*, 69–82.

Layard, R. (2011). *Happiness: Lessons from a new science* (2nd ed.). London: Penguin Books.

Lewis, B. & Ridge, D. (2005). Mothers reframing physical activity: Family oriented politicism, transgression and contested expertise in Australia. *Social Science and Medicine, 60*, 2295–2306.

Lim, C. & Biddle, S. (2012). Longitudinal and prospective studies of parental correlates of physical activity in young people: A systematic review. *International Journal of Sport and Exercise Psychology, 10*, 211–220.

Macdonald, D., Rodger, S., Ziviani, J., Jenkins, D., Batch, J. & Jones, J. (2004). Physical activity as a dimension of family life for lower primary school children. *Sport, Education and Society, 9*, 307–325.

Office for National Statistics (2015). *Families and households, 2014: Statistical bulletin*. London: Crown Copyright.

Ornelas, I., Perreira, K. & Ayala, G. (2007). Parental influences on adolescent physical activity: A longitudinal study. *International Journal of Behavioral Nutrition and Physical Activity, 4*, 3.

Pugliese, J. & Tinsley, B. (2007). Parental socialization of child and adolescent physical activity: A meta-analysis. *Journal of Family Psychology, 21*, 331–343.

Quarmby, T. & Dagkas, S. (2010). Children's engagement in leisure time physical activity: Exploring family structure as a determinant. *Leisure Studies, 29*, 53–66.

Quarmby, T. & Dagkas, S. (2013). Locating the place and meaning of physical activity in the lives of young people from low-income, lone-parent families. *Physical Education and Sport Pedagogy, 18*, 459–474.

Ramanathan, S. & Crocker, P. (2009). The influence of family and culture on physical activity among female adolescents from the Indian Diaspora. *Qualitative Health Research, 19*, 492–503.

Ruseski, J., Humphreys, B., Hallmann, K. & Breuer, C. (2011). Family structure, time constraints, and sport participation. *European Reviews of Aging and Physical Activity, 8*, 57–66.

Thompson, J., Jago, R., Brockman, R., Cartwright, K., Page, A. & Fox, K. (2009). Physically active families – de-bunking the myth? A qualitative study of family participation in physical activity. *Child: Care, Health and Development, 36*, 265–274.

Weed, M. (2016). Evidence for physical activity guidelines as a public health intervention: Efficacy, effectiveness, and harm – A critical policy sciences approach. *Health Psychology and Behavioral Medicine, 4*, 56–69.

Wellard, I. (2014). *Sport, fun and enjoyment: An embodied approach*. London: Routledge.

Wilson, P. & Pahl, R. (1988). The changing sociological construct of the family. *The Sociological Review, 36*, 233–266.

Zecevic, C., Tremblay, L., Lovsin, T. & Michel, L. (2010). Parental influence on young children's physical activity. *International Journal of Pediatrics, 468526*. doi:10.1155/2010/468526.

Ziviani, J., Macdonald, D., Ward, H., Jenkins, D. & Rodger, S. (2006). Physical activity and the occupations of children: Perspectives of parents and children. *Journal of Occupational Science, 13*, 180–187.

22

WORKPLACE PHYSICAL ACTIVITY

Theory, policy and practice

David McGillivray

Introduction

Wellness discourses have become increasingly influential in recent years, particularly in advanced Western societies. Lupton (2014) argues that the movements of human bodies are increasingly monitored, assessed and predicted by digital technologies. Mobile technologies in the form of smartphones, smartwatches, tablet computers and digital self-tracking devices generate endless data about fitness and broader health-related outputs. In this sense, people have become data-emitting nodes, leading to a focus on tracking the self, quantifying performance as part of a calculative rationality that renders the individual in a state of wellness or in need of remedial attention.

In a workplace context, the incursion of wellness narratives is also prevalent, but more difficult to assess in terms of reach, intended outcomes and associated practices. At the level of policy, governments (local and national) now frequently promote the workplace as a site for health promotional activity and national health agencies stress the clinical (and business) benefits of promoting physical activity in the workplace (NICE, 2008, 2015). There is a growing evidence base to suggest that organisational wellness practice (McGillivray, 2005a and b) has permeated the workplace in advanced liberal democracies over the course of the last thirty years but, crucially for this chapter, its form and focus has changed significantly in this time. In this chapter I document the changing emphasis of wellness programmes from their original recreational and social function in the late nineteenth century, to a more explicit health and wellness agenda from the late 1970s onwards. I theorise this shift by building on the work of Michel Foucault (1977, 1978, 1986) and the ideas of governmentality and the subject central to his so-called 'later' period (Moss, 1998). I then draw on policy and practice examples to illustrate current thinking on the role of the workplace as a site for physical activity, before concluding with some implications for future (workplace) physical activity policy and practice. Whilst readers of this book might primarily be interested in finding out 'what works' in relation to physical activity interventions in the workplace, I deliberately locate discussions about organisational wellness in a critical theoretical framework because it is important that readers know about the 'why', as much as 'how' or 'what' associated with these interventions.

Historical perspectives of the workplace as a site for physical activity

In the late 1990s and early 2000s, there was a noticeable increase in the number of academic articles concerned with workplace health promotion, worksite wellness or recreation at work (Atkinson, 2001; Connell and Grainger, 2002; Dishman, Oldenburg, O'Neal and Shephard, 1998; Foley, Maxwell and McGillivray, 2000; Grant and Brisbin, 1992; Grundemann and van Vuuren, 1997; Springett and Dugdill, 1995). I've used the term organisational wellness in my own work to describe the healthy-lifestyle activities promoted by organisations including smoking and alcohol cessation programmes and health eating policies. In this chapter I focus on those activities that can be categorised as involving physical activity available *in* the workplace or facilitated *through* the work organisation.

The workplace has been considered a legitimate space for physical activity interventions for more than two centuries. As early as the seventeenth century, in the UK, with the Clyde shipbuilders (Burton, 1994) and Lanarkshire miners (Campbell, 1979), evidence of employer-sponsored recreational provision was apparent. However, it was during the period of industrial capitalism that paternalistic industrialists started to invest time and resource in providing recreational opportunities for their employees in, or connected to, their workplace. For these employers (e.g. Cadbury's, Rowntrees, Robert Owen), workplace *recreation* provision was a reaction to the emergent middling (or meddling) classes' public health concerns about the mass of workers emerging from rural poverty (Bailey, 1978). Crucially, decisions on 'appropriate' workplace recreational activities were made within a moral framework of Rational Recreation – contrasted with the traditional past-times of the urban working classes. As Holliday and Thompson (2001) have argued, capitalists of this time were concerned with controlling and disciplining unruly working bodies, sugarcoated with a concern for the moral and physical health of workers and delivered through the provision of parklands, public baths, gardens and, latterly, recreational sports teams. Instilling good (moral) habits – inside and outside of work – was of primary concern for employers as they sought to exert influence on workers' behaviour, 'establishing links between the workplace, the home and the cultural milieu' (Rose, 1990: 63). However, although 'health' and 'wellness' in its broadest sense was a feature of the activities of these industrialists, 'health enhancement was neither the primary aim nor outcome' (McGillivray, 2005b: 129). Instead, the focus of investment was on the collective and social dimensions of workplace recreation. As a result, these investments were rarely the subject of an in-depth appraisal of impact, on the 'return' of investment so prevalent in discussions of corporate investments in the contemporary period. Rather, for paternalistic employers, these investments were considered, theoretically, to be the right things to do to create collective solidarity and to foster loyal and committed employees (Moorhouse, 1989).

However, two decades ago, a dramatic shift took place in the way organisations viewed the provision of sites and spaces for physical activity in the North America and the UK which brought about a change in the organisational landscape (Griffiths, 1996: 2):

> by the mid 1970s industrial sports and social clubs had become more commonplace . . . however . . . in North America, a change of emphasis from leisure to fitness programmes in such clubs began to take place in the 1980s . . . rather than helping employees play sports within the social club context, North American employers became increasingly concerned about promoting employee fitness . . . this pattern was followed in the UK.

The creation of workplace sports teams and the maintenance of playing fields to accommodate these activities ceased to be a prevalent feature of workplace provision from the 1980s onwards. Instead, partly as an outcome of the cult of health and fitness that can be traced back to the late 1970s and early 1980s, in the last three decades, we have witnessed a significant shift in discourse from collective solidarity to a focus on what I term the 'project of the self', building on the work of Michel Foucault. There are a number of important features of this shift for how we understand and assess workplace physical activity interventions in the contemporary period. There is both a discursive and a material shift in the emergence of the language of health and fitness, wellness and the body as a target of interventions evidenced by a sizeable growth in the number of organisations providing some sort of programme designed to facilitate the modification of employees' lifestyle behaviour (Chu et al., 2000). Theoretically, at this time it was assumed that investment in holistic organisational wellness initiatives would enhance organisational productivity (Townley, 1994; Holliday and Thompson, 2001) by targeting individual lifestyle behaviours.

Governmentality and the project of the 'fit' (working) self

Conceptually, it is worth drawing on the work of Michel Foucault to help make sense of these emergent discourses of organisational wellness, and workplace physical activity specifically. Foucault's work has been applied extensively in the organisational studies terrain in recent years, especially his writings on governmentality (Moss, 1998). This work extends his analysis of power, focusing less on its (external) disciplinary tendencies, to consider the practices of self-subjectification and technologies of the self. The concept of governmentality refers to the management of populations at both the societal (macro) and individual (micro) levels, linked by an 'overarching rationale of management' (Jackson and Carter, 1998: 49). Taken in the context of organisational wellness, I have been interested for some time in 'the extent to which particular dominant organisational discourses constitute subject positions and how the knowing subject may reflexively interpret and resist particular contingent organisational truths' (McGillivray, 2005b: 127). Here, following Jackson and Carter (1998), I'm interested in how prevailing subject positions (i.e. of the active, healthy worker) are discursively produced, which requires consideration of discourses of resistance and the imperfections of power as much as those that contend that subjects are the *product* of disciplinary power. So, whilst not denying that normalising truths forged around wellness exist, constituting workplace subjects, I'm interested in exploring how local discursivities might also operate. A good place to start is to consider the way a health and fitness discursive formation came to exist and be viewed as a legitimate claim to truth within the work context.

Fitter, happier, more productive workers? Policy pronouncements

When thinking about governmentality, it is crucial to consider the management of populations at both the societal (macro) level as well as the experiences of workplaces and employees themselves. I contend that, since the early 1990s, the workplace has been reconceptualised as a site where 'particular truths and logics about healthy living' (Fullager, 2002: 70) are communicated, especially in the developed western economies where concerns over rising healthcare costs are most pronounced. Workplaces, along with schools and other settings described elsewhere in this book, have been identified and policy prescriptions made to ensure they take on some of the 'burden' of educating the populace in the merits of preventative health interventions.

In terms of policy, in the UK there is a mixed picture in terms of who has responsibility for the workplace arena as a site for the promotion of healthy working lives and the efficacy of these interventions. Numerous health promotion campaigns exist to encourage (and incentivise) employers to embed the promotion of physical activity and associated practices in their operations. In Scotland, there is a dedicated Centre, part of NHS Scotland and funded by the Scottish Government. The Scottish Centre for Healthy Working Lives has been in operation since 1999 and targets mainly those organisations that lack the financial or human resources to invest in the health and fitness and wellness facilities described earlier in this chapter. They work with small and medium sized enterprises (SMEs) to provide support through a network of advisers based across the 14 health boards in Scotland. Although the work of the Centre also includes health and safety advice, being located in the NHS arena, there is an important symbolic emphasis on promoting the improved health of workers, further reinforced in the way they work with employers to register and gain recognition under the Healthy Working Lives Award scheme. Participating companies can secure either Bronze, Silver or Gold awards depending upon their alignment with good practice in providing their employees with an environment (including the provision of physical activity) that promotes health and safety and, crucially, health promotion. The initiative claims that a healthier workforce makes for a healthier business and the benefits listed for engagement with the programme include enhanced reputational capital, reductions in the costs of sickness absence, improved attendance rates, a healthier, more motivated and productive workforce and controlling insurance costs.

Across the rest of the UK there is no equivalent body to the Scottish Centre for Healthy Working Lives. That said, in England, the Workplace Wellbeing Charter is a close equivalent scheme that, though voluntary, provides a framework through which companies can demonstrate their commitment to the health of the people that work for them. Like the Healthy Working Lives Award scheme in Scotland, companies can register and be awarded one of three award categories. A 'Commitment Award' recognises the standards all organisations should meet, putting the building blocks in place. An 'Achievement Award' recognises activity encouraging positive lifestyle choices and addressing health issues, and an 'Excellence Award' recognises fully engaged leadership with a range of programmes and support mechanisms. Again, like Scotland's Centre for Healthy Working Lives, the Workplace Wellbeing Charter is designed to encourage organisations to audit and benchmark themselves against legal (mainly around health and safety) and established standards, help and advise in designing and implementing strategies and plans suitable for the size of the organisation and, finally, the national recognition accruable from possession of an award.

Building on the work of the Workplace Wellbeing Charter, recently the NHS in England has launched a major initiative with £5 million investment to improve the health and wellbeing of its 1.3 million health service staff. Like the other policy developments discussed here, the three pillar strategy seeks to highlight how 'NHS organisations will be supported to help their staff to stay well, including serving healthier food, promoting physical activity, reducing stress, and providing health checks covering mental health and musculoskeletal problems' (NHS, 2015). As the Chief Executive stressed, when launching the new initiative:

> When it comes to supporting the health of our own workforce, frankly the NHS needs to put its own house in order . . . At a time when arguably the biggest operational challenge facing hospitals is converting overspends on temporary agency staff into attractive flexible permanent posts, creating healthy and supportive workplaces is no longer a nice to have, it's a must-do.
>
> *NHS, 2015*

Six actions have been agreed to, including establishing and promoting a local physical activity 'offer' to staff, such as running yoga classes, Zumba classes or competitive sports teams, and promoting healthy travel to work by offering the Cycle to Work scheme. Beyond government and the NHS, the National Institute for Health and Care Excellence (NICE) also provides advice on the importance of the workplace as a site for health promotional activities, including specific advice for employers on the 'business case' for developing policies and plans for the promotion of physical activity within and outside of the workplace. Like the macro-governmental rhetoric around the value of workplace health promotion and organisational wellness, NICE also emphasises the benefits associated with reduced sickness absence, increased loyalty and better staff retention from an investment (in time and resources). NICE also generated guidelines on *Physical Activity in the Workplace* in 2008 and have also recently produced a quality standard for *Physical activity: For NHS staff, patients and carers* (2015).

It is clear that the self-management of risk is now implicated in the economic rationales of private companies (Petersen, 1997) and there is a sense of 'offloading' of responsibility from state to private individuals and other formal and informal structures including work organisations (Jackson and Carter, 1998). More recently, research from the New Economics Foundation (Jeffrey, Mahony, Michaelson and Abdallah, 2014) suggests there is strong evidence of a positive association between good health and wellbeing and that the workplace can play an important role in encouraging physical activity. They go on to suggest that:

> employers should not just help employees avoid ill-health but should support their achievement of good health, by increasing physical activity . . . there are several interventions that employers can take to encourage an ethos of taking regular physical activity at work. This might include sponsored teams of staff to take part in organized walks, runs or cycles; facilitating in-house group exercise sessions, such as lunchtime yoga; participation in schemes that grant employees tax relief on buying a bike . . . or simply encouraging staff to take breaks during the day, during which they can engage in physical activities.
>
> *p. 19*

Whilst work organisations are increasingly likely to be considered part of the wider healthcare solution, the focus on physical activity interventions at work and a health promotion logic aligns closely with what Rose (1993: 3) views as a feature of neo-liberalised governance, which 'embraces the ways in which one might be urged and educated to bridle one's own passions, to control one's own instincts, to govern oneself' (ibid.). It is in the realm of health promotion that workplaces are considered suitable settings for the communication of good habits, as they take on functions outside of their core business (Chu et al., 2000). As I've already argued, this is not a new phenomenon, but over the last two decades there is ample evidence of the intensification in organisational wellness activity – illustrated by the case of Nuffield Health detailed in the practice case in the latter part of this chapter. In some large organisations (the Royal Bank of Scotland HQ provides a good example), the workplace is beginning to mimic a 'surrogate surgery' (McGillivray, 2005b), with not only a range of high-specification health and fitness equipment and activities, but health clinics staffed by medical professionals found on site. Here, discourses of organisational wellness are increasingly legitimated (Foucault, 1980) because of the medicalisation of everyday life. Workers voluntarily sign up to be subject to the medical gaze, willingly accepting their prescriptions to exercise more or eat more healthy food. Whilst the very presence of the wellness programme carries with it a presumed 'good', it is the 'active consent and subjugation of subjects, rather than their oppression, domination or external control' (Clegg, Pitsis, Rura-Polley and Marosszeky, 2002: 317) that is worthy of further scrutiny.

As others have suggested, health promotion logic is based on societal regulation or health risks, alongside self-surveillance, placing the individual in a position of responsibility *vis-à-vis* their own health and wellbeing (Lupton, 2014). Again, we can see governmentality in operation here with 'a subtle, comprehensive management of life drawing both from a top-down exercise of power over conduct . . . with a subjectivity constituted in a sense of personal responsibilities, rights, freedoms and dependencies' (Fox, 1993: 32). As healthcare providers, corporate fitness companies and others come to invade work contexts, so the separation of public and private, worker and patient, becomes more difficult to sustain. The workplace extends its jurisdiction over the lives of its employees.

It is not the intention of this chapter to suggest that all employees are expected to participate in health and fitness or 'body work' (Hancock and Tyler, 2000) whilst at work, or facilitated by their organisation. In reality, relatively few companies can afford to build shiny onsite fitness suites, swimming pools or develop a set of running trails around their workplaces. Yet, there is a growing body of literature suggesting that demonstrating 'disciplinary self improvement' (Petersen, 1997: 198) does carry with it a positive set of connotations in workplaces, whereby in some occupational settings a professional body is also a fit body (Trethewey, 1999) communicating values associated with self discipline, responsibility and willingness to work. Some organisations clearly trade on their employees' aesthetic labour and there is a clearer association between their core business and the demands of a healthy, fit working body (e.g. personal trainers). Yet, those organisations that need no fit and sculpted employees still invest in wellness facilities and activities, or they seek the support of others to design and plan policies for physical activity in the workplace.

Some commentators (e.g. Holliday and Thompson, 2001, Conrad and Walsh, 1992) decry the trend towards the extension of wellness concerns outside of the workplace and into the previously sacrosanct lives of their employees. Health promotional discourses encourage the subtle, comprehensive management of life whether in or outside of the workplace. Participation in health at work schemes provides an avenue for employers to influence the behaviour of their employees as they are provided with free skin caliper readings, weight management tips and the like. Lifestyle incorrectness (Leichter, 1997) is identified in the workplace and remedial action prescribed for the employees' private life. The intensification of wellness discourses illustrates a more generalised omnipresent gaze over the conduct of individuals' lives, where health (and by definition, ill health) is an always-present consideration.

Barriers to workplace physical activity: Resistance at/in work

We have to be careful not to view this extension of wellness discourse as some sort of *fait accompli*. In fact, as I have argued elsewhere, 'there is evidence available to suggest that the employee reception of organisational wellness initiatives is not wholly docile and passive' (McGillivray, 2005b: 133). Contestation, conflict and resistance are, in fact, ever present (as Foucault suggested in his later work) so that the subject cannot be considered a product of the exercise of power. Instead, 'resistance is never in a position of exteriority in relation to power' (Foucault, 1978: 95). As we know from other sites and settings where physical activity is promoted, participation profiles are not uniform or consistent. Contextual factors associated with income, locality, familiarity and social status impact on participation statistics. The same issues confront those proponents of organisational wellness, including the promotion of physical activity interventions in the workplace. Although discourses of organisational wellness align closely with a trend towards enabling individuals to 'make the right choice', this narrative is not recognised by a significant proportion of the workforce in many organisations. The 'powerful norms about what is good and bad; 'healthy' or 'unhealthy'; acceptable or unacceptable; desireable or undesireable' (Duncan and Cribb, 1996: 346) do not result in uniform participation rates across the workforce. In my own previous research, I found that, 'employees bring a project of the self, fostered elsewhere, with them to their work environments' (McGillivray, 2005b: 133) meaning that they responded in different ways to 'external discourses and strategies that attempt to discipline them' (Lupton, 1997: 103).

As with the prevailing literature around physical activity participation, there are some individuals predisposed to invest in their physical capital, and the opportunity to participate at the workplace represents a significant benefit, as they would 'have been mobilising their bodies elsewhere anyway' (McGillivray, 2005b: 134). However, there are also employees who only want to participate in physical activity outside of work, to maintain a clear separation between work and non-work, and those that reject participation discourses outright. For those interested in increasing engagement with and participation in workplace physical activity interventions existing subject positions create both a threat and an opportunity. For the employee that has 'fully assimilated the discourses of wellness and practices a calculable, disciplined and ascetic lifestyle' (McGillivray, 2005b: 134) awareness raising and behavioural change interventions are unlikely to be necessary. They have already bought into the benefits of regular physical activity and provision of facilities and activities either free or at a heavily discounted rate will be viewed as a significant benefit. These individuals are already likely to be accruing distinction from their adherence to health and fitness regimes (Frew and McGillivray, 2005). Those in a transient position, at the contemplation stage in the stages of change model (Prochaska and DiClemente, 1983), are perhaps most open to workplace physical activity promotional information and associated policies and plans. To put it another way, they are listening, weighing up the benefits and the dis-benefits of participation. They can be persuaded to put their decisions into practice or action. At the other end of the spectrum, however, sits the non-participant (or non-user), in the stage of pre-contemplation, expressing passivity towards healthy lifestyle discourses and unwilling or unable to contemplate changing their lifestyle. The non-participant becomes the target of wellness initiatives to initiate change in the 'unproductive' or 'absent' body, subject to hierarchical surveillance and normalising judgment (McGillivray, 2005b: 134).

However, those occupying a pre-contemplation stage related to physical activity participation will also respond to different cues in terms of what motivates them to get involved, whether in a workplace setting or outside of it. As Miller and Rollnick, (1991) have suggested, 'different skills are needed' at 'different stages of readiness for change' (p15). This is why it is important for those charged with the responsibility to encourage companies to play a part in the preventative health project to recognise that employees, like the general population, bring their own subject positions to bear when making choices around participation. In the industrial era, some companies had welfare inspectors who actively intervened in the lives of workers to ensure compliance with puritanical discourses around health (for work); now each individual employee is constituted as being responsible for his or her health and wellbeing.

In some workplaces there have been attempts to address the perception of an invasive organisational gaze and the limitations of prescriptive policies and programmes by co-opting work colleagues as mentors or 'champions' to help promote physical activity. For example, Edmunds and Clow's (2015) research suggests that peer health champions might play an important role in promoting healthy behaviours such as physical activity. Their research found that peer physical activity champions (PPACs) providing direct encouragement and facilitation of wider physical activity supportive social networks within the workplace encouraged behaviour change. Crucially, they found that the PPACs had to provide enthusiastic and persistent encouragement without seeming judgmental. They also conclude that PPACs were deemed acceptable by employees targeted in workplace physical activity programmes but that they need training in managing the sensitivities involved in talking to colleagues about increasing their physical activity and in creating social connections that were valuable in sustaining participation. These findings align closely with NICE's (2008, 2015) advice for the promotion of physical activity in workplaces, where it stresses the importance of being flexible and non-threatening in the action taken. Specifically, NICE suggests an emphasis on accessible physical activity, encourage employees to walk, cycle or use other modes of transport involving physical activity to travel to and from work and as part of their working day accompanied by the dissemination and on-going advice on how to be more physically active and on the health benefits of such activity – including information on local opportunities to be physically active (both within and outside the workplace) tailored to meet specific needs. NICE guidelines are built on the idea that to reach those most at risk from disease associated with the absence of physical activity, voluntary participation in programmes with a low threshold for involvement is necessary.

However, although these guidelines, whether in Scotland, England or via organisations like NICE exist and are part of promotional activity, other than for Health and Safety at Work, there remains no legal obligation for companies to promote health at work. Furthermore, critics argue that the absence of any form of tax incentives to encourage workplaces to commit resources to the promotion of healthy working lives means that only the most enlightened employers will invest in coordinated, strategically embedded schemes. The workplace as a setting for the promotion of physical activity makes sense at a theoretical level, but, in practice, there are numerous obstacles to effective implementation. This is reinforced by recent research from Malik, Blake and Suggs (2014). They conducted a systematic review of workplace physical activity interventions published since 2011 (n=58) and found that though there was evidence that workplace physical activity interventions can be efficacious, many of the studies were inconclusive, especially in terms of the effectiveness of workplace interventions for increasing physical activity and in identifying the *types* of interventions that show the most promise.

A practice perspective: Nuffield Health

So, whilst in theory it appears that workplace physical activity interventions *should* be efficacious with a large, captive audience, supportive policy pronouncements and the macro context of increasing costs associated with sickness absence, there is little evidence in practice of significant gains or successes. In this final section, I highlight the example of an organisation that has invested time and resources in the corporate side of the wellness industry, focusing on interventions across the individual's lifeworld. Nuffield Health is an organisation that has transformed itself from a private health provider focused on hospitals to one that extends its reach into workplaces, educational settings and other sites, taking with it a message of wellness in all its forms. As the company website states, 'your health is at the centre of everything we do. Whether you need prevention or cure, are looking to run your first mile or your first marathon, we want to work with you to ensure your health allows you to lead the life you want' (Nuffield Health, 2015). Nuffield Health has both helped bring about, and become one of the principal beneficiaries, of the reconceptualisation of the workplace as a site for physical activity (and wider health promotional) messages. It has an extensive portfolio of corporate health and fitness facilities operated for large companies as well as a healthy workplace corporate membership clientele using its gyms around the UK. It has recently secured the contract to create a large corporate fitness facility for UBS, the Swiss global financial services company which will include a 100+ gym station and two fitness studios, holding up to 100 classes every week. Like other corporate health and fitness providers in the marketplace, Nuffield Health utilises the evidence base provided by NICE to highlight that workplace illness and absenteeism is a significant cost to business. They position themselves as being able to help companies to build a 'corporate wellbeing' programme that 'actively reduces your employees' health risks, improves quality of life both at work and home, and delivers a tangible benefit to your organisation's bottom line' (Nuffield Health, 2015).

Whilst the company represents a good example of the organisational wellness movement generating corporate opportunities, Nuffield Health is a particularly interesting case because its pitch to clients is that it extends beyond the workplace as a setting to promote health into everyday life. For example, it has developed a mobile application, Nuffield HealthScore, that 'allows your employees to monitor their personal health and to track their progress towards their goals' (Nuffield Health, 2015). Fox (2015, p13) has recently expressed concern over the increasing prevalence of Personal Health Technologies (PHTs), arguing that a

> health app on a mobile phone monetises health and fitness, establishing both a quantified body that competes with others or with itself and a means to further corporatise and monetise daily health activities by gathering data and targeting users for future marketing.

Clearly, for organisations in the corporate healthcare marketplace PHTs like the HealthScore application provide a route into the personal lives of employees. Through engagement with the workplace setting, organisations like Nuffield generate new market possibilities taking employees from a workplace scheme to a more general customer. In the case of Nuffield Health (but by no means the only company operating in this space) there is a strategic imperative to exploit one part of the organisation's core business to benefit the other. So, the corporate wellbeing offer enables access to individuals who may become lifetime customers of the health and fitness business, the hospital or the health clinic. In this sense, these processes reinforce, and extend, an individualising, biomedicalised model of health and illness (Lupton, 2014) subjecting employees to a medical gaze that defines them as individual bodies rather than as parts of social assemblages (Fox, 2015).

Conclusion

In this chapter I've provided a summary of the changes in the purpose and role of workplace physical activity interventions, historically. I've suggested that over the last fifty years, socially-focused, collective leisure and sporting pursuits were replaced with a focus on the 'project of the self', a discursive and a material shift in the emergence of the language of health and fitness, wellness and the body as a target of interventions in (and outside of) the workplace. This shift has led to a greater emphasis being placed on healthy lifestyle improvement policies and practices being promoted by governments and, simultaneously, by a growing (commercial) wellness industry. However, whilst in theory the workplace is an ideal site for physical activity interventions to take place, in practice there is a need to recognise that pre-existing barriers to participation in non-work settings are equally, if not more, difficult to overcome. Individuals bring an existing subject position towards physical activity to their workplace and the evidence available suggests that there is some way to go before those employees most at risk from health-related diseases will view their workplace as a preferable setting for body work.

Implications for future physical activity policy and practice

First, there is a need to better understand the subject positions with which employees arrive at their work if interventions related to physical activity are to be designed effectively and prove efficacious in terms of increasing participation in physical activity, especially for those most 'at risk'. The voluntary nature of advice relating to the workplace as a site for physical activity interventions means that there is a greater need for policy makers and practitioners to generate a robust evidence base for the efficacy of these programmes – otherwise many smaller and medium size employers will simply disregard the opportunity.

Second, macro-level strategies to address societal health need to align with micro-level practices, including resistance to healthy lifestyle messages if they are to be effective at bringing about sustainable change in the behaviour of employees. The workplace is only one element of the physical activity provision in local communities. There is a need for a more holistic, joined up approach to the promotion of physical activity that could lead to some workplaces being opened up for community use and, at the same time, more opportunities for local employers to secure preferential terms to encourage their employees to use local facilities.

References

Atkinson, W. (2001) Is a wellness incentive money well spent?, *Business and Health*, 19 (50), 23–27.

Bailey, P. (1978) *Leisure and class in Victorian England: rational recreation and the contest for control, 1830–1885*, London: Routledge and Kegan Paul.

Burton, A. (1994) *The rise and fall of British shipbuilding*, London: Constable.

Campbell, Alan B. (1979) *The Lanarkshire miners—A social history*, Edinburgh: J. Donald Publishers.

Chu, C., Breucker, G., Harris, N., Stitzel, A., Gan, X., Gu, X., and Dwyer, S. (2000) Health-promoting workplaces—International settings development, *Health Promotion International*, 15 (2), 155–167.

Clegg, S., Pitsis, T.S., Rura-Polley, and Marosszeky, M. (2002) Governmentality matters: Designing an alliance culture of inter-organizational collaboration for managing projects, *Organization Studies*, 23 (3), 317–337.

Connell, J., and Grainger, S. (2002) Exploring attitudes to corporate fitness in Jersey: Employer and employee perspectives, *Managing Leisure*, 7, 176–193.

Conrad, P., and Walsh, D. C. (1992) The new corporate health ethic: Lifestyle and the social control of work, *International Journal of Health Services*, 22 (1), 89–111.

Dishman, R.K., Oldenburg, B., O'Neal, H., and Shephard, R.J. (1998) Worksite physical activity interventions, *American Journal of Preventative Medicine*, 15 (4), 344–361.

Duncan, P., and Cribb, A. (1996) Helping people change—An ethical approach?, *Health Education Research*, 11 (3), 339–348.

Edmunds, S., and Clow, A. (2015) The role of peer physical activity champions in the workplace: A qualitative study, *Public, Environmental and Occupational Health*, Published online before print, September 16, 2015, doi:10.1177/1757913915600741.

Foley, M., Maxwell, G., and McGillivray, D. (2000) UK workplace fitness provision and women: Missing opportunities?, *World Leisure*, 42 (4), 14–23.

Foucault, M. (1977) *Discipline and punish: The birth of the prison*, New York: Pantheon Books.

Foucault, M. (1978) *The history of sexuality, volume 1: An introduction*, New York: Pantheon Books.

Foucault, M. (1980) *Power/knowledge: Selected interviews and other writings 1972–1977* (trans. C. Gordon), Brighton: Harvester.

Foucault, M. (1986) *The care of the self: The history of sexuality, Volume 3*, New York: Pantheon.

Fox, N.J. (1993) *Postmodernism, sociology and health*, Buckingham: Open University Press.

Fox, N.J. (2015) Personal health technologies, micropolitics and resistance: A new materialist analysis, *Health*, Published online before print July 27, 2015, doi: 10.1177/1363459315590248.

Frew, M., and McGillivray, D. (2005) Health and fitness clubs and body politics: Aesthetics and the promotion of physical capital, *Leisure Studies*, 24 (2), 161–175.

Fullager, S. (2002) Governing the healthy body: Discourses of leisure and lifestyle within Australian Health Policy, *Health: An Interdisciplinary Journal for the Social Study of Health, Illness and Medicine*, 6 (1), 69–84.

Grant, C.B., and Brisbin, R.E. (1992) *Workplace wellness: The key to higher productivity and lower health costs*, New York: Van nostrand Reinhold.

Griffiths, A. (1996) The benefits of employee exercise programmes: A review, *Work and Stress*, 10 (1), 5–23.

Grundemann, R.W.M., and van Vuuren, C.V. (1997) *Preventing absenteeism at the workplace: European research report*, Dublin: European Foundation for the Improvement of Living and Working Conditions, p. 195.

Hancock, P., and Tyler, M. (2000) Working bodies, in: P. Hancock, B. Hughes, L. Jagger, K. Paterson, R. Russell, E. Tulle-Winton, and M. Tyler (Eds) *The body, culture and society: An introduction*, pp. 84–100, Buckingham: Open University Press.

Holliday, R., and Thompson, G. (2001) A body of work, in: R. Holliday and J. Hassard (Eds) *Contested bodies*, pp.117–134, London: Routledge.

Jackson, N., and Carter, P. (1998) Labour as dressage, in: A. McKinlay and K. Starkey (Eds) *Foucault, management and organization theory*, pp. 49–64, London: Sage.

Jeffrey, K., Mahony, S., Michaelson. J., and Abdallah, S. (2014) *Well-being at work: A review of the literature*, New Economic Foundation.

Leichter, H.M. (1997) Lifestyle correctness and the new secular morality, in: A.M. Brandt and P. Rozin (Eds) *Morality and health*, London: Routledge, pp. 359–378.

Lupton, D (1997) Foucault and the medicalisation critique, in: A. Petersen and R. Bunton (Eds) *Foucault health and medicine*, pp. 94–112, London: Routledge.

Lupton D (2014) Health promotion in the digital era: A critical commentary. *Health Promotion International*. Epub ahead of print 15 October. DOI: 10.1093/heapro/dau091.

Malik, S.H., Blake, H., and Suggs, L.S. (2014) A systematic review of workplace health promotion interventions for increasing physical activity, *British Journal of Health Psychology*, 19 (1), 149–180.

McGillivray, D (2005a) Governing working bodies through leisure: A genealogical analysis, *Leisure Sciences*, 27 (3), 315–330.

McGillivray, D (2005b) Fitter, happier, more productive: Governing working bodies through wellness, *Culture and Organisation*, 11 (2), 125–138.

Miller, W. R., and Rollnick, S. (1991) *Motivational interviewing: Preparing people to change addictive behaviour*, London: The Guildford Press.

Moorhouse, H.F. (1989) Models of work, models of leisure, in: C. Rojek (Ed.) *Leisure for leisure*, pp. 15–35, London: Macmillan

Moss, J., (ed.) (1998) *The later Foucault: Politics and philosophy*, London: Sage.

NHS (2015) Simon Stevens announces major drive to improve health in NHS workplace www.england.nhs.uk/2015/09/nhs-workplace/ (accessed 31/04/2016).

NICE (2008) *Physical activity in the workplace: Workplace guideline* (May, 2008), Manchester: National Institute for Health and Clinical Excellence.

NICE (2015) *Workplace health: Management practices* (June 2015), Manchester: National Institute for Health and Clinical Excellence.

Nuffield Health (2015) Company Website www.nuffieldhealth.com (accessed 23/10/2015).

Petersen, A. (1997) Risk, governance and the new public health, in: A. Petersen and R. Bunton (Eds) *Foucault, health and medicine*, pp. 189–206, London: Routledge.

Prochaska, J.O., and DiClemente, C.C. (1983) Stages and processes of self change of smoking: Toward an integrative model of change, *Journal of Consulting and Clinical Psychology*, 51, 390–395.

Rose, N. (1990) *Governing the soul: The shaping of the private self*, London: Routledge.

Rose, N. (1993). Government, authority and expertise in advanced liberalism, *Economy and Society*, 22 (3), 283–299.

Springett, J., and Dugdill, L. (1995) Evaluation of workplace health promotion programmes, *Health Education Journal*, 54, 88–98.

Townley, B. (1994) *Reframing human resource management: Power, ethics and the subject at work*, London: Sage.

Trethewey, A. (1999) Disciplined bodies: Women's embodied identities at work, *Organization Studies*, 20 (3), 423–450.

23

PHYSICAL ACTIVITY
IN SCHOOLS

Jordan Smith, David Lubans and Rodney Lyn

Introduction

International data have demonstrated the majority of youth worldwide now fail to meet established physical activity recommendations (Hallal et al., 2012). In light of these findings, there appears to be a clear justification for recent calls to view global inactivity as 'pandemic' (Kohl et al., 2012). Addressing physical inactivity during childhood and adolescence is important not only for the immediate physical and mental health benefits (Janssen and LeBlanc, 2010, Biddle and Asare, 2011), but also as a preventive strategy for future ill-health. Indeed, many of the lifestyle-related chronic conditions that manifest in adulthood have been shown to have their genesis in youth (Srinivasan and Berenson, 1995, Whitaker et al., 1997), and there is growing evidence that physical activity participation during the formative years is protective against future chronic disease risk (Rangul et al., 2012, Ried-Larsen et al., 2013, Gunter et al., 2012). Estimates suggest the proportion of premature mortality attributed to physical inactivity is comparable to that of other established risk factors such as obesity and smoking, making inactivity one of the leading preventable causes of death globally (Lee et al., 2012). In view of this, and considering that inactive youth are likely to become inactive adults (Telama et al., 2014), early intervention should be considered an important preventive health opportunity.

With both immediate and long-term health goals in mind, researchers and public health advocates have increasingly looked to schools as important settings for physical activity promotion. Given the unparalleled access to young people that schools possess, in addition to the availability of valuable infrastructure and qualified personnel, it is not surprising that schools have emerged as attractive settings for tackling this public health issue. Although youth physical activity behaviours are influenced by various sectors of society, schools have been identified as settings with considerable potential to have an impact (Naylor and McKay, 2009). Notably, while some educators may view schools as institutions for learning and not health promotion, emerging evidence of the benefits of physical activity for academic performance (Singh et al., 2012) suggests physical activity promotion in schools may actually help to support the core educational objectives of these institutions.

Given the potential for schools to act as key settings for health behaviour change, there has been a proliferation of school-based physical activity programs in recent decades (Dobbins et al., 2009, Kriemler et al., 2011). Although some evidence has suggested the effects of previous programs have been trivial (Metcalf et al., 2012), a recent comprehensive review of school-based physical activity interventions found that these initiatives can be effective, with successful trials reporting increases in moderate-to-vigorous physical activity (MVPA) of 5 to 45 minutes per week and clinically meaningful improvements in cardiorespiratory fitness (Dobbins et al., 2009). In addition, there is emerging evidence suggesting that intervention effects can be maintained over the longer term (Lai et al., 2014). Of the 60 minutes of MVPA students should accumulate each day (World Health Organization, 2010), it has been recommended that at least half (i.e., 30 mins) should be accrued while at school (BC Ministry for Education, 2008).

Multi-component approaches to physical activity behaviour change appear to have been the most efficacious (Dobbins et al., 2009). Therefore, it is important that future efforts to improve the physical activity levels of students address behavioural determinants across multiple levels (i.e., individual, interpersonal and environmental), and integrate strategies across the entire school day. In recognition of the need for an integrated approach to school-based physical activity promotion, the United States (U.S.) Centers for Disease Control and Prevention (CDC) recommends schools implement a Comprehensive School Physical Activity Program (CSPAP) (Centers for Disease Control and Prevention, 2013). The CSPAP is a coordinated, multi-component strategy for schools to target opportunities for physical activity participation across the following domains: (i) physical education (PE); (ii) physical activity during the school day; (iii) physical activity before and after school; (iv) staff involvement; and (v) family and community engagement. Using the CSPAP as a framework, this chapter will provide an overview of school-based physical activity programs targeting each of these key opportunities. Finally, this chapter will outline the implications of past research for future physical activity policy and practice.

Physical education

In recognition of the important and central role of PE in school-based physical activity promotion, quality PE has been identified as the 'foundation' of any CSPAP initiative (Centers for Disease Control and Prevention, 2013). The centrality of PE within this school-wide approach is based on the capacity for PE to influence students' physical activity behaviours in several unique ways. First, PE provides a direct dose of physical activity during the school day. Indeed, research has clearly demonstrated that students are significantly more active on days in which PE is delivered (Pate et al., 2011, Meyer et al., 2013b). Second, consistent with Hagger and colleagues' (2003) Trans-Contextual Model, positive learning experiences in PE may enhance motivation for physical activity outside of school, leading students to preferentially select physical rather than sedentary activities during their leisure-time. Third, PE may help to develop and refine the foundational movement skills required for successful performance in various sports and physical activities (Lubans et al., 2010a). As proposed by Stodden and colleagues (2008), the development of adequate movement skill competency (both fundamental and lifelong physical activity skills) forms the basis for perceptions of athletic competence which in turn exerts a powerful influence on the motivation to be active. Finally, PE may provide students with valuable behavioural skills that support enjoyment and maintenance of physical activity into adulthood. Skills such as barrier identification, goal setting and self-monitoring may be important for sustaining physical activity levels over time, and learning these skills during the formative years may help support lifelong physical activity participation.

Despite the important influence of PE on students' overall physical activity levels, there is evidence to suggest the provision of regular PE has declined in recent decades (Lowry et al.,

2005, Faulkner et al., 2007). Indeed, the apparent underutilisation of PE as a public health resource has led some to describe school PE as 'the pill not taken' (McKenzie and Lounsbery, 2009), and numerous barriers have emerged to the successful implementation of quality PE programs in schools. For example, elementary school teachers have identified the lack of PE specialists, limited financial resources and a perceived lack of time in the school day as key barriers to the delivery of evidence-based PE programs (Lounsbery et al., 2011). Additionally, while secondary schools typically employ trained PE specialists, low subject status, a crowded curriculum and lack of facilities are commonly cited barriers to the delivery of PE in these settings (Jenkinson and Benson, 2010, Barroso et al., 2005). Exacerbating these largely institutional barriers are philosophical objections to the use of PE for public health aims. Indeed, it has been suggested that 'joy-oriented' and 'health-oriented' PE are incompatible, with any attempt to provide one ultimately undermining the attainment of the other (Kretchmar, 2008). Of course, as aptly noted by Hills and colleagues (2015), this view is based on the flawed assumption that highly active PE lessons cannot also be enjoyable for students. Despite these wide ranging barriers, there have been a number of successful programs targeting activity levels in PE. According to a recent systematic review and meta-analysis, PE-focused interventions can increase physical activity within class (24% relative increase) (Lonsdale et al., 2013a). Clearly, with the right approach PE can support public health goals, as originally advocated by Sallis and colleagues (1991) in their seminal paper on the subject.

The U.S. Sport, Play and Active Recreation for Kids (SPARK) (Sallis et al., 1997) and Child and Adolescent Trial for Cardiovascular Health (CATCH) (McKenzie et al., 1996) programs were two landmark interventions that demonstrated the potential public health value of quality school PE. Both programs targeted within-school physical activity among elementary school students through the provision of enhanced PE curricula and teacher professional learning. These innovative programs resulted in significant improvements in physical activity, with the most pronounced changes found during PE lessons. For example, students involved in CATCH PE increased their in-class MVPA by almost 40 per cent, and by post-intervention were significantly more active during PE than controls (McKenzie et al., 1996). Similarly, as a result of increases in both the frequency and duration of PE lessons, students participating in SPARK accrued more than twice the quantity of MVPA through PE than their control group counterparts (Sallis et al., 1997). Of note, despite increasing the time allocation for PE during the school week, children participating in SPARK also experienced higher achievement in language and reading (Sallis et al., 1999). This important finding provided some of the first evidence that prioritising PE has no adverse impact on students' performance in other academic subjects.

In more recent years, the Swiss Kinder-Sportstudie (KISS) (Zahner et al., 2006) and the Australian Supporting Children's Outcomes using Rewards, Exercise and Skills (SCORES) (Lubans et al., 2012b) programs have provided further insights into the unique ways in which elementary school PE might influence students' physical activity. Similar to SPARK, the KISS intervention increased the frequency and quality of school PE, providing PE lessons daily in accordance with a modified activity-promoting curriculum. SCORES, on the other hand, utilised teacher professional learning to enhance existing mandatory PE lessons, and focused heavily on students' acquisition of fundamental movement skills (FMSs) (e.g., kicking, catching, throwing). Both programs reported beneficial effects for objectively measured physical activity and health-related fitness (Kriemler et al., 2010, Cohen et al., 2015b). In addition, KISS and SCORES reported improvements in students' skeletal health (Meyer et al., 2011, Meyer et al., 2013a) and FMS competency (Cohen et al., 2015b), respectively. While both programs improved students' overall physical activity, there were interesting differences in *when* the additional physical activity was accrued. Unsurprisingly, the increased time allocation for PE in KISS significantly improved MVPA during the school day (mean difference, 13 mins/d, $P < .001$) (Kriemler et al., 2011). However, no significant between-group changes were found for physical activity outside of school (Kriemler et al., 2011). By contrast, the effect on overall physical activity in SCORES was explained by physical activity accrued during the after-school period (mean difference, 4.6 mins/d, $P = .03$) and on weekends (mean difference, 14.5 mins/d, $P = .03$), with no significant changes found during the school day. Interestingly, PE seems to have provided a direct dose of physical activity for students in the KISS program, whereas for SCORES the focus on developing FMSs appears to have given students the competence and motivation to engage in self-directed physical activity during their leisure-time (Cohen et al., 2015a).

Although there is ample evidence to support the value of physical activity programs for elementary school students, there have been fewer school-based physical activity interventions conducted among adolescents (Dobbins et al., 2009). This is surprising considering the recognised influence of this developmental period on future health status (Alberga et al., 2012), and the drastic decline in physical activity levels that occur during the teenage years (Dumith et al., 2011). As a result, the overall effectiveness of programs conducted within secondary schools remains unclear (Dobbins et al., 2009, Waters et al., 2011). There are unique challenges to engaging adolescents in health promotion programs (Steinbeck et al., 2009), and strategies that work with younger children may not be appropriate or effective among this group. Despite mixed findings for programs targeting adolescents, there have been a number of innovative trials conducted in secondary schools.

One of the larger and higher quality trials conducted among adolescents in recent years was the HEALTHY diabetes prevention trial. HEALTHY was a large multi-component school-based intervention conducted in 42 U.S. middle schools (HEALTHY Study Group, 2009). Involving over 4,500 students, this multi-site trial is one of the largest school-based interventions conducted to date. While HEALTHY incorporated a number of intervention components, a key feature of the intervention was an enhanced PE program delivered by teachers (McMurray et al., 2009). As part of the program, teachers were given strategies for optimising MVPA during PE lessons and were allocated a teaching aid to assist with lesson delivery and class management. Example strategies included limiting 'teacher talk' and transition time, using 'instant activities' at the beginning of lessons to get students moving quickly, maximising available equipment, using small group games and integrating vigorous health-related fitness activities (McMurray et al., 2009). In addition, schools were allocated a 'physical activity coordinator' responsible for overseeing program delivery at each school and were provided with funding to purchase sporting equipment. Despite the considerable investment in personnel and resources, no significant improvements in students' physical activity were reported (Jago et al., 2011). However, beneficial effects were observed for measures of body composition and fasting insulin (HEALTHY Study Group, 2010), suggesting that there may have been improvements in students' physical activity that simply weren't captured by the self-report instrument used (Jago et al., 2011). Measurement limitations aside, the lack of a clear positive effect for physical activity in this study further highlights the challenges of influencing adolescents' physical activity behaviours.

Although the class management techniques used in HEALTHY were no doubt useful for creating opportunities for physical activity, the program may have placed insufficient emphasis on students' motivation to be active. PE teachers cite a lack of motivation among the leading obstacles to engaging adolescents in PE lessons (Jenkinson and Benson, 2010), and motivation for PE has been found to decline over the teenage years (Cox et al., 2008). In light of consistent evidence of an association between motivation and physical activity in PE lessons (Aelterman et al., 2012, Lonsdale et al., 2009, Standage et al., 2012, Sebire et al., 2013), interventions specifically targeting students' motivation in PE have begun to emerge in the literature (Chatzisarantis and Hagger, 2009, Lonsdale et al., 2013b). The Motivating Active Learning in Physical Education (MALP) trial (Lonsdale et al., 2013b) was an Australian secondary school PE intervention examining the effects of three separate self-determination theory-based motivational strategies on students' within-class physical activity. Students were randomly allocated to one of four conditions: (i) explaining relevance, (ii) providing choice, (iii) free choice or (iv) control. Interestingly, students in both 'choice' conditions were found to reduce the amount of lesson time spent sedentary, but only the 'free choice' condition resulted in significant improvements in MVPA (Lonsdale et al., 2013b). This finding suggests a benefit to allowing students time during lessons to engage in self-directed activities. However, given that physical activity is only one of a number of outcomes in PE, providing opportunities for choice within structured lessons that link with curriculum content may be more appropriate for future programs. Importantly, aspects of teacher practice can limit opportunities for students to be active, regardless of their motivation (Lonsdale et al., 2013a). Therefore, a promising strategy may be to integrate effective instructional techniques, such as those used in HEALTHY, with evidence-based motivational strategies.

Physical activity during the school day

Children and adolescents spend approximately 6 hours per day at school and there are a number of opportunities to increase physical activity during this time. Such opportunities include break times, classroom-based 'curricular' time, and co-curricular physical activity periods (also known as school sport periods). In many countries, schools dedicate additional time during school hours for physical activity which occurs in addition to scheduled PE. Although the organisation of these periods can differ greatly between schools, they typically involve students selecting from a range of potential sports and activities, many of which would not be offered within traditional PE programs. Previous trials such as ATLAS (Smith et al., 2014a, Smith et al., 2014b) and NEAT Girls (Lubans et al., 2010b, Lubans et al., 2012a), delivered in Australia, represent attempts to use these co-curricular periods for the delivery of evidence-based physical activity and fitness programs.

Unlike PE, school breaks (often known as 'recess' periods) occur daily during the school week for students all around the world. Additionally, schools usually have the facilities to enable students to be active during these periods, albeit that the quality of facilities can vary (Nichol et al., 2009). While the number, length and timing of breaks may differ (Kobel et al., 2015), schools typically provide at least one extended break between lessons for students to eat, rest from classwork and engage in general play. Importantly, school breaks may account for up to 40 per cent of a student's daily physical activity (Ridgers et al., 2006), and the contribution of these periods to overall physical activity levels may increase throughout the elementary school years (Ridgers et al., 2011). Cross-sectional research has identified associations between a range of contextual factors and break-time physical activity (Stanley et al., 2012, Ridgers et al., 2012), highlighting potential targets for intervention. Consequently, school break times are increasingly being viewed as an important component of school-based physical activity promotion (Parrish et al., 2013).

Consistent with much of the cross-sectional research in the area (Ridgers et al., 2012), interventions to increase students' break-time physical activity have predominantly focused on implementing changes to the school physical environment (Parrish et al., 2013). Such changes include the addition of playground markings, modified game spaces (e.g., colour coded areas), providing new fixed play equipment and increasing the availability of non-fixed sports equipment (e.g., balls, bats, skipping ropes, etc.) (Parrish et al., 2013). While less common, prior programs have also implemented organised activities during break-times, such as walking clubs and jump rope (Elder et al., 2011), and at least one study has used active video gaming as a novel way to engage students (Duncan and Staples, 2010). The findings of previous recess interventions have been mixed, with approximately half of trials demonstrating statistically significant improvements in physical activity (Parrish et al., 2013). Of those that have been effective, increases in MVPA have been meaningful and range from 4 per cent to 13 per cent of total break-time (Parrish et al., 2013). These studies demonstrate the potential for school break times to further contribute to students' daily physical activity. However, a number of gaps within the evidence base remain. For example, in the most recent review of recess interventions, none of the included programs were conducted in secondary schools (Parrish et al., 2013). In addition, the methodological quality of most prior studies was rated low to moderate (Parrish et al., 2013).

Although break times have the potential to add to students' daily physical activity, these periods account for only a small portion of the school day. Instead, students spend the majority of their time at school sitting in the classroom. Of concern, the pressure to enhance students' achievement in literacy, numeracy and core academic subjects has led many schools to increase instructional time and, by consequence, decrease time allocated to PE and recess breaks (McMurrer and Kober, 2007). This has a compounding influence on students' daily activity, as students end up spending more time sedentary in the classroom whilst also receiving fewer opportunities to be physically active during the school day. Even in schools that value physical activity, the traditional classroom-based model of teaching and learning has resulted in environments that promote high levels of sedentariness. Consequently, there is a growing body of research focused on the use of curricular time for increasing students' physical activity participation.

Previous 'classroom-based' physical activity interventions have involved two main approaches. The first is the provision of short physical activity breaks during lessons, otherwise known as 'energisers'. Energisers are typically delivered in 5–10 minute blocks and involve students taking a break from classwork to perform a variety of basic movements, such as dance and calisthenics, within the classroom. A number of studies have demonstrated that energisers can be an effective method for increasing students' in-class and daily physical activity (Erwin et al., 2011, Mahar et al., 2006, Carlson et al., 2015, Whitt-Glover et al., 2011). In addition, many of these studies have reported additional benefits to students' concentration and on-task behaviour (Mahar et al., 2006, Whitt-Glover et al., 2011, Carlson et al., 2015). This finding is particularly important, as students' behaviour and engagement during lessons are highly salient outcomes for teachers, which might be leveraged to support adoption of energisers into regular practice (Mahar, 2011). Importantly, a recent economic analysis of school-based physical activity programs showed that the provision of activity breaks during instructional time was among the most cost-effective strategies for increasing students physical activity at school (Babey et al., 2014).

The second main strategy is the integration of physical activity within the school curriculum. Energisers are essentially a temporary respite from lesson content. Conversely, physical activity integration refers to using movement as the medium for teaching and learning. Physical activity integration may be more difficult for teachers to implement, as it requires a substantial change to instructional methods and will therefore add to the many competing demands on teachers' time. This is important, as ease of implementation is a key concern for teachers when considering changes to their teaching practice (McMullen et al., 2014). In addition, perceived lack of time is the most consistently identified barrier to implementing physical activity programs in schools (Naylor et al., 2015). Despite this, teachers often express a desire to contribute to students' wellness and may also value the benefits of active lessons to student engagement in class (Cothran et al., 2010). Considering their preference for classroom-based physical activity to be linked with the curriculum (McMullen et al., 2014), physical activity integration could also be a palatable option for teachers, provided they are given appropriate training and support to aid implementation.

One of the earliest examples of physical activity integration is *Take 10!*, an elementary school program incorporating regular 10 minute physical activity breaks within the classroom (Stewart et al., 2004). Unlike generic energisers the program resources include grade-specific links to the curriculum which reinforce key ideas from mathematics, science, social studies, language arts and general health education (Kibbe et al., 2011). As a result, students engage in movement whilst also consolidating their understanding of academic concepts. The *Take 10!* program, which has now been evaluated in the U.S., China, U.K. and Brazil, has demonstrated positive effects for students' physical activity, BMI, on-task behaviour and academic performance (Kibbe et al., 2011). Additionally, teacher approval and implementation of *Take 10!* has been acceptable, suggesting this can be both an effective and feasible strategy for schools.

More recently, Riley and colleagues (2015) evaluated the 'Encouraging Activity to Stimulate Young Minds' (EASY Minds) physical activity integration intervention. EASY Minds was a six-week program utilising professional learning, email support and lesson observation and feedback to assist Australian elementary school teachers to embed physical activity within their mathematics lessons. Example activities used in the program included reciting multiplication tables while stepping through agility ladders, using heart-rate readings during an aerobics session as data points for graphing and using a jump rope to give the answers to basic arithmetic questions. The program resulted in significant effects for students' overall physical activity, sedentary time and on-task behaviour, while having no adverse impact on mathematics achievement (Riley et al., 2015). Importantly, students involved in the program noted that the active lesson format made their lessons more enjoyable. Moreover, a number of teachers reported that they had begun to apply movement-based learning activities within other curriculum areas (Riley et al., 2015). These positive findings support the feasibility and acceptability of physical activity integration, and provide important insights into how teachers might be encouraged to modify their teaching practice. For example, the high level of teacher satisfaction with the professional learning component (Riley et al., 2015), suggests that meaningful and relevant professional learning experiences may be crucial for effective physical activity integration programs.

Physical activity before and after school

The before and after school periods represent important school-related sources of physical activity for children and adolescents. Active commuting, which refers to the use of active modes of travel such as walking or cycling, can provide a valuable contribution to students' habitual physical activity, as they are required to get to and from school on five days of the week for approximately 40 weeks of the year. Research has demonstrated that active commuters have higher overall physical activity levels than those using passive modes of travel to school (Faulkner et al., 2009). In addition, active commuting may help to improve and maintain students' cardiorespiratory (Lubans et al., 2011) and muscular fitness (Cohen et al., 2014), particularly if cycling is the usual mode of transport. While evidence of an association between active commuting and body composition has been less conclusive (Lubans et al., 2011), some estimates suggest that obesity prevalence among U.S. adolescents could decline by as much as 22 per cent if all students usually walked or cycled to school (Drake et al., 2012). Despite these benefits, there has been a global secular decline in the proportion of children and adolescents using active modes of travel to school (Booth et al., 2015), resulting in a missed opportunity for a type of physical activity that was once commonplace.

There has been a significant body of research investigating the correlates of active commuting among youth. Of the range of correlates that have been identified, parental perceptions of neighbourhood safety (i.e., personal and road safety) (Timperio et al., 2006), social support from friends and family (Hohepa et al., 2007), characteristics of the built environment (e.g., street connectivity) (Giles-Corti et al., 2011) and the presence of active travel infrastructure (e.g., foot and cycle paths) are among the most commonly cited. Perhaps the most consistent correlate of active commuting, however, is the distance from home to school (Panter et al., 2008), with considerable declines in the proportion of students using active transportation after a travel distance of around one to two kilometres (Panter et al., 2013, Timperio et al., 2006, Faulkner et al., 2013). Programs targeting students' active commuting have been varied, and have included a range of different intervention strategies. For example, recognising parents' concerns for children's safety, previous programs have aimed to educate children about road safety (Mendoza et al., 2009), engage parents to plan safe routes to school (McKee et al., 2007), provide supervised commuting groups (i.e., walking school bus) (Sirard et al., 2008) and build safer pedestrian infrastructure (Boarnet et al., 2005).

According to a systematic review of active school commuting interventions, almost all of the included studies reported an increase in the percentage of students using active transport (Chillón et al., 2011). However, the magnitude of change was generally small, and at times trivial (Chillón et al., 2011). Although this finding might seem to undermine the rationale for active commuting programs, it is important to note that the distance from students' home to school was not adopted as an inclusion criteria in any of the reviewed programs, perhaps resulting in an underestimation of their potential effectiveness (Chillón et al., 2011). Given the established influence of travel distance on students' willingness to walk or cycle to school (Panter et al., 2008), a pragmatic approach for future programs may be to focus their efforts only toward students that live within an acceptable distance from the school. In addition, future research should investigate the efficacy of active commuting programs for secondary school students. In the review by Chillón and colleagues (2011), almost all of the included programs targeted elementary school-aged youth. In view of the low prevalence of active commuting in many Western countries (Active Healthy Kids Canada, 2014), engaging even just a small proportion of students could result in significant population health benefits.

As shown, previous school-based physical activity programs have often aimed to enhance or introduce physical activity within defined contexts such as PE, recess breaks or curricular time. Although these approaches have merit, such contexts can be relatively brief (as for recess breaks) or may be inconsistently offered during a typical school week (as for PE). Consequently, their impact on students' overall physical activity participation, at least in isolation, may not always be substantial. By contrast, programs targeting physical activity after school may have greater potential, as this period represents a regular and extended block of uninterrupted time within which youth have the freedom to select from a range of possible leisure activities. Of note, there is larger variability in physical activity levels during the after-school period compared with other parts of the school day (Tudor-Locke et al., 2006). Therefore, this context is particularly useful for distinguishing between high and low active youth (Olds et al., 2011).

Evidence from the published literature supports the important contribution of the after-school period to young people's daily activity. For example, in a study of sixth grade students, Tudor-Locke and colleagues (2006) found that physical activity accrued after school accounted for approximately half of the daily total. In addition, longitudinal research has shown that declines in physical activity occurring during the transition from childhood to adolescence are relatively greater during the after-school period compared with other segments of the school day (Brooke et al., 2014). Finally, in a study of over 1,100 Australian children, unstructured play and structured sports participation were found to account for around 60 per cent of children's daily MVPA (Olds et al., 2011). As noted by the study authors, these activities often occur during the time after school. In light of these findings, the after-school period has been characterised as a 'critical window' for physical activity participation (Atkin et al., 2008, Stanley et al., 2012), providing a strong rationale for interventions targeting these crucial hours.

After-school physical activity programs may be a feasible means of improving students' physical activity, as they fulfil a need of many working parents for after-school childcare. Consequently, these programs may not face the same resistance to recruitment common among programs offered in other contexts and settings (Steinbeck et al., 2009). The after-school period clearly offers potential. However, the effectiveness of previous after-school physical activity programs appears to be mixed. It has been suggested that these programs should enable students to accumulate 30 minutes of MVPA (Beets et al., 2012). Yet, an analysis of physical activity levels within 25 community-based programs in the United States found that most children fell well short of this goal. In the most recent review of after-school interventions (Atkin et al., 2011), only a third of the reviewed programs were found to be effective. Although, the authors did note that programs conducted within the school setting (as opposed to community or home settings) and those focused solely on increasing physical activity (rather than multiple health behaviours) have been the most effective (Atkin et al., 2011).

That *school-based* after-school programs are more effective than those delivered elsewhere is consistent with the findings of an earlier meta-analysis (Beets et al., 2009). Investigating only those programs delivered in schools, Beets and colleagues (2009) reported a moderate pooled effect size for physical activity (mean, 0.44; 95% CI, 0.28 to 0.60), and small but statistically significant effects for cardiorespiratory fitness (mean, 0.16; 95% CI, 0.01 to 0.30). While these findings are encouraging, it is clear that more work needs to be done to realise the potential of after-school programs. Interestingly, a recent review of CSPAPs showed that only one previous program targeted after-school physical activity (Russ et al., 2015), highlighting the fact that after-school programs often occur independent of other school-based strategies. Improving the coordination between after-school and within-school strategies should be a consideration for future physical activity programs.

Staff involvement and staff wellness

School staff can be important role models for students and, as a result, have the capacity to influence school culture and student behaviour. It is therefore sensible, and likely beneficial, to include school personnel in health promotion initiatives. Teachers often play an integral role in school-based physical activity programs, either as primary contacts to assist with logistics and organisation, or as facilitators responsible for delivering the programs in their schools. Indeed, the most recent systematic review of school-based physical activity interventions reported that teachers were the primary intervention providers in 37 of the 44 (84%) included studies (Dobbins et al., 2009). Although it is clear that teachers are heavily involved in the provision of school-based programs, they are far less commonly the recipients of such programs. For instance, in the review of CSPAPs mentioned earlier, staff involvement was a component in all of the reviewed programs, yet staff wellness programs were provided in just two (Russ et al., 2015). This shows the rather stark imbalance between what is asked of and what is offered to teachers.

There are a number of reasons why staff wellness programs should be considered an important aspect of school-based physical activity promotion. First, these programs have the immediate benefit of supporting teachers' health and wellbeing. Stress and burnout are common in 'contact' professions such as teaching (Dollard et al., 2003), and work-related stressors can have adverse effects on teachers' health (Guglielmi and Tatrow, 1998). Encouragingly, previous staff wellness programs have demonstrated positive impacts on teachers' health and wellbeing, including beneficial effects for dietary outcomes, body composition, mental health and physical activity (Osilla et al., 2012). In addition to these important outcomes, staff wellness programs may also help to establish a school culture that values physical activity, as teachers' commitment to supporting students' health needs may improve alongside an enhanced awareness and appreciation of their own (Cullen et al., 1999). Interestingly, schools implementing a CSPAP with a staff wellness component have been found to have a greater impact on students' physical activity (effect size, 0.21; 95%CI, 0.04 to 0.38) than those not including this component (effect size, 0.09; 0.02 to 0.16) (Russ et al., 2015). How and why this occurs are interesting questions for future research. Regardless, this finding provides further support for the idea that the health and wellbeing of school personnel should be an equally valued outcome for future CSPAP initiatives. Clearly, the more widespread implementation of staff wellness programs within schools is warranted.

Family and community engagement

Linking with community organisations, such as local sporting clubs or youth recreation clubs (e.g., YMCA), might be an effective way to enhance school-based physical activity programs. For example, a PE program aiming to improve students' sports skills and physical activity participation might have greater impact if the school also connected with local junior sporting clubs. By linking with such groups, students could discover a pathway into organised sport within their local community. Community organisations often have valuable resources, qualified personnel and the means to deliver before- and after-school programs. Moreover, both schools and community organisations could benefit from the sharing of facilities and resources (Centers for Disease Control and Prevention, 2013). Other community partners could include players from local professional sporting teams, prominent business people or respected elders (as in certain indigenous communities). These partners may or may not offer material support for the program, but could nonetheless help to endorse its objectives. Such an endorsement could help to legitimise the program in the eyes of students and their families, which in itself would be a valuable outcome.

Families, and in particular parents, are a major source of influence in children's lives. As such, they have the power to either reinforce or undermine health promotion efforts. Parents model health behaviours, offer logistic, financial and emotional support to their children and can provide (or fail to provide) a framework of rules that encourages physical activity outside of school (Van der Horst et al., 2007, Trost and Loprinzi, 2011, Tandon et al., 2012). Engaging parents would, therefore, appear to be useful for consolidating the beliefs, attitudes and behaviours being promoted within physical activity programs. In their evaluation of a school-based intervention for adolescents, Haerens and colleagues (2007) found adding a parental support component resulted in greater effects for physical activity than the school-based components alone. In addition, parental engagement strategies have been a feature of a number of other successful multi-component interventions (Cohen et al., 2015b, Williamson et al., 2007). In recognition of these findings, reviews of youth physical activity and obesity prevention interventions have recommended that future programs include both family- and school-based strategies (Dobbins et al., 2009, Waters et al., 2011, Van Sluijs et al., 2007). However, engaging parents in school-based interventions is often challenging (Jones et al., 2014), and there is a lack of consensus regarding the most effective parental engagement approaches (O'Connor et al., 2009, Van Lippevelde et al., 2012). Although more high quality research in this area is needed, a number of promising strategies have been identified (O'Connor et al., 2009).

Often, the easiest way to reach parents is to send newsletters, homework tasks or other educational material to the family home. However, there is no way to ensure that parents attend to this material, and the evidence to date suggests this is not a particularly effective strategy (O'Connor et al., 2009). According to O'Connor and colleagues (2009), face-to-face or telephone contact that provides opportunities for parent training or family counselling may be more effective. Due to the various time demands in parents' lives, gaining their attention and interest can be quite difficult. Therefore, the messages that are used to mobilise parents may also need to be considered more carefully. It is fair to say that parents would be more motivated to participate in a school-based program if they believed that doing so would provide some meaningful benefit to them and their children. Physical activity programs are often predicated on the basis that they can improve health-related quality of life and prevent future chronic disease. Despite being justified in principle, this rationale may not always invoke the desired response from parents, as many fail to recognise that their children's health behaviours are deficient. For example, in a study of 9–10 year old British students 80 per cent of parents with inactive children wrongly believed that their child was sufficiently active (Corder et al., 2010). In light of this, it may be useful to focus on more salient outcomes for parents, including the quality of family relationships, social and emotional wellbeing and academic performance. Recent community-based physical activity programs have utilised this strategy to great effect, resulting in successful recruitment and retention of participants. For example, the Australian 'Healthy Dads, Healthy Kids' program (Morgan et al., 2011) used targeted recruitment strategies that reinforced the unique importance of fathers as role models for their children, and highlighted the opportunity for fathers to spend 'quality time' with their kids while getting fit and losing weight at the same time.

Implications for future physical activity policy and practice

As has been outlined previously, multi-component programs targeting behavioural determinants across various aspects of the school environment appear to be have been the most effective for increasing students' physical activity levels (Dobbins et al., 2009). Consequently, a comprehensive and integrated approach to school-based physical activity promotion is now recommended (Centers for Disease Control and Prevention, 2013). The aims of this chapter were to give an evidence-based rationale for school-based physical activity programs, and to provide a broad overview of past intervention research using the CSPAP target areas as a framework. It is important to note, that although certain intervention programs described within this chapter may have fallen under a specific physical activity context (e.g., PE), many of these programs included multiple components and therefore may have addressed several opportunities. It was, however, beyond the scope of this chapter to describe these programs in detail. Rather, these examples were selected to illustrate the unique ways in which past programs have aimed to enhance students' physical activity participation within the school setting. Importantly, past research has helped to develop our understanding of how schools might be used to tackle the worsening issue of physical inactivity. While comprehensive in some areas, and underdeveloped in others, this research raises some important implications for future physical activity policy and practice.

Physical Education

- Due to the benefits of PE for students' physical activity, PE should be offered to students regularly, and preferably daily. In addition, PE programs should provide opportunities for students to participate in both competitive team sports (e.g., football) and lifelong physical activities (e.g., resistance training) (Hulteen et al., 2015). Competitive team sports are often the focus of traditional PE programs. However, such activities may have little carry over into later life, as many young people drop out of organised sport during adolescence and young adulthood.
- There is a justification for making PE compulsory for the majority of the schooling years. Further, evidence-based PE programs focusing on high levels of active learning time should be implemented into schools' regular practice. Professional learning for teachers may help to support the implementation of such programs.
- Considering that specialist PE teachers deliver better and more active lessons (Davis et al., 2005, Sallis et al., 1997), there is a strong justification for the mandatory employment of PE specialists in elementary schools.
- PE teachers should incorporate, within their teaching practice, evidence-based strategies aimed at maximising physical activity. Teachers should aim for at least 50 per cent of lesson time to be spent in MVPA. In addition, teachers should implement motivational strategies such as autonomy support to enhance students' motivation and physical activity participation in class (Chatzisarantis and Hagger, 2009).
- Pre-service teacher training programs should explicitly address pedagogical techniques for maximising physical activity and motivation during PE lessons (Lonsdale et al., 2013a, Owen et al., 2014).

Physical activity during the school day

- Recess breaks should not be removed or reduced in length in favour of increased curricular time. Opportunities for physical activity during the school day may already be supporting students' academic performance, making such decisions pointless.
- School environments should be designed or modified to promote physical activity. This may have implications for the design of future schools, which could be made to be 'activity-promoting'.
- Schools should provide fixed play equipment and playground markings, and maintain facilities such as sporting fields, hard surface courts and indoor/covered play areas. Schools should also provide loose sporting equipment for students to play with during break times, and could also deliver organised activities (including team games and non-traditional activities) during these periods. It may also be useful to offer gender-segregated areas to support physical activity participation among young girls, who may be intimidated by male students who often dominate school play areas.
- The integration of energisers into regular practice should be encouraged by schools. Energisers are easy to implement and do not require large changes to teacher practice. To

support this, teachers could be required to record or 'register' their delivery of energiser breaks, as they typically do for other aspects of the school curriculum. Face-to-face or online training modules may help to prepare teachers to deliver energisers effectively.

- Resources and training should be provided to pre-service and practicing teachers to support physical activity integration into other subject areas. Physical activity integration could be included within undergraduate teacher training programs. In addition, professional learning workshops on this topic could be offered periodically in schools.
- Future research should investigate the feasibility and efficacy of physical activity integration in secondary schools. Considering the availability of appropriately trained personnel (i.e., PE teachers), cross-faculty collaboration might be a feasible way to train non-PE teachers in physical activity integration.

Physical activity before and after school

- Schools should promote active commuting to school. To support this, schools could: (i) provide secure storage areas for students' bicycles, skateboards or scooters; (ii) create and disseminate safe commuting routes within the local area; (iii) engage with parents to address concerns for student safety; (iv) promote school-wide active commuting events (e.g., walk or cycle to school days); (v) offer a supervised 'walking school bus' service using school staff or community volunteers; and (vi) target parents of students living close to the school as part of an active commuting promotion campaign.
- Future urban design projects within residential areas should consider whether pedestrian safety is being adequately addressed. In addition, such projects could apply a physical activity 'lens' to evaluate whether design features maximise opportunities for active commuting (e.g., good street connectivity, availability of foot and cycle paths).
- Providing after-school programs within the school setting appears to be an effective strategy. This allows for continuous supervision of students from the end of the school day, and negates the need for transport to external venues which might be costly or difficult to organise. After-school programs should be coordinated with other school-based physical activity promotion strategies and should be included more often within CSPAPs.

Staff involvement/staff wellness programs

- Staff may be more willing to be involved in school-based physical activity programs if there are tangible incentives for participation. Schools might offer release time from teaching duties as a reward for involvement. In addition, professional learning experiences that link with existing teacher accreditation requirements may help to attract teachers into these programs.
- Staff wellness programs may support both teachers' and students' health. Therefore, future CSPAP initiatives should include a staff wellness component. This might include health education combined with before or after-school activities (e.g., Yoga, group fitness sessions, walking/running groups).

Family and community engagement

- School-based programs should attempt to connect with community organisations. Community groups could be used to facilitate before- or after-school activities, provide sports-specific coaching to students, or might simply enable pathways into organised sports.

- Schools should consider parents as key partners in school-based physical activity promotion. Information nights at existing school and community events might help to engage parents. In addition, mobilising parents may be most effective when messaging focuses on valued outcomes including students' school performance, social and emotional well-being, and benefits to family relationships.

References

Active Healthy Kids Canada 2014. Is Canada in the running? The 2014 Active Kids Canada report card on physical activity for children and youth. Toronto: Active Healthy Kids Canada.

Aelterman, N., Vansteenkiste, M., Van Keer, H., Van Den Berghe, L., De Meyer, J. & Haerens, L. 2012. Students' objectively measured physical activity levels and engagement as a function of between-class and between-student differences in motivation toward physical education. *Journal of Sport and Exercise Psychology*, 34, 457.

Alberga, A., Sigal, R., Goldfield, G., Prud' Homme, D. & Kenny, G. 2012. Overweight and obese teenagers: Why is adolescence a critical period? *Pediatric Obesity*, 7, 261–273.

Atkin, A. J., Gorely, T., Biddle, S., Marshall, S. J. & Cameron, N. 2008. Critical hours: Physical activity and sedentary behavior of adolescents after school. *Pediatric Exercise Science*, 20, 446–456.

Atkin, A. J., Gorely, T., Biddle, S. J., Cavill, N. & Foster, C. 2011. Interventions to promote physical activity in young people conducted in the hours immediately after school: a systematic review. *International Journal of Behavioral Medicine*, 18, 176–187.

Babey, S. H., Wu, S. & Cohen, D. 2014. How can schools help youth increase physical activity? An economic analysis comparing school-based programs. *Preventive Medicine*, 69, S55–S60.

Barroso, C. S., McCullum-Gomez, C., Hoelscher, D. M., Kelder, S. H. & Murray, N. G. 2005. Self-reported barriers to quality physical education by physical education specialists in texas. *Journal of School Health*, 75, 313–319.

BC Ministry for Education 2008. *Program guide for daily physical activity kindergarten to grade 12*. Victoria, BC: BC Ministry of Education.

Beets, M. W., Beighle, A., Bottai, M., Rooney, L. & Tilley, F. 2012. Pedometer-determined step-count guidelines for afterschool programs. *Journal of Physical Activity and Health*, 9, 71.

Beets, M. W., Beighle, A., Erwin, H. E. & Huberty, J. L. 2009. After-school program impact on physical activity and fitness: A meta-analysis. *American Journal of Preventive Medicine*, 36, 527–537.

Biddle, S. J. & Asare, M. 2011. Physical activity and mental health in children and adolescents: A review of reviews. *British Journal of Sports Medicine*, 45, 886–895.

Boarnet, M. G., Day, K., Anderson, C., McMillan, T. & Alfonzo, M. 2005. California's Safe Routes to School program: Impacts on walking, bicycling, and pedestrian safety. *Journal of the American Planning Association*, 71, 301–317.

Booth, V. M., Rowlands, A. V. & Dollman, J. 2015. Physical activity temporal trends among children and adolescents. *Journal of Science and Medicine in Sport*, 18, 418–425.

Brooke, H. L., Atkin, A. J., Corder, K., Ekelund, U. & Van Sluijs, E. M. 2014. Changes in time-segment specific physical activity between ages 10 and 14 years: A longitudinal observational study. *Journal of Science and Medicine in Sport*. DOI: 10.1016/j.jsams.2014.10.003.

Carlson, J. A., Engelberg, J. K., Cain, K. L., Conway, T. L., Mignano, A. M., Bonilla, E. A., Geremia, C. & Sallis, J. F. 2015. Implementing classroom physical activity breaks: Associations with student physical activity and classroom behavior. *Preventive Medicine*, 81, 67–72.

Centers for Disease Control and Prevention 2013. Comprehensive School Physical Activity Programs: A Guide for Schools. *In:* U.S. Department of Health and Human Services (ed.). Atlanta, GA: U.S. Department of Health and Human Services.

Chatzisarantis, N. L. & Hagger, M. S. 2009. Effects of an intervention based on self-determination theory on self-reported leisure-time physical activity participation. *Psychology and Health*, 24, 29–48.

Chillón, P., Evenson, K. R., Vaughn, A. & Ward, D. S. 2011. A systematic review of interventions for promoting active transportation to school. *International Journal of Behavioural Nutrition and Physical Activity*, 8, 10.

Cohen, D., Ogunleye, A. A., Taylor, M., Voss, C., Micklewright, D. & Sandercock, G. R. 2014. Association between habitual school travel and muscular fitness in youth. *Preventive Medicine*, 67, 216–220.

Cohen, K. E., Morgan, P. J., Plotnikoff, R. C., Barnett, L. M. & Lubans, D. R. 2015a. Improvements in fundamental movement skill competency mediate the effect of the SCORES intervention on physical activity and cardiorespiratory fitness in children. *Journal of Sports Sciences*, 1–11.

Cohen, K. E., Morgan, P. J., Plotnikoff, R. C., Callister, R. & Lubans, D. R. 2015b. Physical activity and skills intervention: SCORES cluster randomized controlled trial. *Medicine and Science in Sports and Exercise*, 47, 765–774.

Corder, K., Van Sluijs, E. M., McMinn, A. M., Ekelund, U., Cassidy, A. & Griffin, S. J. 2010. Perception versus reality: Awareness of physical activity levels of British children. *American Journal of Preventive Medicine*, 38, 1–8.

Cothran, D. J., Kulinna, P. H. & Garn, A. C. 2010. Classroom teachers and physical activity integration. *Teaching and Teacher Education*, 26, 1381–1388.

Cox, A. E., Smith, A. L. & Williams, L. 2008. Change in physical education motivation and physical activity behavior during middle school. *Journal of Adolescent Health*, 43, 506–513.

Cullen, K. W., Baranowski, T., Baranowski, J., Hebert, D., Demoor, C., Hearn, M. D. & Resnicow, K. 1999. Influence of school organizational characteristics on the outcomes of a school health promotion program. *Journal of School Health*, 69, 376–380.

Davis, K. S., Burgeson, C. R., Brener, N. D., McManus, T. & Wechsler, H. 2005. The relationship between qualified personnel and self-reported implementation of recommended physical education practices and programs in US schools. *Research Quarterly for Exercise and Sport*, 76, 202–211.

Dobbins, M., Husson, H., Decorby, K. & Larocca, R. L. 2009. School-based physical activity programs for promoting physical activity and fitness in children and adolescents aged 6 to 18. *Cochrane Database of Systematic Reviews*, 1, CD007651.

Dollard, M. F., Dormann, C., Boyd, C. M., Winefield, H. R. & Winefield, A. H. 2003. Unique aspects of stress in human service work. *Australian Psychologist*, 38, 84–91.

Drake, K. M., Beach, M. L., Longacre, M. R., Mackenzie, T., Titus, L. J., Rundle, A. G. & Dalton, M. A. 2012. Influence of sports, physical education, and active commuting to school on adolescent weight status. *Pediatrics*, 130, e296–e304.

Dumith, S. C., Gigante, D. P., Domingues, M. R. & Kohl, H. W. 2011. Physical activity change during adolescence: A systematic review and a pooled analysis. *International Journal of Epidemiology*, 40, 685–698.

Duncan, M. & Staples, V. 2010. The impact of a school-based active video game play intervention on children's physical activity during recess. *Human Movement*, 11, 95–99.

Elder, J. P., McKenzie, T. L., Arredondo, E. M., Crespo, N. C. & Ayala, G. X. 2011. Effects of a multi-pronged intervention on children's activity levels at recess: The Aventuras para Niños study. *Advances in Nutrition: An International Review Journal*, 2, 171S–176S.

Erwin, H. E., Beighle, A., Morgan, C. F. & Noland, M. 2011. Effect of a low-cost, teacher-directed classroom intervention on elementary students' physical activity. *Journal of School Health*, 81, 455–461.

Faulkner, G., Goodman, J., Adlaf, E., Irving, H., Allison, K. & Dwyer, J. 2007. Participation in high school physical education-Ontario, Canada, 1999–2005. *Morbidity and Mortality Weekly Report*, 56, 52–54.

Faulkner, G., Stone, M., Buliung, R., Wong, B. & Mitra, R. 2013. School travel and children's physical activity: A cross-sectional study examining the influence of distance. *BMC Public Health*, 13, 1166.

Faulkner, G. E., Buliung, R. N., Flora, P. K. & Fusco, C. 2009. Active school transport, physical activity levels and body weight of children and youth: A systematic review. *Preventive Medicine*, 48, 3–8.

Giles-Corti, B., Wood, G., Pikora, T., Learnihan, V., Bulsara, M., Van Niel, K., Timperio, A., McCormack, G. & Villanueva, K. 2011. School site and the potential to walk to school: The impact of street connectivity and traffic exposure in school neighborhoods. *Health and Place*, 17, 545–550.

Guglielmi, R. S. & Tatrow, K. 1998. Occupational stress, burnout, and health in teachers: A methodological and theoretical analysis. *Review of Educational Research*, 68, 61–99.

Gunter, K. B., Almstedt, H. C. & Janz, K. F. 2012. Physical activity in childhood may be the key to optimizing lifespan skeletal health. *Exercise and Sport Sciences Reviews*, 40, 13.

Haerens, L., De Bourdeaudhuij, I., Maes, L., Cardon, G. & Deforche, B. 2007. School-based randomized controlled trial of a physical activity intervention among adolescents. *Journal of Adolescent Health*, 40, 258–265.

Hagger, M. S., Chatzisarantis, N. L., Culverhouse, T. & Biddle, S. J. 2003. The processes by which perceived autonomy support in physical education promotes leisure-time physical activity intentions and behavior: A trans-contextual model. *Journal of Educational Psychology*, 95, 784–795.

Hallal, P. C., Bo Andersen, L., Bull, F. C., Guthold, R., Haskell, W., Ekelund, U. & Lancet Physical Activity Series Working Group 2012. Global physical activity levels: Surveillance progress, pitfalls, and prospects. *Lancet*, 380, 247–257.

HEALTHY Study Group 2009. HEALTHY study rationale, design and methods: Moderating risk of type 2 diabetes in multi-ethnic middle school students. *International Journal of Obesity*, 33, S4.

HEALTHY Study Group 2010. A school-based intervention for diabetes risk reduction. *New England Journal of Medicine*, 363, 443–453.

Hills, A. P., Dengel, D. R. & Lubans, D. R. 2015. Supporting public health priorities: Recommendations for physical education and physical activity promotion in schools. *Progress in Cardiovascular Diseases*, 57, 368–374.

Hohepa, M., Scragg, R., Schofield, G., Kolt, G. S. & Schaaf, D. 2007. Social support for youth physical activity: Importance of siblings, parents, friends and school support across a segmented school day. *International Journal of Behavioral Nutrition and Physical Activity*, 4, 54.

Hulteen, R. M., Lander, N. J., Morgan, P. J., Barnett, L. M., Robertson, S. J. & Lubans, D. R. 2015. Validity and reliability of field-based measures for assessing movement skill competency in lifelong physical activities: A systematic review. *Sports Medicine*, 1–12.

Jago, R., McMurray, R. G., Drews, K. L., Moe, E. L., Murray, T., Pham, T. H., Venditti, E. M. & Volpe, S. L. 2011. HEALTHY intervention: Fitness, physical activity, and metabolic syndrome results. *Medicine and Science in Sports and Exercise*, 43, 1513.

Janssen, I. & LeBlanc, A. G. 2010. Systematic review of the health benefits of physical activity and fitness in school-aged children and youth. *International Journal of Behavioral Nutrition and Physical Activity*, 7, 1–16.

Jenkinson, K. A. & Benson, A. C. 2010. Barriers to providing physical education and physical activity in Victorian state secondary schools. *Australian Journal of Teacher Education*, 35, 1.

Jones, R. A., Lubans, D. R., Morgan, P. J., Okely, A. D., Parletta, N., Wolfenden, L., De Silva-Sanigorski, A., Gibbs, L. & Waters, E. 2014. School-based obesity prevention interventions: Practicalities and considerations. *Obesity Research and Clinical Practice*, 8, e497–e510.

Kibbe, D. L., Hackett, J., Hurley, M., McFarland, A., Schubert, K. G., Schultz, A. & Harris, S. 2011. Ten Years of TAKE 10!®: Integrating physical activity with academic concepts in elementary school classrooms. *Preventive Medicine*, 52, S43–S50.

Kobel, S., Kettner, S., Erkelenz, N., Kesztyüs, D. & Steinacker, J. M. 2015. Does a higher incidence of break times in primary schools result in children being more physically active? *Journal of School Health*, 85, 149–154.

Kohl, H. W., Craig, C. L., Lambert, E. V., Inoue, S., Alkandari, J. R., Leetongin, G. & Kahlmeier, S. 2012. The pandemic of physical inactivity: Global action for public health. *Lancet*, 380, 294–305.

Kretchmar, R. S. 2008. The increasing utility of elementary school physical education: A mixed blessing and unique challenge. *The Elementary School Journal*, 108, 161–170.

Kriemler, S., Meyer, U., Martin, E., Van Sluijs, E., Andersen, L. & Martin, B. 2011. Effect of school-based interventions on physical activity and fitness in children and adolescents: A review of reviews and systematic update. *British Journal of Sports Medicine*, 45, 923–930.

Kriemler, S., Zahner, L., Schindler, C., Meyer, U., Hartmann, T., Hebestreit, H., Brunner-La Rocca, H. P., Van Mechelen, W. & Puder, J. J. 2010. Effect of school based physical activity programme (KISS) on fitness and adiposity in primary schoolchildren: Cluster randomised controlled trial. *BMJ*, 340, c785.

Lai, S. K., Costigan, S. A., Morgan, P. J., Lubans, D. R., Stodden, D. F., Salmon, J. & Barnett, L. M. 2014. Do school-based interventions focusing on physical activity, fitness, or fundamental movement skill competency produce a sustained impact in these outcomes in children and adolescents? A systematic review of follow-up studies. *Sports Medicine*, 44, 67–79.

Lee, I.-M., Shiroma, E. J., Lobelo, F., Puska, P., Blair, S. N. & Katzmarzyk, P. T. 2012. Effect of physical inactivity on major non-communicable diseases worldwide: An analysis of burden of disease and life expectancy. *Lancet*, 380, 219–229.

Lonsdale, C., Rosenkranz, R. R., Peralta, L. R., Bennie, A., Fahey, P. & Lubans, D. R. 2013a. A systematic review and meta-analysis of interventions designed to increase moderate-to-vigorous physical activity in school physical education lessons. *Preventive Medicine*, 56, 152–161.

Lonsdale, C., Rosenkranz, R. R., Sanders, T., Peralta, L. R., Bennie, A., Jackson, B., Taylor, I. M. & Lubans, D. R. 2013b. A cluster randomized controlled trial of strategies to increase adolescents' physical activity and motivation in physical education: Results of the Motivating Active Learning in Physical Education (MALP) trial. *Preventive Medicine*, 57, 696–702.

Lonsdale, C., Sabiston, C. M., Raedeke, T. D., Ha, A. S. & Sum, R. K. 2009. Self-determined motivation and students' physical activity during structured physical education lessons and free choice periods. *Preventive Medicine*, 48, 69–73.

Lounsbery, M. A., McKenzie, T. L., Trost, S. & Smith, N. J. 2011. Facilitators and barriers to adopting evidence-based physical education in elementary schools. *Journal of Physical Activity and Health*, 8, S17.

Lowry, R., Brener, N., Lee, S. & Epping, J. 2005. Participation in high school physical education-United States, 1991–2003. *The Journal of School Health*, 75, 47.

Lubans, D. R., Boreham, C. A., Kelly, P. & Foster, C. E. 2011. The relationship between active travel to school and health-related fitness in children and adolescents: A systematic review. *International Journal of Behavioral Nutrition and Physical Activity*, 8.

Lubans, D. R., Morgan, P. J., Cliff, D. P., Barnett, L. M. & Okely, A. D. 2010a. Fundamental movement skills in children and adolescents: Review of associated health benefits. *Sports Medicine*, 40, 1019–1035.

Lubans, D. R., Morgan, P. J., Dewar, D., Collins, C. E., Plotnikoff, R. C., Okely, A., D., Batterham, M. J., Finn, T. & Callister, R. 2010b. The Nutrition and Enjoyable Activity for Teen Girls (NEAT girls) randomized controlled trial for adolescent girls from disadvantaged secondary schools: Rationale, study protocol, and baseline results. *BMC Public Health*, 10, 652.

Lubans, D. R., Morgan, P. J., Okely, A. D., Dewar, D., Collins, C. E., Batterham, M., Callister, R. & Plotnikoff, R. C. 2012a. Preventing obesity among adolescent girls: One-year outcomes of the nutrition and enjoyable activity for teen girls (NEAT Girls) cluster randomized controlled trial. *Archives of Pediatrics and Adolescent Medicine*, 166, 821–827.

Lubans, D. R., Morgan, P. J., Weaver, K., Callister, R., Dewar, D. L., Costigan, S. A., Finn, T. L., Smith, J., Upton, L. & Plotnikoff, R. C. 2012b. Rationale and study protocol for the supporting children's outcomes using rewards, exercise and skills (SCORES) group randomized controlled trial: A physical activity and fundamental movement skills intervention for primary schools in low-income communities. *BMC Public Health*, 12, 427.

Mahar, M. T. 2011. Impact of short bouts of physical activity on attention-to-task in elementary school children. *Preventive Medicine*, 52, S60–S64.

Mahar, M. T., Murphy, S. K., Rowe, D. A., Golden, J., Shields, A. T. & Raedeke, T. D. 2006. Effects of a classroom-based program on physical activity and on-task behavior. *Medicine and Science in Sports and Exercise*, 38, 2086.

McKee, R., Mutrie, N., Crawford, F. & Green, B. 2007. Promoting walking to school: results of a quasi-experimental trial. *Journal of Epidemiology and Community Health*, 61, 818–823.

McKenzie, T. L. & Lounsbery, M. A. 2009. School physical education: The pill not taken. *American Journal of Lifestyle Medicine*, 3, 219–225.

McKenzie, T. L., Nader, P. R., Strikmiller, P. K., Yang, M., Stone, E. J., Perry, C. L., Taylor, W. C., Epping, J. N., Feldman, H. A. & Luepker, R. V. 1996. School physical education: Effect of the Child and Adolescent Trial for Cardiovascular Health. *Preventive Medicine*, 25, 423–431.

McMullen, J., Kulinna, P. & Cothran, D. 2014. Physical activity opportunities during the school day: classroom teachers' perceptions of using activity breaks in the classroom. *Journal of Teaching in Physical Education*, 33, 511–527.

McMurray, R., Bassin, S., Jago, R., Bruecker, S., Moe, E., Murray, T., Mazzuto, S. & Volpe, S. 2009. Rationale, design and methods of the HEALTHY study physical education intervention component. *International Journal of Obesity*, 33, S37–S43.

McMurrer, J. & Kober, N. 2007. *Choices, changes, and challenges: Curriculum and instruction in the NCLB era*. Washington DC: Centre on Education Policy.

Mendoza, J. A., Levinger, D. D. & Johnston, B. D. 2009. Pilot evaluation of a walking school bus program in a low-income, urban community. *BMC Public Health*, 9, 122.

Metcalf, B., Henley, W. & Wilkin, T. 2012. Effectiveness of intervention on physical activity of children: Systematic review and meta-analysis of controlled trials with objectively measured outcomes (EarlyBird 54). *BMJ*, 345.

Meyer, U., Ernst, D., Zahner, L., Schindler, C., Puder, J. J., Kraenzlin, M., Rizzoli, R. & Kriemler, S. 2013a. 3-Year follow-up results of bone mineral content and density after a school-based physical activity randomized intervention trial. *Bone*, 55, 16–22.

Meyer, U., Romann, M., Zahner, L., Schindler, C., Puder, J. J., Kraenzlin, M., Rizzoli, R. & Kriemler, S. 2011. Effect of a general school-based physical activity intervention on bone mineral content and density: A cluster-randomized controlled trial. *Bone*, 48, 792–797.

Meyer, U., Roth, R., Zahner, L., Gerber, M., Puder, J., Hebestreit, H. & Kriemler, S. 2013b. Contribution of physical education to overall physical activity. *Scandinavian Journal of Medicine and Science in Sports*, 23, 600–606.

Morgan, P. J., Lubans, D., Callister, R., Okely, A. D., Burrows, T., Fletcher, R. & Collins, C. 2011. The 'Healthy Dads, Healthy Kids' randomized controlled trial: Efficacy of a healthy lifestyle program for overweight fathers and their children. *International Journal of Obesity*, 35, 436–447.

Naylor, P.-J. & McKay, H. A. 2009. Prevention in the first place: Schools a setting for action on physical inactivity. *British Journal of Sports Medicine*, 43, 10–13.

Naylor, P.-J., Nettlefold, L., Race, D., Hoy, C., Ashe, M. C., Higgins, J. W. & McKay, H. A. 2015. Implementation of school based physical activity interventions: A systematic review. *Preventive Medicine*, 72, 95–115.

Nichol, M. E., Pickett, W. & Janssen, I. 2009. Associations between school recreational environments and physical activity. *Journal of School Health*, 79, 247–254.

O'Connor, T. M., Jago, R. & Baranowski, T. 2009. Engaging parents to increase youth physical activity: a systematic review. *American Journal of Preventive Medicine*, 37, 141–149.

Olds, T., Ann Maher, C. & Ridley, K. 2011. The place of physical activity in the time budgets of 10-to 13-year-old Australian children. *Journal of Physical Activity and Health*, 8, 548.

Osilla, K. C., Van Busum, K., Schnyer, C., Larkin, J. W., Eibner, C. & Mattke, S. 2012. Systematic review of the impact of worksite wellness programs. *The American Journal of Managed Care*, 18, e68–81.

Owen, K. B., Smith, J., Lubans, D. R., Ng, J. Y. & Lonsdale, C. 2014. Self-determined motivation and physical activity in children and adolescents: A systematic review and meta-analysis. *Preventive Medicine*, 67, 270–279.

Panter, J., Corder, K., Griffin, S. J., Jones, A. P. & Van Sluijs, E. M. 2013. Individual, socio-cultural and environmental predictors of uptake and maintenance of active commuting in children: Longitudinal results from the SPEEDY study. *International Journal of Behavioural Nutrition and Physical Activity*, 10, 83.

Panter, J. R., Jones, A. P. & Van Sluijs, E. M. 2008. Environmental determinants of active travel in youth: A review and framework for future research. *International Journal of Behavioral Nutrition and Physical Activity*, 5, 34.

Parrish, A.-M., Okely, A. D., Stanley, R. M. & Ridgers, N. D. 2013. The effect of school recess interventions on physical activity. *Sports Medicine*, 43, 287–299.

Pate, R. R., O'neill, J. R. & McIver, K. L. 2011. Physical activity and health: Does physical education matter? *Quest*, 63, 19–35.

Rangul, V., Bauman, A., Holmen, T. L. & Midthjell, K. 2012. Is physical activity maintenance from adolescence to young adulthood associated with reduced CVD risk factors, improved mental health and satisfaction with life: The HUNT Study, Norway. *International Journal of Behavioral Nutrition and Physical Activity*, 9, 144.

Ridgers, N. D., Salmon, J., Parrish, A.-M., Stanley, R. M. & Okely, A. D. 2012. Physical activity during school recess: a systematic review. *American Journal of Preventive Medicine*, 43, 320–328.

Ridgers, N. D., Stratton, G. & Fairclough, S. J. 2006. Physical activity levels of children during school playtime. *Sports Medicine*, 36, 359–371.

Ridgers, N. D., Timperio, A., Crawford, D. & Salmon, J. 2011. Five-year changes in school recess and lunchtime and the contribution to children's daily physical activity. *British Journal of Sports Medicine*, 46, 741–746.

Ried-Larsen, M., Grøntved, A., Kristensen, P. L., Froberg, K. & Andersen, L. B. 2013. Moderate-and-vigorous physical activity from adolescence to adulthood and subclinical atherosclerosis in adulthood: Prospective observations from the European Youth Heart Study. *British Journal of Sports Medicine*, 49, 107–112.

Riley, N., Lubans, D., Holmes, K. & Morgan, P. 2015. Findings from the EASY Minds cluster randomized controlled trial: Evaluation of a physical activity integration program for mathematics in primary schools. *Journal of Physical Activity and Health*, 13(2), 198–206.

Russ, L. B., Webster, C. A., Beets, M. W. & Phillips, D. S. 2015. Systematic review and meta-analysis of multi-component interventions through schools to increase physical activity. *Journal of Physical Activity and Health*, 12, 1436–1446.

Sallis, J. F. & McKenzie, T. L. 1991. Physical education's role in public health. *Research Quarterly for Exercise and Sport*, 62, 124–137.

Sallis, J. F., McKenzie, T. L., Alcaraz, J. E., Kolody, B., Faucette, N. & Hovell, M. F. 1997. The effects of a 2-year physical education program (SPARK) on physical activity and fitness in elementary school students. Sports, Play and Active Recreation for Kids. *American Journal of Public Health*, 87, 1328–1334.

Sallis, J. F., McKenzie, T. L., Kolody, B., Lewis, M., Marshall, S. & Rosengard, P. 1999. Effects of health-related physical education on academic achievement: Project SPARK. *Research Quarterly for Exercise and Sport*, 70, 127–134.

Sebire, S. J., Jago, R., Fox, K. R., Edwards, M. J. & Thompson, J. L. 2013. Testing a self-determination theory model of children's physical activity motivation: A cross-sectional study. *International Journal of Behavioral Nutrition and Physical Activity*, 10, 111.

Singh, A., Uijtdewilligen, L., Twisk, J. W., Van Mechelen, W. & Chinapaw, M. J. 2012. Physical activity and performance at school: A systematic review of the literature including a methodological quality assessment. *Archives of Pediatrics and Adolescent Medicine*, 166, 49–55.

Sirard, J. R., Alhassan, S., Spencer, T. R. & Robinson, T. N. 2008. Changes in physical activity from walking to school. *Journal of Nutrition Education and Behavior*, 40, 324–326.

Smith, J. J., Morgan, P. J., Plotnikoff, R. C., Dally, K. A., Salmon, J., Okely, A., D.,, Finn, T. L., Babic, M., Skinner, G. & Lubans, D. R. 2014a. Rationale and study protocol for the 'Active Teen Leaders Avoiding Screen-time' (ATLAS) group randomized controlled trial: An obesity prevention intervention for adolescent boys from schools in low-income communities. *Contemporary Clinical Trials*, 37, 106–119.

Smith, J. J., Morgan, P. J., Plotnikoff, R. C., Dally, K. A., Salmon, J., Okely, A. D., Finn, T. L. & Lubans, D. R. 2014b. Smart-phone obesity prevention trial for adolescent boys in low-income communities: The ATLAS RCT. *Pediatrics*, 134, e723–e731.

Srinivasan, S. R. & Berenson, G. S. 1995. Childhood lipoprotein profiles and implications for adult coronary artery disease: The Bogalusa Heart Study. *American Journal of the Medical Sciences*, 310, S68.

Standage, M., Gillison, F. B., Ntoumanis, N. & Treasure, D. C. 2012. Predicting students' physical activity and health-related well-being: A prospective cross-domain investigation of motivation across school physical education and exercise settings. *Journal of Sport and Exercise Psychology*, 2012, 37–60.

Stanley, R. M., Ridley, K. & Dollman, J. 2012. Correlates of children's time-specific physical activity: A review of the literature. *International Journal of Behavioural Nutrition and Physical Activity*, 9, 50.

Steinbeck, K., Baur, L., Cowell, C. & Pietrobelli, A. 2009. Clinical research in adolescents: challenges and opportunities using obesity as a model. *International Journal of Obesity*, 33, 2–7.

Stewart, J. A., Dennison, D. A., Kohl, H. W. & Doyle, J. A. 2004. Exercise level and energy expenditure in the Take 10!® in-class physical activity program. *Journal of School Health*, 74, 397–400.

Stodden, D. F., Goodway, J. D., Langendorfer, S. J., Roberton, M. A., Rudisill, M. E., Garcia, C. & Garcia, L. E. 2008. A developmental perspective on the role of motor skill competence in physical activity: An emergent relationship. *Quest*, 60, 290–306.

Tandon, P. S., Zhou, C., Sallis, J. F., Cain, K. L., Frank, L. D. & Saelens, B. E. 2012. Home environment relationships with children's physical activity, sedentary time, and screen time by socioeconomic status. *International Journal of Behavioural Nutrition and Physical Activity*, 9, 10.1186.

Telama, R., Yang, X., Leskinen, E., Kankaanpaa, A., Hirvensalo, M., Tammelin, T., Viikari, J. S. A. & Raitakari, O. T. 2014. Tracking of physical activity from early childhood through youth into adulthood. *Medicine and Science in Sport and Exercise*, 46, 1–8.

Timperio, A., Ball, K., Salmon, J., Roberts, R., Giles-Corti, B., Simmons, D., Baur, L. A. & Crawford, D. 2006. Personal, family, social, and environmental correlates of active commuting to school. *American Journal of Preventive Medicine*, 30, 45–51.

Trost, S. G. & Loprinzi, P. D. 2011. Parental influences on physical activity behavior in children and adolescents: A brief review. *American Journal of Lifestyle Medicine*, 5, 171–181.

Tudor-Locke, C., Lee, S. M., Morgan, C. F., Beighle, A. & Pangrazi, R. P. 2006. Children's pedometer-determined physical activity during the segmented school day. *Medicine and Science in Sports and Exercise*, 38, 1732–1738.

Van der Horst, K., Paw, M., Twisk, J. W. & Van Mechelen, W. 2007. A brief review on correlates of physical activity and sedentariness in youth. *Medicine and Science in Sport and Exercise*, 39, 1241.

Van Lippevelde, W., Verloigne, M., De Bourdeaudhuij, I., Brug, J., Bjelland, M., Lien, N. & Maes, L. 2012. Does parental involvement make a difference in school-based nutrition and physical activity interventions? A systematic review of randomized controlled trials. *International Journal of Public Health*, 57, 673–678.

Van Sluijs, E. M., McMinn, A. M. & Griffin, S. J. 2007. Effectiveness of interventions to promote physical activity in children and adolescents: Systematic review of controlled trials. *BMJ*, 335, 703–707.

Waters, E., De Silva-Sanigorski, A., Hall, B., Brown, T., Campbell, K., Gao, Y., Armstrong, R., Prosser, L. & Summerbell, C. 2011. Interventions for preventing obesity in children. *Cochrane Database of Systematic Reviews*, 12, CD001871.

Whitaker, R. C., Wright, J. A., Pepe, M. S., Seidel, K. D. & Dietz, W. H. 1997. Predicting obesity in young adulthood from childhood and parental obesity. *New England Journal of Medicine*, 337, 869–873.

Whitt-Glover, M. C., Ham, S. A. & Yancey, A. K. 2011. Instant Recess®: A practical tool for increasing physical activity during the school day. *Progress in Community Health Partnerships: Research, Education, and Action*, 5, 289–297.

Williamson, D. A., Copeland, A. L., Anton, S. D., Champagne, C., Han, H., Lewis, L., Martin, C., Newton, R. L., Sothern, M. & Stewart, T. 2007. Wise Mind Project: A school-based environmental approach for preventing weight gain in children. *Obesity*, 15, 906–917.

World Health Organization 2010. *Global recommendations on physical activity for health*. Geneva: WHO.

Zahner, L., Puder, J. J., Roth, R., Schmid, M., Guldimann, R., Pühse, U., Knöpfli, M., Braun-Fahrländer, C., Marti, B. & Kriemler, S. 2006. A school-based physical activity program to improve health and fitness in children aged 6–13 years. *BMC Public Health*, 6, 147.

24

PHYSICAL ACTIVITY
IN PRISONS

Mark Norman

There is an inherent paradox in the study of physical activity in prisons, which are institutions built to physically contain certain individuals, yet are also sites for the development and expression of vibrant physical cultures. There are over 10.3 million individuals incarcerated in penal institutions worldwide, a figure that has increased almost 20 per cent since 2000 and that continues to climb as rates of incarceration surpass global population growth (Walmsley, 2016). While males represent the vast majority of these incarcerated individuals, the rates of female incarceration have spiked 50 per cent since 2000 and there are now over 700,000 women and girls imprisoned globally (Walmsley 2015a). Despite the severe restrictions that govern prisoners' daily lives, including their freedom of movement, research shows that physical activity thrives in many correctional institutions around the globe.

Prisons are a prime example of what Goffman (1961) labels *total institutions*—that is, physically and socially isolated places in which groups of people are housed together under the management of a bureaucratic disciplinary regime. Due to the loss of freedom of movement and identity brought on by incarceration in a total institution, inmates have limited opportunities for self-expression and exercising agency. However, research in prison settings around the world reveals that, even in such environments of extreme deprivation and hardship, prisoners engage with a diverse range of physical activities. This chapter reviews this literature and explores key issues relating to prison physical activity.

This chapter begins with a discussion of the concept of the total institution (Goffman, 1961), and a consideration of the significance of physical activity in such an environment. It then discusses policy and practice regarding prison physical activity, including a consideration of international and national correctional policies. Central to this discussion is a recognition of inconsistencies between the requirement of policy and the reality of correctional practice, and the ways that this can affect prisoners' access to physical activity. The bulk of the chapter reviews the literature on prison physical activity, with a focus on six major themes: rehabilitation and therapy; masculinity and violence; women's corrections; race and ethnicity; social control; and alternative forms of physical activity. It then concludes with a discussion of areas for future research and policy development.

Prisons as total institutions

Prisons are a prime example of what sociologist Erving Goffman (1961) labels *total institutions*—that is, physically and socially isolated places in which groups of people (referred to as "inmates") are housed together under the management of bureaucratic disciplinary regimes. In addition to prisons, examples of total institutions described by Goffman include mental hospitals, military bases, concentration camps, and boarding schools; other contemporary spaces that match his descriptions include refugee camps, nursing homes, and religious cults. The cultures of total institutions are shaped by their mutually reinforcing spatial and social characteristics. Spatially, they are separated from the outside world both through physical barriers (e.g., in prisons, high walls and armed guards) and contoured to enable regular surveillance of inmates by staff. Furthermore, total institutions collapse the usual boundaries between spaces of work, leisure, and sleep, forcing inmates to undertake these activities in a single location and in an extremely regimented manner. This spatial construction significantly constrains an inmate's privacy and agency over his or her daily movements.

Socially, total institutions such as prisons create a unique social word by stripping the inmate of his individuality and reinforcing a rigid hierarchy between staff and inmates. Upon entry to a total institution, inmates are usually subjected to humiliating rituals, dispossessed of personal affects, assigned a standard uniform, and, in more extreme cases, given identical haircuts and assigned serial numbers rather than names. Together, these actions serve as *mortifications of the self*, in which key aspects of inmates' previous identities are stripped from them and they are symbolically assigned the lowest status within the institution's social world (Goffman, 1961). Prisoners are given few resources for constructing and presenting a new self (cf. Goffman, 1959), making actions or items that can form the basis of a unique identity extremely coveted by inmates. This perspective helps explain how sport paraphernalia, such as weight belts or yoga mats, and activities that help sculpt muscular bodies can be socially significant resources for prisoners (Norman, 2015c).

It is important to recognize that total institutions are not uniform, and that significant variation exists between them (Goffman, 1961). Even within prisons, there can be significant variation in the day-to-day inmate experience within institutions of different security levels, and even within sections of the same institution. With regard to physical activity, this means that prisoners in different institutions will have access to very different exercise possibilities. A comparison of extreme cases highlights this point. When the modern United States "supermax" prison was developed in late-1970s and early-1980s, it established extreme conditions of confinement: inmates' hands were cuffed and legs were chained before leaving their cells under escort; almost all forms of personal property were banned; and exercise was limited to a small, caged area bereft of exercise equipment (Ward and Werlich, 2003). By contrast, prisoners at Norway's Prison Island, though enduring a variety of pains of imprisonment, enjoy relatively free movement around the island and can participate in a wide range of individual and collective forms of recreation (Shammas, 2014). While it is critical to be sensitive to the specific social contexts of different total institutions, central characteristics of the total institution—such as the bureaucratic handling of batches of inmates, various dehumanizing rituals, and sociospatial isolation from the outside world—are present, to varying degrees, in prisons around the world.

Policy versus practice: What should happen, and what does happen, in prison physical activity?

While each correctional jurisdiction has its own policies concerning imprisonment, the United Nations *Standard Minimum Rules for the Treatment of Prisoners* (United Nations, 1955) offers a broad guideline for respecting inmates' human rights and establishing minimum conditions of confinement. Although the *Rules* have been endorsed by most countries, they are not always effectively implemented (Correctional Service of Canada, 2015). The *Rules* contain the following specific directions concerning physical activity:

> Every prisoner who is not employed in outdoor work shall have at least one hour of suitable exercise in the open air daily if the weather permits. . . .
>
> *Article 21.1*

> Young prisoners, and others of suitable age and physique, shall receive physical and recreational training during the period of exercise. To this end space, installations and equipment should be provided. . . .
>
> *Article 21.1*

> Recreational and cultural activities shall be provided in all institutions for the benefit of the mental and physical health of prisoners.
>
> *Article 78*

While such regulations offer a framework for correctional jurisdictions to build in to prison policy, the reality of day-to-day life in prisons may deviate from the guarantee of physical activity provision. Critical criminologists acknowledge that there can be major gaps between the development of corrections policy and its application in institutions. As Moore and Hannah-Moffat (2005) succinctly summarize:

> Penal policy is best thought of as consisting of two components, rhetoric and practice. The rhetoric . . . does not, however, translate automatically into practice.
>
> *p. 89*

This is an important caveat to the study of penal policy concerning physical activity. In Canada, federal prison policy decrees that, except if it creates a security threat, "every inmate shall be given the opportunity to exercise outdoors for at least one hour every day, or indoors when weather does not permit outdoor exercise" (Correctional Service of Canada, 2008, Article 7). However, there have been numerous situations in which inmates housed in segregation cells have been denied access to exercise time outside of the their cells (Norman, 2015b); furthermore, recent government policy shifts have hinted at a move from the provision sports and physical activity as a prisoner's right to a reward for certain behaviour (Correctional Service of Canada Review Panel, 2007; Jackson and Stewart, 2009). In the US, although prisoners are not considered to have a right to recreation, "courts have come to realize that prolonged idleness can have a distinctly debilitating effect and, consequently, consider such harmful idleness to be a form of [prohibited] cruel and unusual punishment" (Lee, 1996, p. 169). As such, inmates are generally entitled to have access to five hours of recreation time each week—however, there are variations on the interpretation of this requirement, and neither access to specific types of exercise (e.g. weightlifting, a space for running) nor the opportunity to socialize with other inmates is guaranteed (Lee, 1996).

In the European Union, the Council of Europe (2006) lays out basic policies concerning access to exercise and recreation in its *European Prison Rules*. These *Rules* mirror those of the United Nations with regard to minimum access to outdoor exercise, stating that "every prisoner shall be provided with the opportunity of at least one hour of exercise every day in the open air, if the weather permits" (Article 27.1). However, the *European Prison Rules* go further in recognizing the provision of opportunities for physical activity to "form an integral part of prison regimes" (Article 27.3), requiring prison administrations to provide infrastructure and equipment to facilitate these opportunities (Article 27.4), and emphasizing the social importance of physical activity by assuring that inmates are allowed to associate with each other during recreation (Article 27.7). A small number of European Union countries (Greece, Spain, and Italy) allow inmates in certain institutions many hours of outdoor recreation and exercise each day, in excess of Council of Europe guidelines, and have been recognized by the European Prison Observatory as examples of best practice (Crétenot, 2013). However, in many other countries, the minimum level of physical activity provision is not met. For example, the United Kingdom aims to provide inmates with an hour of outdoor recreation each day, yet an inspection into prison conditions "found that, contrary to its expectations, many prisoners in England and Wales did not have the opportunity to spend one hour in the open air every day" (Silvestri, 2013, p. 34). A European Prison Observatory report noted that, in most European Union countries,

> The recommendations of the Council of Europe are . . . not respected with regard to the possibility to spend many hours outside the cell and benefit from a balanced programme of [physical] activities. Activities provided in detention are generally insufficient to cover the period of a normal day and allow prisoners to spend at least eight hours a day out of cell. Moreover, in most countries, prisons generally operate under a closed door regime, so that inmates are sometimes forced to stay in their cells for 22 or 23 hours a day.
>
> *Crétenot, 2013, p. 13*

As these few examples demonstrate, correctional policy and practice can vary between and within correctional jurisdictions. It is of paramount importance for researchers of prison physical activity to attend to these possible divergences and to understand the reasons for them. Furthermore, there is great scope for research on how prisoners cope with correctional practices that offer inadequate physical activity provision, and how they find ways of engaging in physical activity in spite of excessive confinement or lack of recreational opportunity (Norman, 2015b). Such research will help deepen the understanding of the ways in which prison physical activity is designed, implemented, and experienced.

Major themes in prison physical activity research

It is important to distinguish between the different types of physical activity in which prisoners may partake, as these can range from punitive physical labour to pleasurable recreational exercise. For the purposes of this chapter, the definition of physical activity is limited to recreational and rehabilitative or therapeutic physical activities. The first category includes organized or informal forms of sport and exercise undertaken in leisure time. The second category refers to physical activities, such as yoga, that are provided to prisoners as part of a formalized rehabilitation or therapy program. This section reviews six major themes that emerge from the literature on prison physical activity.

Rehabilitation and therapy

Offender rehabilitation and therapy are major aims of many corrections systems, and many studies discuss the possible contribution of physical activity to achieving these goals (e.g.

Martos-García, Devís-Devís, and Sparkes, 2009; Meek, 2014; Meek and Lewis, 2014b; Norman, 2015a; Williams, Walker, and Strean, 2005). Rehabilitation focuses on transforming the behaviour of a criminal offender through treatment, so that he or she is less likely to reoffend upon release (Davis, 2002; Hollin, 2004). Therapeutic programming, meanwhile, uses targeted interventions in an attempt to address a specific issue, such as addiction or anger, that is linked to engaging in criminal behaviour (Moore and Hannah-Moffat, 2005). Both concepts, while often contrasted with punitive approaches to corrections, are problematic. Both can operate from the assumption that criminal behaviour can be "cured" (Cullen and Johnson, 2011), and thus ignore structural reasons for crime and imprisonment. Furthermore, discourses of rehabilitation can discursively hide the ways in which therapeutic programming can itself be punitive (Moore and Hannah-Moffat, 2005). The degree to which studies of physical activity grapples with these problematic issues in rehabilitation and therapy is mixed.

Policymakers commonly view sport and physical activity as tools for crime deterrence, in spite of limited evidence to support this link (Coalter, 2007). In a related vein, many studies have sought to determine whether participation in sport and physical activity inside prison can contribute to an inmate's rehabilitation or therapy. There is some support for this outcome. Research by Meek (Meek, 2014; Meek and Lewis, 2014a, 2014b) has suggested that structured sport and recreation programs can allow prisoners to acquire skills that will aid their societal reintegration and reduce the likelihood that they will reoffend. Williams, Walker and Strean (2006), while careful to avoid overstating its benefits, suggest that physical recreation can contribute to healing-focused and strengths-based rehabilitation efforts for prisoners: "[correctional recreation], if planted from within the empirically fertile soil of offender rehabilitation and rooted in concepts of restorative justice, may yet prove to be a critical and underutilized component of offender rehabilitation and subsequent reduced recidivism" (p. 53). Meanwhile, other studies have considered the therapeutic value of physical activity to prisoners. Research on programs that combine yoga and meditation has offered confident assertions about their therapeutic potential in increasing self esteem (Duncombe et al., 2005), improving mood (Bilderbeck et al., 2013), and combating addiction (Bowen et al., 2006, 2007; Simpson et al., 2007). Some inmate participants in a Spanish study (Martos-García et al., 2009) stated that physical activity programs provided benefits such as mental escape, stress release, and increased feelings of social inclusion, while staff members also suggested that physical recreation provided prisoners with mental health benefits.

Other research problematizes a straightforward relationship between prisoners' participation in physical activity and potential rehabilitative or therapeutic outcomes. Andrews and Andrews (2003) conducted a long-term participant observation in an English youth prison, and found that participation in sport had multiple meanings for inmates: for some, it was an important contributor to the rehabilitative goal of social development, while for others it could be an inconsequential or socially damaging practice. Some studies note that many prisoners, though aware that physical activities may be offered with the understanding that they will achieve certain outcomes, reject the belief that their participation will contribute to their rehabilitation (Caplan, 1996; McIntosh, 1986). Norman (2015a) cautioned that, despite statements from yoga teachers and inmate participants about the rehabilitative impact of yoga participation, it is difficult to determine if such statements are accurate:

> Despite the reported impacts of yoga for prisoners, particularly the belief that it allows them to reduce violent behaviour and effectively channel their frustrations, extreme caution should be exercised in determining whether yoga is an effective alternative form of rehabilitation. While yoga appears to offer various benefits to some prisoners,

it is not at all clear that this will translate into long-term behaviour change or reduced rates of recidivism upon release.

Clearly, the relationship between physical activity, rehabilitation, and therapy is mixed. There is certainly compelling evidence that participating in various forms of physical activity may contribute to inmate's rehabilitation or offer him or her therapeutic benefits. However, such outcomes are not inevitable, and prisoners may have diverse experiences with sport and physical activity programs. Future research on this topic needs to be attuned to such differences, and to explore how physical activity can have diverse social meanings and outcomes in various correctional settings.

Masculinity and violence

In all countries and territories around the globe, men make up the vast majority of prisoners; in fact, in 80 per cent of countries men comprise 91 per cent to 98 per cent of the prison population (Walmsley, 2015b). Given this overwhelming representation of men in prisons, it is not surprising that an examination of physical activity and masculinity is prominent in many studies on physical activity in prisons. Research suggests that male prison culture is often characterized by a hegemonic masculinity—that is, an idealized set of characteristics that men in a given culture are expected to possess and display—premised upon physical domination and strict adherence to an *inmate code* that informally regulates acceptable masculine behaviour (Ricciardelli, 2013, 2014; Sabo, Kupers and London, 2001). Sabo (2001) argues that, in a prison environment, "masculine identity is earned, rehearsed, refined, and relived through each day's activity" (p. 63), with sport acting as a major site for the expression of masculinity.

Various studies suggest that sports and physical activities, such as weightlifting, boxing, or martial arts, can be important contributors to the performance of hegemonic masculinity in both youth and correctional settings. Specifically, various physical activities can be used by male prisoners to construct social hierarchies through the development of muscular bodies and assertion of physical dominance over other boys or men (Martos-García et al., 2009; Ricciardelli, 2014, 2015; Sabo, 2001). Martos-García et al. (2009) and Sabo (2001) both describe a mental and physical "hardness" that prisoners attempt to develop through participation in activities such as weightlifting and martial arts. The celebration of this hardness celebrates "particular kinds of masculinity over others that provide a limited script for those men choosing to enter the arena of sport and physical activity within the prison" (Martos-García et al., 2009, p. 93). These findings dovetail with the broader ways in which sport and physical activity contribute to the construction of hegemonic masculinity (McKay, Messner, and Sabo, 2000).

There is a relationship between the social construction of prison masculinity, physical activity, and the cultures of violence that characterize many men's prisons. Physical activities that develop strength or fighting skills can be used by prisoners as a strategy to mitigate the threat of violent attacks or sexual assaults (Abrams et al., 2008; Kupers, 2001; Ricciardelli, 2014, 2015; Sabo, 2001). Ricciardelli's (2014, 2015) research on the culture of Canadian men's prisons effectively demonstrates that inmates use the activity of weightlifting to build muscular physiques that make them appear more intimidating. This form of self presentation is an important part of prisoners' masculinity, as "the more 'dangerous' a prisoner is perceived to be, the more respect, status and dominance he is awarded" (Ricciardelli, 2015, p. 188). Meanwhile, sport and other forms of physical recreation can be sites for the enactment of physical violence between inmates. For example, Norman (2015b; 2015c) found that male Canadian inmates engaged in both instrumental (i.e. tactical and premeditated) and expressive (i.e. unplanned) violence during physical recreation. Instrumental violence involved serious attacks during recreation periods, such as using weight bars as weapons, and was a tactic for settling scores, asserting gang dominance, or presenting a tough persona. Expressive violence occurred during heated sport matches, such as boxing and full-contact floor hockey, and was tolerated by staff and inmates. There is thus a complex relationship between physical activity in men's prisons, the social construction of prison masculinity, and both instrumental and expressive forms of violence.

Women's corrections

Most research on physical activity in prisons has focused on male institutions, meaning that the experiences of women prisoners have not been explored in as much depth. However, the recent publication of studies on leisure and recreation for women prisoners suggests that scholars are increasingly seeking to address this imbalance. The research that exists tends to focus on benefits of or barriers to physical activity participation. In terms of benefits, a study of sport programs in English women's prisons (Meek and Lewis, 2014a) found that women gained a variety of health and psychosocial benefits from participation, including: improving self-esteem and physical health, coping with the challenges and frustrations of imprisonment, providing opportunities for positive relationship building with staff, and even teaching skills that assisted with social and employment challenges upon release. Meanwhile, studies by Canadian scholars (Granger-Brown, et al., 2012; Pedlar, Yuen, and Fortune, 2008; Yuen, Arai, and Fortune, 2012) offer insight into incarcerated women's experiences of prison leisure and therapy, including physical activity. Among the significant findings were the value of culturally sensitive leisure programming for Aboriginal women, and the potential for these to offer a space for collective healing and challenging colonial legacies (Pedlar et al., 2008); the possibility for physical activities, led by volunteers from the outside community, to be sites for women inmates to build relationships and enjoy humanizing and pleasurable recreation opportunities (Pedlar, Yuen, and Fortune, 2008); and the value of therapeutic recreation programs, which improve women's physical and mental health and "permit women to acquire skills, explore aspects of themselves and the world, and have fun" (Granger-Brown, et al., 2012, p. 510).

The literature also highlights some specific issues hindering the physical activity participation of women prisoners in specific correctional contexts, including the lack of female supervising staff (Meek and Lewis, 2014a); symbolic violence enacted on the bodies of women prisoners through inadequate food and the excessive use of psychotropic drugs as a tool of social control (Norman, 2015b); competing duties, such as work or (in mother-child facilities) parenting (Meek and Lewis, 2014a); and the challenges for women former prisoners engaging in physical leisure practices after reentering the community (Yuen, Arai, and Fortune, 2012). Martos-García et al.'s (2009) research in a Spanish prison, which housed in separated units both men and women, offered a nuanced analysis of how gender can contour physical activity participation amongst women prisoners. In particular, the study argued that low rates of participation amongst women inmates reflected broader cultural attitudes toward gender in Spanish society, and that the prison administration adhered to stereotypical understandings of femininity that unfairly assumed that women have little interest in sport. Meanwhile, Andrews and Andrews's (2003) study in a British youth prison highlights the need for careful consideration of the social and emotional needs of adolescent female inmates when designing physical activity programming for this population.

Overall, the limited research on physical activity in women's prisons suggests that it has great potential to provide prisoners with a variety of health and social benefits, but that institutional and structural barriers can inhibit their participation. Studies by Martos-García et al. (2009) and Yuen and Fortune (2008) offer valuable examples of how researchers can connect the experiences of women prisoners in physical activity with broader social constructions of gender (and other intersecting structures) in a specific cultural context. Given the recent scholarly interest in physical activity for women's prisoners, there will hopefully be more studies in this vein in the near future.

Race and ethnicity

Reflecting broader structures of social inequality and marginalization, racial and ethnic minorities are typically overrepresented in prison populations around the world (King, 2008). However, despite their significance, race and ethnicity feature in a limited manner in research on prison physical activity. Certainly some studies of carceral physical activity recognize the significance of race to prison culture, but they rarely grapple deeply with the implications. For example, McIntosh (1986) used surveys to examine how Black, Hispanic, and Native American prisoners in the United States viewed recreation and rehabilitation. The study's treatment of race is not very critical—the three groups were chosen because they represented the largest racial minority groups in United States prisons, without consideration of *why* these groups were overrepresented—but it does demonstrate that underlying assumptions about prison physical activity having rehabilitative benefits are not necessarily shared by inmates from minority groups. Rather, prisoners from diverse backgrounds may choose to engage or not engage with physical activity programming for cultural reasons.

Research in Canada and Australia has touched upon physical activity and leisure for Aboriginal Peoples and Indigenous Australians, respectively. In Canada, where Aboriginal people make up four percent of the population and nearly one quarter of federal prisoners (Sapers, 2014), some efforts have been made to create leisure and therapeutic activities programs that use Aboriginal knowledge and cultural practices to assist prisoners. Yuen et al.'s (2009) participatory research with incarcerated Aboriginal women suggested that culturally specific and meaningful forms of leisure can be a site for the development of an Aboriginal identity that had been erased by colonialism. An example of such a program is a horse-assisted therapy program, run by the Nekaneet First Nation, that was offered to Aboriginal women in a federal prison. The program taught prisoners "traditional lessons about the horse from a Nekaneet perspective, and allow[ed] them to master the basics of equine care and horseback riding. Horses are often used for healing in Aboriginal culture" (Amellal, 2006, section 3, para. 7). Such programs suggest the importance of physical activities, such as horseback riding, in the leisure and therapy practices of Aboriginal prisoners. Meanwhile, Gallant, Sherry, and Nicholson's (2015) research on sport in Australian prisons was careful to acknowledge the overrepresentation of Indigenous Australians in the prison population, including in their participant group. However, the authors only presented a small amount of data on Indigenous prisoners' participation, in part because of language barriers. The researchers did report that Indigenous prisoners saw football skills, which they improved through the prison's sport programs, as offering an opportunity to connect with and serve as a role model in Indigenous communities upon release.

Clearly, given the severe overrepresentation of minorities in prisons, there is a need for much deeper research about the experiences of racial and ethnic minorities with prison physical activity. Topics for exploration could include consideration of if and how prison regimes accommodate diverse populations; whether physical activity might dovetail with other social or therapeutic programming for specific populations; if an expansion of recreation programming should include forms of culturally significant physical activity; and whether physical activity plays a part in exacerbating or reducing racial or ethnic tensions amongst inmates.

Social control

Prisons, as total institutions, are sites of social control in which inmates have little agency over when and where they can move, work, play, and sleep (Goffman, 1961). Prison physical activity plays a role in administrations' efforts to control prisoners, reflecting the broader ways in which sport and physical activity can be sites for the exertion of social control (Eitzen, 2000). In prisons, physical activity is offered by administrations as a means of exercising control over the behaviour of inmates: as a number of studies demonstrate, prison staff often believe that inmates' participation in physical activity will reduce their boredom and allow them to work off excess energy that may otherwise be directed toward violence (Caplan, 1996; Frey and Delaney, 1996; Gallant et al., 2015; Martos-García, et al., 2009; Meek, 2014; Pawelko and Anderson, 2005; Truss and Hunter, 2004). As Truss and Hunter (2004) summarize, these viewpoints help to underpin the rationale for prison physical activity programming:

> For their supporters, prison recreation programs provide constructive ways for inmates to use their spare time while also endowing them with skills that may help prevent them from reoffending. When inmates are completely idle, like anyone else, they will become bored. They may also feel frustrated or aggressive, and become violent toward themselves or others. A number of activities like football, softball, and basketball are specifically designed to help reduce the stresses of incarceration by providing physical stimulation.
>
> *p. 827*

However, such assumptions about the impact of physical activity as a form of social control provide a limited understanding of this phenomenon. By adhering to a catharsis hypothesis of violence, which understands exercise to be a safety valve for releasing aggression, they are supporting an inaccurate interpretation of the causes of violence in sport and physical activity (Young, 2012). As Young (2012) notes, research has shown that participation in sports may increase, rather than reduce, violence, calling into question the legitimacy of the catharsis theory as a rationale for controlling prisoners through physical activity. For example, Norman (2015b) found that, although former prisoners described physical activity as having cathartic effects, the culture of prison sport and physical activity was, in fact, extremely violent and exclusionary. Furthermore, prisoners do not automatically achieve the outcomes of participation that are assumed by staff, nor do they accept passively attempts at social control. Research on the experiences of Canadian prisoners (Norman, 2015b; 2015c; Yuen et al., 2009) suggests that recreation and leisure can be activities through which prisoners resist administrative attempts to control them. For example, Yuen et al. (2009) suggested that leisure practices of female Canadian Aboriginal prisoners "served as a context where women could understand and resist the marginalizing and oppressive structures related to their colonization" (p. 559). Norman (2015b, 2015c), drawing on Goffman's (1961) theorization of the total institution, argued that inmates use physical activity as a site for small acts of individual and collective resistance against the aims of the prison administration. There is a great need for further research on the tensions between prison physical activity's potential to serve as both a tool for social control and a vehicle for resistance.

Alternative forms of physical activity

The activities highlighted in the literature on prison physical recreation tend to reflect dominant forms of European or American activity, especially team sports or individual activities such as weightlifting. However, some research examines non-dominant physical activities, such as dance (Milliken, 2002; Seibel, 2008), animal-assisted interventions (Dell and Poole, 2015; Furst, 2007), and yoga (Bilderbeck et al., 2013; Bowen et al., 2006; Duncombe et al., 2005; Norman, 2015a; Simpson et al., 2007). Research on dance programs suggests that they can help prisoners cope with stress, build trust, and develop communication skills (Seibel, 2008), and that they may be deployed as a form of arts-based therapy (Milliken, 2002). Literature on animal-assisted interventions demonstrates their potential to assist with healing from trauma, provide opportunities for social development, and create change in the broader prison environment (Dell and Poole, 2015; Furst, 2007). Meanwhile, participation in yoga has been associated with a wide range of psychosocial therapeutic outcomes (Bilderbeck et al., 2013; Bowen et al., 2006; Duncombe et al., 2005; Simpson et al., 2007).

These alternative physical activities are usually part of a carefully designed therapeutic or rehabilitation program, often operated in concert with prisons' social work or chaplaincy departments. As such, they may be more explicitly structured to achieve prosocial outcomes than many mainstream recreational or leisure activities. However, Norman's (2015a) research on prison yoga in Canada offers a cautionary approach to overstating the positive outcomes from such alternative physical activities. He found that, while it is a meaningful practice for individual inmates and offers an alternative to violent and hierarchical forms of physical activity, yoga is also a form of institutional control used to induce behavioural change and monitor inmates (Norman, 2015a). There is thus need for caution in analyzing the impact of such alternative activities. Deeper research on their social potential and problematic aspects will contribute to an understanding of their impacts in prison cultures.

Conclusion

This chapter has examined the ways of prisons' total institutional characteristics make various physical activities significant practices for inmates as they construct new identities, as well as the potential disjuncture between policy and practice related to prison physical activity. It also reviewed six key themes and issues in research about prison physical activity: rehabilitation and therapy; masculinity and violence; women's corrections; race and ethnicity; social control; and alternative forms of physical activity. Emerging from these discussions are some important implications for research and policy concerning prison physical activity.

In terms of future research, there is a clear need for deeper qualitative research on the experiences of prisoners with formal, informal, and alternative forms of physical activity. Such research will highlight the experiences of prisoners and deepen scholarly understanding of the complex social meanings of physical activity in various corrections settings. Of course, conducting qualitative research in prisons is more easily suggested than accomplished— Wacquant (2002) has noted the difficulties facing researchers attempting to get inside prisons, which he describes as "opaque organizations that can be difficult and sometimes nearly impossible to penetrate" (p. 387). Nonetheless, as some of the studies cited in this chapter highlight, persistent researchers have had success in gaining access to correctional institutions and examining their physical cultures. Where access is not permitted, researchers may be forced to employ a creative mixed methods approach that uses available data to piece together an interpretive understanding of physical activity in a particular prison setting (Norman,

2015b). A continued effort by scholars to shed light on correctional institutions will allow for stronger analysis of how physical activity relates to issues such as rehabilitation, gender, race, violence, and social control. Further, a deeper consideration of the alternative forms of physical activity highlighted here will help how they differ from dominant forms of activity, and the implications of this for the social environment of the prison. While this chapter is focused exclusively on prisons, the concept of the total institution (Goffman, 1961) may allow researchers to make meaningful comparisons between the social meaning of physical activity in correctional institutions and in other social settings, such as refugee camps, military institutions, and boarding schools.

One area of research that should be a high priority for researchers, especially those concerned with the potential for physical activity to contribute to rehabilitation, is the (dis) continuity of participation for former prisoners upon release. Former prisoners may face considerable challenges when attempting to reintegrate into the community, including in the way they move in public spaces and physically present themselves in public settings (Caputo-Levine, 2013). If participation in prison physical activity can provide inmates with physical and social benefits, it is paramount to determine if similar opportunities exist and outcomes can be achieved in a community setting. Research that explores these questions, even if it is difficult to carry out, will provide important insight into whether physical activity remains a long term feature in the lives of former prisoners, and what, if any, impact this has on their likelihood of reoffending.

In terms of policy development, the literature offers a number of suggestions for improving physical activity in correctional institutions. The physical activity guidelines presented in the UN's (1955) *Standard Minimum Rules for the Treatment of Prisoners* should be immediately implemented as a baseline by all nations and territories, as these are the basic levels to which world governments have agreed. This is an especially important consideration in situations of extreme deprivation, such as segregation units and "supermax" institutions. The examples provided by Norway (Shammas, 2014) and certain European Union countries (Crétenot, 2013) make clear that more liberal approaches to relative freedom of movement are possible in correctional settings. The research on race and/or ethnicity and prison physical activity highlights that the needs and interests of diverse inmate populations may not be met by physical recreation offerings. Taking steps to determine and implement culturally sensitive programming for minority inmate groups could be extremely important in engaging them in physical activity. Similarly, the physical activity needs and interests of women inmates may differ from men, and should be considered when designing policy in women's corrections. Meanwhile, although physical activity can contribute to a violent and exclusionary prison masculinity, yoga, dance, and animal-assisted interventions appear to have potential to construct physical activity in radically different ways. The potential of these activities should be explored in more depth, and it would behoove correctional jurisdictions to consider implementing such programs in their prisons.

Finally, as prisons are unhealthy and damaging places, a major reconsideration should be undertaken in various societies of the underlying causes of crime, the overrepresentation of minorities and the poor in prison populations, and the social role of correctional institutions. A wide body of research calls into question the effectiveness of prisons for reducing crime, yet in many societies mass incarceration is relied upon for punishment and deterrence (Garland, 2013; Wacquant, 2002). Returning to the paradox that introduces this chapter, such an overreliance on prisons means that numerous individuals are incarcerated and have their freedom of movement severely curtailed. While changes to prison physical activity can certainly make it more accessible or enhance its potential benefits, incarceration by its definition results in a restriction of the range of physical movement open to a person. Imprisoning fewer people would, therefore, be the most expedient way of increasing criminal offenders' access to healthy physical activity.

References

Abrams, L.S., Anderson-Nathe, B., and Aguilar, J. (2008) Constructing masculinities in juvenile corrections. *Men and Masculinities.* 11(1). pp. 22–41.

Amellal, D. (2006) No walls, no wire, but I will never run away: Enhanced capacities to provide effective interventions for First Nations, Métis and Inuit Offenders. *Let's Talk.* 31(1). Retrieved May 14, 2015 from www.csc-scc.gc.ca/publications/lt-en/2006/31-1/7-eng.shtml.

Andrews, J.P., and Andrews, G.J. (2003) Life in a secure unit: The rehabilitation of young people through the use of sport. *Social Science and Medicine.* 56(3). pp. 531–550.

Bilderbeck, A.C., Farias, M., Brazil, I.A., Jakobowitz, S., and Wikholm, C. (2013) Participation in a 10-week course of yoga improves behavioural control and decreases psychological distress in a prison population. *Journal of Psychiatric Research.* 47(10). pp. 1438–1445.

Bowen, S., Witkiewitz, K., Dillworth, T.M., Chawla, N., Simpson, T.L., Ostafin, B.D., . . . and Marlatt, G.A. (2006) Mindfulness meditation and substance use in an incarcerated population. *Psychology of Addictive Behaviors.* 20(3). pp. 343–347.

Bowen, S., Witkiewitz, K., Dillworth, T.M., and Marlatt, G.A. (2007) The role of thought suppression in the relationship between mindfulness meditation and alcohol use. *Addictive Behaviors.* 32(10). pp. 2324–2328.

Caplan, A. (1996) *The Role of Recreational Sports in the Federal Prison System.* (Unpublished Master's thesis). Acadia University: Wolfville, NS.

Caputo-Levine, D.D. (2013) The yard face: The contributions of inmate interpersonal violence to the carceral habitus. *Ethnography.* 14(2). pp. 165–185.

Coalter, F. (2007). *A Wider Social Role for Sport: Who's Keeping the Score?* New York: Routledge.

Correctional Service of Canada. (2008) *Commissioner's Directive Number 760: Leisure Activities.* Retrieved November 18, 2014 from www.csc-scc.gc.ca/text/plcy/cdshtm/760-cde-eng.shtml.

Correctional Service of Canada. (2015) United Nations Standard Minimum Rules For the Treatment of Prisoners 1975. Retrieved August 29, 2017 from www.csc-scc.gc.ca/text/pblct/rht-drt/07-eng. shtml.

Correctional Service of Canada Review Panel. (2007) *A Roadmap to Strengthening Public Safety.* Ottawa: Minister of Public Works and Government Services Canada.

Council of Europe. (2006) *European Prison Rules.* Strasbourg: Council of Europe Publishing. Retrieved August 29, 2017 from www.coe.int/t/DGHL/STANDARDSETTING/PRISONS/PCCP%20 documents%202015/EUROPEAN%20PRISON%20RULES.pdf.

Crétenot, M. (2013) *From National Practices to European Guidelines: Interesting Initiatives in Prison Management.* Rome: European Prison Observatory. Retrieved August 29, 2017 from www.prisonobservatory.org/upload/EPOinterestinginitiatives.pdf.

Cullen, F.T., and Johnson, C.L. (2011). Rehabilitation and treatment programs. In Wilson, J.Q., and Petersilia, J. (eds.). *Crime and Public Policy.* New York: Oxford University Press.

Davis, M.S. (2002) *The Concise Dictionary of Crime and Justice.* Thousand Oaks, CA: SAGE.

Dell, C.A., and Poole, N. (2015). Taking a PAWS to reflect on how the work of a therapy dog supports a trauma-informed approach to prisoner health. *Journal of Forensic Nursing.* 11(3). pp. 167–173.

Duncombe, E., Komorosky, D., Wong-Kim, E., and Turner, W. (2005) Free inside: A program to help inmates cope with life in prison at Maui Community Correctional Center. *Californian Journal of Health Promotion.* 3(4). pp. 48–58.

Eitzen, D.S. (2000) Social control and sport. In Coakley, J., and Dunning, E. (eds.). *Handbook of Sports Studies.* Thousand Oaks, CA: SAGE Publications.

Frey, J.H., and Delaney T. (1996) The role of leisure participation in prison. *Journal of Offender Rehabilitation.* 23(1). pp. 79–89.

Furst, G. (2007). Without words to get in the way: Symbolic interaction in prison-based animal programs. *Qualitative Sociology Review.* 3(1). pp. 96–109.

Gallant, D., Sherry, E., and Nicholson, M. (2015) Recreation or rehabilitation? Managing sport for development programs with prison populations. *Sport Management Review.* 18(1). pp. 45–56.

Garland, D. (2013). Punishment and social solidarity. In Simon, J., and Sparks, R. (eds.). *The SAGE Handbook of Punishment and Society* (pp. 23–40). London: SAGE.

Goffman, E. (1959) *The Presentation of Self in Everyday in Life.* Garden City, NY: Doubleday Anchor Books.

Goffman E. (1961) *Asylums: Essay on the Social Situation of Mental Patients and Other Inmates.* Garden City: Anchor Books.

Granger-Brown, A., Buxton, J.A., Condello, L.L., Feder, D., Hislop, G., Martin, R.E., . . . and Thompson, J. (2012) Collaborative community prison programs for incarcerated women in BC. *BC Medical Journal.* 54(10). pp. 509–513.

Hollin, C.R. (2004) To treat or not to treat? An historical perspective. In Hollin, C. (ed.). *The Essential Handbook of Offender Assessment and Treatment.* Chichester, UK: Wiley.

Jackson, M., and Stewart, G. (2009) *A Flawed Compass: A Human Rights Analysis of the Roadmap to Strengthening Public Safety.* Retrieved January 28, 2015 from http://papers.ssrn.com/sol3/Delivery.cfm/SSRN_ID1881036_code746470.pdf?abstractid=1881036andmirid=1.

King, R.D. (2008). Prisons and jails. In Shoham, S.G., Beck, O., and Kett, M. (eds.). *Penology and Criminal Justice.* Boca Raton, FL: CRC Press.

Kupers, T. (2001) Rape and the prison code. In Sabo, D., Kupers, T.A., and London, W.J. (eds.). *Prison Masculinities.* Philadelphia: Temple University Press.

Lee, R.D. (1996) Prisoners' rights to recreation: Quantity, quality, and other aspects. *Journal of Criminal Justice.* 24(2). pp. 167–178.

Martos-García, D., Devís-Devís, J., and Sparkes, A.C. (2009) Sport and physical activity in a high security Spanish prison: An ethnographic study of multiple meanings. *Sport, Education and Society.* 14(1). pp. 77–96.

McIntosh, M. (1986) The attitudes of minority inmates towards recreation programs as a rehabilitative tool. *International Journal of Comparative and Applied Criminal Justice.* 10(1–2). pp. 107–113.

McKay, J., Messner, M.A., and Sabo, D. (2000) *Masculinities, Gender Relations, and Sport.* Thousand Oaks, CA: SAGE.

Meek, R. (2014) *Sport in Prison: Exploring the Role of Physical Activity in Correctional Settings.* New York: Routledge.

Meek, R. and Lewis, G.E. (2014a). Promoting well-being and desistance through sport and physical activity: The opportunities and barriers experienced by women in English prisons. *Women and Criminal Justice.* 24(2). pp. 151–172.

Meek, R., and Lewis, G.E. (2014b) The impact of a sports initiative for young men in prison: Staff and participant perspectives. *Journal of Sport and Social Issues.* 38(2). pp. 95–123.

Milliken, R. (2002) Dance/movement therapy as a creative arts therapy approach in prison to the treatment of violence. *The Arts in Psychotherapy.* 29(4). pp. 203–206.

Moore, D., and Hannah-Moffat, K. (2005) The liberal veil: Revisiting Canadian penality. In Pratt, J., Brown, D., Brown, M., Hallsworth, S., and Morrison, W. (eds.). *The New Punitiveness: Trends, Theories, Perspectives.* Portland, OR: Willan Publishing.

Norman, M. (2015a) Prison yoga as a correctional alternative? Physical culture, rehabilitation, and social control in Canadian prisons. In Crichlow, W., and Joseph, J. (eds.). *Alternative Offender Rehabilitation and Social Justice: Arts and Physical Engagement in Criminal Justice and Community Settings.* New York: Palgrave.

Norman, M. (2015b) *Sport and Physical Recreation in Canadian Federal Prisons: An Exploratory Study of Carceral Physical Culture.* (Unpublished doctoral thesis). University of Toronto: Toronto, Canada.

Norman, M. (2015c) Sport in the underlife of a total institution: Social control and resistance in Canadian prisons. *International Review for the Sociology of Sport.* DOI: 10.1177/1012690215609968.

Pawelko, K.A., and Anderson T.K. (2005) Correctional recreation, weightlifting in prison, and rehabilitation: A comparison of attitudes. *11th Canadian Congress on Leisure Research,* Nanaimo, BC, 17–20 May 2005. Retrieved September 22, 2010 from http://lin.ca/Uploads/cclr11/CCLR11-109.pdf.

Pedlar, A., Arai, S., Yuen, F., & Fortune, D. (2008). Uncertain futures: Women leaving prison and re-entering community. Retrieved 8 September 2017 from: http://www.ahs.uwaterloo.ca/uncertainfutures/.

Pedlar, A., Yuen, F., and Fortune, D. (2008) Incarcerated women and leisure: Making good girls out of bad? *Therapeutic Recreation Journal.* 42(1). pp. 24–36.

Ricciardelli, R. (2013) Establishing and asserting masculinity in Canadian penitentiaries. *Journal of Gender Studies.* 25(2), 170–191.

Ricciardelli, R. (2014) *Surviving Incarceration: Inside Canadian Prisons*. Waterloo: Wilfred Laurier University Press.

Ricciardelli, R. (2015) Establishing and asserting masculinity in Canadian penitentiaries, *Journal of Gender Studies*, 24:2, 170–191.

Sabo, D. (2001) Doing time, doing masculinity: Sport and prison. In Sabo, D., Kupers, T.A., and London, W.J. (eds.). *Prison Masculinities*. Philadelphia: Temple University Press.

Sabo, D., Kupers, T.A., and London, W.J. (2001) Gender and the politics of punishment. In Sabo, D., Kupers, T.A., and London, W.J. (eds.). *Prison Masculinities*. Philadelphia: Temple University Press.

Sapers, H. (2014) *Annual Report of the Office of the Correctional Investigator 2013–14*. Ottawa: The Correctional Investigator of Canada.

Seibel, J. (2008) Behind the gates: Dance/movement therapy in a women's prison. *American Journal of Dance Therapy*. 30(2). pp. 106–109.

Shammas, V.L. (2014) The pains of freedom: Assessing the ambiguity of Scandinavian penal exceptionalism on Norway's Prison Island. *Punishment and Society*. 16(1). pp. 104–123.

Silvestri, A. (2013) *Prison Conditions in the United Kingdom*. Rome: European Prison Observatory. Retrieved August 29, 2017 from www.crimeandjustice.org.uk/sites/crimeandjustice.org.uk/files/Prison%20conditions%20in%20the%20UK.pdf.

Simpson, T.L., Kaysen, D., Bowen, S., MacPherson, L.M., Chawla, N., Blume, A., Marlatt, G.A., and Larimer, M. (2007) PTSD symptoms, substance use, and vipassana meditation among incarcerated individuals. *Journal of Traumatic Stress*. 20(3). pp. 239–249.

Truss, G., and Hunter, W.T. (2004) Recreation programs. In Bosworth M. (ed.). *Encyclopedia of Prisons and Correctional Facilities*. Thousand Oaks, CA: SAGE.

United Nations. (1955) *Standard Minimum Rules for the Treatment of Prisoners*. Retrieved June 30, 2012 from www2.ohchr.org/english/law/treatmentprisoners.htm.

Wacquant, L. (2002) The curious eclipse of prison ethnography in the age of mass incarceration. *Ethnography*. 3(4). pp. 371–397.

Walmsley, R. (2015a) *World Female Imprisonment List* (3rd edition). London: International Centre for Prison Studies.

Walmsley, R. (2015b) *World Prison Population List* (11th edition). London: International Centre for Prison Studies.

Walmsley, R. (2016) *World Prison Population List* (12th edition). London: International Centre for Prison Studies.

Ward, D.A., and Werlich, T.G. (2003) Alcatraz and Marion: Evaluating super-maximum custody. *Punishment and Society*. 5(1). pp. 53–75.

Williams, D.J., Walker, G.J., and Strean, W.B. (2005) Correctional recreation on death row: Should pardon be granted? *Journal of Offender Rehabilitation*. 42(2). pp. 49–67.

Young, K. (2012) *Sport, Violence and Society*. New York: Routledge.

Yuen, F., Arai, S., and Fortune, D. (2012) Community (dis)connection through leisure for women in prison. *Leisure Sciences*. 34(4). pp. 281–297.

Yuen, F., Pedlar, A., Arai, S., and Kivel, B.D. (2009) Leisure as a context for justice: Experiences of ceremony for Aboriginal women in prison. *Journal of Leisure Research*. 41(4). pp. 547–564.

THEME E INTRODUCTION
Understanding and evaluating practices and programmes

This section presents a variety of programmes and practices that have sought to enhance physical activity provision for different population groups. More specifically, this section explores the issues and challenges in attempting to develop positive outcomes from interventions, judged by both formal evaluations and more personal and political unintended outcomes. All of the programmes and practices face a number of challenges to be successful. Further, readers will come to appreciate that many of these settings require diligent evaluation and critical reflection on the part of those intervening, and not simply evangelical promotion of physical activity.

In their chapter examining the Swedish sports system and its connection with public health, Anna Aggestål and Josef Fahlén develop our understanding about the complexities involved when government agencies work with voluntary sports clubs to achieve health outcomes. In the Swedish case, ideas about democracy, equality and physical activity are used to legitimise the Swedish Sport Confederation's role in public health promotion. While this might seem an excellent example of partnerships in action, there are important challenges for organised sport becoming increasingly beholden to public health objectives. The authors discuss their use of a 'critical discourse analysis' approach, which involves a close critical examination of the ideas which inform policy.

In the case of hard to reach groups such as those designated as 'inactive' or living in areas of deprivation, intervention programmes often rely on precarious and limited external funding. Carolynne Mason's chapter examines a charity programme running for over a decade in the UK. With hopes of changing change lives and communities, StreetGames goes beyond provision of accessible sport and physical activity. It also attempts to encourage leadership, increase employability and decrease offending rates of young people. By emphasising gathering good data and involving the right people, StreetGames shows what can be achieved in terms of providing PA to young people in difficult situations.

Undoubtedly children are the focus of the majority of physical activity interventions, and many of these take place in schools. As Darren Powell and Michael Gard show, however benevolent sponsors may seem, there are serious ethical issues related to sponsored physical activity educational initiatives. In many countries, it is clear that corporations are eager to promote health (and their own brands) in school settings. Powell and Gard interrogate the apparently charitable interventions of companies in schools, and show these schemes may well be problematic, especially when sponsoring companies are those often criticised for promotion of unhealthy food and drink.

Paul Bretherton and Billy Graeff provide a comparative analysis of the most recent two Summer Olympic Games in London and Rio in order to consider how much (or how little) effort is put into implementing physical activity legacy goals. Calling these policies problematic, the authors highlight the complexity of the settings, the range of actors, and the practical issues that have twice meant that there has been not been any significant physical activity legacy from these mega sport events. The authors also note problems with measuring any purported legacy effect. Questions about measurement continue in three chapters. Abby Foad and Michelle Secker discuss how there has been a need to generate good evidence for policy change, and they explain how this was achieved – through on-going systematic collection of a range of data about a school sport programme. Nonetheless the authors note that even though good evidence might exist, physical activity interventions are always shaped by social, political and economic factors.

The need for rigorous evaluations is considered in detail by Andy Pringle, Jim McKenna and Stephen Zwolinsky. They examine the credibility and impact of a number of physical activity interventions and offer a number of powerful practices and shortcomings in evaluations. Acknowledging and mitigating the shortcomings will be useful for anyone involved in programme implementation and evaluation. Nana Anokye continues this evaluation theme by comparing the costs and consequences of various health interventions in the UK. Anokye describes the application of economic evaluation techniques to evaluate two physical activity interventions – the General Practitioner (GP) brief advice and Exercise referral schemes – highlighting the associated challenges and how they have been addressed to date.

Richard J. Buning and Heather J. Gibson discuss cycling, a popular activity in the vast majority of countries around the world, and an activity which is lauded for its health and sustainability related benefits. The authors discuss the interplay between benefits and challenges. Successful cycling systems will inevitability disrupt traditional motor vehicle infrastructure, and victories for cycling advocacy groups are often hard fought. This chapter examines the place of cycling in urban environments and the potential for cultural habits and priorities to change in favour of cycling-friendly cities.

Our final chapter in this section on practices and programmes moves away from the official, explicit PA interventions and considers a case where physical activity poses specific problems. In a case study on elite sport Jenny McMahon demonstrates that ideas about achievement, athleticism come with the potential for severe and devastating unintended consequences. Given that organised sport is one of the most popular sites for physical activity intervention, it is pertinent to consider possible unintended consequences of physical activity in connection with achievement and performance. The chapter provides an opportunity to reflect on the ideas that we imbue physical activity and performance with.

It is clear that there is no one best way to understand the vast array of practices and programmes and which involve physical activity, not is it easy to account for the multitude of meanings and values attributed to it. There is both a need for rigorous evaluation of PA programme claims as well as a need for understanding how practices encouraged and enforced by dominant institutions may not always be in the best interest of the intervention's recipients. We hope therefore that readers will be inspired to view physical activity interventions with equal amounts of scrutiny and sympathy.

25

EMPLOYING VOLUNTARY SPORTS ORGANISATIONS IN THE IMPLEMENTATION OF PHYSICAL ACTIVITY POLICY

Anna Aggestål and Josef Fahlén

Introduction

The approach of utilising sport with the intention of contributing to fundamental change and transformation in society has received much attention within the field of "sport for development" over the last decade (Coalter, 2013; Schulenkorf & Adair, 2014). In particular, interventions to promote physical activity and health have been studied in many different forms and settings (for an extensive review, see Baker, Dobbins, Soares, Francis, Weightman, & Costello, 2015). Taking a departure in this literature, this text reports a study of this phenomenon, though not with the interventionist approach dominating much of the contemporary research efforts (Hartmann & Kwauk, 2011). Instead, it seeks to problematise interventions employing organised sport for public health, in this case, by posing questions about voluntary sports organisations' will, ability, readiness and propensity to act as a counteracting force against differences in sport participation and health between groups in society. As such, this chapter explores how public health is being constructed, implemented and given meaning within organised sport. Departing from the fact that civil society's involvement in attaining government objectives on physical activity participation is often carried out by voluntary sport organisations, the chapter examines the Swedish Sports Confederation's (SSC) role and position in this work. By interviewing SSC representatives and national sport organisations' (NSO) general managers and drawing on a critical discourse approach (Fairclough & Fairclough, 2012), this chapter will explore how discourses on democracy, equality and physical activity are used to legitimise the SSC's role in public health promotion and how such discourses pose challenges for organised sport in meeting public health objectives.

In Sweden, which is used in this chapter as an empirical example of the growing phenomenon of employing voluntary sport organisations in the implementation of physical activity policy, sport and physical activity have received a prominent position in welfare policy and are, as such, governed through the national objectives on public health, including those pertaining to physical activity (SOU, 2000, p. 91). The SSC, a voluntary and membership-based non-profit organisation, has, since receiving its first government grant in 1913 (Norberg, 2004), been granted permanent annual state subsidy for sport activities as the main provider of sport for the people and has, as such, been included in the government's welfare policy objectives regarding physical activity. With a relationship more of a partnership balancing rights and obligations in a way that has been described as an *implicit contract*, the SSC has been assigned a government mandate to act towards objectives of physical activity and public health (Norberg, 2011). In the SSC's policy document (Riksidrottsförbundet, 2009) on recreational sport it is stated that health, comfort and well-being are the norm, although performance and competition often serve as a spur. Furthermore, the SSC pledges in its strategy document on public health (Riksidrottsförbundet, 2007) to undertake health-related development work within the frames of all of its regular sports activities and also to make targeted efforts (such as, for example, exercise on prescription, adapted activities for overweight children and activities for adults on long-term unemployment or sick leave) to reach new groups with inclusion as the main goal.

During the last decade, two large, nationwide sports development programmes, the Handshake (Handslaget) and the Sports Lift (Idrottslyftet), have been launched to further pursue this ambition and, more specifically, to strive towards the ambition of including more children and youth in voluntary and membership-based club sport activities (Fahlén & Karp, 2010; Fahlén, Eliasson, & Wickman, 2015). Similar to their Nordic counterparts in Denmark (Ibsen, 2002), Finland (Vuori, Lankenau, & Pratt, 2004) and Norway (Skille, 2009; Skille & Waddington, 2006), the basic idea behind the programmes has been the government commissions to national umbrella organisations for sport to develop their activities so that more children and youth (especially underrepresented and underprivileged groups) choose to participate in sports club activities, as well as to develop their activities so that children and youth choose to participate longer into their teens and early adulthood (with the underlying ambition to increase physical activity levels in the population). While these programmes, and similar interventions in other countries (cf., Friis Thing & Ottessen, 2010, for a study of civil society's involvement in welfare policy on public health; Wickman, 2011, for equal opportunity; Theeboom, Schaillée, & Nols, 2012, for integration; Morgan, 2013, for democracy; Mutz & Baur, 2009, for criminality; Stenling, 2014, for youth delinquency; Grix & Carmichael, 2012, for national identity; and Thorpe, 2014, for individual identity), have been valuable for social inclusion—and in extension for increased physical activity levels—some evidence indicates difficulties in relying on civil society organisations on the one hand and in confusing physical activity with voluntary and membership-based club sport on the other hand.

Regarding the first and in relation to the empirical example in this chapter, many studies (e.g., Adams, 2011; May, Harris, & Collins, 2012; Nichols, Padmore, Taylor, & Barrett, 2012; Skille & Solbakken, 2011; Stenling & Fahlén, 2014) have explored the propensity, ability, readiness and will of sport organisations to fulfil policy aims formulated by external stakeholders such as the state. These studies have found that sport organisations' existing ideas, norms and values act as strongholds against policy initiatives differing too much from their core activities. Regarding the latter, critics have found that most studies cited to support the notion that sport is beneficial for public health actually refer to physical activity or exercise (and not to sport) and that sport and physical activity are not the same (Coalter, 2007). However, as noted by Bloyce and Smith (2010), Collins (2010) and Coalter (2007), less is known about how sport and health policy are enacted in practice.

Paying heed to the claim by Collins (2010) that the promotion of health through physical activity with the use of voluntary and membership-based sport organisations has not been explored sufficiently, the study this chapter uses as an illustration explores the promotion of public health in the context of Swedish sport. Answering the call made by Hylton and Bramham (2001) to direct research focus at the gap between formulation and implementation of strategies, the aims of the study were to analyse how public health is being constructed, implemented and given meaning on a strategic level within voluntary and membership-based club sport, as well as to discuss implications in relation to society and public health objectives— to understand organised sport's potential as a national physical activity promoter. In order to do so, we begin by sketching the outlines of Swedish voluntary and membership-based club sport and its connection to government policy on physical activity.

Contextual background

The SSC is, as mentioned in the introductory section, appointed by the government to act towards the national objectives of physical activity and public health, and has since 1970 been given the mandate to distribute government funds to sport organisations (Norberg, 2002). Government funds to voluntary organised and membership-based club sport have been granted since 1913 and today amount to some €210 million (Centrum för idrottsforskning, 2013). Public funding to sport also comes in the form of municipal support of €490 million (€360 million to facilities and €130 million to activities and leaders; Bergsgard & Norberg, 2010). This extensive public funding is provided as means for implementing social policy and is distributed to 3,300,000 sport club members in 20,164 Swedish sport clubs (Centrum för idrottsforskning, 2013), but it is also distributed to some 1,000 district sport organisations (DSOs, with regional authority over one specific sport), 21 regional sports organisations (RSOs, with regional authority over all sports) and 70 national sport organisations (NSOs, with national authority over one specific sport) for coordination, administration and support. These organisations are federated under one large umbrella organisation with almost a monopoly on competitive sports (Bairner, 2010; Bergsgard & Norberg, 2010). The monopoly is based on the fact that the SSC holds the roles as the highest authority in voluntary organised and membership-based club sport and as the public authority in sport policy (Norberg, 2011).

The role of the government has traditionally been limited to decisions on the extent of funding and its overarching goals, while the SSC has had the mandate to decide on the means for reaching such goals. This state-SSC relationship has enabled the government to control its expenditures and the SSC to preserve its self-determination in a corporative collaboration. The confederation's main tasks include representing voluntary and membership-based club sport in communication with authorities, officials and the surrounding society; supporting and servicing affiliated organisations; administering and distributing government funds to affiliated organisations; stimulating sport development and research; coordinating social and ethical issues; leading and coordinating anti-doping work; coordinating international cooperation; protecting sport's historical legacy; and acting as the governmental authority for the 51 upper-secondary elite sport schools with some 1,200 students in 30 sports. The defining character of and main organising principle for contemporary voluntary and membership-based club sport in Sweden is that of individuals forming and/or taking part as members in voluntary and membership-based sport clubs. To understand how public health is being constructed, implemented and given meaning on a strategic level within this organisational complex, in the following we will outline the theoretical approach used to analyse the reasoning expressed by SSC representatives and NSOs' general managers.

Theoretical approach

In the study this chapter uses as an empirical example of the growing phenomenon of employing voluntary sport organisations in the implementation of physical activity policy, critical discourse analysis (CDA) was employed to understand the relationship between discursive representations of public health and sport practice. CDA involves normative critique of discourse and the existing social reality focussed upon dialectical relations between discourse, social practice and social structure—all being conditions for, and effects of, each other (cf., Fairclough, 1992). CDA aims at evaluating societies in order to understand possibilities for changing them to make them better, in terms of cultivating the well-being of their members rather than undermining it. In the most recent variant of CDA (Fairclough & Fairclough, 2012), discourse is viewed primarily as *practical argumentation* for (or against) particular ways of acting, a deliberative form of argumentation that can ground decisions. Representations of actions enter as premises in arguments, and arguments based on such representations can be critically evaluated. The authors claim that an analysis and evaluation of arguments can increase the capacity of CDA to extend the critique of discourse, moving from normative critique (representations) to explanatory critique (practical arguments). This statement was put to the test in the study this chapter uses as an empirical example by using it to understand the SSC's possibilities in and obstacles for acting as the national physical activity promoter.

In trying to make use of the proposed framework, practical reasoning and practical argumentation were employed. Practical arguments for, as well as against, certain actions (*means premises*) are understood in this approach as taking *circumstances* and *goals* as premises, and the circumstances (which are described in a way that fits with the claim of action) are understood as being informed by the agents' *values* premises. In the study and from an argumentative perspective, statements about strategies, procedures, working methods and actions employed in fulfilling ideas of public health were treated as representations that enter as premises in the arguments of how sport contributes to public health. In a similar way, means premises were deconstructed to identify inherent goals, circumstances and values. Finally, arguments were evaluated in terms of whether the actions were reasonable and sufficient in view of the goal and of the consequences of action. The methodological details of this approach are provided below.

Methodological approach

CDA provided the methodology for both data collection and analysis. Capturing agents' practical reasoning required qualitative interviews (Kvale & Brinkmann, 2009) and capturing the construction, implementation and sense-making of public health through voluntary organised and membership-based sport required a purposeful sampling (cf., Patton, 2002) of respondents, together representing the collective reasoning of the SSC. Thus, respondents were chosen on the basis of their assumed knowledge about and possible influence on decisions made in relation to the object of study (Bryman, 2008). Following this notion it was deemed important to select key actors with formal power and mandate to govern the confederation towards the public health aims provided by the government. Thus, key actors from the SSC and its federated NSOs, with national authority over their respective sport, were selected.

Selection of SSC representatives was guided by an ambition to capture the strategic dimensions of policy enactment. The selection resulted in six representatives: the chairperson of the confederation, the director of sports policy, the director of sports development, the director of economy, the director of recreational sport for children and youth and recreational sport for adults. The purposeful selection of NSOs aimed at providing information-rich examples. Therefore, a sample of NSOs was made on each organisation's merits of distinguishing itself as being more public health oriented. Four NSOs, out of the total of 70, were selected: company sports, gymnastics, school sports and academic sports. Each NSO was represented by its general manager with the formal power and mandate to govern the organisation.

The semi-structured interview guide departed from the key objectives in state sport policy and public health policy, resulting in six themes: emphasising sport's significance for public health; encouraging participation, physical activity and recreational sport in the population; offering sport "for all"; reducing societal differences in sport participation and health; targeting efforts for public health; and collaborating between sectors. The semi-structured format of the interviews enabled the respondents to talk about how they are implementing the above-mentioned public-health-related objectives in their everyday practice within their organisations. This, in turn, allowed for the conversation to move beyond common (political) rhetoric and discourse towards richer knowledge about how "sport for public health" is implemented and why (Kvale & Brinkmann, 2009).

Data were analysed in several careful reviews, marking and sorting out arguments about the meaning of public health and in what way sport is valuable for and promotes better overall health. With the CDA perspective employed, these arguments were collected into themes that can be seen as representations of the respondents' understanding and ideas of sport's significance for public health. The themes are: democracy, equality, recreation and physical activity. In order to take the analysis a step further beyond those representations and to explore how the respondents are putting them into practice within their respective organisations, the interviews were analysed using an argumentative perspective on discourse (Fairclough & Fairclough, 2012), as outlined under the Theoretical Approach section.

Findings

Aiming at understanding the SSC's potential as a national physical activity promoter, the findings are presented thematically, following the respondents' lines of argumentation.

The significance of sport for public health

When asked about what significance sport has for the public health of the Swedish population, the respondents claimed that sport's role in public health is important in several ways. The statements about sport's significance for and contribution to public health are very much in line with the key objectives in state sport policy. A common argument among the respondents was that the sport movement already delivers public health through its regular activities and that sport is entitled to government support for doing just that and that alone, without having to perform further specific actions such as, for example, those connected to the government programmes presented in the introduction or other targeted efforts such as exercise on prescription, adapted activities for overweight children and activities for adults on sick leave. This line of reasoning is exemplified by one respondent: "The good in sport is sport itself, so to speak . . . just the fact that sport exists makes it a health perspective".

When scrutinising the arguments within this line of reasoning—that sport is inherently beneficial for public health—four main discourses come to the fore: *democracy, equality, recreation* and *physical activity*. The first discourse is about how sport participation fosters democracy and suggests that being offered opportunities to exercise influence is key to public health. Schooling in democratic values is a cornerstone in Swedish voluntary and membership-based organisations, and by offering members voting rights, influence and power, members are included and empowered. Connected to the democracy discourse is the argument that sport promotes equality. By stating that sport is an activity for all, regardless of age, gender, ethnicity, religion, sexual orientation or social/financial background, it is again argued that sport is intimately connected to public health due to its inclusive nature. The inclusiveness, by extension, brings about the third argument: recreation. Since all are included, sport makes up an arena for social interaction, which in turn promotes a sense of community and belonging. Community and belonging, it is asserted, are instrumental for public health. The argument of recreation is also based on the view of sport as something one does simply because it is fun, not based on goals for performance improvement or competition. Fourth and finally, it is argued, sport is healthy based upon the merits of its physical character. Thus, this particular argument contains little else than the first statements given about sport's significance for and contribution to public health, which in turn are little more than echoes of the key objectives in state sport policy. By that it shows how cemented the hegemonic discourse about the value of sport is and how the sport–public health relationship is constructed through circular arguments.

The implementation of sport for public health

When discussing how sport for public health is implemented in practice within the respondents' respective organisations, the circular arguments remain. This is visible in the general opinion among the respondents: that their main responsibility is to provide support for and create the best possible conditions for their organisations and their members to do sport. In an attempt to move beyond this seemingly self-evident argument, respondents were asked to specify what they as professionals do in their day-to-day operations to meet the goals of sport for public health. Their descriptions were oriented around activities such as advocacy for sport and lobbying government agencies and community representatives such as policy makers, national and local politicians, business leaders and school leaders. The lobbying of public officials is specifically focussed on arguing for a more open and free distribution of public funds for sport with less regulation and control. By that, it is claimed, sport is better equipped to act as a public health promoter.

Respondents also talked about taking internal measures to further facilitate the implementation of public health through sport—to influence the organisation for public health from within. The measures referred to are the on-going restructuring of the organisations, spurred by a shared argument that voluntarily organised and membership-based club sport needs to change and broaden its activities and, thereby, its target groups. It is, however, simultaneously emphasised that Swedish sport organisations are in fact part of a voluntary and democratically governed popular movement acting on behalf of its members, who are in the end those in charge of the what, how, when and why of sport clubs' activities: "It's not like a company with subsidiaries that one can say what they should do". Thus, the concept of *democracy*, which was one of the arguments given by the respondents for sport's importance for public health, resurfaces but seems to be a double-edged sword. On the one hand, voluntariness and active membership are pointed to as vehicles for public health, as members can exercise their democratic rights in an organisation and thereby be empowered, which is argued to contribute to public health. On the other hand, it is complicated from the point of view of the limited possibility to influence or control an organisation in any direction since the respondents are acting on behalf of the members.

Nevertheless, several of the means employed to promote public health aim to influence and change the organisations' culture in a top-down manner. In order for sport to be more inclusive and open to all, as well as to be able to fulfil the function as *the* national physical activity promoter, respondents claimed that the organisations' inherent logic of competition and performance needs to change: "We are trying to get the NSOs to review their operations and to consider what they might need to change to get people outside the sport movement to want to join". This quote indicates that promoting public health is thought to be best realised by making efforts to reach new groups of people, such as the inactive or sedentary, and at the same time striving against "sport for all". The practical argumentation for how these efforts are implemented shows how increasing the number of members is a means to receive more legitimacy and funding, which may benefit competitive sports in the end. The goal to increase membership, and not necessarily to even out differences in health, is identified by examples of recruitment activities that target former members or individuals that have previously been physically active. There are also examples of the contrary, for instance, the NSO of school sports that cooperates with other NSOs organising so-called non-traditional sports (boule petanque is given as one example) in an attempt to attract children not interested in regular club sports such as soccer or gymnastics. The respondent representing the NSO for school sports explained:

> If we are serious about making a better sports movement that more people feel they want to be a part of, it is necessary to influence sport clubs to stop thinking in terms of the logic of competition and performance and to broaden their perception of for whom they exist.

Thus, similar to the double-edged nature of the concept of *democracy*, *equality* is equally being used both as an argument for sport's significance for public health *and* as a measure taken to implement ideas for public health.

However, including new groups of people in the pursuit of realising sport for all was also problematised by the respondents. While the ambition is very much on the agenda in the on-going development work, it was argued by some of the SSC representatives that reaching new groups involves more than just offering more or perhaps non-traditional sport activities. They claimed that the whole organisational structure of sport has to change in order for sport to be able to move away from the priority on competition and ranking of performance. As an example, they pointed to the most recent and still on-going sport development programme, the Sports Lift (alluded to in the introduction of this paper), in which actions are taken aiming at broadening the sport movements' uptake. While such programmes are argued to be valuable and referred to as means to fulfil public health objectives, they cannot be expected to repair the mechanisms behind the problem: "We cannot just make these additional investments all the time; we have to change internally, and there really is no quick fix." Since regular club sport activities, the respondents elaborated, are not organised with *recreation* and *physical activity* for the participants as their main aim, it is far-fetched to expect participants who are first and foremost interested in physical exercise. In addition, it appears as if that particular type of participant is not very interesting for a sport club to attract either: "The sport movement has traditionally not been interested in people who are not interested in competing in sports but only to move for the sake of exercise."

The NSO representatives also seemed to be aware of how the sporting activities they provide and the groups of people they attract fit in with contemporary societal public health ambitions. The NSO representative for company sports concluded that their organisation seems to attract many leaders with specific skills and interest in delivering recreational physical activities for young people and adults, a direction that happens to fit well with a public health profile. This particular NSO has, in recent years, involved all its affiliated sport clubs in extensive strategic planning activities and development work, which has resulted in a business strategy of taking a stand for concepts such as health and public health. Some factions within the NSO have voiced opinions to further include various kinds of public health activities (such as smoking prevention, dietary advice and physical activity on prescription), but the strategy work has resulted in a more consolidated offering of activities: "Our contribution to public health is to improve the physical health of our members by physical activity." There are still affiliated sport clubs working towards specific target groups (for example, overweight children and people on sick leave) and in cooperation with county and municipality administrations, but experiences of such efforts have shown that such activities are often afflicted with problems of coordination and tend to require additional funding in addition to regular government grants. The NSO representative for gymnastics expanded on the difficulties in implementing physical activity on prescription. Since activities for people granted a prescription are to be provided during the day and most voluntary leaders are available in the evenings after work, it has proven difficult to coordinate supply and demand, resulting in a decline in interest from the activity leaders to perform such duties. The NSO representative for academic sports reported being more successful and exemplified this with a large externally funded project aiming at recruiting physically inactive students, which has resulted in the development of a model for getting young people started with physical activity. In conclusion, with regards to implementing sport activities for public health, the strategies of the four NSOs represented in this study seem to be in line with public health objectives. However, and importantly, it appears difficult to provide activities that are disconnected from the logic of competition and performance: "In the traditional sport club the focus is naturally on improvement of per-formance, on the next game or next competition."

Potential of sport for public health

While the respondents argued that sport already delivers public health through its existing and regular activities, they also highlighted that sport holds a big potential for contributing to public health even more in the future. The potential is argued to lie within the reorientation of the larger sport movement, which has been initiated and which is hoped to bring about a change of direction, making the sport movement more inclusive and open to all. At the same time, the respondents argued strongly that it is completely voluntary for sports clubs to take on health promotion activities, and that the organisation is, by no means, to be perceived as a public health supplier for the government—it simply has no obligation to take responsibility for public health. While the respondents all painted a picture of an organisational willingness to be an advocate for health and to strive towards contributing to public health, at the same time they pointed to the fact that willingness, advocacy and perseverance are all in the hands of the existing members. In relation to the latter, the respondents were not too optimistic since the existing priority in most sport clubs appears to be to preserve the longstanding tradition of *sport* activities: "Too much focus on public health interventions can make us lose focus on sport, which is the core and foundation." This overemphasised focus was seen as problematic in other ways too by one of the respondents, claiming that there are leaders within the organisation who, on their own initiatives, "take on too much responsibility for public health and put in too much work without getting paid for it". Such an argument is particularly interesting in light of the ascribed value of grassroots-anchored initiatives and the experienced problem of leaders being guided too much by the logic of competition and performance. Simultaneously, it is argued that it is difficult to design activities with a public health perspective, instead of with the traditional competition and performance perspective; it requires a different kind of leadership and competence that cannot be expected of the voluntary leaders in Swedish sport, even if the respondents acknowledge that leaders holding such competence do exist. The internal education system does not seem equipped to prepare leaders for such leadership, as the health aspects included in these programmes are restricted to basic knowledge in relation to the specific sport in question and are often reduced to injury prevention and treatment.

In conclusion, with regards to the potential of sport for public health, the respondents appeared to be somewhat ambivalent. On the one hand, they claimed that sport is, in its existing form, promotive of public health and has the potential to be even more so in the future. On the other hand, they saw obstacles in the form of self-determining members and leaders guided by traditions and the logic of competition and performance. One of the respondents elaborated on the latter and highlighted the importance of the sports movement to be built on voluntary initiatives—that possible public-health-related activities carried out within the organisation must be based on the members' own desires and interests. However, the focus of the local sport clubs, as another representative concluded, is not to remedy various social problems: "One probably should not overestimate the capacity of sport to play the role of public health promoter."

Conclusions

The ambitions of this chapter were to show how public health is implemented and given meaning within Swedish sport and to add to the broader understanding of voluntarily organised and membership-based sport's potential as a physical activity promoter. The evaluation of SSC and NSO representatives' practical arguments on how ideas on public health are implemented within their respective organisations shows how stated health-related goals are being compromised by other values underlying the described means taken. Thus, actions can be viewed as insufficient in view of the goal of public health since the values and concerns, such as sport performance enhancement and competitive sport, informing the actions taken differ in stance. These findings are in line with previous studies showing how the main convention in sport is competitiveness and that sport representatives' arguments for health "seem to be manifested in rhetoric, symbolic or legislative processes" rather than being regulative for social practice (Skille, 2011, p. 250) and sport's difficulties to change in order to act on ideas that are not in line with its organisational self-identity (Stenling, 2014). Similarly, actions taken to reach new target groups (in the name of equality) can be seen as insufficient when the values and concerns informing the actions are about increasing membership and gaining legitimacy and funding for traditional competitive sports. A consequence of gaining more members on such basis would possibly imply a continued imbalance in terms of sport participation and distribution of health between different social groups in society. A consequence of lobbying and advocating for sport in the name of public health could result in continued support for the sport movement for actions not prioritised in practice. As shown in aforementioned research (Skille, 2011; Stenling, 2014), health issues may not necessarily be the regulating concern for the actions taken in practice in the name of public health. Allocating grants to short-term efforts and specific "inclusion-targeted projects" could allow regular competitive sport activities to remain unchanged. This conclusion is supported by previous studies (Fahlén & Karp, 2010; Fahlén, Eliasson, & Wickman, 2015) that have shown that targeted efforts to develop alternative sport activities in order to attract new target groups have not only been unsuccessful but also contribute to consolidate dominating logics in regular activities. On that particular note, some argue for the need for a cultural and structural change from within sport organisations in order for change to occur (Coalter, 2007). The respondents in the study used as an empirical example in this chapter all referred to an on-going restructuring of their organisations in order to change and broaden their activities and, thereby, their target groups; but as is shown in the results, the actions taken to work internally on influencing the organisations to review their operations and activities (in the name of democracy) have resulted in a more limited range of targeted public health activities, possibly limiting the organisations' abilities to contribute to a more equal distribution of health between different social groups.

Implications for future physical activity policy and practice

The findings of the study used as an empirical example in this chapter indicate some implications for future physical activity policy and practice. In relation to the latter, a limitation in the SSC's potential to promote participation and inclusion from a public health perspective is its duty to act on the members' behalf. Thus, even if the sport movement at the strategic level would have the ambition to broaden the uptake of members based on the goal of reaching vulnerable groups in society (with regards to public health), it is the members at the operative level who determine the actions and activities—and ultimately the prioritised target groups. At the core of the problem lies the fact that public health demands a population perspective per se, while the sports movement's obligation, as a voluntary and membership-based organisation, is first, foremost and exclusively towards its constituting members. Consequently, if the inherent values and concerns of the SSC's members support traditional competitive sport ideals, it is difficult to design and carry out actions and activities that are effective in relation to public-health-related goals. Another finding with implications for the sport for public health practice is the taken-for-granted argument that sport equals physical activity. As also problematised by Coalter (2007), we argue that if sport is intended to improve citizens' health, more thought should be given to *what kinds* of physical activities should be encouraged.

In relation to the former (physical activity policy), we see problematic contradictions between the representatives' normative discourse on how sport is significant for and contributes to public health and the practical arguments on the actions and means taken in practice. These contradictions are possibly due to the space of freedom enabled by the way sport is governed by the state, referred to by researchers as the *implicit contract* (Norberg, 2011). These circumstances raise questions about governments' use of voluntary and membership-based non-profit organisations to achieve public health goals. Also, it demonstrates a need for further studies on how public health promotion is put into practice on a strategic and operative sport level—in order to better understand the potential for sport to act as a counteracting force against differences in sport participation and health between groups in society.

Acknowledgements

The authors would like to give thanks to the Swedish National Centre for Research in Sports for its financial support of the research on which this chapter is based. A version of this text was originally published in *Social Inclusion*, 3, 108–117, under a Creative Commons license: Attribution 4.0 International (CC-BY).

References

Adams, A. (2011). Between modernization and mutual aid: The changing perceptions of voluntary sports clubs in England. *International Journal of Sport Policy and Politics*, *3*(1), 23–43.

Bairner, A. (2010). What's Scandinavian about Scandinavian sport? *Sport in Society*, *13*(4), 734–743.

Baker, P. R., Dobbins, M., Soares, J., Francis, D. P., Weightman, A. L., & Costello, J. T. (2015). Public health interventions for increasing physical activity in children, adolescents and adults: An overview of systematic reviews. *The Cochrane Library*, DOI: 10.1002/14651858.CD011454.

Bergsgard, N. A., & Norberg, J. R. (2010). Sports policy and politics—The Scandinavian way. *Sport in Society*, *13*(4), 567–582.

Bloyce, D., & Smith, A. (2010). *Sport policy and development. An introduction.* New York: Taylor & Francis.

Bryman, A. (2008). *Samhällsvetenskapliga metoder* [Methods in social science]. Malmö: Liber.

Centrum för idrottsforskning (2013). *Statens stöd till idrotten—uppföljning 2012* [Government support to sport—follow up 2012]. Stockholm: Centrum för idrottsforskning.

Coalter, F. (2007). *A wider social role for sport. Who's keeping the score?* New York: Routledge.

Coalter, F. (2013). *Sport for development: What game are we playing?* London: Routledge.

Collins, M. (2010). *Examining sports development.* New York: Taylor & Francis group.

Fahlén, J., Eliasson, I., & Wickman, K. (2015). Resisting self-regulation: An analysis of sport policy programme making and implementation in Sweden. *International Journal of Sport Policy and Politics*, *7*(3), 391–406.

Fahlén, J., & Karp, S. (2010). Access denied: The new "Sports for all"—programme in Sweden and the reinforcement of the "Sports performance"—logic. *Sport & EU Review: The Review of the Association for the Study of Sport & the European Union*, *2*(1), 1–48.

Fairclough, I., & Fairclough, N. (2012). *Political discourse analysis. A method for advanced students.* London: Routledge.

Fairclough, N. (1992). *Discourse and social change.* UK: Polity press.

Friis Thing, L., & Ottessen, L. (2010). The autonomy of sports: Negotiating boundaries between sports governance and government policy in the Danish welfare state. *International Journal of Sport Policy*, *2*(2), 223–235.

Grix, J., & Carmichael, F. (2012). Why do governments invest in elite sport? A polemic. *International Journal of Sport Policy and Politics*, *4*(1), 73–90.

Hartmann, D., & Kwauk, C. H. (2011). Sport and development: An overview, critique, and reconstruction. *Journal of Sport and Social Issues*, *35*(3), 284–305.

Hylton, K., & Bramham, P. (2001). *Sports development. Policy, process and practice.* New York: Taylor & Francis group.

Ibsen, B. (2002). *Evaluering af det idrætspolitiske idéprogram* [Evaluation of the ideaprogramme sport policy]. Copenhagen, Denmark: Københavns Universitet and Institut for forskning i Idræt og Folkelig Oplysning.

Kvale, S., & Brinkmann, S. (2009). *Den kvalitativa forskningsintervjun* [The qualitative research interview]. Lund: Studentlitteratur.

May, T., Harris, S., & Collins, M. (2012). Implementing community sport policy: Understanding the variety of voluntary club types and their attitudes to policy. *International Journal of Sport Policy and Politics*, *5*(3), 397–419.

Morgan, H. (2013). Sport volunteering active citizenship and social capital enhancement: What role in the big society. *International Journal of Sport Policy and Politics*, *5*, 381–395.

Mutz, M., & Baur, J. (2009). The role of sports for violence prevention: Sport club participation and violent behaviour among adolescents. *International Journal of Sport Policy*, *1*(3), 305–321.

Nichols, G., Padmore, J., Taylor, P., & Barrett, D. (2012). The relationship between types of sports club and English government policy to grow participation. *International Journal of Sport Policy and Politics*, *4*(2), 187–200.

Norberg, J. R. (2002). Idrottsrörelsen och staten. In J. Lindroth and J. R. Norberg (Eds.), *Riksidrottsförbundet 1903–2003* [The Swedish Sports Confederation 1903–2003]. Stockholm: Informationsförlaget, 181–231.

Norberg, J. R. (2004). *Idrottens väg till folkhemmet—studier i statlig idrottspolitik 1913–1970* [Sport's road to the welfare state: Studies in Swedish government policy towards sport, 1913–1970]. Stockholm: SISU Idrottsböcker.

Norberg, J. R. (2011). A contract reconsidered? Changes in the Swedish state's relation to the sports movement. *International Journal of Sport Policy and Politics*, *3*(3), 311–325.

Patton, M. Q. (2002). *Qualitative research and evaluation methods* (3rd ed.). London: SAGE.

Riksidrottsförbundet (2007). *Idrott hela livet. Strategisk plan för idrottsrörelsens folkhälsoarbete* [Sports throughout life. Strategic plan for the sport movement's public health work]. Stockholm: Riksidrottsförbundet.

Riksidrottsförbundet (2009). *Idrotten vill [What sport wants]*. Stockholm: Riksidrottsförbundet.

Schulenkorf, N., & Adair, D. (2014). *Global sport-for-development: Critical perspectives*. London: Palgrave Macmillan.

Skille, E. Å. (2009). State sport policy and voluntary sport clubs: The case of the Norwegian sports city program as social policy. *European Sport Management Quarterly, 9*(1), 63–79.

Skille, E. Å. (2011). The conventions of sport clubs: Enabling and constraining the implementation of social goods through sport. *Sport, Education and Society, 16*(2), 241–253.

Skille, E. Å., & Solbakken, T. (2011). Sport as a vehicle for health promotion—An analysis of Norwegian policy documents. *Critical Public Health, 21*(2), 191–202.

Skille, E. Å, & Waddington, I. (2006). Alternative sport programmes and social inclusion in Norway. *European Physical Education Review, 12*(3), 251–271.

SOU (2000). *Hälsa på lika villkor. Nationella mål för folkhälsan [Health on equal terms. National targets for public health]*. Stockholm, Sweden: Statens offentliga utredningar.

Stenling, C. (2014). Sport programme implementation as translation and organizational identity construction: The implementation of Drive-in sport in Sweden as an illustration. *International Journal of Sport Policy and Politics, 6*(1), 55–69.

Stenling, C., & Fahlén, J. (2014). Same same, but different? Exploring the organizational identities of Swedish voluntary sports: possible implications of sports clubs' self-identification for their role as implementers of policy objectives. *International Review for the Sociology of Sport*, DOI: 1012690214557103.

Theeboom, M., Schaillée, H., & Nols, Z. (2012). Social capital development among ethnic minorities in mixed and separate sport clubs. *International Journal of Sport Policy and Politics, 4*(1), 1–21.

Thorpe, H. (2014). Action sports for youth development: Critical insights for the SDP community. *International Journal of Sport Policy and Politics*, DOI: 10.1080/19406940.2014.925952.

Vuori, I., Lankenau, B., & Pratt, M. (2004). Physical activity policy and program development: The experience in Finland. *Public Health Reports, 119*, 331–345.

Wickman, K. (2011). The governance of sport, gender and (dis)ability. *International Journal of Sport Policy and Politics, 3*(3), 385–399.

26

PHYSICAL ACTIVITY OPPORTUNITIES FOR YOUNG PEOPLE

A case study of StreetGames

Carolynne Mason

Context: Inequality in participation in youth sport

This chapter examines the work of the organisation StreetGames, which is a UK-based charity launched in 2007. StreetGames aims to bring sport to the doorstep of young people living in disadvantaged communities and in so doing 'change sport, change lives and change communities'. The author has been involved with the organisation as an external evaluator on a number of different StreetGames programmes over a period of more than five years. The insight documented in this chapter is based on this experience viewed through a lens informed by broader debates around young people's participation and active citizenship (Percy-Smith, 2008 & 2010; Tisdall, 2008; Mason et al., 2011). Such debates indicate that, despite considerable efforts, children and young people are still excluded from much of the formal decision-making that impacts on their lives.

StreetGames targets its work at young people aged 14–25 living primarily within the 20 per cent most deprived communities. In England these areas are identified by use of the English Index of Multiple Deprivation (IMD) calculated in England by the Department for Local Government and Communities (similar IMD are calculated in Scotland, Wales and Northern Ireland facilitating regional variation). The English IMD includes seven domains: income, employment, education, health, crime, barriers to health and services and living environment with the greatest weightings being applied to income and employment.

The term 'disadvantaged communities' is one which attempts to encapsulate the complex ways in which people experience living in households in poverty whilst simultaneously living in communities which reflect the divisive impact of widespread and persistent poverty. Whilst the term disadvantage is one that is much broader than the term poverty the two concepts cannot be isolated from each other – that is families that experience poverty typically experience a range of additional challenges beyond limited fiscal resources which leave them disadvantaged when compared to people living in more affluent households.

Rather than relying on absolute measures poverty has become increasingly recognised as being a relative term (currently positioned as living below a threshold of 60 per cent of median income). This approach highlights that those who experience poverty are excluded from activities that those from more affluent communities consider basics of life. In the UK around 2.3 million children were living in relative low income households and 2.6 million in absolute low income households in 2013/14 (Department for Work and Pensions, 2015).

The pervasive impact of poverty (and disadvantage) on people's everyday lives has been documented for many decades. Townsend's seminal work on poverty in the UK stated:

> Individuals, families and groups in the population can be said to be in poverty when they lack the resources to obtain the types of diet, participate in the activities, and have the living conditions and amenities which are customary, or at least widely encouraged or approved, in the societies to which they belong. Their resources are so seriously below those commanded by the average individual or family that they are, in effect, excluded from ordinary patterns, customs and activities.
>
> *Townsend, 1979:31*

More recently Darton et al. noted:

> Poverty in Britain is inextricably intertwined with disadvantages in health, housing, education and other aspects of life. It is hard for people who lack resources to take advantage of the opportunities available to the rest of society.
>
> *Darton et al., 2003:9*

As Darton et al. (2003) note low-income is also linked to educational under-achievement. It is known, for example, that 11-year-olds eligible for free school meals because of low income are twice as unlikely to achieve basic standards in literacy and numeracy as other 11-year-olds (Palmer et al., 2008). The challenges faced by children and young people in childhood have implications which continue to disadvantage them as they progress into adulthood. Additionally, the lower a child's socio-economic group at birth, the greater the probability they will experience multiple deprivation in adulthood (Feinstein et al., 2007).

It is perhaps not surprising then that people living in disadvantaged communities are less likely to take part in sport than their more affluent peers. The Active People survey reveals that since the first survey was conducted in 2005–2006 (APS1) the rate of participation (one session of 30 minutes per week) amongst people aged 16 years and over is greater amongst people from higher socio-economic groups than those from lower socio-economic groups (Sport England, 2015). It also shows that rates of participation have decreased amongst the lowest socio-economic groups since 2005–2006.

StreetGames network

StreetGames was originally established as a result of a small number of neighbourhood sports projects, all experienced in community regeneration projects, working in collaboration. They aimed to make sport more widely available for disadvantaged young people and to maximise the power of sport to change young lives and communities. Following a successful two year pilot StreetGames secured funding from the Sport England Lottery and officially launched in January 2007.

StreetGames continues to work to ensure that more young people living in disadvantaged communities take part in sport than have done previously. Despite its focus on sports participation it is important to note that StreetGames is not a sports delivery organisation. Instead the charity works with more than 700 local partners (community organisations) who deliver a range of sports-based activities to young people living in disadvantaged communities utilising a doorstep approach. StreetGames projects are therefore more accurately visualised as being sports-based activities delivered by a network of organisations using a doorstep approach. The network of organisations is supported by the infrastructure that the charity StreetGames has developed since 2007. The support on offer to the network organisations includes financial resources, monitoring and evaluation, training and opportunities for young people to participate in a range of sports and volunteering activities.

Whilst StreetGames has always sought to increase participation in sport their remit is much broader as they also aim to impact positively on young people's lives and on the communities in which these young people live. These ambitious aims are articulated by the charity as a desire to 'change lives, change communities and change sport' (StreetGames, 2015a). This chapter examines each of these three ambitions for change beginning with the aspiration to change sport which also includes an outline of the doorstep approach that is intrinsic within StreetGames' delivery.

Changing sport

From the outset StreetGames recognised that attempting to redress inequality in sports participation in disadvantaged communities required a new approach to sports delivery. Whilst lack of financial resources was clearly a pervasive barrier to sports participation StreetGames recognised it was not the only barrier that disincentivised young people in disadvantaged communities taking part in sport. Another, possibly equally pervasive barrier, impacting on participation in sport by young people in disadvantaged communities was the belief that the sporting offer that was typically available was not reflective of the aspirations and preferences of many young people.

StreetGames recognised that even within disadvantaged communities there existed various school- and community-based sports opportunities on offer for young people who were already enthusiastic about sport and could afford to take part. However StreetGames also believed that there were many young people within these communities who were excluded from sport either through financial constraints or who were not attracted to the existing sporting offer within their communities. StreetGames believed that lack of enjoyment was an important reason why the traditional sporting offer was not engaging more young people from disadvantaged communities. Fun and enjoyment is therefore a key element of StreetGames sports delivery.

In addition it was recognised by StreetGames that the opportunities for 14–25 year olds in particular were limited, and perhaps non-existent, within disadvantaged communities. This was particularly the case when there was a need for the opportunities to also be affordable and accessible. In response StreetGames developed a new sporting offer which was often in direct contrast to existing provision for young people. The alternative approach was named 'doorstep sport' which reflected a desire reduce the barriers to participation by bringing sport (and physical activity) to young people – on their doorstep – in a style that better reflected their lifestyles and aspirations.

Doorstep sport – The StreetGames approach

The doorstep approach was developed by StreetGames in order to address some of the barriers that impact specifically on young people's participation in sport in disadvantaged communities. The term doorstep describes sports delivery which is offered to young people living within disadvantaged communities in the 'right place, at the right time, for the right price, in the right style and by the right people'. The doorstep approach is not prescriptive in terms of the sports and activities that are offered and instead deliberately seeks to ensure that the sporting offer is developed with young people's preferences as its starting point. The approach recognises that different groups of young people, who may all share an experience of living in disadvantaged communities, may not share their expectations of sport and for this reason the sporting offer therefore needs to be very different in different locations and within different communities within those locations. The StreetGames Strategic Plan 2013–2017 describes doorstep sport as follows:

> Doorstep sport provides a vibrant and varied sporting offer that keeps young people coming back for more. Doorstep sport has very few of the costs, social expectations and rules that shape a traditional sports club. Instead it is informal, fun and designed to suit young people's lifestyles and expectations.
>
> *StreetGames Strategic Plan, 2013–2017:4*

Whilst doorstep sport varies significantly in terms of individual projects at a local level StreetGames has developed programme strands which focus on particular target groups of young people. These programmes utilise the learning that has been gained through adapting and refining projects across the UK. An example of such a programme is Us Girls.

Us Girls

Engaging more young girls and women aged in sport has been recognised as a particularly challenging aspiration for many years. StreetGames developed their own response to this challenge in 2011 in the form of the Us Girls programme. This was initially designed as a two year programme targeted young women aged 16–25, and it was funded with a grant of £2.3 million of National Lottery investment via Sport England. The programme engaged 34,000 young women, exceeding its initial target of 30,000, from 50 different disadvantaged areas. In 2013 the success of the programme was recognised as it won the public vote for Best Sports Project awarded by the National Lottery (StreetGames, 2015b).

The Us Girls programme illustrates the importance (and effectiveness) of the 'right place, right time, right price, right style and by the right people' principles. The programme responds to many of the challenges which have been identified as being particularly relevant to teenage girl's disengagement from sport. These challenges include fear of judgement, wanting to participate with friends in social and fun activities and lack of confidence to attend generic sessions. Us Girls was promoted on the basis of a sports-based session, specifically targeted at girls, which offered 'fun, fitness and friends'. An Us Girls session would typically be located near to the girls' home, take place at a convenient time for them, involve incentives for regular attendance and be delivered by a staff team (supported by volunteers) experienced with working this target group. This is not to say, however, that all Us Girls sessions will look and feel the same. Each project will reflect the local context in which it is located resulting in unique projects which evolve over time.

Impact on national governing bodies

As outlined in their 2013–2017 strategy, by 2013 StreetGames had 'helped 200,000 young people to broaden their horizons onto a pathway towards a healthy, active lifestyle' (StreetGames,

2013:1) and they aimed to have enabled 10,000 young people to become volunteer coaches and encourage 250,000 new participants to enjoy sport on their doorstep by 2017.

As a result of the success of doorstep sport StreetGames were funded by Sport England to work with 12 priority NGBs in order develop their sports offer within disadvantaged areas. This work involved researching young people's aspirations and developing new sports offers in order to meet these aspirations. Young people within the doorstep sports clubs trialed the new offers and groups of StreetGames Young Advisors worked with a number of NGBs to help co-create new offers and ensure that these appeal to young people in disadvantaged communities. Examples of new offers that were developed with the support of StreetGames were StreetGolf, Smashup! Badminton and Instant Ping Pong. These new formats all addressed particular barriers to participation that prevented young people in disadvantaged communities engaging in more traditional sports offers.

Changing lives

The aspiration for StreetGames to help change the lives of young people living in disadvantaged communities recognises that there is a widely held belief that participation in sport can result in a range of positive outcomes for young people. Despite successive UK governments seeking to capitalise upon this potential the National Children's Bureau (2013) recently concluded that very little has changed over the last 50 years for children and young people living in poverty. In 1969 the National Children's Bureau (NCB) completed a major study of the experiences of children from poor, disadvantaged backgrounds in the UK and concluded that children from poorer backgrounds were 'Born to Fail' as a direct result of poverty due to poor health, under-achievement at school and lack of opportunities to fulfil their potential. Fifty years later, in 2013, the NCB re-examined 12 key factors and found that children in the UK still experience inequality and disadvantage and found no evidence to suggest that the position has improved in the intervening decades. Other studies have also concluded that poverty in childhood and youth has an impact on achievement at school which also impacts on their upon aspirations and future life-chances (Hirsch, 2007; Menzies, 2013; Raffo et al., 2007).

The evidence relating to young people aged 16–24 is equally concerning. Job prospects for young people without or with low level qualifications are poor and without support for young people continue to deteriorate (Wilson and Bivand, 2014). More than one in five young people experiencing long-term unemployment believe they have nothing to live for, and that 40 per cent of jobless young people have experienced symptoms of mental illness (The Prince's Trust, 2014). Evidence such as this supports the case that there is a need to change the lives (and life chances) of those living in disadvantaged communities. As Darton et al. (2003) note:

> A wide range of disadvantages in childhood and youth – from mental health problems to low educational attainment – are experienced more by people with worse-off parents. Therefore, strategies to fight poverty and to combat wider social disadvantage need to go hand in hand.
>
> *Darton et al., 2003:16*

The legitimacy of the claims made for sporting participation to positively impact on young people's lives have however been contested as a result of the inconclusive evidence base underpinning the claims arising, in part, from poor or unsystematic monitoring and evaluation processes (Coalter et al., 2000; Coalter, 2007). This critique does not necessarily mean that the claims made for participation in sport and physical activity are not appropriate but instead indicates that there is a need for a more nuanced understanding of which outcomes are realised, by which young participants in sport and under what circumstances (Coalter et al., 2000; Coalter, 2007).

The StreetGames aspiration to 'change lives' recognises that regular and sustained participation in sport can provide a range of benefits for those taking part including impacts on health, wellbeing and psycho-social outcomes. Lower rates of participation in sport by young people in disadvantaged communities potentially result in a range of missed opportunities for these young people to reap a range of potential benefits of sporting participation including improved health (physical and mental), development of psycho-social skills, improved educational outcomes and enhanced employability. In addition taking part in sport that young people can enjoy is important given that young people in the UK experience greater levels of life dis-satisfaction than young people living in many other countries around the world.

Some of the ways in which StreetGames have helped to change young people's lives include encouraging sustained sports engagement, increasing employability and reducing youth offending.

Sustained sports engagement

In 2012, *Creating a Sporting Habit for Life – A New Youth Sport Strategy* was published by DCMS. This strategy marked a change in approach to youth sport that recognised that individuals' involvement in sport across the life course is not uniform. As they progress through their lives the sporting habits of individuals change in response to changes in their lives. Working with Sport England, DCMS aimed to increase the proportion of 14–25 year olds engaged in sport and to establish a network of links between schools and sports clubs in local communities with the aspiration of keeping young people playing sport up to, and beyond, the age of 25. The strategy also recognised that in order to engage more young people in sport there needed to be a broader sporting offer. As a result Sport England worked with StreetGames, and other partners, to extend the reach of doorstep sport by creating 1,000 sustainable Doorstep Sport Clubs (DSCs), taking sport to where young people live. Each project is unique and more than 30 sports feature in StreetGames projects with around 20 per cent of projects using multi-sport delivery. Sessions take place in a range of different venues including leisure centres, parks, schools, youth centres and less conventional sites such as beaches and car parks in order to ensure 'doorstep' provision.

The doorstep approach was developed specifically in order to engage young people in disadvantaged communities in sport, and importantly to keep them engaged in the longer term, and this was clearly in keeping with the ethos of *Creating a Sporting Habit*. Because enjoyment is intrinsic to the perceived success of doorstep sport this approach specifically aims to retain young people in the long term. Importantly if a StreetGames project is found to no longer be meeting the needs of local young people it changes. The project adapts to ensure the offer is still offered in the 'right place, at the right time, for the right price, in the right style and by the right people' even if this means changing the day, time, venue or sport that is offered. In this way doorstep sport evolves with the young people it aims to serve. It is not static or restricted by a particular pre-existing infrastructure.

StreetGames has a number of different work strands which impact on changing the lives of young people. In addition to locally based sporting opportunities StreetGames provides a range of opportunities for young people to take part in residential activities including attending major sports events such as the London 2012 Olympics and the Glasgow 2014

Commonwealth Games. Other residential opportunities include a series of annual regional sports-based activity camps and also competition finals where young people attend as participants or as volunteers. The impact of residential experiences on young people have been well-documented and yet young people in disadvantaged communities typically have less opportunity to participate in residentials due to a lack of financial resources.

Increasing employability

In addition to the sporting offer available through the StreetGames network young people also have the opportunity to develop other skills through their involvement. Coaches who deliver doorstep sport are trained and experienced in meeting the needs of young people, and they seek to enhance the development of the young participants through sport. Young people are supported to develop their soft skills (e.g. confidence, self-esteem, resilience, team working) in a supportive environment. More than 13,900 young people have volunteered through the StreetGames network and they have collectively gained 7,400 qualifications which helps sustain their involvement further. This approach helps to ensure that the sports offer is delivered in the 'right style' and by the 'right people' as these young volunteers have strong connections with the communities the projects are located within and they are visible role models for their younger peers.

Reducing youth offending

The government's ten year strategy for young people introduced in 2007 (Department for Children, Families and Schools/HM Treasury, 2007) emphasised the role of sport and other positive activities in promoting a range of favourable outcomes for young people including reducing involvement in crime and anti-social behaviour and improving attainment. One of the priorities for community safety in addressing crime and anti-social behaviour is the provision of youth sport and activities in local communities within a multi-agency approach (Sport England, 2008).

The Sport and Recreational Alliance (2013) identified four main ways in which sport can be utilised in order to reduce crime and anti-social behaviour. At the simplest level sport can be used as a diversionary activity to keep young people away from trouble. Sport is also used as a 'hook' for other interventions and opportunities which help young people to develop positively. Additionally, some sports experiences are believed to provide opportunities for personal transformation which results in behaviour modification through the activity itself (e.g. Outdoor Education). Finally engagement in sport is characterised as providing an opportunity for the promotion of social inclusion which then has favorable impacts on young people and the communities they live in. Whilst the processes through which youth sport participation enhances youth crime prevention remain poorly understood (Kelly, 2011) there is still a strong commitment to developing better insight. A recent study by New Philanthropy Capital (NPC) suggests that sport is most successful when it is linked to other educational opportunities and support:

> When sport is used as part of a wider programme of education and support, it can be highly effective at tackling youth crime, and can provide excellent value for money. Given the huge costs associated with youth crime, there is a compelling case for government and other funders to support such projects.
>
> *New Philanthropy Capital, 2012:8*

StreetGames have taken up the challenge of utilising sport to reduce youth crime and enhance community safety. For example, in 2015, in collaboration with the Police and Crime Commissioner for Derbyshire, they began a Youth Crime Reduction and Sport programme after securing funding from the Home Office Police Innovation Fund. The project will test, explore and build an evidence base to show the most effective ways to maximise the value of appropriately designed sport interventions to policing and youth crime reduction. As with other StreetGames programmes this endeavour involves delivery partners utilising a doorstep sport approach to engage young people in targeted areas in disadvantaged communities in, and through, sport.

Changing communities

The third aspiration identified by StreetGames for their work is to change communities. This is clearly an extremely ambitious aim but nonetheless it is one that recognises the inherent structural inequalities that exist within the disadvantaged communities where StreetGames delivery takes place. The previous discussion has identified some of the ways in which StreetGames projects deliver outcomes that have the potential to impact favourably on the wider community by enhancing the health, well-being and employability of young people engaged in doorstep sport living within these communities. As noted above a key way in which StreetGames aim to positively impact on changing communities is through young people volunteering in sport and therefore being 'active' citizens.

Volunteering in sport

The aspiration to engage young people in volunteering remains a visible aspiration for successive governments. Examples within the UK include Millennium Volunteers (2000), Active Citizens in Schools (2001), Giving Campaign and Giving Nation (2006), Young Volunteers Challenge (2003–2005) and V Inspired (2006). More recently the current government's National Citizens Service programme seeks to engage young people in volunteering across a range of community and education sectors. Underpinning these efforts is a belief in a range of positive outcomes that can arise both for young people and for their communities through such experiences. Young people, employers, HE staff and volunteering organisations agree that volunteering allows young people to develop transferable skills including communication and team working skills (V, 2008).

Inequality in sports participation is also reflected in volunteering participation. Bennett and Parameshwaran (2013) found higher classes were more likely to volunteer than lower classes but social class effects become insignificant once social and cultural capital measures were included. However, young people not in education, employment and training (NEET) were the most sceptical about the benefits to be derived from volunteering (V, 2008) thus indicating that those with potentially the most to gain from volunteering were those least convinced about the benefits of volunteering.

Morgan (2013) examined the links between sport volunteering, active citizenship and social capital enhancement within a political context which promotes a 'Big Society' (an aspiration of the 2010 UK coalition government whereby a significant amount of responsibility for the running of a society is devolved to local communities and volunteers). Drawing on previous studies Morgan questioned whether community sports clubs – a site where much sports volunteering is located – are well positioned to be able to enhance individuals' social capital. Morgan suggests that social capital enhancement through voluntary involvement is most likely to be achieved when:

- Individuals are deeply involved and engaged
- Individuals are involved in the longer term

Working with local partners the StreetGames network offers those involved in doorstep sport the chance to undertake a range of volunteering opportunities through programmes including the StreetGames Young Volunteers (SYV), Coca Cola Training Academy and the Pre Apprentice programme. Through such opportunities young people access training, undertake qualifications, take part in residential experiences and volunteer at a range of events including high profile events such as the Commonwealth Games. This investment in young people helps ensure that the network retains 'the right people' within the StreetGames network as some volunteers go on to become employed within the StreetGames network.

The StreetGames doorstep approach offers opportunities to young people who may not have previously been engaged in sport to become involved in volunteering opportunities that suit their individual preferences. Some volunteers will be involved in stand-alone events and festivals in roles such as marshalling, assisting delivery of activities and social media interaction. Other volunteers will be engaged over a longer duration in weekly sports/activity sessions in roles such as assisting in the delivery of sessions, leading a session, mentoring other volunteers, administrative support and social media coordination. Some of the regular volunteers also take on 'Young Advisor' roles and work on the design and delivery of national StreetGames programmes. In addition StreetGames provides a small number of full-time, intensive, social action opportunities where volunteers contribute 25–30 hours per week for 13 weeks to 24 weeks.

Keys to success

StreetGames is an ambitious organisation that has a clear mission to bring about change for disadvantaged young people and their communities utilising a doorstep approach which offers sport 'right place, at the right time, for the right price, in the right style and by the right people'. In order to be able to do this StreetGames works with a wide range of partners who know what the challenges and opportunities are locally. This partnership approach is integral to the success of StreetGames delivery.

The approach is a flexible one which means that doorstep sport sessions will be extremely varied in terms of location, time, venue and sports offer and these may all change within one location over the duration of the project in response to the preferences of the young people involved. The element that all successful doorstep projects share however is that they are built on the recognition that young people need to enjoy the sessions otherwise they will not come back and none of the other additional potential benefits (on health, well-being and employability) will therefore be realised in the longer term.

In addition to the network of partners StreetGames has developed another vital ingredient of their success is the human infrastructure that supports StreetGames delivery. Developing sport in the 'right style' demands that those who deliver the sport understand not only sport but also young people and their preferences and are therefore 'the right people'. For this reason StreetGames invest heavily in the coaches and volunteers who make doorstep sport a reality. This investment includes a training academy which enables coaches and volunteers to develop their skills and seek accreditation and also opportunities for progression. The

StreetGames Training Academy offers workshops, coaching courses and resources which have been developed in order to prepare the doorstep sport workforce to provide high-quality sporting opportunities in a style suited to the particular community.

Another area which StreetGames prioritises is insight. The organisation takes monitoring and evaluation seriously and continually seeks to improve the processes through which it evaluates its own successes (and failures). Additionally StreetGames invests resources into gathering insight, knowledge and understanding which will help to ensure that decisions that are made at both operational and strategic levels are evidence-based. They also have a willingness to share that knowledge and understanding with others as exemplified by their website (with a section devoted to 'knowledge and insight') and by their willingness to engage with numerous partners and organisations in the UK and beyond in order to share insight.

Implications for future physical activity policy and practice

This chapter has examined the StreetGames offer to young people in disadvantaged communities. The work of StreetGames is extremely significant in terms of implications for future physical activity policy and practice and this is recognised by the charity which lobbies vigorously to try and ensure that disadvantaged and socially marginalised young people are visible within sport and physical activity policy across the UK. This was exemplified as doorstep sport was showcased within the 'Creating a Sporting Habit' strategy where it was noted that NGBs have adapted their practice – and sporting offer – as a result of the success of doorstep sport in disadvantaged communities. With its ethos of meaningful engagement in sport, and its focus on people who tend not to participate in sport, the StreetGames network is also well placed to contribute to realising the vision contained within *Sporting Future – A New Strategy for an Active Nation* (DCMS, 2015). The new strategy also recognises the importance of broader engagement in sport, in particular through volunteering in sport, and this is another strength of the existing StreetGames network.

As a charity, however, StreetGames is reliant on the support of external funding partners in order to maintain and extend the reach of doorstep sport. The organisation is necessarily required to make decisions about how to balance the desire to create opportunities for young people within disadvantaged communities with the ethical dilemmas that surround con-tributing to the corporate social responsibility agendas of commercial business. In a broader context of austerity and fiscal constraint these tensions look unlikely to be resolved within the short term.

Whilst StreetGames have a mission to bring about greater equality for young people in terms of their access to sport and physical activity their work also highlights that there are additional possibilities for all young people in terms of providing alternative offers that meet their preferences. Some young people may not experience fiscal constraints but they will still have their own preferences for sport and physical activity. Using young people's preferences as the starting point for changing practice and prioritising opportunities that are enjoyable may challenge the notion that young people are 'sporty' or 'not sporty' and instead be characterised as 'having their physical activity preferences met' or 'not having their physical activity preferences met'.

As noted in the introduction to this chapter this discussion has been informed by wider debates around young people's participation and citizenship which argue that young people are largely excluded from decision-making that impacts on their lives – particularly young people living within disadvantaged communities. In order to bring about change Percy-Smith (2010:119) argues that:

We need to move away from the current emphasis on participation in formal, institutionalised public decision making processes and instead focus more on the multiplicity of ways which people act, contribute to and realise their own sense of agency in everyday life contexts.

Percy-Smith provides a timely reminder that young people from disadvantaged communities must influence the future of physical activity and sports policy and practice directly if these are to be effective in delivering positive outcomes for these young people. Doorstep sport provides an example of how this aspiration can be realised for young people living within disadvantaged communities.

References

Bennett, M. and Parameshwaran, M. (2013) *What Factors Predict Volunteering Among Youths in the UK?* Briefing Paper 102, Third Sector Research Centre.

Coalter, F. (2007) Sports Clubs, Social Capital and Social Regeneration: Ill-Defined Interventions with Hard to Follow Outcomes?, *Sport in Society*, 10(4), 537–559.

Coalter, F., Allison, M. and Taylor, J.A. (2000) *The Role of Sport in Regenerating Deprived Urban Areas.* Scottish Executive Unit.

Darton, D., Hirsch, D. and Strelitz, J. (2003) *Tackling Poverty: A 20-year Enterprise.* York: Joseph Rowntree Foundation.

Department for Children, Families and Schools/HM Treasury (2007) *Aiming High for Young People: A Ten Year Strategy for Positive Activities* [Online] Available at: http://webarchive.nationalarchives.gov. uk/20130401151715/http://www.education.gov.uk/publications/eOrderingDownload/PU214. pdf (Accessed 7th March 2016).

DCMS (2015) *Sporting Future – A New Strategy for an Active Nation* [Online] Available at: www.gov. uk/government/publications/sporting-future-a-new-strategy-for-an-active-nation (Accessed 7th March 2016).

DCMS (2012) *Creating a Sporting Habit for Life – A New Youth Sport Strategy* [Online] Available at: www. sportengland.org/media/130949/DCMS-Creating-a-sporting-habit-for-life-1-.pdf (Accessed 7th March 2016).

Department for Work and Pensions (2015) *Households Below Average Income (HBAI)* An analysis of the income distribution 1993/4 – 2013/14 [Online] Available at www.gov.uk/government/uploads/ system/uploads/attachment_data/file/437246/households-below-average-income-1994-95- to-2013-14.pdf (Accessed 7th March 2016).

Feinstein, L., Hearn, B. and Renton, Z. (2007) *Reducing Inequalities: Realising the Talents of All.* London: National Children's Bureau.

Hirsch, D. (2007) *Experiences of Poverty and Educational Disadvantage.* York: Joseph Rowntree Foundation.

Kelly, L. (2011) 'Social inclusion' through sports-based interventions? *Critical Social Policy*, 31(1), 126–150.

Mason, C., Cremin, H., Warwick, P. and Harrison, T. (2011) learning to (dis)engage ?: the socialising experiences of young people living in areas of socio-economic disadvantage, *British Journal of Educational Studies*, 59(4), 421–437.

Menzies, L. (2013) *Educational Aspirations: How English Schools Can Work with Parents to Keep Them on Track.* York: Joseph Rowntree Foundation.

Morgan, H. (2013) Sport volunteering, active citizenship and social capital enhancement: What role in the 'Big Society'?, *International Journal of Sport Policy and Politics*, 5(3), 381–395.

National Children's Bureau (2013) *Greater Expectations: Raising Aspirations for our Children.* London: National Children's Bureau.

New Philanthropy Capital (2012) Teenage Kicks – The value of sport in reducing youth crime [Online] Available at: www.thinknpc.org/wp-content/uploads/2012/09/Teenage-Kicks.pdf (Accessed 7th March 2016).

Palmer, G., Macinnes, T. and Kenway, P. (2008) *Monitoring Poverty and Social Exclusion 2008.* York: Joseph Rowntree Foundation, and New Policy Institute.

Percy-Smith, B. (2008) *Evaluating the Development of Children's Participation Plans in Two Children's Trusts. Year One Report.* Leicester: National Youth Agency.

Percy-Smith, B. (2010) Councils, consultations and community: Rethinking the spaces for children and young people's participation, *Children's Geographies,* 8(2), 107–122.

Raffo, C., Dyson, A., Gunter, H., Hall, D., Jones, L. and Kalambouka, A. (2007) *Education and Poverty: A Critical Review of Theory, Policy and Practice.* York: Joseph Rowntree Foundation.

Sport England (2008) Creating safer communities: Reducing anti-social behaviour and the fear of crime through sport [Online] Available at: www.sportengland.org/media/91502/creating-safer-communities.pdf (Accessed 7th March 2016).

Sport England (2015) Overall APS9 Factsheet [Online] Available at: www.sportengland.org/media/875700/1x30_overall_factsheet_aps9q2v2.pdf (Accessed 7th March 2016).

StreetGames (2013) *The StreetGames Strategic Plan 2013 – 2017.* Manchester: StreetGames.

StreetGames (2015a) *About StreetGames* [Online] Available at: www.streetgames.org/about-us/about-streetgames (Accessed 7th March 2016).

StreetGames (2015b) *US Girls* [Online] Available at: www.streetgames.org/our-work/us-girls (Accessed 7th March 2016).

StreetGames Strategic Plan (2013–2017) *Changing Lives, Changing Sport, Changing Communities:* [Online] Available at: www.streetgames.org/sites/default/files/StreetGames-Strategic-Plan-2013-2017.pdf (Accessed 7th March 2016).

The Prince's Trust (2014) *The Prince's Trust Macquarie Youth Index 2014.* London: The Prince's Trust.

Tisdall, K. (2008) Is the honeymoon over?: Children and young people's participation in public decision making, *International Journal of Children's Rights,* 16(3), 419–429.

Townsend, P. (1979) *Poverty in the United Kingdom.* London: Allen Lane and Penguin Books.

V (2008) *Youth Volunteering: Attitudes and Perceptions.* London: V.

Wilson, T. and Bivand, P. (2014) *Equitable Full Employment: Delivering a Jobs Recovery For All.* London: TUC.

27

SCHOOLS, CORPORATIONS AND PROMOTION OF PHYSICAL ACTIVITY TO FIGHT OBESITY

Darren Powell and Michael Gard

Childhood obesity is a complex problem driven by multiple social, economic and environmental factors . . . If we are to tackle this major public health issue effectively we need a multi-sector response and Nestlé firmly believes industry has a vital role to play in this. We are convinced the best way to leverage our capabilities and expertise is by working in partnership with other organisations to help promote healthy nutrition and physical activity through community-based programmes.

Nestlé, 2012a, para.7–9

To avoid public criticism and forestall government intervention, the food and beverage industry hopes that self-regulation is sufficient and also seeks to establish public-private partnerships.

Koplan & Brownell, 2010, p.1487

In the global war against childhood obesity 'everyone' has been called upon to be part of the solution. A shared 'interest' in the shared 'problem' of childhood obesity and children's unhealthy lifestyles has helped to forge alignments between corporations, schools, government agencies, non-governmental organisations (NGOs), sporting organisations, charities, and a mishmash of other for-profit and 'not-for-profit' organisations. What follows is an interrogation of how the notion of *partnership* is deployed as a tactic to bring together the ambitions of corporations, charities, the state, and schools; a strategy used to translate a collective 'will to improve' (Li, 2007a) children's bodies and behaviours into policies and programmes that shape physical activity practice in schools.

However, given that a number of organisations that work in partnership have competing, sometimes contradictory, aims and values, there are tensions that require critical examination. Perhaps the most obvious tension is when the commercial interests of the private sector compete with the educational interests of schools, teachers, and principals. With this in mind, we draw on documentary evidence (educational resources, websites, annual reports, advertising) gathered from a New Zealand-based research project (see Powell, 2015) to demonstrate how the various 'solutions' to children's fatness and sedentary lives are promoted by a number of key partners, and how they are closely connected to business strategies (such as public relations, marketing, and branding). The assemblage of disparate players is complex and requires interrogation in order to understand how organisations employ, even exploit, partnerships in order to re-establish themselves as 'obesity fighting', physical activity promoting, and profitable.

Shared interests in being 'part of the solution' to childhood obesity

In most societies, the political, social, cultural, and economic agenda for children to be shaped into certain types of citizens cannot be achieved by a single sector or institution alone. As Rose (2000, p.323) argued, government can only be achieved 'through the actions of a whole range of other authorities, and through complex technologies, if they are to be able to intervene upon the conduct of persons'. The war on childhood obesity is a good example of this 'multiple-authority' approach to government. A 'panoply of players' (Coveney, 2008, p.208) has been recruited to 'fix' this urgent public health imperative, including children, teachers, principals, external providers, politicians, lobbyists, parents, corporate employees, celebrities, corporations, industry groups, government departments, philanthropists, corporate foundations, sporting bodies, charities, and advocacy groups.

Bringing together these disparate authorities and maintaining the connections between them is by no means a simple task. As Li (2007a, p.268) notes, the 'will to govern' acts as both 'a point of convergence and fracture'. One practice that works to attract various parties to one another *and* resolve any tensions and potential fractures that occur is *forging alignments*: 'the work of linking together the objectives of the various parties . . . both those who aspire to govern conduct and those whose conduct is to be conducted' (Li, 2007a, p.265). Alignments are forged in order to unite the *interests* of different sectors (public, private, voluntary or 'third sector'), as well as institutions within and across these sectors (e.g. schools, corporations) and individual subjects (e.g. children, shareholders). As Miller and Rose (2008, p.34) state, for multiple parties to align they must first convince each other 'that their interests are consonant, that each can solve their difficulties or achieve their ends by joining forces or working along the same lines'. Forging alignments by sharing interests and working together is, therefore, a key element of forming successful partnerships. This is also a practice of assemblage that does not occur in isolation, but interweaves and interconnects with other practices of assemblage, such as containing critiques, managing contradictions, anti-politics, and problematisation (for a discussion, see Li, 2007a). Drawing on the work of Li (2007a, 2007b) and Miller and Rose (2008), we argue that there are four key components of 'shared interests' that make it possible for alignments to be forged between institutions with different, sometimes competing, aims: a shared interest based on an 'urgent need' to fix a problem (e.g. obesity or poor public relations); a shared interest in and agreement on who requires governing (e.g. children); a shared interest in solving the problem (for example, using physical activity programmes in schools); and, a shared interest in certain thoughts, actions, and bodies that need to be governed (e.g. children's fat and inactive bodies).

At a macro level we can see how alignments have been made through a shared interest in the 'urgent need' to fight childhood obesity. The World Health Organization (2015a, para.3–5, emphasis added), for instance, argues it is 'essential' for people and institutions to share a common interest and play a partnership role in fighting childhood obesity:

> Curbing the childhood obesity epidemic requires sustained political commitment and the *collaboration of many public and private stakeholders*. Governments, International Partners, Civil Society, NGO's and the Private Sector have vital roles to play in shaping healthy environments and making healthier diet options for children and

adolescents affordable, and easily accessible. It is therefore WHO's objective to mobilize these partners and engage them in implementing the Global Strategy on Diet, Physical Activity and Health. WHO supports the designation, the implementation, the monitoring and the leadership of actions. A *multisectoral approach is essential* for sustained progress: it mobilizes the combined energy, resources and expertise of all global stakeholders involved.

The World Health Organization has now 'mobilized' multiple stakeholders across all sectors of society to engage, collaborate, and partner with one another in the global war against childhood obesity.

One stakeholder that has mobilised its resources, energy, and 'expertise' in diet, physical activity, health, and obesity with particular vigour is the food and beverage industry. This is perhaps not surprising given that the World Health Organization has singled out this industry (as well as sporting-goods manufacturers) to play a greater role in promoting physical activity and healthy diets, to develop and implement physical activity programmes for children, and to review their marketing practices (see also World Health Organization, 2015b, 2015c). However, corporations and other supporters of 'Big Food' (e.g. advertisers, food industry groups, lobbyists) have not only aligned their obesity goals with the public health aspirations of the World Health Organization (and national governments), but formed collaborative relationships *with each other*. This is a startling move. Corporations who have been and continue to be fierce competitors in the marketplace (for example, the 'Cola Wars' between PepsiCo and The Coca-Cola Company) have now taken a public and political stance to work together to help solve childhood obesity. For instance, a number of competitive food and beverage companies have became partners in organisations, such as the Partnership for a Healthier America and the Healthy Weight Commitment Foundation in the United States, Companies Committed to Kids (formerly the Concerned Children's Advertisers) in Canada (see also Powell, 2014), and the International Food and Beverage Alliance (IFBA), a global group of CEO's represeting Nestlé, General Mills, Ferrero, Kellogg's, Grupo Bimbo, Mondelēz International, Mars, PepsiCo, The Coca-Cola Company, Unilever, and McDonald's.

However, it is worth pointing out that it is not solely the food and beverage industry and its multi-national corporations who have expressed an interest in fighting childhood obesity. Globally there are now a range of 'for profit' and 'not-for-profit'[1] organisations that have formed relationships with each other through a shared interest in children's fatness, health, and physical activity. For instance, at the time of writing this chapter, the Partnership for a Healthier America (see http://ahealthieramerica.org/) had a total of 116 partners, including a number of universities (e.g. Arizona State University, Florida State University), sportswear and sporting goods companies (e.g. NIKE, Reebok, FirstBIKE), 'non-profit' organisations (e.g. Boys and Girls Clubs of America, National Recreation and Parks Association), medical organisations (e.g. Children's Mercy Hospitals, Kaiser Permanente), education organisations (e.g. Sesame workshop), physical activity companies (e.g. GoNoodle), and large corporations (e.g. Subway, Walmart, Mercedes-Benz USA, Bird's Eye). Indeed, as Huxham and Vangen (2000, p.303) described at the turn of the millennium, the explosion of multi-sector partnerships in contemporary societies is like a form of 'partnershipitis', a phenomenon that shows little sign of being quelled.

Physical activity partnerships

Within the regime of practices that constitute anti-obesity programmes, physical activity initiatives, and healthy lifestyles education resources, corporations are forming partnerships with multiple authorities and actors at 'epidemic' proportions. Partnerships are visible across a range of sites and spaces of government. In the realm of public health, for instance, King (2006, p.8) argues that corporations have created 'partnerships with community groups, local governments, and other companies that share a common interest in a particular concern', including breast cancer and childhood obesity. Global reforms of public education, described by Sahlberg (2006) as the Global Education Reform Movement or GERM, have also been facilitated by the proliferation of multi-sector partnerships, such as public-private partnerships (see Ball, 2007).

In terms of school-based anti-obesity/physical activity initiatives, an epidemic of partnerships is also evident across the globe (for discussion and examples, see Hawkes & Buse, 2011; Kraak & Story, 2010; Powell, 2014; Powell & Gard, 2015). For instance, Darren's (Powell, 2015) ethnographic research examining healthy lifestyles education programmes in just three New Zealand primary schools demonstrated there were almost fifty different partner organisations (also described as sponsors) who were *directly* involved in the implementation of only twelve programmes and resources. Of these, twenty-five partners were private sector companies, eighteen 'not-for-profit' organisations, and only four state-funded 'public' agencies (although it is not always easy or even possible to demarcate the difference between public, private, and 'not-for-profit'). Further to this, there were also numerous other organisations that were *indirectly* connected to these programmes, as 'partners of the partners' or 'funders of the funders'. For example, Nestlé New Zealand produces a healthy eating/physical activity resource called *Be Healthy, Be Active* with partners AUT Millennium and the New Zealand Nutrition Foundation (see www.behealthybeactive.co.nz). AUT Millennium is a charitable, sport science organisation funded by the New Zealand Government, philanthropic donors (both individual philanthropists and charitable trusts), AUT University, High Performance Sport New Zealand (a government-funded organisation), as well as Nestlé New Zealand, Speedo, and *ActivePost*. In short, the formation of partnerships is a rather messy business and the relationships made are rarely clearly defined or articulated.

National governments and international governing bodies (such as the World Health Organization) continue to position multi-sector partnerships as an integral component of the global war on obesity. Unsurprisingly, the food and beverage industry has been particularly motivated to align their business interests with the interests of international and national public health organisations and policy-makers. For instance, the IFBA (2013, p.1) pledged their support of the *World Health Assembly's Global Action Plan on the Prevention and Control of Noncommunicable Diseases* by stating: 'We believe – and experience has shown that multisectoral actions represent one of the most cost-effective means to address public health challenges.' In the following quote, Janet Voûte, Global Head of Public Affairs for Nestlé S.A., demonstrates how the world's wealthiest food company embraces and publicly supports public health policies and multi-sector partnerships:

> Childhood obesity is a complex problem driven by multiple social, economic and environmental factors . . . If we are to tackle this major public health issue effectively we need a *multi-sector response* and Nestlé firmly believes industry has a vital role to play in this. We are convinced the best way to leverage our capabilities and expertise is by *working in partnership* with other organisations to help promote healthy nutrition and *physical activity* through community-based programmes.
>
> *Nestlé, 2012a, para. 7–9, emphasis added*

The desire of multi-national corporations like Nestlé to engage in multi-sector 'responses' to the childhood obesity 'problem' means that a number of other organisations are drawn into 'their' global and local solutions. For example, Nestlé (2016, para.1) promotes its *Healthy Kids Global Programme*, an initiative based on the simple idea that '[g]etting active and acquiring healthy eating habits can help children achieve and maintain a healthy body weight'. The overall objective of the programme is 'to raise nutrition and health knowledge and promote physical activity among school-age children around the world', which Nestlé claims it achieves because their various national programmes are 'based on multi-partnership approaches: we work with almost 300 partners worldwide, including national and local governments, NGOs, nutrition health institutes and sport federations' (Nestlé, 2016, para.1–2).

One example of the *Healthy Kids Global Programme* 'in action' is *Be Healthy, Be Active*, a healthy eating/physical activity programme (and educational resource) devised and implemented by the New Zealand division of Nestlé and a few key partners:

> Nestlé New Zealand has funded the new *Be Healthy, Be Active* programme as part of the Nestlé Global Healthy Kids Programme [sic]. The materials that make up *Be Healthy, Be Active* have been developed in conjunction with Nestlé New Zealand's partners, the Millennium Institute of Sport and Health [now AUT Millennium] and the New Zealand Nutrition Foundation. The content of the programme is not commercial in nature. We hope that teachers and students will enjoy *Be Healthy, Be Active* and that New Zealand as a whole will benefit from the programme, creating a happier, healthier nation.
>
> *Nestlé New Zealand, 2011, para.3–4, italics in original*

As evident in this quote, Nestlé clearly positions itself as a key player in the war on obesity. By forming partnerships with numerous other 'players' to fight childhood obesity and make children (in fact, a whole country) healthier, for-profit organisations such as Nestlé are able to align their interests – financial, philanthropic, public relations, health, educational – with other organisations and individuals who shared *similar* interests. However, these same organisations also have incongruent interests and desired outcomes. Alleviating the tensions that occur when for-profit and 'not-for-profit' organisations partner with one another is critical for those disparate organisations with the 'will to govern' to achieve their aims. This is particularly true when multi-sector partners wish to work in and with schools.

School-business partnerships and the 'problem' of physical (in)activity

Problematising childhood obesity is a significant aspect of forming and re-forming physical activity policy communities, as it successfully works to unite the interests and activities of multiple partners. There are a number of programmes implemented in schools all over the world that connect different organisations together through the idea that there are dual *crises* of childhood obesity and children's unhealthy lifestyles – especially physical (in)activity – that need immediate attention (see Jette, Bhagat & Andrews, 2014; Powell, 2014; Powell & Gard, 2015). These are crises that can be 'solved' through school-based interventions that focus on 'improving' children's physical activity.

Like corporations, charities, and government agencies, schools too demonstrate an interest in children's fatness and physical activity. This is not that shocking given that schools have for a long time been encouraged or instructed to solve various moral and public health crises (see Gard & Pluim, 2014). Schools and teachers continue to be frequently lambasted for contributing to a so-called 'obesogenic' environment, such as selling or providing 'junk' food to children, restricting physical activity experiences, or providing inadequate health and physical education lessons (for examples, see Gordon, 2014; Grant & Bassin, 2007; Taylor, 2007).

Employing crisis discourses and available 'solutions' is a critical part of being able to build and maintain relationships between corporations, 'not-for-profits', CEOs, schools, principals, and teachers, and is especially effective when the proposed 'part of the solution' to obesity is perceived or promoted as both *healthy* and *educational*. The discourses of education and health form relay points – points of connection between parties – and are a key strategy for the private sector to connect their interests (for example, in solving obesity, promoting physical activity, improving brand image and their bottom line) with the educational interests of schools. For instance, in 2012 the stated aim of the Nestlé *Healthy Kids Global Programme* was:

> to *raise nutrition, health and wellness awareness of school-age children* around the world, we intend to implement the scheme in all countries where we operate . . . We believe that regular physical activity and establishing healthy eating habits help children achieve and maintain a healthy body weight. *Education is therefore a powerful tool* for ensuring that children understand the value of nutrition and physical activity, and continue leading healthy lives as they get older.
>
> *Nestlé, 2012b, para. 1–3, emphasis added*

Similarly, a number of organisations 'connect the dots' between themselves, children's education, (ill)health, and physical (in)activity. New Zealand physical activity/athletics programme *Get Set Go* is one example of a programme that formed partnerships under the impression that there were dual crises of childhood obesity and physical inactivity that needed immediate attention. These were crises that were positioned as 'solvable' through a particular intervention, in this instance, a physical activity programme.

Get Set Go was promoted in a national newspaper by the headline: 'Initiatives to help our kids with alarming obesity stats' (Thornton, 2011, p. B2). The article began with journalist Thornton aligning his own concerns about the obesity 'crisis' with concerns raised by state-owned corporation and main sponsor/partner/funder of *Get Set Go*, New Zealand Post: 'Almost a third of Kiwi kids are considered overweight or obese, compared with only 10% in 1977. NZ Post has launched *ActivePost* to address this problem' (*ActivePost* is the corporate social responsibility/community wellness programme of New Zealand Post). These concerns about children's fatness were reinforced by the 'expert' enlisted by New Zealand Post to 'help shape the programme': Mike Hall-Taylor, the CEO of private sports consultancy firm HTC Sportsworld.[2] In the article, Hall-Taylor said he was surprised by New Zealand's obesity statistics, arguing that although New Zealand adults were active in sport and recreation activities, 'there are clearly some issues amongst kids':

Thornton: Why do you think the problem of obesity is a problem here?

Hall-Taylor: It's a problem in every developed nation, and is primarily a factor of over-nutrition and under-exercising. It's a complex issue . . . but the *ActivePost* programme can try to help get kids, and adults, more active.

Hall-Taylor did not only connect the 'complex' 'problem' of obesity with what he described as 'over-nutrition and under-exercising', but positioned the *ActivePost* initiative as being part of the solution.[3] In other words, he represented a position on obesity, inactivity, and lifestyles that enabled his company to connect with (and assumingly, profit from) New Zealand Post,

Athletics New Zealand, the *Get Set Go* programme, and primary schools. In a similar vein, the main partner to New Zealand Post – national sports organisation Athletics New Zealand – drew on 'recent studies' about children's physical activity and fatness to make a link between fundamental movement skills and obesity, and to justify their involvement this programme:

> Research highlights that children in early childhood and early primary school are not mastering the fundamental movement skills. (Sanders & Kidman, 1998). This has very serious implications . . . Research also shows that New Zealand children appear to be following the global trends of increasingly being more overweight and suffering obesity problems (Ministry of Health 2003). Changes in lifestyle and technology are all contributing factors of these trends, leading to a negative impact on the overall health and wellbeing of our children, and affecting the capability for enjoyable participation and lifelong interest in sport and an active lifestyle.
>
> *Athletics New Zealand, 2013, p.6*

The research that Athletics New Zealand (and New Zealand Post) refers to in the quote above does not demonstrate any empirical connections between children's fundamental movement skills and fatness, or physical activity and fatness, or fundamental movement skills and health. Instead, it employs tenuous connections between obesity, physical activity, lifestyles, sport, skills, and health. Through the juxtaposition of multiple crises – overweight and obesity, fundamental movement skills, physical inactivity and technology, health and wellbeing, lifelong sports participation and lifelong active lifestyles – the various partners rationalise their support for the *Get Set Go* programme as a solution; a somewhat certain solution to an uncertain problem.

Other organisations and individuals, such as teachers, coaches, families, children, and CEOs, are also drawn into *Get Set Go* by the rationale of crises. In the introduction to the *Get Set Go teachers* [sic] *resource*, the Chief Executive of the New Zealand Post Group, Brian Roche, signalled how the twin 'problems' of childhood obesity and children's reduced fitness could be solved when different parties share an interest in his company's solution:

> Children today have access to a wider range of activities and entertainment options than any previous generation. Unfortunately many of those options are sedentary, and there are worldwide growing trends in childhood obesity and reduced physical fitness. . . . *With the support* of teachers, coaches and families, Get Set Go has the potential to instil an environment where children can experience success, develop skills and learn positive attitudes towards sport and recreation. . . . *By partnering with* Athletics New Zealand and Regional Sports Trusts, New Zealand Post can help young people to develop a love of sport and recreation that leads to lifelong participation.
>
> *Athletics New Zealand, 2012, p.2, emphasis added*

The assumption that schools were an appropriate 'environment' for this particular 'solution' to children's problematic bodies and behaviours meant that teachers (and the externally provided *Get Set Go* coaches) were positioned as fitting agents and key partners who would 'teach' positive attitudes towards physical activity, aspects that adults assumed would lead children to being physically active and non-fat for the rest of their lives.

The process of assembling these partnerships and programmes together was sometimes problematic, particularly when a perceived 'unhealthy' corporation (e.g. McDonald's) or product (e.g. Coca-Cola) was partnered with a so-called 'healthy' educational activity, such as McDonald's *My Greatest Feat,* a national pedometer physical activity programme for primary schools. However, this is a tension that tended to be resolved when schools deemed it appropriate to endorse 'healthy' (or at least *healthier*) corporate products within a programme. For instance, as Darren's research (Powell, 2015) with primary schools demonstrated, teachers and principals justified using programmes that were sponsored by multi-national corporations by focusing on a particular product promoted in the programme that they deemed to be 'healthy' (e.g. fruit juice), rather than the company itself (e.g. a company that not only made fruit juice, but sugar-sweetened beverages and caffeine-based energy drinks). Resolving this tension by focusing on the 'healthy' products promoted in a physical activity or healthy lifestyles programme obscured the 'less healthy' products and business practices of a particular corporation or industry.

A so-called healthy (or even just 'more healthy') product acted not only as a buffer between the corporation, its public reputation, its products, and its physical activity programmes, but also as a way of connecting these elements. Teachers and 'not-for-profit' physical activity providers (such as a local sports club or a national sporting organisation, such as Hockey New Zealand), seemed to find themselves having to do one of two things: either choosing the lesser of two 'evils' (such as Powerade® or Coca-Cola®, MILO® or Pepsi®), or not having any partner, sponsor, or physical activity programme at all.

Furthermore, partnerships and the associated 'healthy' branding work to encourage teachers and principals to 'consume' the corporatised solutions to childhood obesity and unhealthy lifestyles. The fact that for most physical activity initiatives, certainly in the New Zealand context, it is not the private sector player physically delivering the programmes, teachers, principals, and children's attention is diverted away from *who* is funding, *who* is shaping, and *who* is profiting from these physical activity programmes and policies. We are not suggesting that individuals in schools are easily duped by these private sector business strategies. Indeed, Darren's research clearly demonstrates the ways in which some children are able to negotiate and challenge the corporate commercialism of various healthy eating and physical activity programmes. However, the nature of partnerships appears to 'muddy the waters' and ameliorate concerns that people might have about the educative value of these programmes or their effectiveness in making children more active. That is, the relationships between corporations and schools, between for-profit and not-for-profit organisations, work to maintain the *status quo*. Private sector players continue to attempt to reform public education and public health policies and practices in ways that best meet their own interests.

Profiting from partnerships

There is little doubt that the partnerships formed in the name of fighting childhood obesity and promoting physical activity are part of an overall business strategy for corporations and industries (and governments) to improve their bottom line. As Vander Schee (2005, p.20) argued, '[c]orporations would not be involved in schools were it not for the promise of increased profits and market share'. So how does the private sector 'profit' from their physical activity partnerships with not-for-profits and schools?

Given the public and political concerns about childhood obesity, promoting physical activity has become a key corporate social responsibility strategy (Herrick, 2009). More so, it is crucial for food and beverage corporations to *be seen* to be trying to reduce childhood obesity and promote physical activity. In this way, 'socially responsible' physical activity programmes in schools and partnerships with schools and not-for-profits act as a particularly useful form of public relations, what MacDonald (2008, p.71) describes as 'reputation insurance'. Kenway and Bullen (2001, p.100) pointed this out over fifteen years ago: 'Not only do schools offer a way to establish and maintain a high public profile, but an opportunity for businesses with doubtful reputations or bad publicity to practice some reverse psychology.' In short, partnerships help to serve two key functions: diverting public attention from 'less agreeable' practices (e.g. marketing of 'junk' food to children) *and* re-shaping consumers' image of the corporation (e.g. as an altruistic, socially-responsible, health-promoting organisation).

The profit-seeking motives for corporations to build partnerships and be more socially responsible, even philanthropic, are therefore also closely tied to their marketing strategies. As Blanding (2010, p.136–137, emphasis in original) writes:

> The danger of CSR initiatives is that they have become such a branding tool that they make it seem like the opposite is true – that companies are somehow investing in causes out of a motive of self-sacrifice, rather than *partnering* with causes for mutual benefit. And as branding has become the primary reason for CSR, the appearance of doing something can overshadow the benefits of doing it.

In other words, the *marketing* of social responsible physical activity programmes in schools is a business strategy in itself. For instance, McDonald's *My Greatest Feat* pedometer programme in New Zealand received much acclaim from its advertising partners when 'McDonald's brand trust scores took a giant leap seeing increases up to 50%', a great feat given that 'McDonald's had been the whipping boy for everything big and bad about America and fast food. Brand trust scores were in decline' (Tribal DDB, 2009, para.1–5). By combining corporate social responsibility with partnerships (including the New Zealand Olympic Committee and a number of advertisers), McDonald's was able to merge its business strategies into its own physical activity initiative and re-invent the 'big and bad' McDonald's as responsible and health-promoting.

The perceived threat of obesity to national economies and individual health has also resulted in a threat of increased regulatory controls and potential litigation (see Mello, Pomeranz, & Moran, 2008). This is, of course, also a threat to profit. Corporations and industries are increasingly protective – and pro-active – in ensuring that *they* remain in control of regulations. The current policy environment for the food and beverage industry (and their advertisers) is dominated by self-regulation (see Mello et al., 2008), in particular 'government-approved forms of self-regulation' (International Association for the Study of Obesity, 2010, p.6), where self-regulation has been developed either in collaboration with government, at the request of government, or at least 'encouraged' by government.

Partnerships play an important role in shaping policies and regulatory controls. They are used as 'evidence' to policy and lawmakers that corporations and industries are socially responsible, helping promote physical activity, are 'part of the solution' to childhood obesity, and therefore do not require stricter regulatory controls. For instance, the United Kingdom's *Public Health Responsibility Deal* is a multi-sector partnership (with associated physical activity pledges and commitments) that was described by erstwhile Minister for Health Andrew Lansley as a 'response to challenges which we know can't be solved by regulation and legislation alone. It's a partnership between Government and business that balances proportionate regulation with corporate responsibility' (Department of Health, 2011, p.2). However, as Mello et al. (2008, p.601) point out, the benefit of self-regulation is mostly for the private sector as it creates 'the perception of cooperation with a seemingly binding agreement. However, unlike law, regulations, or settlements reached in litigation, an agreement is not binding'. In other words, the various policies, promises, pledges, and commitments to promote physical activity and fight obesity are not only self-regulated and non-binding, but are self-concocted and specifically designed to meet the profit-seeking interests of corporations. The threat of regulation has therefore become an opportunity for industry to shape international, national, and regional policies on physical activity, as well as marketing to children (see Powell, 2016); to form partnerships with schools and other trustworthy (or at least trusting) organisations; to build relationships with teachers, parents, politicians, and children; to improve public relations, brand image, and of course, the bottom line – profit.

Conclusions

School-based solutions to childhood obesity and physical inactivity are made possible by a number of partnerships, policies, and private sector practices that encourage corporations, charities, industry groups, state agencies, and schools to 'work together'. Given the disparate, even opposing interests, within this messy mix of authorities and actors, clear tensions arise. These tensions are especially evident when an industry or company with a reputation problem attempts to align themselves with schools and notions of health and education. However, tensions are often resolved by the idea that cross-sector relationships in the name of promoting of physical activity (and fighting obesity) are a 'win-win' situation for everybody involved – especially 'for the kids'.

Multi-sector physical acitvity partnerships also illuminate a practice that Li (2007a) describes as *anti-politics*. Rather than challenging the idea that the private sector has any role to play in improving children's diet, physical activity or obesity levels, the food and beverage industry works to close down political (and public) debate about the food and beverage industry being responsible for obesity. After all, the partnerships are sold to both the public and policymakers on the basis that corporations are *genuinely* and *meaningfully* being 'part of the solution' to obesity. Discussions about possible political actions, including regulatory and legislative actions to reduce obesity (e.g. stricter controls on marketing to children) are subdued. The responsibility for children's health, fatness, and access to food is transformed from an issue that corporations (and governments) should take responsibility for, to a problem that 'everyone' (i.e. everyone else, including children) must take a shared interest in solving (see also Jette et al., 2014; Ken, 2014).

'Partnerships' between schools, 'not-for-profits', and the private sector are not benign. They help to re-assemble certain organisations and individuals to be seen as philanthropic, responsible, healthy, and even educational. They endeavour to mask private sector players' self interests: branding, public relations strategies, avoidance of stricter regulations and legislation, and profit. They attempt to transfer the responsibility of governments to provide physical activity funding for students, teachers, and schools to the food and drink industry (and a number of other for-profit and not-for-profit organisations and individuals). And they also try to shape the thoughts, actions, and identities of those targeted in the school-based physical activity programmes: children (see Powell, 2016). In this way, public health and public education partnerships have become 'big business' for 'Big Food'. Childhood obesity and the promotion of physical activity in schools has become a big opportunity for the private sector to make a fat profit. The question that remains though is: If these are the ways that the private sector 'wins', what are the ways others – schools, children, teachers – may 'lose'?

Notes

1 The term 'not-for-profit' (also 'non-profit') should be understood with a degree of caution. Although these organisations are often seen as part of the voluntary sector (or 'third sector') and referred to as non-governmental organisations (NGOs), they are not necessarily autonomous entities, separate from and unconnected to the state or for-profit organisations.

2 According to the HTC Sportsworld website (www.htcsportsworld.com) they are 'global consultants in sport', with expertise in sponsorship management, brand development and licensing, and strategic consultancy. Hall-Taylor's interests are listed as business strategy, development, investments, marketing, and sponsorship. Nowhere on the website is there mention of HTC Sportsworld's experience or interest in obesity, education, or schools. Neither *Get Set Go* nor *ActivePost* are promoted on the website as clients or partners.

3 Interestingly, only a few years prior to *Get Set Go* being implemented, a national physical activity survey reported that New Zealand children aged 5–9, on average, particpated in 190.5 minutes of moderate-to-vigorous intensity physical activity *per day,* over three times the amount of physical activity recommended in national guidelines. Contrary to this evidence, the various partners involved with *Get Set Go* continued to reproduce the assumption that New Zealand children are inactive (see Maddison, Turley, Legge, & Mitchelhill, 2010).

References

Athletics New Zealand. (2012) *Get Set Go: Teachers manual.* [Online] Available from: www.zeus-sport.com/Athletics/Resource.aspx?ID=15789.

Athletics New Zealand. (2013) *Get Set Go: Teachers manual.* Wellington, Athletics New Zealand.

Ball, S. J. (2007) *Education plc: Understanding private sector participation in public sector education.* New York, Routledge.

Blanding, M. (2010) *The Coke machine: The dirty truth behind the world's favorite soft drink.* New York, Penguin.

Coveney, J. (2006) *Food, morals and meaning: The pleasure and anxiety of eating.* 2nd ed. Abingdon, Oxon, Routledge.

Coveney, J. 2008. The government of girth. *Health Sociology Review*, 17 (2): 199–214.

Department of Health. (2011) *Public Health Responsibility Deal.* [Online] London, Department of Health. Available from: www.dh.gov.uk/prod_consum_dh/groups/dh_digitalassets/documents/digitalasset/dh_125237.pdf.

Gard, M. & Pluim, C. (2014) *Schools and public health: Past, present and future.* Lanham, MD, Lexington Books.

Gordon, B. (2014, August 6) Healthy lifestyle as important a lesson as reading. *The Dominion Post.* [Online] Available from: www.stuff.co.nz/dominion-post/.

Grant, B. & Bassin, S. (2007) The challenge of paediatric obesity: More rhetoric than action. *The New Zealand Medical Journal,* 120 (1260), 61–68.

Hawkes, C. & Buse, K. (2011) Public health sector and food industry interaction: It's time to clarify the term 'partnership' and be honest about underlying interests. *European Journal of Public Health.* [Online] 21 (4), 400–401. Available from: doi:10.1093/eurpub/ckr077.

Herrick, C. (2009) Shifting blame/selling health: Corporate social responsibility in the age of obesity. *Sociology of Health & Illness.* [Online] 31 (1), 51–65. Available from: doi:10.1111/j.1467-9566.2008.01121.x.

Huxham, C. & Vangen, S. (2000) What makes partnerships work? In S. Osbourne (ed.) *Public-private partnerships: Theory and practice in international perspectives.* London, Routledge, pp. 293–310.

International Association for the Study of Obesity. (2010) *The Polmark Project: Policies on marketing food and beverages to children: Final project report, executive report.* [Online] London, International Association for the Study of Obesity. Available from: www.worldobesity.org/what-we-do/policy-prevention/projects/marketing-children/polmarkproject/.

International Food & Beverage Alliance. (2013) *IFBA statement on the adaption by member states at the 66th World Health Assembly of the Resolution on the Follow-up to the Political Declaration of the High-level Meeting of the General Assembly on the Prevention and Control of Non-communicable Diseases.* [Online] Available from: www.ifballiance.org/sites/default/files/IFBAStatementontheAdoptionoftheResolutionofthe66thWHAonthepreventionandcontrolofNCDs28May2013.pdf.

Jette, S., Bhagat, K. & Andrews, D. L. (2014) Governing the child-citizen: 'Let's Move!' as national biopedagogy. *Sport, Education and Society.* [Online] 21 (8), 1109–1126. Available from: doi:10.108 0/13573322.2014.993961.

Ken, I. (2014) A healthy bottom line: Obese children, a pacified public, and corporate legitimacy. *Social Currents.* [Online] 1 (2), 130–148. Available from: doi: 10.1177/2329496514524927.

Kenway, J. & Bullen, E. (2001) *Consuming children: Education-entertainment-advertising.* Buckingham, UK, Open University Press.

King, S. (2006) *Pink ribbons, inc.: Breast cancer and the politics of philanthropy.* Minneapolis, MN, University of Minnesota Press.

Koplan, J. P. & Brownell, K. D. (2010) Response of the food and beverage industry to the obesity threat. *JAMA: The Journal of the American Medical Association.* [Online] 304 (13), 1487–1488. Available from: doi:10.1001/jama.2010.1436.

Kraak, V. I. & Story, M. (2010) A public health perspective on healthy lifestyles and public-private partnerships for global childhood obesity prevention. *Journal of the American Dietetic Association.* [Online] 110 (2), 192–200. Available from: doi: 10.1016/j.jada.2009.10.036.

Li, T. M. (2007a) Practices of assemblage and community forest management. *Economy and Society.* [Online] 36, 263–293. Available from: doi: 10.1080/03085140701254308.

Li, T. M. (2007b) *The will to improve: Governmentality, development, and the practice of politics.* Durham, NC, Duke University Press.

MacDonald, C. (2008) *Green Inc.: An environmental insider reveals how a good cause has gone bad.* Guilford, CT, The Lyons Press.

Maddison R., Turley M., Legge N. & Mitchelhill G. (2010) *A national survey of children and young people's physical activity and dietary behaviours in New Zealand: 2008/09.* [Online] Auckland, New Zealand: Clinical Trials Research Unit. Available from: www.health.govt.nz/publication/national-survey-children-and-young-peoples-physical-activity-and-dietary-behaviours-new-zealand-2008.

Mello, M. M., Pomeranz, J. & Moran, P. (2008). The interplay of public health law and industry self-regulation: The case of sugar-sweetened beverage sales in schools. *American Journal of Public Health.* [Online] 98 (4), 595–604. Available from: doi:10.2105/AJPH.2006.107680.

Miller, P. & Rose, N. (2008) *Governing the present.* Cambridge, UK, Polity.

Nestlé. (2012a) *Nestlé joins call for more community-based programmes to prevent childhood obesity.* [Online] Available from: www.nestle.com/media/newsandfeatures/global-obesity-forum.

Nestlé. (2012b) *Nestlé Healthy Kids Global Programme.* [Online] Available from: www.Nestlé.com/CSV/NUTRITION/HEALTHYKIDSPROGRAMME/Pages/HealthyKidsProgramme.aspx.

Nestlé. (2016) *Nestlé Healthy Kids Global Programme.* [Online] Available from: http://pub-staging.nestle.com/nutrition-health-wellness/kids-best-start/children-family/healthy-kids-programme.

Nestlé New Zealand. (2011) *Be Healthy, Be Active: Teachers' resource.* Wellington, Learning Media.

Powell, D. (2014) Childhood obesity, corporate philanthropy and the creeping privatisation of health education. *Critical Public Health.* [Online] 24 (2), 226–238. Available from: doi:10.1080/09581596.2013.846465.

Powell, D. (2015) *'Part of the solution'?: Charities, corporate philanthropy and healthy lifestyles education in New Zealand primary schools.* (Unpublished doctoral dissertation). Bathurst, Australia, Charles Sturt University.

Powell, D. (2016) Governing the(un)healthy child-consumer. *Sport, Education and Society.* Available from: doi:10.1080/13573322.2016.1192530.

Powell, D. & Gard, M. (2015) The governmentality of childhood obesity: Coca-Cola, public health and primary schools. *Discourse: Studies in the Cultural Politics of Education.* [Online] 36 (6), 854–867. Available from: doi: 10.1080/01596306.2014.905045.

Rose, N. (2000) Government and control. *British Journal of Criminology.* [Online] 40, 321–339. Available from: doi:10.1093/bjc/40.2.321.

Sahlberg, P. (2006) Education reform for raising economic competitiveness. *Journal of Educational Change.* [Online] 7 (4), 259–287. Available from: http://link.springer.com/article/10.1007/s10833-005-4884-6.

Taylor, R. (2007) Obesity in New Zealand children: A weighty issue. *Journal of the New Zealand Medical Association,* 120 (1260), 1–3.

Thornton, R. (2011, August 6) Initiatives to help our kids with alarming obesity stats. *Weekend Herald,* p. B24.

Tribal DDB. (2009) *My Greatest Feat.* [Online] Available from: www.tribalddb.co.nz/tribalog/?paged=64.

Vander Schee, C. (2005) The privatization of food services in schools: Undermining children's health, social equity, and democratic education. In D. R. Boyles (ed.), *Schools or markets?: Commercialism, privatization, and school-business partnerships.* Mahwah, NJ, Lawrence Erlbaum, pp. 1–30.

World Health Organization. (2015a) *Global Strategy on diet, physical activity and health: What can be done to fight the childhood obesity epidemic?* [Online] Available from: www.who.int/dietphysicalactivity/childhood_what_can_be_done/en/.

World Health Organization. (2015b) *Global Strategy on diet, physical activity and health: The role of the private sector.* [Online] Available from: www.who.int/dietphysicalactivity/childhood_private_sector/en/index.html

World Health Organization. (2015c) *Global strategy on diet, physical activity and health: Marketing of foods and non-alcoholic beverages to children.* [Online] Available from: www.who.int/dietphysicalactivity/marketing-food-to-children/en.

28

THE OLYMPIC GAMES
AND PHYSICAL ACTIVITY
PROMOTION

Paul Bretherton and Billy Graeff

The hosting of the Olympic Games is increasingly being justified in part because of the event's perceived capacity to increase physical activity (PA) participation in the host nation. This chapter critically reviews the PA policies and initiatives delivered in association with both London 2012 and Rio 2016. Attention is given here to a range of social factors that render mass participation-based legacy objectives of this nature particularly problematic. These include the respective roles and responsibilities of the multitude of different organisations and actors that co-operate around PA participation, the practical difficulties that must be overcome in order to increase PA and the challenge of proving the effect of the Games on PA conclusively. The interaction between these factors and the respective social contexts of the UK and Brazil therefore offers a useful vantage point from which to consider an increasingly prominent aspect of contemporary rationales for hosting the Olympic Games.

Following the addition of ideas about "legacy" to the Olympic Charter in 2002 (International Olympic Committee, 2013), there is now a growing expectation that hosts of the Olympic Games demonstrate that the event will leave a positive social legacy in the host community. This requirement is increasingly managed in part by drawing upon the event's perceived capacity to increase physical activity (PA) participation in the host nation, primarily under the assumption that the elite sport on show during the event will encourage – or "inspire" – more people to become permanently involved in regular exercise or sport participation. However, a range of social factors suggests mass participation-based PA legacy objectives of this nature to be particularly problematic. These include the respective roles and responsibilities of the multitude of different organisations and actors that must co-operate in order to increase PA participation, the practical difficulties that must be overcome in order to encourage and accommodate previously inactive individuals to turn to exercise, and the empirical challenge of proving the effect of the Games on PA.

This chapter provides a critical examination of the PA participation legacy policies and rhetoric employed in relation to London 2012 and Rio 2016 – the first two summer Olympic host cities to be selected following the formal incorporation of legacy into the Olympic Charter in 2002. The interaction between the practical factors discussed above and the respective social and cultural contexts of the UK and Brazil offers a useful vantage point from which to consider an increasingly prominent aspect of contemporary rationales for hosting the Olympic Games – as well as the broader implications that the case of PA participation legacies may have for all forms of legacy that are emphasised by contemporary Olympic hosts.

Following this introduction, the chapter is therefore organised into two main parts. First, the PA participation legacy of London 2012 is reviewed, starting with the bidding and preparation stages and finishing with the time that has passed since the staging of this event. Second, the same approach is taken in relation to the way PA has been articulated and approached in the lead-up to Rio 2016. Finally, the concluding section draws these two cases together in order to demonstrate the broader significance of these approaches to PA legacy strategies in relation to both the broader concept of Olympic legacy as well as the need to consider the specific cultural and political dimensions of different host cities and nations.

London 2012: "Inspire a Generation"

From the UK Government's official decision to support a London bid for the 2012 Summer Olympic Games in 2003 onwards, the event's potential to bring about a national increase in sport and physical activity (PA) participation was repeatedly emphasised. In a January 2004 publication of the London 2012 Bid Company, the breadth of this potential was articulated by then Prime Minister Tony Blair:

> A London Olympics would be an unparalleled boost for sport throughout the UK. By encouraging the young and the not-so-young to take up sport, it would help us to produce the champions of the future and, importantly, a healthier and fitter population.
>
> *cited in London 2012, 2004a*

This ambition was the central pillar of an attempt to distinguish London "from both previous editions of the Games and from its bid competitors" (Weed, 2013, p. 87), and as "the first major sporting event to have broad and ambitious commitments to healthy living and inclusion" (Commission for a Sustainable London 2012, 2011, p. 4). Indeed, Blair's sentiments epitomised the London bid's early rhetoric: a London Games in 2012 would encourage sport participation and therefore health across all of society, regardless of age or competitive aspiration.

However, by the submission of the official London Candidate File in November 2004, this all-encompassing focus had given way to the more specific claim that "mounting excitement in the seven years leading up to the Games will inspire a new generation of youth to greater sporting activity" (London 2012, 2004b, p. 19), an emphasis on young people's participation that was echoed by London Bid Company Chair Lord Coe on the basis that Olympic success requires "millions of young people around the world to be inspired to choose sport" (London 2012, 2005). While this lack of consistency around participation legacy focus is perhaps inevitable in the bidding stage, attempts to formalise these grand visions became increasingly problematic following London's selection as host in 2005. Indeed, citing London 2012 as the "best chance in a generation to encourage people to be more physically active" (DCMS, 2008, p. 22) the UK Government's official plans for the legacy of the Games stated that:

> The first priority of the Games is to make the UK a world-leading sporting nation. We hope to see people becoming increasingly active, with a goal of seeing two million people more active by 2012 through focused investment in our sporting infrastructure and better support and information for people wanting to be active.
>
> *DCMS, 2008, p. 3*

This target of 2 million was to be achieved through a range of measures including cooperation with a range of local and national organisations, tackling barriers to participation and ensuring a conducive environment for activity participation. Progress was to be monitored by Sport England's Active People Survey and the DCMS Taking Part Survey. Within this overall plan, both the Department of Health (2009a) and LOCOG (2009) published separate documents detailing their respective roles in promoting physical activity participation around the Games.

However, in line with Girginov and Hills's (2008) warning that pursuing participation on this scale required "deeply rooted social structures" (p. 2091) to be successfully addressed, academic evidence increasingly began to cast these targets as more accessible to the fantasist than the realist. For example, multiple authors concluded that the evidence to support the use of London 2012 as a means of promoting sport or PA participation was insufficient (Mahtani et al., 2013; McCartney et al., 2010; Department of Health, 2009b), and that any attempt to do so would require a broader coordinated effort with the Games representing one part of a wider PA and sport promotion strategy (Department of Health, 2009b). To even approach the intended increase of 2 million people more active by 2012 would therefore have required a phenomenal collective effort by both the event's organisers and a considerable range of other sport, health and local organisations.

Such a supernatural effort did not materialise, and Sport England Chief Executive Jennie Price announced the abandonment of the 2008 participation targets in 2011:

> I am very disappointed that we have only got 111,000 more people into sport when we were counting on 1 million people, but we have to be realistic about the climate in which we are working. Jeremy Hunt [the Culture Secretary] has already said he does not believe that the one million target is the right measure of participation immediately after the Olympics, though I do think we will get a good measure of participation in the year or two after and we will get a bounce from the Olympics.
> *cited in Kelso, 2011, para. 9–10*

Price's rationale here touches upon two important factors cited for the failure of the mass participation legacy. Firstly, the reference to "the climate" refers to the financial crisis of the late 2000s, with the assumption that that this had a direct impact on the accessibility of sport and PA. Secondly, the questioning of the timescale against which the 2008 participation targets were set highlights the broader issue of Olympic legacy measurement, which for some authors requires a period of 15–20 years to be judged satisfactorily (Gratton & Preuss, 2008). The foremost implication here is that any potential sport or PA participation legacy from the Games must be regarded as inherently problematic given its susceptibility to external influences that act well beyond the control of a specific OCOG or host government.

With the 2008 mass participation targets officially abandoned, the focus of the proposed sporting legacy was narrowed to young people. Once again, the role of the wider economic context was central to the explanation provided by then Culture Secretary Jeremy Hunt:

> I do think it's reasonable to ask whether, with resources as constrained as they are, if it's an appropriate use of taxpayers' money to be focusing on adult participation when really what we want is to be getting young people into a habit for life.
> *cited in Gibson, 2011, para. 3*

This rationale was soon formalised in January 2012, when the DCMS (2012) published its new sporting legacy plans. The aim of this was to use London 2012 to "inspire the nation and help young people in particular to start a sporting habit for life" and thus "make good on the original promise" (Hunt, cited in DCMS, 2012, p. 2) that Lord Coe and the bid team set out in 2005. This promise was supposed to be fulfilled via an approach featuring increased emphasis on grassroots links between schools and clubs and a reward-based system of cooperation with national sport organisations. While this focus on youth and the future may appear laudable, a longer term approach of this nature poses significant problems for accountability, attribution and measurement. As noted by Wellings, Datta, Wilkinson and Petticrew (2011), determining the extent to which Olympic-based policy initiatives can be judged to have made a measurable difference is complex. Moreover, the timescale required for this attempt to foster a "sporting habit" over a lifetime to take effect suggests that any conclusive assessment will prove exceptionally difficult.

Further confusion is apparent when setting this policy emphasis of the DCMS against the public proclamations of government figures. For example, in the same month as this youth sport focus was formalised, then UK Prime Minister David Cameron (2012) claimed that:

> The whole country can benefit from the legacy of the Games because of the inspiration that these Games will bring to people young and old right across the country about getting involved, taking exercise, learning to swim, learning to dive, and all the rest of it.

Cameron's contradiction of the strategy developed by the DCMS demonstrates the difficulty of viewing the overall participation legacy strategy without suspicion. More broadly, the need for Olympic legacy to be coordinated across all of the event's organising bodies as well as an inherently capricious host government demonstrates the problematic nature of the entire process.

In addition to these concerns, it is important to recognise that the host government is liable to change over the period of preparation for hosting the Games. In 2010, the Labour (traditionally left leaning) government that had overseen the initial bidding and planning stages was replaced by a Conservative-led coalition. Although many aspects of the Government's approach to the Games were consistent with those of its predecessor, a notable difference was its emphasis upon reducing public spending and seeking to transfer responsibilities to both the *private* and *voluntary* sectors. In terms of the sport and PA participation legacy, this approach was most directly demonstrated by then Education Secretary Michael Gove's reported intention to reduce funding for school sport partnerships – although this was eventually not fulfilled (Helm, 2010). More broadly, the Coalition's advocacy of business's role in society had important implications for the provision of health:

> The strength of the Deal lies in the diversity of organisations that it brings together
> – public sector, commercial, non-governmental, and academic – to determine things business can do to accelerate the progress towards public health goal . . . Put simply, commercial organisations can reach individuals in ways that other organisations, Government included, cannot.
>
> *Lansley, cited in DH, 2011, p. 2*

This attitude towards the role of business in promoting health is consistent with the growing conviction that sport's social potential should be exploited by Corporate Social Responsibility (CSR) schemes (e.g. Smith & Westerbeek, 2007). In relation to the sport and PA participation legacy of London 2012, several Olympic sponsors – under the supervision of LOCOG – coordinated social initiatives involving sport, health or PA in various forms. Lloyds TSB's

National School Sport Week, Cadbury's *Spots v Stripes, Coca-Cola's* partnership with *StreetGames* were all examples of participation-based local events that prioritised specific populations such as schoolchildren or deprived communities. Other initiatives such as McDonald's *Champions of Play* and GE's *Design My Break* also sought to contribute towards health or PA awareness by encouraging young people to engage more with these issues while adidas installed exercise facilities called *adiZones* in local parks for the public to use for free.

While this corporate activity may appear nobly intended, it must be squared with the assertion that business may simply attempt to exploit the "value and altruistic nature of sport to fulfil their own goals" (Carey et al., 2011, p. 259). Where sponsors of London 2012 were concerned, Lloyds TSB's Head of Olympic Marketing and Group Sponsorship Gordon Lott (2012, para. 3) acknowledged that:

> Becoming a partner of the Games was a brand-led decision. Sponsorship sits within our marketing portfolio alongside other channels – advertising, branches and social media and so on – to communicate our messages and values in the round.

The risk of Olympic-based sponsor CSR schemes being secondary to commercial objectives is exacerbated by the fact that while certain sponsors sought to associate themselves with London 2012's sport and PA participation targets, corporate organisations were not directly involved in this aspect of the legacy, and therefore beyond accountability for its abandonment. For example, in May 2011 a representative of Adidas claimed that their attempt to overcome "major barriers to taking up sports" and engage "the whole community in sport" via the adiZone initiative formed "part of our pledge to inspire participation in sport and create a legacy" from the Games (Craggs, cited in London Borough of Hackney, 2011, para. 9). This claim must be seen as particularly problematic given that it was published two months after Jeremy Hunt's (Gibson, 2011) admission that the mass participation legacy was doomed to failure and that focussing on youth participation was the best solution.

By lacking a formal link to official legacy targets, corporations are ultimately able to exploit the altruistic rhetoric contained within host government policies without finding themselves accountable for their realisation. Although evaluation of sport and PA-based CSR activity exists, this is typically organised or funded by the sponsor itself (e.g. Cadbury, 2011). With corporate involvement in the Games increasing in tandem with the pro-business attitudes exemplified by the UK government here, it can therefore be seen that the proclaimed contributions of sponsors to legacy targets should be treated with similar scrutiny to the rhetoric of the government and organisational bodies that organise the Games.

Upon the conclusion of the Games in August 2012, then Mayor of London Boris Johnson (2012, para.10) declared that:

> They will say there will be no increase in sporting participation, and no economic benefits, and that we will not succeed in regenerating east London. Well, just remember one thing, everyone. These Olympo-sceptics were proved decisively wrong about the Games. They will be proved wrong about the legacy as well.

Johnson's enthusiasm here typified both the dominant media discourse during and immediately after the Games themselves and the way that this celebratory tone was frequently taken as evidence that "positive" legacy outcomes such as increased sport (and PA) participation would naturally follow. However, by 2013, then Sport Minister Hugh Robertson could be seen to be taking a more cautious stance:

I think that we will need at least five years, and probably a decade, before we can make an authoritative judgement on the success of the London 2012 sports legacy but the foundations are incredibly strong. Britain's reputation in world sport has certainly been transformed. Everywhere I have gone since London 2012 people have congratulated this country for hosting [a] wonderful Games.

cited in UK Government/Mayor of London, 2013, p. 22

Although Robertson's recognition of the need for a longer term assessment is consistent with academic recommendations for Olympic legacy measurement (Gratton & Preuss, 2008), he can be seen here to conflate the issue with the international acclaim received by the UK for its hosting of the Games. In the same document, it is noted that despite a recent decrease, 2013 saw 1.4 million more people playing sport at least once a week than in 2005 when London was chosen as host for 2012 (UK Government/Mayor of London, 2013). "Positive underlying trends" (p. 25) are also noted in the participation of groups such as young people, women and the disabled. While these statistics may appear positive, it must firstly be noted that the comparison with 2005 is limited given that no formal attempt to increase participation was announced until 2008. Secondly, the singular focus upon sport participation here conflicts with the earlier commitment to encourage participation in broader PA simultaneously. Thirdly – and finally – any increase measured by 2013 would need to be proven to be more sustainable than the short term increases in participation that have been observed at previous events (Department of Health, 2009b).

In relation to these concerns, it is worth noting Weed and colleagues' (2015) systematic analysis of the potential of a "demonstration effect" (wherein an elite sport event "inspires" increased sport participation). These authors conclude that while such a "demonstration effect" may both increase sport participation "frequency" and encourage lapsed participants to return to sport, there remains no evidence that it can attract new participants – and conclude that increasing participation alone is insufficient to justify the hosting of a major sport event. In terms of the official proclamations around the participation legacy of London 2012, these conclusions are particularly problematic. Most apparently, the fact that statements about legacy became intertwined with immediate responses to the overall staging of the Games suggests a heavy dependence on a presumed demonstration effect that is unlikely to attract the new participants that are required for an overall increase. Beyond this, even a minor sustained increase in participation would remain difficult to consider a success given the lofty rhetoric of the bidding stage and the initial target of two million more people becoming active by 2012.

Although the current discussion portrays a legacy objective that was enthusiastically advocated by Government and LOCOG representatives from the bidding stage onwards, empirical evidence both shows that genuine progress has thus far been negligible and that the early visions will ultimately go unfulfilled. Furthermore, the one-off nature of the Games, the prompt disbanding of LOCOG and the subsequent turnover of relevant governmental ministers suggests that accountability for its failure will ultimately never be established. This is not to conclude that a sustained and tangible increase in sport and PA participation via an Olympic Games is impossible, but that any attempt to prove otherwise will require a far more comprehensive and coordinated effort than has been reviewed here in relation to London 2012.

Rio 2016 – It is Brazil's turn

In contrast with the published aims of the London 2012, PA was not a priority for Brazilian Governments in general (Federal, State and City spheres were involved with the bidding and hosting) regarding the 2016 Olympics and its bidding process – as the emphasis had been put upon the potential of the Games to enhance *socio economic* development from the beginning. Before the final vote in which Rio was ultimately selected as host for the 2016 Games, then President Luiz Inácio "Lula" da Silva stated to the International Olympic Committee that the Olympic Games should be taken to South America for the first time (Maranhão, 2009). He stressed that such a decision would correct a historical distortion and that it would help in the economic development of both the country and even the continent (Aquino, 2009). Thus it was not surprising to those who follow the political economy of international sport that an underdeveloped nation had been chosen as a sport mega event host, after Football World Cups and Olympics were being allocated in the Global South and in poor countries for a period that seems to have started prior Athens 2004 and that extends at least to Qatar 2022. Additionally, it can be argued that Brazil's candidacy fitted well with the narrative of Olympics as catalysts for development, which could have helped the bid to be victorious (Darnell, 2010) in a context in which this had became part of the official discourse (International Olympic Committee, 2013).

In 2010, Brazilian presidential candidate Dilma Rousseff emphasised the aspects that were part of her plans in relation to sport and the Olympics – without mentioning PA:

> The commitment we would like to reiterate here today is to make the Olympics a tool to transform Brazil into one of the largest and best sports powers in the world. We want a country with high sports and social performances, to form and train athletes and at the same time that we form citizens with good education, training, and quality jobs.
>
> *Viga & Bulcão Pinheiro, 2010*

Following her election as president, Dilma Rousseff promoted an executive act to release R$1 billion for the Program Plan Brazil Medals 2016 (Previdelli, 2012). The Brazilian government's website shows that not only R$1 billion would be spent in trying to ensure Brazil finished among the top 10 nations in the Rio 2016 Olympic Games and in the top 5 in the Rio 2016 Paralympics Games medal tables, but that R$2.5 billion was allocated for other investments in high-level sport (Ministério do Esporte, 2012).

In turn, the candidacy dossier (BRASIL, 2009) stressed the fact that Brazil would invest billions in a program for development acceleration as well as creating an Olympic Public Authority with a division for Olympic Traffic and Transport and an Olympic Division for Sustainability. Thus it can be said that issues related to the historical deficit in terms of economic and urban development as well as in terms of democracy increase were the most important for the Rio 2016 project.

The same document also accentuates the celebratory aspects of the Games and focuses on the participation of young people and the potential for social transformation through sport. Further, the document reveals that the strategy would be to invest in school and elite sports in order to produce a sporting legacy. Additionally, a number of articles published on the official website of the event outlined how such a policy would be developed (RIO2016, 2013a; 2013b; 2015). Meetings with teachers from the municipal and state school systems were the main tools used by the ROCOG. However, a study of Physical Education teachers living in Rio de Janeiro showed that they "had hardly any knowledge of the candidature file for Rio 2016" or "soft" legacies as possible PA legacies (Reis et al., 2013, p. 444). Additionally, the teachers claimed that they "had never been informed of any attempt to leverage the Olympic Games for increasing sport/physical activity participation" (Reis et al., 2013, p. 449). Another strategy towards this end would be the realisation of School Olympics (RIO2016, 2008).

On the other hand, considerable resources have been invested in the acquisition of high-tech equipment and the hiring of technical staff in the preparation of Brazilian athletes in order to improve the Brazil Olympic team's performance in its own Olympics (Brum, 2014). This is a strong tendency for the area of sports funding, meaning that it was specifically targeted at high level sports with an emphasis on Olympic sports. Thus it can be said that despite the rhetoric, health and PA are not the highest funding priority within the field of sports in general and that it seems to be the same when sport mega events are considered (Hogan and Norton, 2000) and that apparently Rio 2016 was consistent with this tendency.

Together with the discourse concerning the economic, social and urban development, some attention was given by stakeholders to the sporting potential in terms of social mobility. Although it has been part of official discourse in relation to wider issues (Chahad, 2009), with reference to PA and the possibility of bringing it to disadvantaged strata of the population, the discourse supposedly has not been repeated. For instance, the findings of Reis and Sousa-Mast (2012, p. 42) indicated that:

> The initiatives ... proposed and executed by the different levels of the Brazilian Government as well as the OCOG (LOCOG) have not been extensively felt or successful in reaching the people who are in most need: those children and youth living in low income communities and therefore more vulnerable and at-risk.

Nonetheless, as stated earlier, recent studies focused on the health legacy of sport mega events have been inconclusive (e.g. Mahtani et al., 2013). In support of this evidence, a specific study conducted in relation to RIO 2016 echoed the "current lack of evidence about the Olympic legacy regarding health promotion" (Demarzo et al., 2014, p. 8). Despite this, the subject of PA is present in the initial report to measure the impacts and the legacy of the Rio 2016 Games produced by the Olympic Games Impact Study – RIO 2016 (OGI 2016, 2014), localised in the Socio-Cultural Sphere part of the report, among 22 other different sub-themes. However, PA is not one of the main focuses in the area of health within the report, which are:

> Birth rate, life expectancy at birth, the infant mortality rate, percentage of hospital beds per capita, percentage of health professionals per capita and the dengue fever incidence rate in the state of Rio de Janeiro; the expenditure of the Ministry of Health with health care per capita at the federal level; and the prevalence of smoking at the municipal level.
>
> *OGI 2016, 2014, p. 124*

The report includes a note which states that "the practice of physical activity of at least 150 minutes of mild or moderate intensity, per week; or, at least 75 minutes of physical activity per week of vigorous-intensity volume" (OGI 2016, 2014, p. 137) would be the target of the investigation. These guidelines would be used by the authors of the report in order to "monitor physical activity, through an 'Index of physical activity'" (OGI 2016, 2014, p. 137). The report highlights an initiative called:

> Rio em Forma Olímpico, a municipal Programme created in 2009, [that] aimed at improving access to sports practiced by offering free physical activity of high quality, with the support of qualified professionals, from Monday to Friday, across urban areas of the city of Rio de Janeiro. Currently, there are more than 24,000 people being assisted in 436 units.
>
> *OGI 2016, 2014, p. 139, emphasis added*

Nevertheless, little publicly available information has been found on the practical effects of the creation of the initiative and the instruments to be used in order to "recommend practice" within the context suggested by the report. Further, the report also gives importance to Physical Education and School Sport and presents a list of indicators to be observed when focussing on the area:

> Weekly workload destined to sport in schools; Percentage of students who engage in physical activity at school counter-shift; Number of schools with sports facilities; Investment in sports equipment; Relationship between the budget and in construction/maintenance of sports facilities and equipment in schools; Physical education professionals.
>
> *OGI 2016, 2014, p. 140*

Notwithstanding that this is only the first version (the research group aims to publish 3 more reports), the report could not present results regarding the indicators due to problems related to federal sphere difficulties in gathering data. Additionally, it can only be expected that the monitoring part of the report can be sustained. Also, even if this is considered the most ambitious study in the context of the RIO2016, it seems to fail in tackling the fact that "there is currently a dearth of well-designed studies that support the notion that hosting an Olympic Games leads to improvements in health or an increased participation in physical activity and sports" (Demarzo et al., 2014, p. 9) once its main feature is to monitor studies to be performed by other institutions. Also, it partially fails to consider the International Olympic Committee consensus statement on the health and fitness of young people through physical activity and sport (Mountjoy et al., 2011), which apparently has not been considered within the research project that supports the rationale for the reports.

Additionally, the literature suggests that the Games in general "generated a negative perception in the population", for political or administrative reasons, which can also have "in turn, . . . a negative effect on physical activity and possibly for the health levels of the population" (Demarzo et al., 2014, p. 8; Mahtani et al., 2013). Also, plenty of evidence could be related to negative perception of recent sport mega events in recent in Brazil and especially in Rio de Janeiro (Saad-Filho & Morais, 2014; Saad-Filho, 2013; Braga, 2013; Ruediger et al., 2014). Consequently it can be said that in addition to the general tendency that sport mega events present to decreasing in PA, the Brazilian context could have had this situation aggravated by the size, relevance and social impact of the "June Journeys" and subsequent demonstrations (Harvey et. al., 2013).

Furthermore RIO2016 seems to be another opportunity missed by stakeholders in general which insist in assuming that sport, health and physical activity would have levels increased and generate life conditions improvements by the simple fact of holding a sport mega event (Murphy & Bauman, 2007) relegating specific planning, funding and assessment for the specific area to other parts, the private sector or simply ignoring this need.

Recently, the governments involved in the initiatives described before and the ROCOG apparently lowered their investments in the PA part of the programs and decided to use the opportunities presented to reinforce Olympic and Paralympic Values, which are defined as "excellence, respect, friendship, courage, determination, inspiration and equality" (RIO2016, 2013b).

Moreover, the timing could not be more dramatic for the country to fail to seize an opportunity with great potential that the proponents of such an idea suggest. In June 2015, the Brazilian Sports Ministry revealed part of an ambitious project called National Sport

Diagnosis. The research aims to look into a number of relevant factors in the context of sports practices, and its first part deals with the levels of physical activity practice of the national population. However the results are not the best that could be expected: "It reveals that nearly half of the population between 14 and 75 years, about 45.9%, does not practice any physical activity" (Portal Brasil, 2015).

Nevertheless, another indication of how issues related to public health have been addressed in the context of the Rio 2016 Olympic Games comes from the treatment given to the waters that will host rowing competitions, for example. After participating in the Junior Rowing World Championships in Rodrigo de Freitas Lagoon in Rio de Janeiro, a preparatory event for the Olympics, 13 of the 40 rowers of the United States team returned home with stomach problems. The North Americans had vomiting and diarrhoea. The doctor Kathryn Ackerman, who was responsible for delegation, suggested that the contamination happened due to water pollution, in the water that will be used during the Rio 2016 Olympic Games (ZERO HORA, 2015).

Conclusion

The two cases presented in this chapter demonstrate that whilst PA legacies are regarded as an increasingly important part of the Olympic Games, their translation into practice (or policies) is still a challenge for governments, bid teams, corporate stakeholders, Olympic Games organisers and to the Olympic Movement itself. Also, this analysis lays bare the challenges for researchers seeking to establish protocols in order to assess PA initiatives within the context of Olympic legacies.

One of the first issues to consider seems to be the fact that PA can be and (in the cases studied) indeed has been given different levels of emphasis by different bid teams in the context of the broader political role played by the process of bidding, planning and hosting the event. Additionally, the political, economic and cultural context of the host nation is crucial in determining the desired series of outcomes from events of such magnitude, including the amount of resources dedicated to PA increasing policies, either practically or rhetorically. Referring to the case of Brazil, for example, we could not consider here that the country also hosted the 2014 FIFA World Cup, which certainly had some effect upon the process of Olympic legacy planning for the 2016 Games.

Regarding the latter, it is important to highlight that whereas the United Kingdom is a highly developed nation, Brazil is a former European colony struggling to overcome difficulties in most of the basic areas of human development. This contrast was apparent in the differences in which PA was treated in the political discourse. While for the UK, with one of the most developed health systems in the world, PA was central to Olympic legacy discourse and planning, for Brazil it was not given any serious attention as more fundamental needs were emphasised instead.

Specifically considering the field of studies, research designs capable of reaching a good understanding of the complex and changeable contours of the social phenomenon of PA measurement, assessment and improvement can be considered one of the foremost challenges to be overcome. Also the lack of more comprehensive and agreed designs in order to assess PA legacies in relation to sport mega events such as the Olympic Games could be considered one of the few consensuses among researchers. This could perhaps be done more conveniently if PA promotion could take a more integrated and prominent role within sport mega events and Olympic planning and hosting.

This leads to at least two main concerns: attribution and resources. Although legacy has become a constant in the discursive resources of sport mega events and the Olympic Games,

PA promotion is neither unified nor consolidated within it. Consequently, roles are not yet clear and responsibility and accountability are diffused amongst several actors. The practical implication here is that PA planning, promotion, assessment and funding are also diffused across numerous actors and this is indeed a factor that can be considered as central for the failure of the cases cogitated. Moreover it must be said that in addition to the claims made for specific planning, funding and assessment for PA promotion in the context of sport mega events and Olympic Games earlier, it seems that considering the historical and apparently omnipresent imbalance in favour of elite sports is necessary in order to increase the effectiveness of PA legacies from future Games.

References

Aquino, Y. (2009). Lula: Olimpíadas serão oportunidade única para o Brasil. [online] Available at: www.redebrasilatual.com.br/esportes/jogos-olimpicos/lula-olimpiadas-seraooportunidade-unica-para-o-brasil [Accessed 19 Oct. 2015].

Braga, R. (2013). As jornadas de junho no Brasil: Crônica de um mês inesquecível. OSAL Observatorio Social de América Latina Año XIV N° 34 / publicación semestral / noviembre de 2013. Available at: http://biblioteca.clacso.edu.ar [Accessed 14 Dec. 2014].

BRASIL (2009). Dossie de candidatura. [online] Available at: www.rio2016.com/sites/default/files/parceiros/dossie_de_candidatura_v1.pdf [Accessed 9 Oct. 2015].

Brum, A. (2014). Sonho do top 10 no Rio faz Brasil se curvar a gringos. *Gazeta do Povo*. [online] Available at: www.gazetadopovo.com.br/esportes/olimpiadas/2016/sonho-do-top-10no-rio-faz-brasil-se-curvar-a-gringos-96cwl6gdq43ec0fvql0wwl6by [Accessed 9 Oct. 2015].

Cadbury (2011). Cadbury Spots v Stripes community impact report 2011. Great Britain: Cadbury.

Cameron, D. (2012). Cameron hails Olympics legacy as cabinet meets at site. Online video, retrieved 9/1/2012 from www.bbc.co.uk/news/uk-politics-16460572.

Carey, M., Mason, D.S., & Misener, L. (2011). Social responsibility and the competitive bid process for major sporting events. *Journal of Sport and Social Issues*, 35(3), 246–263.

Chahad, A. (2009). "Sim, nós podemos e vamos realizar essa Olimpíada", diz Lula. *Terra*. [online] Available at: http://esportes.terra.com.br/sim-nos-podemos-e-vamos-realizar-essa-olimpiadadiz-lula,404872b4b13ba310VgnCLD200000bbcceb0aRCRD.html [Accessed 9 Oct. 2015].

Commission for a Sustainable London 2012 (2011). *Fit for purpose? A review of inclusion and healthy living across the 2012 programme*. Great Britain: Commission for a Sustainable London 2012.

Darnell, S. C. (2010). Mega sport for all? Assessing the development promises of Rio 2016. In *Rethinking matters Olympic: Investigations into the socio-cultural study of the modern Olympic movement, 10th international symposium for Olympic research* (pp. 498–507). London, Ontario, Canada.

Demarzo, M.M.P., Mahtani, K.R., Slight, S.P., Barton, C.A., Blakeman, T., & Protheroe, J. (2014). The Olympic legacy for Brazil: Is it a public health issue?. *Cad. Saúde Pública, Rio de Janeiro*, 30(1), 8–10.

DCMS (2008). *Before, during and after: Making the most of the London 2012 Games*. London: DCMS.

DCMS (2012). *Creating a sporting habit for Life: A new youth sport strategy*. London: DCMS.

Department of Health (2009a). *Be active be healthy: A plan for getting the nation moving*. London: DH.

Department of Health (2009b). A systematic review of the evidence base for developing a physical activity and health legacy from the London 2012 Olympic and Paralympic Games. London: DH.

Department of Health (2011). *The public health responsibility deal*. London: DH.

Gibson, O. (2011, March 29). Jeremy Hunt admits London 2012 legacy targets will be scrapped. *The Guardian*. Retrieved from www.theguardian.com/sport/2011/mar/28/jeremy-huntlondon2012-legacy.

Girginov, V. & Hills, L. (2008). A sustainable sports legacy: Creating a link between the London Olympics and sports participation. *International Journal of the History of Sport*, 25(14), 2091–2116.

Gratton, C. & Preuss, H. (2008). Maximizing Olympic impacts by building up legacies. *The International Journal of the History of Sport*, 25, 1922–1938.

Harvey, D., Vainer, C., Zizek, S. et al. (2013). *Cidades rebeldes: Passe Livre e as manifestações que tomaram as ruas do Brasil*. Sao Paulo: Boitempo Editorial.

Helm, T. (2010, Dec 5). School sports: Half a million pupils protest against Michael Gove's cuts. *The Guardian*. Retrieved from www.theguardian.com/education/2010/dec/05/school-sportpartnerships-protests-michael-gove.

Hogan, K. & Norton, K. (2000). The 'price' of Olympic gold. *Journal of Science and Medicine in Sport*, 3(2), 203–218.

International Olympic Committee (2013). Olympic Charter. Retrieved from www.olympic.org/Documents/olympic_charter_en.pdf.

Johnson, B. (2012, Aug 12). London 2012 Olympics: London and Team GB – take a bow. You've dazzled the world. *The Telegraph*. Retrieved from Johnson, B. (2012). London 2012 Olympics: London and Team GB – take a bow. You've dazzled the world. Available at: www.telegraph.co.uk/comment/columnists/borisjohnson/9471567/London-2012-Olympics-London-and-Team-GB-take-a-bow.-Youve-dazzled-the-world.html.

Kelso, P. (2011, Dec 8). London 2012: Sport England to miss legacy target as Games fail to inspire youngsters. *The Telegraph*. Retrieved from www.telegraph.co.uk/sport/olympics/news/8944428/London2012-OlympicsSportEngland-to-miss-legacy-target-as-Games-fail-to-inspire-youngsters.html.

LOCOG (2009). *Towards a one planet 2012*. London: London 2012.

London 2012 (2004a). *London 2012: A vision for the Olympic Games and Paralympic Games*. London: London 2012.

London 2012 (2004b). *London 2012 candidate file*. London: London 2012.

London 2012 (2005). *Singapore presentation*. Presented at 117th International Olympic Committee Session, 6 July 2005.

London Borough of Hackney (2011). Ian Thorpe visits London 2012 legacy project. Retrieved from http://apps.hackney.gov.uk/servapps/newspr/NewsReleaseDetails.aspx?id=2029.

Lott, G. (2012). Olympic sponsorship: ROI. Retrieved from www.sportbusiness.com/sportbusinessinternational/olympic-sponsorship-roi.

Mahtani, K., Protheroe, J., Slight, S., Demarzo, M., Blakeman, T., Barton, C., Brijnath, B., & Roberts, N. (2013). Can the London 2012 Olympics 'inspire a generation' to do more physical or sporting activities? An overview of systematic reviews. *BMJ Open*, 3(1), pp.e002058e002058.

Maranhão, R. (2009). Com reforço de Lula, 'seleção' brasileira usa a emoção na cartada final por2016. [online] Available at: http://globoesporte.globo.com/Esportes/Noticias/Olimpiadas/ [Accessed 19 Oct. 2015].

McCartney, G., Thomas, S., Thomson, H., Scott, J., Hamilton, V., Hanlon, P., Morrison, D.S., & Bond, L. (2010). The health and socioeconomic impacts of major multi-sport events: Systematic review (1978–2008). *British Medical Journal*, 340, c2369.

Ministério do Esporte (2012). Plano Brasil Medalhas 2016. [online] Available at: www.esporte.gov.br/index.php/institucional/alto-rendimento/plano-brasil-medalhas [Accessed 19 Oct. 2015].

Mountjoy, M., Andersen, L., Armstrong, N., Biddle, S., Boreham, C., Bedenbeck, H., Ekelund, U., Engebretsen, L., Hardman, K., Hills, A., Kahlmeier, S., Kriemler, S., Lambert, E., Ljungqvist, A., Matsudo, V., McKay, H., Micheli, L., Pate, R., Riddoch, C., Schamasch, P., Sundberg, C., Tomkinson, G., van Sluijs, E., & van Mechelen, W. (2011). International Olympic Committee consensus statement on the health and fitness of young people through physical activity and sport. *British Journal of Sports Medicine*, 45(11), 839–848.

Murphy, N.M. & Bauman, A. (2007). Mass sporting and physical activity events: Are they bread and circuses or public health interventions to increase population levels of physical activity? *Journal of Physical Activity and Health*, 4, 193–202.

OGI 2016, The OGI – SAGE/COPPE/UFRJ Research Team For: The Organising Committee for the Rio 2016 Olympic and Paralympic Games (Rio 2016™) (2014). *Olympic Games Impact (OGI) Study – RIO 2016 Initial report to measure the impacts and the legacy of the Rio 2016 Games*. [online] Available at: www.rio2016.com/sites/default/files/parceiros/ogi_rio_2016_r1_engl.pdf [Accessed 9 Oct. 2015].

Portal Brasil (2015). Diagnóstico Nacional do Esporte mapeia atividade física. [online] Available at: www.brasil.gov.br/esporte/2015/06/diagnostico-nacional-do-esporte-mapeia-atividadefisica-no-pais [Accessed 17 Oct. 2015].

Previdelli, A. (2012). O plano do Brasil para ganhar medalhas nas Olimpíadas. *Exame*. [online] Available at: http://exame.abril.com.br/brasil/noticias/o-plano-do-brasil-para-ganhar medalhas-nas-olimpia-das [Accessed 19 Oct. 2015].

Reis, A.C. & Sousa-Mast, F.R. (2012). Rio 2016 and Sport Legacies The legacies of the Olympic Games for youth at-risk in Rio de Janeiro. (IOC Olympic Studies Centre Postgraduate Research Grant Programme 2012).

Reis, A., de Sousa-Mast, F. & Gurgel, L. (2013). Rio 2016 and the sport participation legacies. *Leisure Studies*, 33(5), 437–453.

RIO2016 (2008). Projeto das Olimpíadas Escolares é apresentado em congresso mundial. [online] Available at: www.rio2016.com/noticias/noticias/projeto-das-olimpiadas-escolares-eapresentado-em-congresso-mundial [Accessed 9 Oct. 2015].

RIO2016 (2013a). Rio 2016™ comemora marco de três anos para os Jogos de olho na educação. [online] Available at: www.rio2016.com/noticias/noticias/rio-2016-comemora-marcode-tres-anos-para-os-jogos-de-olho-na-educacao [Accessed 9 Oct. 2015].

RIO2016 (2013b). Rio 2016 video festival spreads Olympic and Paralympic values in city's schools. [online] Available at: www.rio2016.com/en/news/news/rio-2016-video-festival-spreadsolympic-and-paralympic-values-in-citys-schools [Accessed 17 Oct. 2015].

RIO2016 (2015). Transforma, programa de educação Rio 2016, é ampliado e vai chegar a 19 municípios do Rio. [online] Available at: www.rio2016.com/noticias/noticias/transforma-programa-de-educacao-rio-2016-eampliado-e-vai-chegar-a-19-municipios-d [Accessed 9 Oct. 2015].

Ruediger, M., de Souza, R., Grassi, A., Ventura, T., & Ruediger, T. (2014). June Journeys in Brazil: From the Networks to the Streets. *SSRN Journal*. Available at: http://papers.ssrn.com/sol3/papers.cfm?abstract_id=2475983. [Accessed 14 Dec. 2014].

Saad-Filho, A. (2013). Mass Protests under 'Left Neoliberalism': Brazil, June–July 2013. *Critical Sociology*, 39(5), 657–669.

Saad-Filho, A. and Morais, L (2014). Mass protests: Brazilian spring or Brazilian malaise?. *Socialist Register*, V. 50. Available from: http://socialistregister.com [Accessed: 12th December 2014].

Smith, A.C.T. & Westerbeek, H.M. (2007). Sport as a vehicle for deploying corporate social responsibility. *Journal of Corporate Citizenship*, 25, 43–54.

UK Government & Mayor of London (2013). Inspire by 2012: The legacy from the London 2012 Olympic and Paralympic Games. London: UK Government & Mayor of London.

Viga, R. and Bulcão Pinheiro, L. (2010). Dilma visita COB e ganha agasalho de equipe brasileira. *Terra*. [online] Available at: http://esportes.terra.com.br/jogos-olimpicos/2016/dilma-visitacob-e-ganha-agasalho-de-equipe brasileira,3b8872b4b13ba310VgnCLD200000bbcceb0aRCRD.html [Accessed 19 Oct. 2015].

Weed, M. (2013). London 2012 legacy strategy: Ambitions, promises and implementation plans. In V. Girginov (Ed.) *Handbook of the London 2012 Olympic and Paralympic Games (Volume One)* (pp. 87–98). Great Britain: Routledge

Weed, M. E., Coren, E., Fiore, J., Wellard, I., Chatziefstathiou, D., & Suzanne, D. (2015). The Olympic Games and raising sports participation: A systematic review of evidence and an interrogation of policy for a demonstration effect. *European Sport Management Quarterly*, 15(2), 195–226.

Wellings, K., Datta, J., Wilkinson, P., & Petticrew, M. (2011). The 2012 Olympics: Assessing the public health effect. *The Lancet*, 378(9797), 1193–1195.

ZERO HORA (2015). Treze atletas americanos adoecem após evento-teste de remo no Rio. [online] Available at: http://zh.clicrbs.com.br/rs/esportes/olimpiada/noticia/2015/08/treze-atletasamerica-nos-adoecem-apos-evento-teste-de-remo-norio4821554.html?utm_source=&utm_medium=&utm_campaign= [Accessed 17 Oct. 2015].

29

THE ROLE OF EVALUATION IN SCHOOL SPORT POLICY, PROVISION AND PARTICIPATION

Change4Life School Sports Clubs

Abby Foad and Michelle Secker

In this chapter we show how independent evaluations of the Change4Life School Sports Club programme over the four year period from 2010 to 2015 has contributed to the evidence base for policy-makers, provided a rationale for investment and informed programme improvement, in turn impacting positively on young people's engagement and physical activity levels. We also examine the wider socio-political context of 2010 to 2015 to consider how the research has both contributed to and been shaped by social, political and economic factors.

> Not on the team? Then no more sport for you . . . we were united – and not in a good way. Within moments, the mood turned indignant, then ugly. The netball coach, the rowing crew, the trampolining squad, the football team, no one was spared our venom. Why? Not because our kids hadn't made the team (well, maybe a bit because our kids hadn't made the team), but mostly because not making the team meant that they were no longer able to take part in the sport they loved. Instead, the school's focus was concentrated entirely – and I do mean entirely – on nurturing the best and ignoring the rest.
>
> *Woods, 2015*

Background

The National Curriculum for Physical Education (NCPE), developed under the Conservative Government in 1992 and revised since, had at its focus elite sport and competitive team games. It was developed during an era in which an estimated 10,000 school playing fields were sold by schools to raise funds (1979–1997). In the early 2000s, the Labour Government adopted a more interventionist approach to physical education and school sport policy, and in 2002 it introduced the Physical Education and Sport Strategy (PESS) and PE, School Sport and Club Links strategy (PESSL). Successive UK governments have largely maintained the commitment of PESS to the provision of a minimum of two hours a week (high quality) physical education in schools. While schools are not obliged to allocate a fixed time to physical education, the average amount of provision in primary and secondary schools is approximately two hours a week (Ofsted, 2013). The Department for Education (DfE) provides guidance to schools on the aims and targets for the national curriculum for physical education, with specific content at the discretion of schools. Activities undertaken typically include the development of fundamental movement skills and introduction to sports in primary schools and at secondary level include activities such as dance and aerobics in addition to more 'traditional' sports such as football, netball, hockey and rugby. While the terms physical education and school sport are closely associated, physical education refers to delivery within the school curriculum time. School sport is used to describe the delivery of physical activity and sporting opportunities outside of curriculum time, such as that offered during after-school clubs and through links with community clubs. However, the two are not mutually exclusive; many schools employ external providers and private coaches to deliver sessions both within curriculum PE and in extra-curricular time. The role of links between schools and community providers has been recognized by policy makers of all political persuasions in recent years, as providing expertise and enhancing sustainability of participation, though the contracting out of PE to external providers is perhaps more controversial. At the time of PESSL a network of 450 School Sport Partnerships (SSPs) – linking Specialist Sports Colleges, secondary and feeder primary schools – was established to provide a delivery framework and the PE and Sport Survey was introduced in order to monitor participation and progress. The network was seen by stakeholders (including the Association for Physical Education, the Youth Sport Trust, and Community Providers of Physical Education and Sport) as largely successful and there was widespread criticism of the Coalition Government's announcement in 2010 to end ring-fenced funding of SSPs and schools' obligation to complete the Survey, effectively marking the demise of both structures. Following an era of relative high profile for physical education and school sports, policy changes were met with 'confusion, disgruntlement and disenchantment' among physical education teachers (Keech, 2012), and underpinned by an uncertain economic climate. The Coalition Government instead focused on the introduction of a new School Games framework for competitive school sport and, while practice is varied and nuanced in schools, the resounding rhetoric of 'bringing back competition' continues under the Conservative Government of the day.

Policy and evidence

In her article for the *Telegraph* at the beginning of this chapter, Woods calls for competition for all, in place of what she sees as the current elitism in school sports. There is a paradox in this to the extent that competition necessitates the success of the few. The subject of this chapter is the evaluation of a physical activity and healthy lifestyle school programme with a broad range of outcomes achieved through an inclusive, largely non-competitive, approach. In this regard Woods is perhaps quoted out of context here. But her article demonstrates that on both the political left and right there is dissatisfaction with current physical education and school sport policy and she highlights the emotive nature of debate in this area. It would be reassuring to think that all policy was evidence-based, well-advised and not based on such emotions. Consideration of recent policy in relation to school sport, physical education and physical activity, however, suggests this is not always the case. A wealth of recent reports highlight the dearth of robust evidence for physical activity programmes and initiatives amidst socio-political calls for action to address obesity and inactivity 'epidemics' (All-Party Commission on Physical Activity, 2014; Cabinet Office, 2014; Public Health England, 2014; ukactive, 2014; Future Foundation, 2015; UNESCO, 2015). In this context, physical education and school sport have become assimilated into a 'crowded and contested policy space' (Penney, 2008) in which increasing young people's physical activity is seen as the panacea for reducing obesity, facilitating physical literacy, increasing academic attainment, reducing crime, developing citizenship, enhancing health and wellbeing and reducing future burdens on the NHS. The irony perhaps is that, in the face of widening demands on the outcomes of physical education and school sport, policy-makers have significantly narrowed the inputs with diminished funding and a focus on competition.

Arguments about the 'truth' of these 'epidemics' aside, what is clear is that effective policy in this area must be guided by valid, reliable, robust evidence. There is clearly an appetite for such evidence and for government action in response, with calls in 2014/15 from ukactive, Future Foundation, UNESCO and the All-Party Commission on Physical Activity; the latter stating:

> The UK . . . lags behind other countries in evaluating the quality of physical activity interventions. We lack a coherent picture of what 'good' looks like . . . it is almost impossible to tell which interventions to increase levels of physical activity have been successful and which have failed as the majority are not objectively assessed or evaluated over a sufficient time-frame . . . Progress is dependent on a shifting to a position of objective and comprehensive evaluation of all interventions, using standardized measures of physical activity and literacy . . . Funders, both statutory and charitable, are in a strong position to drive change.
>
> *All-Party Commission on Physical Activity, 2014: 15*

Similarly, Baroness Tanni Grey-Thompson, Chair of the ukactive Board, points to the deficiencies of evidence in relation to children's physical activity:

> At best we are measuring solely the inputs into a system, as opposed to having any regard for the outcome, even though the outcome we seek is a healthy childhood that sets young people up for a healthy life. It is the equivalent of measuring the impact of maths lessons by counting the number of hours in the timetable, rather than whether a child can count.
>
> *2014: 5*

In 2015–2016, Sporting Future (Department for Digital, Culture, Media and Sport) and Towards an Active Nation (Sport England) strategies have recognized and raised awareness of the need for high standards of evidence in order to establish 'what works' and to guide funding for programmes of activity in this area.

Change4Life research

In 2010, the Centre for Sport, Physical Education and Activity Research (*spear*) – an academic research centre based at Canterbury Christ Church University – was contracted by the Youth Sport Trust (YST) to undertake an independent evaluation of the Change4Life School Sports Club programme. YST is a charity that aims to enhance children's physical activity and wellbeing through quality PE and school sport. The Change4Life School Sports Club programme has received government funding and is managed by YST. It is currently delivered in primary schools (initially being delivered in secondary schools) by teachers and the school workforce, using resources distributed by YST and supported by Schools Games Organizers.

Year 1 Findings: 61,000 participants in secondary schools;

90% choosing to play every week and positive attitude to sport;

Social, emotional wellbeing outcomes, especially among non-sporty.

- **Recommendations:**
  - Target non-sporty/less active
  - Utilise schools' internal workforce and young people in leadership
  - Develop participation destinations

- **Outcomes:**
  - DH funding
  - Inclusion of wider health and social emotional wellbeing outcomes
  - Development of primary school programme and targeting of non-sporty/less active

Year 2 Findings: Successful targeting of non sporty and less active;

Clubs increase physical activity of least active and social-emotional changes taking longer;

Use of external coaches for delivery in secondary schools

- **Recommendations:**
  - Deliver for minimum of 12 weeks to impact on attitudes and physical activity
  - Recognise role of self-esteem, confidence and respect in increasing physical activity
  - Develop leadership opportunities and participation pathways

- **Outcomes:**
  - YST guidance to schools on targeting least active
  - Investment in CSPs (training young leaders and establishing community club links)
  - Focus on primary programme as route to participation in School Games

Year 3 Findings: Secondary school clubs moving away from Change4Life model;

50% primary clubs running for more than 12 weeks;

Primary clubs provide safe space for children without confidence to join traditional sports clubs.

- **Recommendations:**
  - Maintain focus of 3 key aspects to maximise outcomes:
  - Provision of safe space for less active; opportunities to contribute to club delivery; encourage small steps to increase physical activity

- **Outcomes:**
  - Continued investment in primary programme
  - Systematic controlled experimental research funded
  - Increase opportunities for young people to run clubs

Year 4 Findings: Clubs reaching target group;

Increased physical activity levels and self-efficacy among least active;

Activities, ownership, fun and incentives key to engaging children and achieving outcomes

- **Recommendations:**
  - Articulate how clubs support whole school agenda and Ofsted expectations
  - Sustain clubs through training and mentoring
  - Continue programme evaluation to establish impact of support networks, assess programme alignment with public health priorities and explore economic impact

- **Outcomes:**
  - YST able to demonstrate 'return on investment' to funders and schools
  - Encouraged broad whole school approach to physical education
  - Programme positioning in public health context

Figure 29.1 spear's evaluation of Change4Life School Sports Clubs

SGOs are funded by the Department for Digital, Culture, Media and Sport (DCMS) and the Department of Health (DH) and work with schools and partners nationally to support sporting opportunities. Resources include a programme of physical and educational activities, equipment and 'logbooks' which include questionnaires for participating children to complete at regular intervals. The Change4Life School Sports Club programme forms part of the national Change4Life campaign (DH) and shares its aim to increase and enhance engagement in physical activity and knowledge and understanding of healthy lifestyles.

Year 1: Programme, evaluation and impact

In 2010 the rationale for government funding of the Change4Life Schools Sports Clubs was embedded in the wider context of the build-up to Britain hosting the 2012 Olympic and Paralympic Games and its policy ambitions to use the 2012 Games to 'inspire a generation of young people' through sport, 'make the UK a world-leading sporting nation' and 'get people more active' (DCMS, 2008). Research had already highlighted the potential for Games-related 'festival' and 'celebration effects' to inspire increased physical activity among primary-aged children (*spear* 2009, 2010). However, such evidence was not available for secondary-aged young people, at whom the Change4Life School Sports Club programme was initially targeted.

The original aims of the programme were to increase participation and improve attitudes to sport and physical activity through Olympic and Paralympic themes and sports (boccia, wheelchair basketball, volleyball, table tennis, badminton, fencing and handball), delivered in secondary schools through Change4Life School Sports Clubs. Funding was provided through DCMS and was allocated in the final round of the Comprehensive Spending Review just prior to the Labour Government leaving office. YST was responsible for the development, implementation and management of the programme.

The research (an independent process and outcome evaluation) was commissioned prior to the programme being implemented. The evaluation comprised a mixed methods design including secondary analysis of monitoring returns on participation from YST; telephone interviews with lead teachers responsible for delivery of the programme in schools; surveys of participants, young leaders and lead teachers; site visits to schools delivering the programme; and telephone interviews with representatives from DH, DCMS, YST, Sport England and National Governing Bodies of sport (NGBs).

As the evaluation was commissioned during the final stages of programme development, it was possible to incorporate research tools into the programme resources; specifically children's 'quizzes' (surveys) were developed and included in the children's 'logbooks' alongside activities which children completed at regular intervals as part of their participation in the programme. In this way, the research was embedded in the programme; the activity of completing the quizzes was an integral part of participation and served to increase children's self-awareness of their physical activity and knowledge of healthy lifestyles as well as informing the research.

The findings of the evaluation in the opening year of the Change4Life School Sports Clubs showed that over 61,000 young people participated in the programme in 2010/11. Perhaps more significantly, at the end of 2010/11, 90 per cent of participants were *choosing* to play sport every week and had a positive attitude towards sport – an increase of 40 per cent since joining the clubs. While less than 4 per cent of schools had directly targeted girls to participate in the programme (girls comprised one third of participants), the increase in the number of girls choosing to play sport at least once a week (36%) was more than two and a half times that of boys (14%), and the increase in the number of girls with a positive attitude to sport (31%) was almost three times as high. *spear's* evidence-based recommendations for development of the programme included encouraging schools to clearly target the 'non-sporty', as such targeting had the potential to double the reach of the impact of the Change4Life Clubs. The research also highlighted the ways in which schools were employing external coaches to deliver the Clubs. It was recommended that schools be encouraged and guided to utilize their internal workforce and recognize the informal leadership contributions of young people to enhance the programme's sustainability. Further recommendations included the development of destinations for participants in community sports clubs and the development of support networks between SGOs, schools, Clubs and NGBs.

By 2011, armed with independent evaluation data, YST was able to demonstrate the impact of the Change4Life School Sports Club programme to the new Coalition government and to secure continued funding, now from DH. The programme was to focus on primary schools, using new themed resources relating to 'Target', 'Adventure' and 'Creative'. In secondary schools the programme continued with the seven sports themes. Evaluation in the first year had shown that, despite the focus of the programme on increasing participation in Olympic and Paralympic sports, it had significant impact on wider outcomes relating to social and emotional wellbeing, particularly among the 'non-sporty'. Over 90 per cent of this group reported that they had 'been proud of their achievements', 'felt respected' and 'respected people regardless of their ability', and the research found that these wider outcomes had been a key factor in the success of the Change4Life School Sports Clubs. In line with DH priorities, the outcome indicators for the programme widened and participation was now aligned to social and emotional wellbeing, eating habits, obesity and healthy lifestyle in addition to enhancing participation and attitudes to physical activity.

In the political sphere, the emphasis was firmly on competitive sport. The Secretary of State for Education, Michael Gove, called for a re-focusing of physical education on competitive sport and caused outcry when he proposed the disbanding of the School Sport Partnerships (SSPs), which had been widely acknowledged as successful in bringing together a network of schools and community clubs to encourage participation among young people and increase opportunities for all. Gove decided to 'give schools the time and freedom (from the requirements of the previous Government's PE and Sport Strategy) to focus on competitive sport' (DfE, 2010). Schools would no longer be required to complete the School Sport Survey, effectively sealing the fate of this method of collecting evidence around the efficacy of school sports provision. In the place of PESSL and PESS, the School Games was introduced as the government's flagship policy, replacing the UK school games.

Year 2: Programme, evaluation and impact

In 2011/12, *spear's* evaluation of the Change4Life School Sports Clubs continued with the inclusion of the primary programme evaluation. The research found that over 62,000 primary children participated in over 4,000 Change4Life School Sports Clubs in 2011/12. One of the main aims of the programme was to increase the number of children achieving the Chief Medical Officers' recommendations for physical activity of 60 minutes per day (DH, 2011) and, in line with recommendations arising from the previous year's evaluation, the clubs were targeted at the 'less active' (the change in terminology here from 'non-sporty' to 'less active' primarily reflective of the shift in programme funding from DCMS to DH). The Change4Life School Sports Clubs were seen as a vehicle to both increase physical activity and to give children the confidence and skills to take part in competitive school sports (the School Games).

The Clubs were found to be reaching the target group of less active children, with over 85 per cent of participants not achieving at least 60 active minutes every day at the start of the programme. However, after 12 weeks, 30 per cent of participants were achieving at least 60 active minutes on more days than they did previously. Moreover, 46 per cent of participants who were achieving at least 30 active minutes per day 'less than half the time' on joining the clubs were doing so 'more than half the time' when they finished the programme. Increases across all levels of activity demonstrated that the Change4Life School Sports Clubs were effective mechanisms for increasing physical activity levels among less active primary children, regardless of the extent of their initial activity. The research found that while positive behavioural changes occurred quickly (within the first 6 weeks of participation), changes in self-esteem took longer to develop. Evidence also suggested that while the programme had yet to have a substantive impact on children's confidence to try new things (indicative of confidence, motivation, aspiration, creativity, all of which play a role in sustained physical activity participation), changes in such confidence may develop if participation occurred over a longer period. Recommendations arising from the research therefore included that primary schools be strongly encouraged to run the Change4Life School Sports Clubs with the same group of children for as much of the school year as possible and for a minimum of 12 weeks, because attitudinal changes associated with a subsequent increase to at least 60 active minutes every day (such as liking to learn new skills and helping others to improve) were shown to occur later in the programme.

In the secondary programme, the Change4Life School Sports Clubs had almost 47,000 participants in the second year, of whom two thirds were new members and 45 per cent were in the non-sporty target group. Approximately one third of the non-sporty target group who were in their second year of club membership (1,600 young people) reported being positive about sport and choosing to play once a week. The research suggested that seeking to move the non-sporty target group who had chosen to remain in Change4Life Clubs onto other physical activities without a similarly supportive exit route would risk reducing the positive impact of the programme on this group by up to 20 per cent. The proportion of schools paying external coaches to contribute to club delivery had fallen from 46 per cent to 40 per cent, though this was still equivalent to almost 1,000 clubs buying in deliverers rather than building their internal delivery capacity. The previous year's evaluation had recommended the utilization of schools' internal workforce in order to enhance sustainability; the continued use of external coaches in delivery implies that this internal capacity building was not taking place. The programme in secondary schools continued to focus on competitive sport, with the evaluation report urging that care must be taken to ensure that competitive sport outcomes did not eclipse the key programme priorities of encouraging participation (particularly among the 'non-sporty'), engendering respect and increasing knowledge of healthy lifestyles. Recommendations relating to the secondary programme included a reiteration of the strong encouragement needed to ensure clubs were targeted at the non-sporty and that clubs should be driven by the needs of this group. The recommendations in 2011/12 advised that to be effective (both in primary and secondary settings) an element of competition must be delivered in tandem with, and not in place of, themes shown to be associated with increased physical activity and sport participation, namely building self-esteem, confidence and respect.

Year 3: Programme, evaluation and impact

By 2012 the sporting landscape had changed considerably from that of the previous Labour government, with the SSP network, aimed at increasing opportunities and participation for all, nearly demolished, the School Sport Survey scrapped and a revised PE curriculum in which competitive school sport was, at least in rhetoric, to have priority over the provision of inclusive participatory experiences for young people. The Coalition continued to emphasize competition as the key policy objective. With competition at its heart, the School Games was likely to attract and encourage the already 'sporty' rather than the 'non-sporty' and this 'bias' towards the already 'sporty' was emphasized by the selection processes of the four levels of competition therein (within school, between schools, at county/area level and national finals). Further the School Games policy failed to establish exit routes and pathways for continued participation (Keech, 2013) and many schools chose not to sign up to it in any case; in 2011 Hugh Robertson, Minister for Sport, stated that 11,000 schools had signed up, representing approximately 60 per cent of schools participating (Hansard, 2011).

Within this context, evaluation of the Change4Life School Sports Clubs in secondary schools in 2012/13 considered whether the impact shown in previous years was being sustained, and assessed the extent to which the programme was able to develop appropriate links to community clubs in order to enhance school club provision and create sport pathways for young people. The context of dismantled SSPs, diminished funding and confusion in schools about policy, what was required and how they could deliver it, added to the significance of school-club links in achieving increased participation of young people in sport and physical activity. Further, operating in the wider policy drive for increased competition, the clubs potentially offered a means of meeting broader objectives in schools, despite the policy focus on competition – increasing participation, particularly among the 'non-sporty', embracing inclusion, enhancing self-efficacy and contributing to physical literacy and the formation of lifelong participation habits. Informed by the 2011 research, YST provided guidance and advice to schools participating in the programme in the following year which resulted in improved targeting of the Change4Life School Sports Clubs programme at the less active (YST, 2012). In 2012/13, the proportion of less active young people joining the clubs doubled and the clubs reached an additional 125,000 of the least active young people. In 2011, recommendations of the research also included the development of leadership opportunities and participation pathways and the £575,000 subsequently invested in County Sport Partnership (CSP) activities led to a further 8,000 young leaders being trained and an additional 787 community clubs linking to schools (*spear,* 2011). This is not to say that there was by any means perfect implementation of all recommendations arising from the research. Funders, delivery agents, schools all have their own agendas, timeframes, budgetary constraints and priorities. Rather, the evidence garnered support for the programme where it met these objectives and the programme itself evolved to aid the achievement of desired outcomes.

The research in 2012/13 found that, while the clubs in secondary schools attracted nearly 20,000 new participants (of a total 37,000 participants), the number of new members recruited in Change4Life School Sports Clubs had fallen by 10,000 since 2011/12. However, the clubs continued to attract the non-sporty, this target group comprising one third of members (though this had fallen from 40% in the previous year), of whom 46 per cent were positive about sport and choosing to play sport at least once a week by the end of the year. The research also suggested that for some young people the Change4Life Clubs were seen as a supportive participation destination, rather than a stepping-stone to participation elsewhere. The number of Change4Life Clubs fell by 26 per cent from the previous year, though the number of school-club links remained at a similar level at just over 4,000 (the number of links per club having increased slightly). The research suggested that approximately half of the 1,434 new links established in 2012/13 had resulted from investment through the CSPs; however almost half of Change4Life Clubs reported that they had not developed any new links with community clubs in 2012/13 with the key barrier being lack of local infrastructure. The objectives and delivery in secondary schools were found to have evolved, as schools 'moved away' from the Change4Life ethos, aims and resources in attempts to access alternative sources of funding and equipment. The most cited reason for secondary schools choosing not to run a Change4Life Club was lack of staff time, while the closure of clubs was widely attributed to the lack of a community club to link to.

The research had shown that, while behavioural changes (such as increased activity levels) tended to occur within the first 6 to 12 weeks of participation, attitudinal and emotional changes (such as enjoyment and confidence) sometimes took longer to achieve. To enhance programme impact, in 2012/13 primary schools were therefore encouraged to run the programme for as much of the school year as possible and the children's logbooks were extended to include surveys to be completed at weeks 18 and 24. The 2012/13 primary evaluation found that 75 per cent of participants were new to the clubs, representing over 52,000 new club members, 80 per cent of whom were not achieving at least 60 active minutes every day on joining. Thus the primary clubs were effectively being targeted at the less active. The number of children achieving 60 active minutes every day increased by 71 per cent over 12 weeks of the programme, representing 7,000 additional children newly achieving the Chief Medical Officers' guidelines for physical activity. Increases in self-efficacy and confidence to make up new games were positively linked to the development of a sense of belonging and the opportunity to contribute to club delivery, and once again, took longer to occur than behavioural changes. While the research in 2012/13 included children's survey returns for weeks 18 and 24, YST did not include content or activities in the logbooks beyond 12 weeks, resulting in a small sample of survey returns beyond the 12 week period. As such, data relating to longer-term impact needed to be collected over a longer timeframe and this aspect of the research was extended into 2013/14. Nevertheless, teacher survey data showed that 51 per cent of existing clubs ran for 13 weeks or more compared with 13 per cent of clubs in 2011/12. Only 13 per cent of schools used external coaches to deliver their clubs and the involvement of primary pupils in delivery more than doubled from the previous year, enhancing the sustainability of the programme. In addition to targeting less active children, teachers reported that the clubs had also targeted those with low confidence and/ or self-esteem (46%) and children who did not join other clubs (41%). The research showed how children joining the clubs enjoyed being active but did not have the confidence to take up the traditional sport club opportunities available in schools, and that the Change4Life Clubs gave these children a 'safe space' to increase their physical activity which they would not otherwise have had. Among schools choosing not to run Change4Life School Sports Clubs, the most significant factors in their decision remained lack of staff time and lack of funding. Recommendations arising from the 2012/13 primary evaluation included maintaining the focus of the clubs on three key aspects of delivery shown to maximize outcomes: the provision of a safe space for less active children to play and be active; the opportunity to contribute to club delivery; and the encouragement of small steps toward increasing activity levels.

Year 4: Programme, evaluation and impact

In 2013/14 the Change4Life School Sports Club programme continued in primary schools, the secondary clubs having transitioned to the NGBs. The programme in 2013/14 included the development of 'support networks' (hubs of expertise to support and share effective practice among schools and local authority health and wellbeing boards) in 'priority areas'

(areas of greatest health inequalities). Data was collected for the final year programme evaluation in 2013/14 and in 2015 *spear* examined the lifetime impact of the Change4Life School Sports Club programme (2011–2015) in primary schools. In this third evaluation of the primary programme, *spear* adopted a systematic, controlled experimental methodology. In addition to the aspects included in previous evaluations, repeated measures analysis was undertaken on surveys completed at weeks 1 and 12 by a 'control group' of non-participating schools. For the lifetime impact analysis, survey returns were analysed from 7,573 children participating in 512 Change4Life Clubs and from 489 children in 15 control schools, as well as 2,047 survey completions from SGOs and club deliverers, and data from 20 site visits.

The research showed that Change4Life Primary School Sports Clubs have a significant, positive and sustained impact on the activity levels, health and wellbeing of participating children. The clubs were shown to effectively reach the target group of less active children, with 82 per cent of participants (approximately 222,000) not achieving at least 60 active minutes every day on joining the clubs. However, by week 12, 30 per cent of members were achieving 60 active minutes every day (an increase of 69%); this level of participation consistent with the control condition and with the 30 per cent of children reported nationally to be achieving 60 daily active minutes. Evidence showed that children join the clubs with positive attitudes to sport and games and that participation in 30 and 60 active minutes increases in tandem with positive changes in self-efficacy. The research found that children yet to achieve at least 60 active minutes could benefit from continued engagement in the clubs, however, children achieving at least 60 active minutes every day by week 12 were likely to regress unless they were transitioned into more challenging activity opportunities. The evaluation also highlighted that continuous monitoring at school level was vital to determine the appropriate turnover of club members.

Interviews with club leads suggested that the clubs were seen as 'safehouses' where children could play, developing creativity, aspirations, resilience and empathy to engage in wider school life. Deliverers reported that the clubs enhanced positive attitudes to being active and to sport, improved physical skills, increased confidence and knowledge of healthy lifestyles and developed a sense of belonging among members. The research also found that there were four key elements to a club that engage children and achieve programme outcomes: activities, ownership, fun and incentives. Incentives (such as wristbands and stickers included in the resources) supported the learning process and complemented the provision of fun activities in an environment that allowed children ownership of their developmental journey. In 2013/14 almost a quarter of schools were found to be providing opportunities for young people to help run the clubs, more than double the figures for 2011/12, and almost half of schools ran clubs for more than 12 weeks.

The ownership element of activities is particularly relevant within the context of the introduction of the PE and Sport Premium in 2013/14. The DfE found that in this period (the first year of the Premium), the percentage of schools using external sport coaches to deliver curricular PE had risen from 37 per cent to 82 per cent (DfE, Nov. 2014); a figure which is likely to be even higher for extra-curricular activities. Suggestive of wider pedagogical issues, specifically minimal physical education training and guidance for teachers, many schools are using the Premium to buy in expertise, which raises questions regarding ownership and sustainability of physical education and physical activities in schools (Griggs & Ward, 2013). While the DfE found that 79 per cent of responding teachers thought that the Premium had increased participation of all children, including those less engaged/least active (38%), it is unclear what this reported rise is attributed to. While it may be that sport coaches are able to offer something different, and possibly innovative ways to both increase physical activity and meet broader social and emotional outcomes, enhancing the pedagogy of existing schools staff through training is likely to offer a more sustainable means of achieving these outcomes.

Conclusions

The broad scope of the Change4Life School Sports Club programme has been found to be key to its appeal and *spear* has recommended that YST should clearly articulate to schools how Change4Life Clubs can support whole school agenda and help meet Ofsted expectations. Recommendations also include schools' transitioning children achieving 60 active minutes every day into more challenging activity opportunities to sustain their participation, and advice to schools to embed continuous monitoring into delivery of the clubs to ensure appropriate turnover of participants and maximize impact, as well as evidence the value of their investment in the programme.

It is reasonable to suggest that school sport policy over the timeframe of the Change4Life evaluation has largely been based on an assumption that competitive school sport was in decline, and that as a result, a re-focusing of physical education in schools was required. However, there was evidence to the contrary; the 2009/10 PE and School Sport Survey found that the proportion of pupils participating in intra-school competitive activities (Years 1–11) had risen from 69 per cent to 78 per cent between 2008/09 and 2009/10, that inter-school competition participation was also on the rise (49% Years 1–11 in 2009/10) and that regular participation had increased substantially in the same period (Years 3–13) from 28 per cent to 39 per cent (Quick et al., 2010). With the School Sport Survey discontinued, more recent comparable data is not available. Political focus on competition appears to have rejected evidence that a) competition was not in decline and b) increasing competition in 'traditional' sports does little to increase participation overall and may in fact have the adverse effect of disengaging a substantial proportion of pupils from school sports, physical education and physical activity (Keech, 2013). Such evidence seems to have been largely ignored or rejected in favour of the instinctual/ideological preference of Conservative ministers for 'competition':

> There seems to be no underlying rationale for the preference/prejudice in favour of competitive team sports and no explanation of how competitions relate to participation and the Olympic legacy for the vast majority of young people.
>
> *Keech, 2013: 186*

When in 2011 Michael Gove, Secretary of State for Education, 'freed' schools from collecting data by scrapping the School Sport Survey, he not only removed a key data source, but implied that such evidence was not even necessary. In 2015, DCMS produced the 'A Living Legacy: 2010–2015 sport policy and investment' report, highlighting the importance of sport in education. However, while recognizing the contribution of sport to wider psycho-social aspects, from the outset the report shows a certain naivety:

> Sport makes a real difference – in many different ways. For children just starting school, physical education provides them with the physical literacy they take with them through childhood and beyond into adulthood. We know too of the positive effects of sport on education more broadly, with regular participation resulting in improved attainment, lower absenteeism and drop-out, and increased progression

> to higher education . . . Physical activity including sport, is linked to reduced risk
> of over 20 illnesses . . . can reduce depression, anxiety and psychological distress.
>
> *DCMS, 2015: 6*

The recognition of the important role of physical education, physical activity and sport is cautiously welcomed (there are risks associated with a panacea approach), but the policy fails to recognize the need for continuous physical literacy development throughout the lifecourse; it does not demonstrate understanding of the complex ways in which physical education and physical activity impacts upon confidence, self-esteem, motivation, knowledge and understanding; all aspects which effect levels and sustainability of participation. Nor does it adequately examine the complex relationships between social, economic and cultural capital/ deprivation and inequalities in levels of physical activity, health and wellbeing and educational achievement. The document highlights the way in which policy and investment has been guided by assumptions, rather than evidence, and the government's focus on competitive sport is implicit but pervasive.

There is government recognition of the significance of physical activity in its broader terms at policy level and, in particular, of the economic costs of inactivity. In 2014–2016, the All-Party Commission on Physical Activity, DCMS, Sport England, DH and Public Health England have all highlighted the need to increase levels of physical activity in the UK: Sporting Future; Towards an Active Nation; Moving More, Living More; Everybody Active, Every Day; Tackling Physical Activity; Five Year Forward View. And some funding has been directed this way: the government committed £150 million per year towards Physical Education and Sport via the PE and Sport Premium, Sport England continues to provide funding through Get Healthy, Get Active and investment in CSPs has supported school-club links and the training of young leaders (albeit at the expense of the £162 million ring-fenced funding for SSPs abolished in 2010). However, evidence of the impact of such investment will not be forthcoming unless sufficient attention is paid to the need for robust research. While data from the Public Health Outcomes Framework, Active Lives Survey and Health Survey for England is widely used to measure physical (in)activity among adults, the continued measurement of children's Body Mass Index via the National Child Weight Measurement Programme seems woefully insufficient as a means of measuring impact and its potential to inform policy is surely minimal.

The participation of children and young people in sport and physical activity is increasingly linked to education and seen as the schools' responsibility, yet schools' ability to shape and influence policy in this area has decreased in recent years (Smith, 2012). Moreover, austerity has meant that the cost of enhancing sport and physical activity opportunities for young people in schools has become daunting to head teachers, and while investment in the PE and Sport Premium has been welcomed by schools (DfE, Nov. 2014), the lack of investment in infrastructure since the dismantling of the SSPs has left many unsure of how to use it wisely. Further, the marginalization in the policy making process of organizations with specialist knowledge, such as YST, and of (Junior) Sports Ministers (McMaster, 2011) in favour of broader more powerful policy sectors, such as education (Ball, 2012; Houlihan & Lindsey, 2012), risks a loss of expertise, experience and evidence in this process. With a widening remit for physical education and physical activity in schools, it has become increasingly difficult to define who is actually responsible for policy in this area – sport, health, social inclusion, community safety, education? Not only is robust evidence vital in such a complex and unstable policy environment, but it needs to consider much more than participation statistics; it needs to examine the multifarious and byzantine aspects of young people's experiences. The Change4Life research showed the positive effects of 'ownership' on young participants and it may further be helpful, as the Future Foundation suggests, to involve young people themselves in the policy-making process (Future Foundation, 2015). There is certainly growing evidence that the involvement of young people in decisions about what and how they participate in physical activity can offer effective means of engaging the disengaged and least active and that concomitantly the 'one size fits all' approach of competitive sports is not effective at encouraging lifelong participation among all (*spear*, 2014/15; Griggs & Ward, 2013; Sandford et al., 2008; Holroyd & Armour, 2003).

The Change4Life School Sports Club evaluations have shown that across primary and secondary clubs, participation increases are linked to children and young people being respected and respecting others regardless of ability, increases in self-esteem and confidence, provision of a safe and inclusive space for less active children to play and be active, the opportunity to contribute to club delivery, and the encouragement of small steps toward increasing physical activity levels. Overall, the research concluded that a club-style model delivered in schools with a focus on processes shown to engage the least active in participation and leadership is an effective mechanism for physical activity behaviour change in less active young people.

The research has been key to evidencing the Change4Life Clubs impact, thereby securing programme funding. In 2013, Jane Ellison, the Minister for Public Health, noted that the research 'demonstrates the value of these clubs', highlighting the data on increased physical activity levels to justify continued investment. Similarly, Ann Sourby, the previous Minister for Public Health, had noted that the research demonstrated Change4Life Clubs were 'an effective way of making sport and physical activity a lifelong habit' (2012) and therefore formed part of the rationale for £8.4m government investment in the programme. In addition, DH included the research findings in their submission to the House of Commons Select Committee on School Sport (2013) in relation to investment in school sport targeting children who are disengaged with sport. Evidence of the efficacy of the club model delivered in schools shown by the research also informed Sport England's 'Creating a Sporting Habit for Life' strategy (2012–2017). In these times of fiscal austerity, such evidence and justification are particularly necessary, even if the evidence supports current policy direction and especially where it does not. The Change4Life research has helped to secure funding, despite the programme's focus on engagement of the 'non-sporty' running somewhat counter-intuitively to perceived policy wisdom of the time. Indeed, increasing activity levels among the less active now forms one of DCMS's key performance indicators in Sporting Future, though in relation to physical education and school sport policy the mantra remains competition.

Despite budgetary constraints in recent years, physical (in)activity has become a top tier public health priority. Local authorities have doubled the amount allocated to physical activity from their public health grant in the last year, albeit from just 2 per cent to 4 per cent (the smallest proportion of public health grants), integrating physical activity within public health services such as health checks, smoking cessation and weight management (ukactive, 2014). Government focus and investment in physical activity and the commissioning of physical activity interventions will demand evidence of impact. In 2014, ukactive produced the report 'Steps to Solving Inactivity' which highlighted the 'lack of robust, clinically relevant and academically sound evidence to show the value and importance' (2014: 4) of what is being done. It provides examples across the UK of physical activity interventions alongside the evidence these have collated and the Nesta Standards of Evidence rating achieved, and recommends that government improves data collation with such a single framework. The report further recommends increased government investment in physical activity research; and that the activity sector design programmes with a focus on engaging the inactive, routinely collect data to demonstrate impact and use this data to refine these programmes. Although not listed in the report, *spear*'s evaluations of the Change4Life School Sports Club programme achieved Level 4/5 Nesta rating (with Level 5 being the highest evidence rating possible). While we recognize the methodological limitations of social science research in this area (isolating control variables, validity of self-report data, reliability of perceptual responses), this chapter has shown the ways in which the research has informed programme development to maximize impact on the physical activity of young people, and contributed to the evidence base for policy makers and funders.

Initially designed to increase physical activity participation and provide a route into competitive School Games, the Change4Life School Sports Club programme evolved to reflect wider health and education policy objectives, including educational attainment, attendance, social and emotional aspects, healthy lifestyles, obesity and 'closing the gap' (reducing inequalities in these areas). In the face of declining resources and wider policy objectives, the need for evidence of programme impact has increased, while schools express uncertainty in relation to delivering and measuring these aspects. Aided by the research findings, YST was able to position the programme, the role of school sport and the SGOs within the public health context and secure continued funding, despite the non-competitive focus of the clubs in the context of the political focus on competitive sports in schools. Similarly, with the introduction of the Primary Sport Premium, YST was able to demonstrate with evidence from *spear*'s evaluations that Change4Life School Sports Clubs could help schools to deliver the health and sport outcomes required.

The independent, controlled, empirical evaluations of the Change4Life School Sports Clubs have informed programme development and enabled YST to demonstrate return on investment, not only to policy-makers and funders, but to teachers. It has enabled YST to offer a viable business case to schools by demonstrating the impact on their pupils. It has placed the Change4Life programme in a strong position moving forward, gaining support at Ministerial level at a time of significant cuts in public sector funding, reflected across sport and education. Following *spear*'s recommendations in 2015, the research has provided YST with the means to evidence the benefits of a broader whole-school approach to physical education and activity moving forward.

In the wider context of policy development, the Change4Life evaluations offer key insights into improving the motivation and means of participation for pupils in physical activity. Ofsted has highlighted that where secondary schools offer a wider range of games, performing arts and alternative sports this has increased participation in after school clubs by pupils of all ages, interests and abilities and had a significant impact on improving pupils' confidence, self-esteem and attitudes towards learning in other subjects (Ofsted, 2011: 7). It has further commented that in the 'best' schools, 'good' provision is tailored to attract previously uninterested or disenchanted pupils by increasing the number of leisure-based and contemporary sporting activities which encourages more pupils to engage in PE, reduces disaffection and improves engagement particularly among vulnerable groups (Ofsted, 2009: 38). The Change4Life evaluations have highlighted the significance of pupil involvement in delivery to maximize impact and the aspects of the programme which have most engaged pupils. If the proportion of 'gifted and talented' 9 to 16 year olds is around 8 per cent of pupils in schools (Quick et al., 2010: 4), physical education policy needs to encourage participation and engagement among the other 82 per cent also and be mindful of the risk of deterring the vast majority of pupils who are not going to become elite athletes. There are many mixed messages in the Government's vision for physical education and physical activity in schools;

among them the need for inclusion and increasing levels of physical activity for all young people alongside the focus on competitive sport. Increasing the evidence base for policy makers within this complex and confusing arena will be key to achieving desired outcomes and will enable the interrogation of policy to ensure its direction is itself desirable.

References

All-Party Commission on Physical Activity (2014). *Tackling Physical Inactivity – A Coordinated Approach* www.sportsandplay.com/upload/public/APCOPA%20Final.pdf.

Ball, S. J. (2012). *Politics and Policy Making in Education: Explorations in Sociology*. Abingdon, Oxon Routledge.

Cabinet Office (2014). *Moving More, Living More: The Physical Activity Olympic and Paralympic Legacy for the Nation* www.gov.uk/government/uploads/system/uploads/attachment_data/file/279657/moving_living_more_inspired_2012.pdf.

Department for Education press release (Oct 2010). In Keech, M (2013) *Sport Policy, Physical Education and Participation*, 181 in Stidder, G. & Hayes, S. eds. (2013). *Equity and Inclusion in Physical Education and Sport*. London: Routledge.

Department for Education press release (Nov 2014). www.gov.uk/government/news/150-million-to-boost-primary-school-sport.

Department for Education research brief (Sept 2014). *PE and Sport Premium: An Investigation in Primary Schools* www.gov.uk/government/uploads/system/uploads/attachment_data/file/369080/DFE-RB385_-_PE_Sport_Premium_Research_Brief.pdf.

DCMS (Dec 2015). *Sporting Future: A New Strategy for an Active Nation* www.gov.uk/government/uploads/system/uploads/attachment_data/file/486622/Sporting_Future_ACCESSIBLE.pdf.

DCMS (2008). *Before, During and After: Making the Most of the London 2012 Games* http://webarchive.nationalarchives.gov.uk/+/http:/www.culture.gov.uk/images/publications/2012LegacyAction Plan.pdf.

Department of Health (DH) (2011). *Start Active, Stay Active; A Report on Physical Activity from the Four Home Countries' Chief Medical Officers, Department of Health, Physical Activity, Health Improvement and Protection* www.gov.uk/government/uploads/system/uploads/attachment_data/file/216370/dh_128210.pdf.

Ellison J., MP (Nov 2013). Speech at ukactive Summit www.ukactive.com/downloads/managed/Jane_Ellison_MP_Parliamentary_Under-Secretary_of_State_for_Public_Health_ukactive_Summit.pdf.

Future Foundation (2015). *The Class of 2035; Promoting a Brighter and More Active Future for the Young of Tomorrow* www.youthsporttrust.org/media/24072132/the_class_of_2035_report.pdf.

Grey-Thompson, T. (2014) In *Generation inactive: An analysis of the UK's childhood inactivity epidemic and tangible solutions to get children moving*. London, UK: Active.

Griggs, G. & Ward, G. (2013). The London 2012 Legacy for Primary Physical Education: Policy by the Way? *Sociological Research Online*, 18(3), 13 www.socresonline.org.uk/18/3/13.html.

Hansard (2011). Column 907, in Stidder, G. & Hayes, S. eds (2013). *Equity and Inclusion in Physical Education and Sport*. London: Routledge.

Holroyd, R. A. & Armour, K. M. (2003). *Re-engaging disaffected youth through physical activity*. Paper presented at British Educational Research Programmes Association Annual Conference www.leeds.ac.uk/educol/documents/00003304.htm.

Houlihan, B. & Lindsey, I. (2012). *Sport Policy in Britain*. New York: Routledge.

House of Commons Select Committee (Jul 2013). *School Sport Following London 2012* www.publications.parliament.uk/pa/cm201314/cmselect/cmeduc/164/164vw.pdf.

Keech, M. (2012) Sport policy, physical education and participation: inclusive issues for schools? In Stidder, G. and Hayes, G., eds. *Equity and inclusion in physical education and sport*. Abingdon, Oxon: Routledge, pp. 176–189.

McMaster, A. (2011). Junior Ministers in the UK: The Role of the Minister for Sport, *Parliamentary Affairs*, 65(1), 214–237.

Ofsted (2009). *Physical Education in Schools 2005/08: Working Towards 2012 and Beyond*, 38 http://dera.ioe.ac.uk/318/1/Physical%20education%20in%20schools%202005_08.pdf.

Ofsted (Jun 2011). *School Sport Partnerships: A Survey of Good Practice*, 7 www.gov.uk/government/uploads/system/uploads/attachment_data/file/413538/School_Sport_Partnerships.pdf.

Ofsted (Feb 2013). *Beyond 2012 – Outstanding Physical Education for All* www.gov.uk/government/uploads/system/uploads/attachment_data/file/413190/Beyond_2012_-_outstanding_physical_education_for_all_-_report_summary.pdf.

Penney, D. (2008). Playing a Political Game and Playing for Position: Policy and Curriculum Development in Health and Physical Education. *European Physical Education Review*, 14(1), 33–50.

Public Health England (2014a). *Everybody Active, Every Day: An Evidence-Based Approach to Physical Activity* www.gov.uk/government/uploads/system/uploads/attachment_data/file/374914/Framework_13.pdf.

Public Health England (2014b). *National Child Measurement Programme Operational Guidance* www.gov.uk/government/publications/national-child-measurement-programme-operational-guidance.

Quick, S., Simon, A. & Thornton, A. (2010). *PE and Sport Survey 2009/10, Department for Education Research Report* www.gov.uk/government/uploads/system/uploads/attachment_data/file/181556/DFE-RR032.pdf.

Sandford, R. A., Duncombe, R. & Armour, K. M. (2008). The Role of Physical Activity in Tackling Youth Disaffection and Anti-Social Behaviour. *Education Review*, 60(4) https://dspace.lboro.ac.uk/dspace-jspui/bitstream/2134/15184/3/EdReviewpaper_revisedFINAL.pdf.

Smith, A. (Sept 2012). *Youth Sport and Evidence-Based Policy in England: The Case for School Sport Partnerships and School Games*. Presentation to European Sports Development Network Symposium, Shefffield Hallam University www.shu.ac.uk/ad/sport-symposium/AndySmith.pdf.

Sourby, A., MP (Nov 2012). Speech at ukactive Summit.

spear (2009–2013). *The Olympic Physical Activity, Sport and Health (OPASH) Legacy Project; Active Celebration: Using the London 2012 Games to get the Nation Moving; National School Sports Week* www.canterbury.ac.uk/social-and-applied-sciences/human-and-life-sciences/spear/research-projects/research-projects.aspx.

spear (2011, 2012, 2013, 2014/15). *Change4Life School Sports Clubs Evaluation Reports to Youth Sport Trust* www.canterbury.ac.uk/social-and-applied-sciences/human-and-life-sciences/spear/research-projects/change-4-life-school-sports-club.aspx.

spear (2014/15). *Skills2Play/Sport Evaluation; Physical Literacy Programme for Schools Evaluation* www.canterbury.ac.uk/social-and-applied-sciences/human-and-life-sciences/spear/research-projects/research-projects.aspx.

Sport England (2016). *Towards an Active Nation* https://www.sportengland.org/media/10629/sport-england-towards-an-active-nation.pdf.

ukactive (2014). *Steps to Solving Inactivity* www.ukactive.com/downloads/managed/Final_Final_Final_Steps_to_Report.pdf.

UNESCO (2015). *Quality Physical Education; Guidelines for Policy-Makers* http://unesdoc.unesco.org/images/0023/002311/231101E.pdf.

Woods, Judith. (17 Jan 2015). Not on the team? Then no more sport for you. *The Telegraph* www.telegraph.co.uk/education/educationopinion/11350940/Not-on-the-team-Then-no-more-sport-for-you.html.

Youth Sport Trust (2011, 2012, 2013). *Celebrating Success: Change4Life Clubs Evaluation Summaries*. London.

30

LINKING PHYSICAL ACTIVITY AND HEALTH EVALUATION TO POLICY

Lessons from UK evaluations

Andy Pringle, Jim McKenna and Stephen Zwolinsky

Introduction

Evaluation is an important component of contemporary physical activity (PA) interventions, although it is a relative newcomer on the policy scene. In this chapter we comment on a number of issues and debates on the role of evaluation in PA policy and interventions, based on our experiences of assessing the impacts and outcomes of PA-led interventions that originated in local and or national policy. Mostly these accounts are available in the peer-review literature, making them readily available for independent scrutiny. At the risk of being accused of collective self-promotion, we agreed on this approach from the outset because we want to contribute an account that only we could. As cases, they provide applied, insightful, contextual and – hopefully – informative, practical examples of partnership evaluations in both PA intervention and policy. To identify them, we applied two key criteria, set elsewhere (Pringle, Hargreaves, Lozano et al., 2014): (I) *Credibility*: Cases represent real world illustrations of the place of evaluation in a policy context. (II) *Impact*: Cases report their effects. Notwithstanding the differences that the technological era brings to daily life, many of these themes appear timeless, i.e., they recur. For that reason, we hope that sharing them will inform current and future practice. Therefore in this chapter we discuss:

1 Key examples of evaluation linking to PA policy
2 Key lessons for PA evaluation

Key examples of evaluation linking to PA policy

We start by looking at key examples of evaluating PA interventions and their link to policy. Position of the evaluator is an important consideration (Gattenhoff, 2017) and it is important to consider the different evaluation designs. For example, external contracting involves independent evaluation specialists who perform all aspects of evaluation work. In contrast, within in-house evaluation designs, this responsibility lies with deliverers. Finally, partnership evaluation designs combine specialist evaluators working alongside programme staff (Pringle,

Hargreaves, Lozano et al., 2014). These designs are popular for a number of reasons. First, a scarcity of resources means PA providers have to make existing funds stretch further. Second, many deliverers have pre-existing alliances with local evaluation partners, such as consultants and local Universities. Third, in the case of the latter, some of these partners have a strategic agenda to support local professional communities of practice and the communities where they operate. Central to decisions to intervene on PA and Public Health (PH) issues are a series of questions. (i) What is the problem? (ii) Why is action needed? (iii) Who is responsible? (vi) Who is generating pressure to act? (v) When does this need to happen? (vi) How can the problem/issue be best addressed?

Responding to these questions and using frameworks from the literature, we provide a suite of partnership evaluation case studies as examples. They illustrate interventions with foundations set in policy for PA and/or health improvement. In doing so, we discuss how monitoring and evaluation interact with policy across two different scenarios.

I   Evaluation used to inform policy and policy decisions
II Evaluation leading to policy formation and the case for intervention

Evaluation used to inform policy and policy decisions

Evaluation can be used to inform policy which supports investment in PH resources. In our first case study, and being mindful of our point that many themes here are recurrent, we refer back to 2004–05 and Choosing Activity (CA), a PA Action Plan (Department of Health, 2005). CA was a subsidiary of the Choosing Health (CH) the former PH white paper. CA set out government plans to encourage and co-ordinate the action of a range of departments and organisations to promote increased participation in PA across England (Department of Health, 2005). The CH white paper reported intentions to establish evidence on which interventions were effective in increasing PA. This was achieved through commissioning the Local Exercise Action Pilots (LEAP) (Department of Health, 2007; Pringle, Marsh, Gilson et al., 2010).

LEAP was a national programme and evaluation of PA interventions; it is useful for our account, not least because it spans different forms of PA, different methods of delivery and local political agendas. Findings from the LEAP programme were intended to inform how £50.7 million (set aside for PA and nutrition promotion through CH) could be used most effectively and efficiently. In its own right LEAP was a £2.6 million Government funded intervention and was a seminal programme as one of England's first multi-site evaluations of community interventions aimed at increasing PA levels. Centred in local communities, LEAP subsumed a suite of PA interventions delivered in 10 primary-care trusts (PCTs), with at least one pilot site in each of nine NHS regions of England (Sport England, 2006; Pringle, 2011). Pilots aimed to develop primary-care led approaches for PA promotion to secure outcomes for health care priority areas and groups previously detailed in key health policy documents, including the then National Service Frameworks (NSF) (Department of Health, 1999; 2001a, 2001b). With no obvious awareness of the scientific standards that this would require – in terms of deploying randomised controlled trial designs – the Department of Health (2007 p.1) reported that LEAP aimed to establish:

> the most effective types of interventions for getting the general population, including people from priority groups to initiate and maintain regular moderate intensity PA, and to reduce the numbers of sedentary adults and children.

To pursue this aim, an independent evaluation was commissioned which set out to:

> Evaluate both qualitatively and quantitatively the overall effectiveness of the LEAP programme and individual pilots at increasing PA levels of both the general population and target groups.
>
> *Department of Health, 2002 p.2*

There are conflicting reports on the effectiveness of LEAP. Pringle, Marsh, Gilson et al. (2010) reported that LEAP interventions had a positive impact on PA levels within an initial intervention period. Conversely, Bagot (2013) suggested that the LEAP pilots had little impact on PA, but provided a useful test-bed for PA interventions. In implementing both LEAP interventions and the evaluation, a number of substantial challenges were encountered and reported in the evaluation reports (Department of Health, 2007; Sport England, 2006). These provide important guidance on conducting the evaluation of PA interventions; many remain relevant today.

To ensure that the widest audience is exposed to research outcomes, dissemination is typically achieved through multiple methods and channels (Eldredge et al., 2016). Thus, it is important to link evaluation to policy so that policy supports and informs subsequent provision. Even though LEAP included a final evaluation report published on the commissioners websites (Department of Health, 2007), publication of a summary of findings (Sport England, 2006), a major launch event supported by Government Cabinet Ministers and their Departments, as well as dissemination at five Regional PA Networks, it is not clear how it was used to inform specific decisions in the white paper. This is important because £50m had been set aside in CA for PA and nutrition – arguably 'a *raison dêtre*' for implementing the LEAP pilots (Department of Health, 2002). While we are not aware of any co-ordinated evaluation which subsequently assessed how findings from LEAP informed policy formation for PA across all PCTs, there are many examples of influences on local policy for PA promotion and subsequent investment decisions. For example, in Nottingham, East Midlands, one of original LEAP pilots, where PH officials invested in activities and intervention designs based on the outcomes of the evaluation. Resources and responsibility were devolved to community-facing agencies who could reach local populations, including the Nottingham YMCA community motivators programme (Carnegie Research Institute, 2010). While in Kirklees, West Yorkshire, once effectiveness of LEAP had been confirmed, staff in the pilot charted an early course to subsume PA interventions in four priority areas in local PA provision (Department of Health, 2007). Sustainable programmes reflected a strategic fit based on locally identified health priorities and needs. Moreover, on-going interventions were underpinned by local partnerships and resourced by mainstream budgets recommended in national (Sport England, 2006) and the PH literature (Eldredge et al., 2016).

Findings from this case study suggest that monitoring and evaluation did inform the direction of local PH and PA promotion. At the same time, and perhaps because of the diffuse nature of the LEAP pilots, its three-year time-scale and the inevitable changeability of PH policy, it remains unclear which, if any, evidence from it was most influential for directing future policy decisions and investments. This means that, using LEAP, commissioners of subsequent programmes will remain unsure of how to use local level evaluation to inform national level policy.

Evaluation leads to policy formation and the case for intervention

In this scenario, evaluation of the intervention leads to the generation of policy which (i) supports decisions to invest within interventions and (ii) the production of policy guidance on how interventions should be implemented, so they are effective. For illustration, we refer to the role of professional sports clubs as settings for local-based health improvement (Baker, Loughran, Crone et al., 2016; Lewis, Reeves and Roberts, 2016) and specifically our experience of evaluating a bespoke men's health improvement service within professional football clubs (Zwolinsky, McKenna and Pringle, 2016). Research across the 27 European member states identifies men's health as a PH concern; this supports calls for a co-coordinated political and strategic approach for improving men's health (European Commission, 2011). Yet, 'despite overall improvements in life expectancy, rates of premature male mortality, particularly for men in areas of socioeconomic deprivation, remain an important issue of concern in the United Kingdom' (Robertson and Baker, 2016 p.102). There is a particular need to identify how best to engage those men who are unhealthy by conventional standards, but who don't see themselves as unhealthy; this scenario leaves them unresponsive to conventional approaches aiming to connect with these men over their health and lifestyle behaviours (White, de Sousa, de Visser, et al., 2011; Robertson, Woodall, Henry et al., 2016). In response, sports clubs, recreation groups, workplaces and religious settings all represent non-traditional channels with the potential to reach the many men at the wrong end of the social gradient of disease (Curran, Drust, Murphy et al., 2016; Zwolinsky, McKenna, Pringle et al., 2016a). While these men did not routinely use Primary Care services (Pringle, Zwolinsky, McKenna et al., 2013a; 2013b; Zwolinsky, McKenna, Pringle et al., 2016), these non-traditional channels reflected their powerful pre-existing interests and hobbies reported elsewhere (Lozano, Pringle, Carless et al., 2016; Curran, Drust, Murphy et al., 2016). Capitalising on these pre-existing behavioural pathways is regarded as a key strength of sport-led health improvement provision (McKenna, Quarmby, Kime, et al., 2016; Martin, Morgan, Parnell et al., 2016).

With football and PH leaders making the case for the power of professional football in connecting previously unresponsive groups to health interventions (Martin, Morgan, Parnell et al., 2016) we discuss *Premier League Health* (PLH). PLH was a three-year programme of men's health promotion delivered through 16 English Premier League football clubs (Zwolinsky, McKenna, Pringle et al., 2016a). Interventions were delivered by professional football clubs' Community Trusts alongside their local health partners. Partners included Primary Care Trusts, local authorities and local charitable organisations. Interventions were led by Health Trainers, allied health professionals with specific training and education in behaviourally based health improvement (Pringle, Zwolinsky, McKenna et al., 2014).

In line with specific policy guidance (NICE, 2007) and the extant literature (Eldredge et al., 2016), PLH interventions addressed the needs of local men even though this varied club-by-club. Activities were typically PA-centred and for many – but not all – clubs, football was at the heart of the programmes (Pringle, Zwolinsky, McKenna et al., 2014; Zwolinsky, McKenna and Pringle, 2016a). PLH interventions reflected the CDC (1999) classification of informational, behavioural and social change approaches based on three modes of delivery, (i) match day activities (ii) regular weekly classes and (iii) outreach work (Sinclair and Alexander, 2012; Curran, Drust, Murphy et al., 2016).

Also in line with PH guidance (NICE, 2007) an independent evaluation was commissioned – at the same time as the clubs were selected. Here the aim was to assess the impact and processes that generated programme outcomes (Eldredge et al., 2016). The resulting multi-method evaluation (Pringle, Zwolinsky and McKenna et al., 2014; Zwolinsky, McKenna, Pringle et al., 2016a) identified that the programmes were effective in reaching and encouraging men to adopt health improvement interventions (Zwolinsky, McKenna, Pringle et al., 2016a). Moreover, the process evaluation helped to identify which components worked more effectively than others (Arends, Bode, Taal and Van de Laar, 2017; Pringle and Zwolinsky, 2016). The evaluation – based on a pre-post design – identified an array of improvements in CVD risk factors and other health outcomes within an initial intervention period (Pringle, Zwolinsky, McKenna et al., 2014; Zwolinsky, McKenna, Pringle et al., 2016a). As men's awareness of health issues can incubate over time (Lozano et al., 2016) the PLH programme focussed on issues and solutions, as defined by men themselves, an important ingredient of effective health improvement with this group (Robertson, Woodall, Henry et al., 2016). Importantly, this signalled the potency of maintaining a specific delivery approach rather than of specific programme content. Partly because PLH actively recruited hard-to-reach groups, the evaluation outcomes informed (i) the case for future investment, (ii) the development of policy on men's health improvement in football settings and (iii) PH guidance on how interventions could be implemented to be effective (White, Zwolinsky, Pringle et al., 2012; Zwolinsky, McKenna and Pringle, 2016).

An evaluation report (White, Zwolinsky, Pringle et al., 2012) supported the case for further rounds of funding for similar football-led health interventions, including interventions with men (Curran, Brook, Lozano et al., 2015; Lozano et al., 2016). Subsequently, funding was made through charities (Curran, Brook, Lozano et al., 2015), statutory services and the charitable arms of football including the Premier League's 'Creating Chances' programme within the specific 'Health' theme (Pringle, Zwolinsky, and McKenna et al. 2013a; 2013b). Creating Chances uses positive associations with the football 'brand' to support the health improvement of individuals and communities (Premier League, 2011; Pringle, Zwolinsky and McKenna, 2013; Zwolinsky, McKenna, Pringle et al., 2016a) in line with policy objectives for health improvement (Department of Health, 2011).

In line with the literature on evaluation (Eldredge et al., 2016; Estabrooks et al., 2016), findings from the PLH evaluation also provided programme guidance of how best to implement interventions delivered by professional football club Community Trusts. With those considerations in mind, three criteria for supporting investments were especially important (i) demonstrating an impact on health profiles and behaviours (ii) working strategically with local health partners to part fund interventions and (iii) demonstrating an exit strategy to sustain activities once start-up funding had expired.

As a result of these strong outcomes, evidenced by the PLH evaluation, community foundations and charities increasingly operate within professional football clubs to deliver on the PH agenda (Martin et al., 2016). This, in part, reflects steps in the right direction of a shift in the policy and intervention context, toward providing acceptable, affordable and accessible (Fineberg, 2012) health improvement opportunities for men at the local level (Robertson and Baker, 2016). That said, reflecting the on-going challenge of making the case for PA and PH resources more generally, our recent review of health improvement provision across the second tier of professional football – the 72 clubs outside the Premier League – has identified difficulties in persuading local policy makers through the Community Commissioning Groups (CCGs) to invest in longer term provision of men's health interventions. Being unable to anchor these programmes in local health plans has meant that funding has been reduced or even cut completely (Pringle and Zwolinsky, 2016).

On a different track, and reflecting post-recessionary policy and thinking, we next report the more contemporary case of *Leeds Let's Get Active* (LLGA). Building on the evidence which supports the role of 'sport' to engage those who are least active, Sport England initiated the Get Healthy Get Active Fund in 2014. This approach was grounded in one of the core notions of PH policy; do more to help the least healthy. With the distinctive power of addressing inactivity – the best returns for PA programmes are often found when improvements are achieved in these least active groups (Blair, Kampert, Kohl et al., 1996) – engaging inactive individuals became an on-going PA and PH priority (Department of Health, 2011).

In LLGA the aim was to improve the evidence base for the role that 'sport' can play in engaging inactive people, i.e., those undertaking <30 minutes of PA per week, and to generate evidence that is sufficiently compelling to support further PH commissioning (Gardner, 2014). LLGA emerged as part of a national programme (macro) to encourage people who do not do any PA to do at least 30 minutes of PA, once a week (Leeds City Council, 2015). To achieve this aim, recruits were provided with free citywide (meso) access to unused leisure centre and community sport provision within a supportive and welcoming environment. LLGA provided around 150 separate hour-long gym and swimming sessions free to registered participants at 17 different venues across the city at a variety of times each week. In addition, a parallel 'community' offer provided a range of group- and family-based activities in local community venues and parks.

In the 20 months since launching, LLGA recruited and captured baseline data from over 64k participants (Zwolinsky and McKenna, 2015). Almost half (48%) of these recruits were classified as inactive and 87 per cent were not meeting the current PA guidelines, suggesting the potential for effective targeting of this group. These powerful recruitment figures were supplemented by intentionally promoting engaging and enjoyable individual/group experiences, and encouraging participants to share these experiences with other potential recruits. These seem to be fundamental approaches for realising successful interventions, especially among previously inactive individuals (Pringle, Zwolinsky, McKenna et al., 2013a; 2013b). Importantly, intervention data revealed substantial increases in PA levels (Zwolinsky and McKenna, 2015), suggesting the importance of powerful induction experiences for sustaining involvement. Using automatic registers of attendance, over a quarter of a million visits to leisure centre gym and swim sessions were undertaken by LLGA participants; over 135k were made by participants classified as inactive at baseline. Crucially, over 80 per cent of participants who provided follow-up data that were classified as inactive at baseline were no longer inactive at follow-up.

Based on these findings, LLGA was able to secure further PH funding, to examine the potential of the programme for impacting wider lifestyle behaviours. In Leeds alone, a considerable proportion of the adult population failed to achieve the current PA recommendations. Combined with a poor diet, smoking and excessive alcohol consumption, these lifestyle risk factors (LRFs) are the most proximal risk factors for non-communicable diseases (Mozaffarian, Wilson and Kannel, 2008). These behaviours account for a 14 year gap in life expectancy between those presenting all four LRFs compared to those with none (Khaw et al., 2008). Although many Leeds residents were likely to harbour multiple concurrent LRFs, little was known about how these behaviours co-occur and many residents – typically those who are most at risk – were reached by this new approach whereas existing approaches had left them (mostly) unreached. Indeed, widespread, community-focused promotion of LRFs is consistent with calls to shift societal attention toward successful and sustainable 'health systems' and away from ineffective and unaffordable 'health care systems' (Fineberg, 2012); removal of the word 'care' is used to denote how health is a universal concern, whereas health care lies in the orbit of medical professionals.

Data from N=13,579 participants revealed that 90 per cent did not do enough PA for health each week, 82.3 per cent did not consume enough fruit and vegetables each day, 19.3 per cent currently smoked and 45.7 per cent reported hazardous and/or harmful alcohol consumption. Moreover, 87 per cent of all participants reported two or more of these LRFs in combination. Insufficient PA combined with a lack of fruit and vegetables was the most prevalent cluster. Nevertheless, at follow-up, there were significant improvements in PA levels from baseline to follow-up; participants were doing the equivalent of an additional 30 minutes each week. Follow-up data showed a 60 per cent relative reduction in the number of inactive participants and a 50 per cent relative increase in the proportion of participants achieving the PA guidelines. Moreover, a quarter of participants improved their LRF profile and there was a reduction in the proportion of participants reporting LRFs in combination. There were also beneficial changes in smoking levels and alcohol risk status, even though neither was a target within LLGA (Zwolinsky and McKenna 2016).

LLGA highlights the need for continued PA and lifestyle improvement opportunities across Leeds. Based on UK health recommendations, these data showed the alarming prevalence of LRFs and how these risks cluster in specific combinations. Nonetheless, LLGA was able to reach a large proportion of health-needy individuals whose social status had left them unreached by other services and interventions. None of these services had the aspiration to intersect multiple behaviours. Yet, LLGA helped to improve and stabilise several of the most important lifestyle behaviours impacting mortality and morbidity. These findings highlight the potential benefits of LLGA-type approaches, supported by an imaginative approach to delivery and to evaluation, to provide a rationale for its integration into long-term sustainable programmes. These programmes can clearly help to prevent and manage the foundational risk factors for non-communicable disease incidence (Zwolinsky, McKenna, Pringle et al., 2016b).

To achieve this, LLGA foundations were set in localism, aiming to meet the needs of local communities across the city. Local policy aspires for Leeds to be an active city and LLGA offers value for money by using spare capacity in local authority sports and leisure provision. In post-recessionary times, these are powerful policy-related issues. Interventions with similar aspirations for targeted effectiveness are most likely to do so when they can be built into the philosophies and cultural practices of the targeted communities. Crucially, they must form part of on-going community activities that incrementally and discreetly mould norms and values.

Key lessons for PA evaluation

While evaluation frameworks are helpful, they are guidelines. Real life is different. Our experience of performing evaluations of interventions at the local and national level leads us to two firm conclusions. First, for a host of reasons, evaluation is not always possible, which proposes the idea of *evaluability*. Evaluability refers to the capacity and amenability of an intervention for monitoring and evaluation (Wholey, Hatry and Newcomer 2004). Second, evaluations can only rarely be delivered in the ways anticipated by stakeholders. While guidance routinely recommends 'good practice' (Dugdill and Stratton, 2007; MRC, 2008; Dugdill, Stratton and Watson, 2009; NOO, 2012; Eldredge et al., 2016), a number of factors can conspire to impact on evaluability.

To understand these points, it is helpful to refer to evaluation definitions. For example, the CDC (2011) refer to evaluation as the *systematic investigation of the merit, worth or significance of an object* (Scriven, in CDC, 1999 p.3). In our experience many organisations undertaking evaluation fail with the first word – systematic. Their institutional habits, and therefore those of their agents, are wholly more reactive than pro-active and planful. This makes anything systematic unlikely, yet they still assume evaluability. Why? Responses depend on the stakeholders' foci, but here are a common set of problematic assumptions we have encountered (Department of Health, 2007):

- Evaluation is simple and uncomplicated with few steps
- Organisations house ample numbers of staff with the skills and resources to do it

- Existing staff (and/or volunteers) will want to do an evaluation and already know how and when to do it
- Existing staff (and/or volunteers) will actually do it alongside higher priority tasks.

Collectively, and worryingly, these assumptions confirm that the inherent nature of human behaviour change is poorly understood in these organisations. This is ironic given that the interventions focus on changing PA behaviour in clients and participants.

At any stage, it is unwise to assume that every programme can be effectively evaluated. Indeed, this is something that should be explored with key stakeholders and confirmed both at the outset and during the evaluation process (Dwyer, Hansen, Barrera et al., 2003; Chapel and Lang, 2009; Eldredge et al., 2016). This is particularly the case in partnership evaluation designs, where specialist evaluators and programme deliverers collaborate to work on shared tasks (Pringle, Zwolinsky, McKenna et al., 2014). Given that health researchers, investigators and funders place importance on collaboration between communities and academic institutions (Corbie-Smith, Bryant, Walker et al., 2015; Simmons, Klasko, Fleming et al., 2015) it is important to get this approach right from the outset (Eldredge et al., 2016; Pringle, 2011).

Indeed, Pringle, McKenna, Whatley et al., (2006) and Pringle, Hargreaves, Lozano et al., (2014) have suggested that those tasked with implementing evaluations will require personal and collective *commitment*, *capacity* and *capabilities* while undertaking and completing evaluations. Using these notions to guide our discussion, *Capability* refers to the skills and expertise that stakeholders can deploy while performing evaluations, including tasks associated with the design, implementation, analysis and dissemination of evaluations. *Capacity* refers to the resources – human or financial – that stakeholders can use to complete evaluation tasks. *Commitment* refers to the strength and direction of motivation that stakeholders have for implementing specific evaluation tasks. In the understanding that stakeholders have other important and concurrent roles, it will come as no surprise that performing the evaluation will be low on most deliverer's list of priorities (Department of Health, 2007). Referring to our previous point, what applies to behaviour change in clients is just as likely to apply to the behaviour change of deliverers (Kok et al., 2015; Eldredge et al., 2016), when it applies to the new behaviours accompanying evaluation. Part of the success of LLGA and the attendance behaviour it helped to identify was that all that data captured was automated, contrast this with the manual processes deployed in the National Evaluation of LEAP (Pringle, 2011).

It is also important to address the experiences of researchers who have completed detailed and informative evaluations. Often they report feeling frustrated that their research has neither been applied to the health promotion context (Blinkhorn and Gittani, 2009) nor translated into practice (Ballhew, Brownson, Joshu et al., 2010). On the other hand, this is hardly surprising; evaluators have been criticised for providing health promoters with more problems than solutions (Blinkhorn and Gittani 2009; Eldredge et al., 2016); our experience in the LEAP programme often drove that point home (Department of Health, 2007; Pringle, 2011). Indeed, evaluations are often seen by practitioners as lacking real-world utility (Wilson, Basta, Bynum et al., 2010), which has given rise to concerns to progress under the aegis of a new 'implementation science' (Lobb and Colditz, 2013; Kok et al., 2015; Eldredge et al., 2016).

Instrumentation is a recurrent problem area. Using instrumentation that is not only inappropriate for the setting (Learmonth and Griffin, 2007; Pringle, Zwolinsky, McKenna et al., 2014), but also for the groups with who they are performed (Judd, Frankish and Moulton, 2001) seem widespread. Instead, addressing all notions health literacy – not least because it so often subsumes shortfalls in literacy – should be standard practice for developing evaluation instruments. Assessing any paperwork for readability and for using plain English is helpful in all cases (Pringle, Zwolinsky, McKenna et al., 2014).

Criticism is not only reserved for evaluators, but also for commissioners who procure evaluations, including the procuring government departments (Chambers, 2009; Whitehead, 2009). Moreover, it is not uncommon for political influences to impact on decisions about whether or not to commission evaluations (Benzeval, 2009; Evans, Hall, Jones et al., 2007; Pringle, 2011), as well as the type of evaluations that are procured (Sowdon and Raine, 2008). Like evaluators, commissioners have also been criticised for failing to appreciate the practicalities associated with implementing evaluations, including those undertaken in community settings, where diverse factors impact on intervention delivery and outcomes (Kryiacou, 2009; South and Phillips, 2014). Indeed, such factors play out even more during evaluations located in the community settings (McKenna, Davis and Pringle, 2005; Donaldson, Patton, Fetterman et al., 2010), including those in areas of high health need and low SES (Hind, Scott, Copeland et al., 2010; Curran, Drust, Murphy et al., 2016). With those thoughts in mind, we propose five considerations aimed at facilitating evaluability in partnership evaluation designs, where specialist evaluators work with delivers to evaluate PA interventions. These considerations are intended to contribute to the body of guidance and evidence on performing evaluations (Pringle, 2011).

- Partnerships require early, timely and on-going dialogue

Green and Tones (2010) and Eldredge et al. (2016) recommend that stakeholders are engaged in dialogue with evaluators at an early stage in the planning process. Such activities generate agreements on evaluation matters, including the choice of instrumentation and roles and responsibilities for evaluation (Dugdill, Stratton and Watson, 2009). Agreeing on the measurements that manage participant burden while also assessing population and programme attributes, stakeholders should be mindful that compromise may be a key consideration when confirming evaluation arrangements (Bauman, Phongsavin, Schoeppe et al., 2006; Wozniak et al., 2016). This is a particular issue within PA promotion where many divergent, and potentially conflicting, messages may be promoted; think of the possible combinations between the elements of the exercise prescription (frequency, intensity, time and type) overlain by programme themes such as 'do less sitting', 'walk more', play sport, exercise at work and so on and the complications become clear.

Further, when stakeholders commit to early dialogue they send powerful messages about the nature of partnership working and of future intentions (Parnell, Pringle, Widdop et al., 2015; Eldredge et al., 2016), as well as enhancing the quality of the evaluation design (Wozniak et al., 2016). Moreover, these pre-emptive actions aimed at identifying potential issues and realistic solutions (Wozniak et al., 2016) are a more effective and efficient use of resources than those actions centred on salvaging and recovering a fractured partnership at a later date (Pringle, 2011). Dissatisfaction is likely when one group, or key individuals within a group, assumes superiority over others or when these dominant agents demonstrate unexplained mission creep for the project, the evaluation or both. Studies confirm that with the right course of actions, damaged or malfunctioning partnerships can be repaired (Moldon and Finkel, 2010; Pringle, 2011), but the resources required can be substantial.

- Partnerships require effective planning and clear goals

With partnership evaluation arrangements being relatively commonplace (Lozano et al., 2016; Zwolinsky, McKenna, Pringle et al., 2016a), we set out a series of considerations for facilitating evaluability and then being more effective in doing evaluations. This now shifts our attention from 'knowing that' to 'knowing to'; this has much to say about routines and practices around day-to-day evaluation. Problematically, 'know that' is often rated as more important than 'know to' in many organisations; our experience is that both are needed in equally high amounts and that organisational habits have much to do with the problems that surround even the most elegant evaluation approaches.

Green and Tones (2010) and Eldredge et al. (2016) recommend that partnerships need to plan, set out and work to clear aims and objectives. However, we have often found that mission creep can affect commissioners as much as deliverers and/or evaluators. This can be helped by establishing a written plan, which becomes reference point for charting progress and activity; it is especially helpful for identifying loss of momentum (Eldredge et al., 2016). Often this loss of focus occurs mid-evaluation.

By combining the efforts of the key constituents, anticipated problems can be identified and potentially offset before they become harmful. By viewing strengths and difficulties together and straightforwardly, potentially, this makes another statement of intent for future working arrangements. It can help to create events where stakeholders repeatedly confirm their commitment to evaluation (Chapel and Lang, 2009; Eldredge et al., 2016). Further, with different perspectives, evaluations can become truly bespoke; this can be important because stakeholders attach different levels of worth to evaluation (Blamey and Mutrie, 2004; Deehan and Wylie, 2010), and hold different ideas on how evaluation should be performed (South and Tilford, 2000; Green and Tones, 2010). Consistent with our experience, the CDC (1999) evaluation framework identified that coming together around the evaluation can help ameliorate some of the inherent challenges it brings (Pringle, Zwolinsky, McKenna et al., 2014; Eldredge et al., 2016).

- Partnerships require common agreements

Agreement between partners provides a powerful signal that partnerships are centred on building effectiveness (Green and Tones, 2010; Parnell, Pringle, Widdop et al., 2015). It has been recommended that individuals and teams within the community must engage around collectively negotiated aims (McDonald, Viehbeck, Robinson et al., 2008;) and procedures. Too often procedures are overlooked in the pursuit of more lofty aspirations (Pringle and Zwolinsky, 2016). As noted previously, decisions around evaluation instrumentation and timing are key areas that are most contested by stakeholders in partnership evaluations (Pringle, Zwolinsky and McKenna, 2013; Parker, Meiklejohn, Patterson et al. 2006). Timely appointment of evaluators will help prioritise key tasks, such as developing a workable evaluation design and securing ethical approval, where necessary (Eldredge et al., 2016). It will also help to ensure that the evaluation instrumentation is piloted and ready for use when the programme begins (Zwolinsky, McKenna, Pringle et al., 2016a). Without that, many participants will be excluded from the evaluation; burdensome evaluations can 'signal' that programmes are unappealing to target audiences. This mistake can be fatal for change-oriented programmes relying on evaluations examining pre-post differences. Collectively, these avoidable evaluation mistakes can undermine claims that programmes meet policy aspirations. That they continue to happen offers an indication of how far there is to travel to ensure that evaluators, commissioners and respective stakeholders work to develop and then use evaluation outcomes to improve on-going programme performance.

- Partnerships should prioritise key tasks

Evaluation partnerships become more effective when they prioritise activities that are the linchpins of what produces programme outcomes (Pringle, Parnell, Rutherford et al., 2016). This should not only include those who deliver, but also those who evaluate and commission programmes (Benzeval, 2009). While commissioned evaluations may be prominent in any level of policy documentation, only rarely does this assure evaluability (Pringle, 2011). Instead, commissioners may focus on the planning or publicising the programme, even though longstanding (CDC, 1999) guidance recommends developing evaluations alongside interventions. An unfavourable start to an evaluation can contribute to accumulating dissatisfaction between stakeholders over a host of seemingly mundane and ordinary issues (Pringle, 2011). Moreover, such feelings may develop long-term enmities that add difficulty to what is already challenging (Pringle, 2011).

• Choosing evaluation instrumentation

Evaluation is often poorly performed, using methods for collecting data that are seen locally as inappropriate to the intervention and the context (Nutbeam, 1998; Freeman, 2009; Glasgow, 2009; Green and Tones, 2010; Eldredge et al., 2016). Dugdill, Stratton and Watson (2009) provide a useful framework for considering instrumentation for evaluating PA interventions. Debates and disagreements often arise over the different yardsticks being used to assess effectiveness of interventions (Pringle, 2011). Tensions can arise between preferences for adopting non-validated 'quick and dirty' methodologies that count heads and ask people what they liked and for using validated instrumentation, in its fullest form, but which lacks relevance to the local setting and people. Indeed, evaluations conducted in interventions in areas of high health need and low SES can be difficult (Sport England, 2006; Department of Health, 2007; Hind, Scott, Copeland et al., 2010). Issues regarding literacy and concerns about civil 'surveillance' have been commonly reported (Pringle, Marsh, Gilson et al., 2010; Pringle, 2011). Unresolved sensitivities about specific evaluation tools – even specific questionnaire items – can end with a general rejection of the evaluation and poor working relationships (Pringle, 2011). Because of these issues, it is important that timely discussions are held between evaluators, deliverers and participants to select and to pilot instruments, and to plan the timing of data collection, submission and review (Dugdill, Stratton and Watson, 2009; Eldredge et al., 2016; Wozniak et al., 2016). In unreached communities, the issues that prick such sensitivities may be subtle and unfamiliar to many evaluators, so responding to local knowledge and insight is important. The engagement of key stakeholders throughout the evaluation is fundamental (Eldredge et al., 2016), not least when enhancing preparedness and building capacity to deliver evaluations (Pringle, Zwolinsky, McKenna et al., 2014; Zwolinsky, McKenna, Pringle, 2016; Wozniak et al., 2016).

Conclusion: Implications for future PA policy and practice related to the chapter topic

Our experience is that enacting and then evaluating policy is complex and it is wise to acknowledge this. This complexity is inextricably linked to the interconnectedness of influences between policy, evaluation, delivery, politics and the people and constituencies involved in these domains. Even so, simplicity can be found beyond this complexity and an array of useful frameworks and guidance are available for putting order around how policy can be enacted and assessed in evaluations. It is rarely mentioned, yet still helpful, to acknowledge that this complexity may parallel the behaviour change that underpins becoming more active. That justifies paying closer attention on the people involved with any of these activities; they are different to the people who engage with programmes and what seems easy (or difficult) from the outside can be seen very differently on the inside.

The recurrence of familiar themes suggests that learning about them – including those affecting evaluation – is often temporary and ephemeral. This underlines why it is important to emphasise the important messages that can be drawn both from current and historical examples. Yet, the difficulties and challenges of executing evaluations are often left unexpressed even though timely and open dialogue of what worked, and didn't, can be a substantial resource in its own right. In any organisation where evaluation is likely to be an on-going issue it makes good sense to maintain a record of in-house learning. We have learned that it is unwise to assume that positive evaluation habits exist, let alone prevail, in any organisation. Neither are resources (human, material or financial) readily or willingly deployed to support evaluation.

The many powerful practices – and shortcomings – we report have been seen while delivering evaluations of community programmes in single and multiple locations, with varying PA content and with distinctive target groups. The powerful practices are replicable and shortcomings are (mostly) recoverable. For reasons of effectiveness and efficiency there is considerable advantage in revisiting and reconsidering them throughout every evaluation. Crucially, it is the behaviours of evaluation staff and their partners – not what they 'know' or claim to know to do – that makes any evaluation work, or not. These are the behaviours that are imperative for generating better PA policy.

Acknowledgments

The authors would like to thank both the participants and organisations who supported research presented in this chapter and performed by the Centre of Active Lifestyles at Leeds Beckett University.

References

Arends, R.Y., Bode, C., Taal, E. and Van de Laar, M.A. (2017) A mixed-methods process evaluation of a goal management intervention for patients with polyarthritis. *Psychology & Health*, 32(1), pp. 38–60.

Bagot, P. (2013) *Diet, nutrition and obesity. Public health policy and politics*. London, Palgrave.

Baker, C., Loughren, E., Crone, D., Tutton, A. and Aitken, P. (2016) 23 Contemporary lifestyle interventions for public health – Potential roles for professional sports clubs. *Sport and Exercise Psychology*: Practitioner Case Studies, p. 417.

Ballhew, P., Brownson, R., D., Joshu, D., Health, G., and Gregory, M. (2010) Dissemination of effective PA interventions: Are we applying the evidence? *Health Education Research*, 25(2), pp. 185–198.

Bauman, A., Phongsavin, P., Schoeppe, S. and Owen, N. (2006) Physical activity measurement: A primer for health promotion. *Promotion and Education*, 13(2), pp. 92–103.

Benzeval, M. (2009) *Designing and evaluating policy effectively*. House of Commons Health Inequalities Health Select Committee, London, HMSO.

Blair, S. N., Kampert, J. B., Kohl, H. W., Barlow, C. E., Macera, C. A., Paffenbarger, R. S., J. R. and Gibbons, L. W. (1996) Influences of cardiorespiratory fitness and other precursors on cardiovascular disease and all-cause mortality in men and women. *JAMA*, 276, pp. 205–210.

Blamey, A. and Mutrie, N. (2004) Changing the individual to promote health enhancing physical activity: The difficulties of producing evidence and translating it into practice. *Journal of Sports Science*, 22(8), pp. 741–754.

Blinkhorn, A and Gittani, J. (2009) A qualitative evaluation of the views of community workers on the dental health education material available in New South Wales for culturally and linguistically diverse communities. *Health Education Journal*, 68(4), pp. 314–319.

Carnegie Research Institute (2010) *Evaluation of the Nottingham YMCA exercise referral pathway*, Leeds, Centre for Active Lifestyles Leeds Metropolitan University.

Centre for Chronic Disease Prevention and Health Promotion (1999) *Physical activity evaluation handbook*. Atlanta, USA, Centre for Disease Control and Prevention.

Centre for Chronic Disease Prevention and Health Promotion (2011) Programme Evaluation. Available from: www.cdc.gov/eval/framework/index.htm [accessed 31 October 2011].

Chambers, J. (2009) *Designing and evaluating policy effectively*. House of Commons Health Inequalities Health Select Committee, London, HMSO.

Chapel, T. and Lang, J. (2009) Practical programme evaluation: Ensuring findings are used for programme improvement. In N. Pronk, *ACSM's Worksite Handbook: A guide to guiding healthy and productive companies*. Champaign, Illinois, Human Kinetics, pp. 127–139. ISBN-13: 9780736074346.

Corbie-Smith, G., Bryant, A. R., Walker, D. J., Blumenthal, C., Council, B., Courtney, D. and Adimora, A. (2015) Building capacity in community-based participatory research partnerships through a focus on process and multiculturalism. Progress in community health partnerships. *Research, Education, and Action*, 9(2), pp. 261–273.

Curran, K., Brook, K., Lozano, L., Parnell, D., Zwolinsky, S. and Pringle, A. (2015) *An independent evaluation of 'Fit Reds'; a football-led health improvement programme for men delivered at Barnsley Football Club*. Institute of Sport, Physical Activity and Leisure, Centre for Active Lifestyles, Leeds UK, Leeds Beckett University.

Curran, K., Drust, B., Murphy, R., Pringle, A. and Richardson, D. (2016) The challenge and impact of engaging hard-to-reach populations in regular physical activity and health behaviours: An examination of an English Premier League 'Football in the Community' men's health programme. *Public Health*, 135, pp. 14–22.

Deehan, A. and Wylie, A. (2010) *Health promotion in medical education*. Oxford, Radcliffe.

Department of Health (1999) *National service framework for coronary heart disease*. London, HMSO.

Department of Health (2001a) *National service framework for older people disease*. London, HMSO.

Department of Health (2001b) *National service framework for diabetes disease*. London, HMSO.

Department of Health (2002) *The local exercise action pilots: An evaluation scoping paper*. London, Department of Health.

Department of Health (2005) *Choosing activity: A physical activity action plan*. London, Crown.

Department of Health (2007) National Evaluation of the Local Exercise Action Pilots. Available from: www.dh.gov.uk/en/Publicationsandstatistics/Publications/PublicationsPolicyAndGuidance/DH_073600 [Accessed 6 June 2008].

Department of Health (2011) Health Lives Healthy People: Our Strategy for Public Health in England, London, Department of Health. Available from: www.dh.gov.uk/en/Publicationsandstatistics/Publications/PublicationsPolicyAndGuidance/DH_121941 [Accessed 25 October 2013].

Donaldson, S., Patton, I., Fetterman, M. and Scriven, M. (2010) Claremont debates: The promise and pitfalls of utilisation-focused and empowerment evaluation. *Journal of Multi-Disciplinary Evaluation*, 6(13), pp. 15–57.

Dugdill, L. and Stratton, G. (2007) *Evaluating sport and physical activity interventions: Guide for practitioners. A report commissioned by Sport England and the North West Public Health Team*. Salford, University of Salford.

Dugdill, L., Stratton, G. and Watson, P. (2009) Developing the evidence base for physical activity interventions. In L. Dugdill, C. Crone and R. Murphy (Ed.), *Physical activity and health promotion: Evidence-based approaches to practice*. Chichester, Wiley-Blackwell, pp. 60–84.

Dwyer, J., Hansen, B., Barrera, N., Allinson, K., Ceolon-Celestini, S., Koenig, D., Young, D., Good, M. and Rees, T. (2003) Maximising children's physical activity: An evaluability assessment to plan a community-based, multi-strategy approach in an ethno-racially and socio-economically diverse city. *Health Promotion International*, 18(3), pp. 199–208.

Eldredge, L. K. B., Markham, C. M., Kok, G., Ruiter, R. A. and Parcel, G. S. (2016) *Planning health promotion programs: An intervention mapping approach*. London, John Wiley & Sons.

Estabrooks, P., Stoutenberg, M., Galaviz, K., Lobelo, F., Joy, J., Heath, G. and Hutber, A. (2016) *Adapting the RE-AIM framework for the pragmatic evaluation of exercise is medicine*. 65th annual meeting American College of Sports Medicine. Boston, MA, May 28–31.

European Commission (2011) *State of men's health in Europe*. Available from: http://ec.europa.eu/health/population_groups/docs/men_health_report_en.pdf [Accessed 31 October 2011].

Evans, L., Hall, M., Jones, C. and Neiman, A. (2007) Did the Ottawa Charter play a role in the push to assess the effectiveness of health promotion? *Promotion & Education*, 14(28), DOI: 10.1177/10253823070140020901x.

Fineberg, H. (2012) Shattuck Lecture. A successful and sustainable health system--how to get there from here. *The New England Journal of Medicine*, 366(11), pp. 1020–1027.

Freeman, R. (2009) Health promotion and the randomised controlled trial: A square peg in a round hole? *BMC Oral Health*, 9(1). Available from: www.biomedcentral.com/1472-6831/9/1 [Accessed 7 July 2010].

Gardner, S. (2014) *Get Healthy Get Active what we've learnt so far April 2013–July 2014.* Available from: https://www.sportengland.org/media/397773/FINAL-Get-Healthy-Get-Active-what-we-ve-learnt.pdf [Accessed 20 October 2015].

Gattenhof, S. (2017) Reframing the position of the evaluator. In *Measuring impact: Models for evaluation in the Australian arts and culture.* UK, Palgrave Macmillan, pp. 33–37.

Glasgow, R. (2009) RE-AIMing research for application: Ways to improve evidence for family medicine. *Journal American Board Family Medicine*, 19(1), pp. 11–19.

Green, J. and Tones, K. (2010) *Health promotion: Planning and strategies.* 2nd edition. London, Sage.

Hind, D., Scott, E., Copeland, R., Breckon, J., Crank, H, Waters, S., Brazier, J., Nicol, J., Cooper, C. and Goyder, E. (2010) A randomised controlled trial and cost effectiveness evaluation of 'booster' interventions to sustain increases in physical activity in middle-aged adults in deprived urban neighbourhoods. *BMC Public Health*, 10(3). Available from: www.biomedcentral.com/1471-2458/10/3 [Accessed 9 October 2010].

Judd, J., Frankish, J. and Moulton, G. (2001) Setting standards in the evaluation of community-based health promotion programmes: A unifying approach. *Health Promotion International*, 16(4), pp. 367–380.

Khaw, K. T., Wareham, N., Bingham, S., Welch, A., Luben, R. and Day, N. (2008) Combined impact of health behaviours and mortality in men and women: The EPIC-Norfolk prospective population study. *PLoS Med*, 5(1), p. e12.

Kok, G., Gottlieb, N. H., Peters, G. J. Y., Mullen, P. D., Parcel, G. S., Ruiter, R. A., Fernández, M. E., Markham, C. and Bartholomew, L. K. (2015) A taxonomy of behaviour change methods: An intervention mapping approach. *Health Psychology Review*, 10(3), pp. 1–16.

Kryiacou, C. (2009) Bridging theory and practice: Design and implementation of the NORC-SSP linkage. *International Journal of Integrated Care*, 9, Annual Conference Supplement.

Learmonth, A. and Griffin, B. (2007) Research and evaluation. In J. Merchant, B. Griffin and A., Charnock (Ed.), Sport *and physical activity: The role of health promotion.* London, Palgrave, pp. 45–59.

Leeds City Council (2015) Leeds Let's Get Active. Available from: www.leedsletsgetactive.co.uk/ [Accessed 20 October 2015].

Lewis, C. J., Reeves, M. J. and Roberts, S. J. (2016) Improving the physical and mental well-being of typically hard-to-reach men: An investigation of the impact of the Active Rovers project. *Sport in Society*, 20(2), pp. 258–268.

Lobb, R. and Colditz, G. A. (2013) Implementation science and its application to population health. *Annual Review of Public Health*, 34, pp. 235–251.

Lozano-Sufrategui, L., Pringle, A., Carless, D. and McKenna, J. (2016) 'It brings the lads together': A critical exploration of older men's experiences of a weight management programme delivered through a Healthy Stadia project. *Sport in Society*, 20(2), pp. 303–315.

Martin, A., Morgan, S., Parnell, D., Philpott, M., Pringle, A., Rigby, M., Taylor, A. and Topham, J. (2016) A perspective from key stakeholders on football and health improvement. *Soccer & Society*, 17(2), pp. 175–182.

McDonald, P. W., Viehbeck, S., Robinson, S. J., Leatherdale, S. T., Nykiforuk, C. I., Jolin, M. A. (2009) Building research capacity for evidence-informed tobacco control in Canada: A case description. *Tobacco Induced Diseases*, 5(1), pp. 1–12.

McKenna, J., Davis, M. and Pringle, A. (2005) Scientists within community research. *The Sport and Exercise Scientist*, 4, p. 67.

McKenna, J., Quarmby, T., Kime, N., Parnell, D. and Zwolinsky, S. (2016) Lessons from the field for working in Healthy Stadia: Physical activity practitioners reflect on 'sport'. *Sport in Society*, 20(2), pp. 316–324.

Medical Research Council (2008) *Developing and evaluating complex interventions: New guidance.* London, Medical Research Council. Available from: www.mrc.ac.uk/Utilities/Documentrecord/index.htm?d=MRC004871 [Accessed October 7 2013].

Moldon, D. and Finkel, E. (2010) Motivations for promotion and prevention and the role of trust and commitment in inter-personal forgiveness. *Journal of Experimental and Social Psychology*, 46(2), pp. 244–268.

Mozaffarian, D., Wilson, P. W. and Kannel, W. B. (2008) Beyond established and novel risk factors: Lifestyle risk factors for cardiovascular disease. *Circulation*, 117(23), 3031–3038.

National Institute for Health & Clinical Excellence (2007) *The most appropriate means of generic and specific interventions to support attitude and behaviour change at the population and community level*. London, NICE. Available from: www.nice.org.uk/nicemedia/pdf/PH006guidance.pdf [Accessed 5 July 2010].

National Obesity Observatory (NOO) (2012) *Standard evaluation framework for physical activity interventions*. London, National Obesity Observatory. Available from: www.noo.org.uk/uploads/doc/vid_16722_SEF_PA.pdf [Accessed 20 February 2014].

Nutbeam, D. (1998) Evaluating health promotion: Progress, problems and solutions. *Health Promotion International*, 13(1), pp. 27–44.

Parker, E., Meiklejohn, B., Patterson, C., Edwards, K., Preece, C., Shuter, P. and Gould, P. (2006) Our games our health: A cultural asset for promoting health in indigenous communities. *Health Promotion Journal of Australia*, 17(2), pp. 103–108.

Parnell, D., Pringle, A., Widdop, P. and Zwolinsky, S. (2015) Research partnership to understand football as a vehicle for social inclusion delivered within Burton Albion Community Trust. *Social Inclusion*, 3. ISN 2183-2803.

Premier League (2011) *Creating chances*. London, Premier League. Available from: http://addison.ceros.com/premier-league/creating-chances-2011/page/1 [Accessed 25 January 2013].

Pringle, A. (2011) *A national evaluation of the local exercise action pilots: Effectiveness, efficiency and evaluability*. Doctor of Philosophy, Leeds Metropolitan University.

Pringle, A., Hargreaves, J., Lozano, L., McKenna, J. and Zwolinsky, S. (2014) Assessing the impact of football-based health improvement programmes: Stay onside, avoid own goals and score with the evaluation! *Soccer & Society*, 15(6), pp. 970–987.

Pringle, A., Marsh, K., Gilson, N., McKenna, J. and Cooke, C. (2010) Cost-effectiveness of interventions to improve moderate physical-activity: A study in nine UK sites. *Health Education Journal*, 69(2), pp. 211–224.

Pringle, A., McKenna, J., Whatley, E. and Gilson, N. (2006) Qualitative perspectives on evaluability of community physical activity interventions. From Education to Application: Sport, Exercise and Health Proceedings of the British Association of Sport & Exercise Science, 2006, Wolverhampton University, UK. Leeds, British Association of Sport & Exercise Science, September 11–13.

Pringle, A., Parnell, D., Rutherford, Z., McKenna, J., Zwolinsky, S. and Hargreaves, J. (2016) Sustaining health improvement activities delivered in English professional football clubs using evaluation: A short communication. *Soccer & Society*, 17(5), pp. 759–769.

Pringle, A. and Zwolinsky, S. (2016) Health Improvement Programmes for Local Communities Delivered in 72 Professional Football (Soccer) Clubs: 1562 Board# 215 June 2, 8:00 AM-9:30 AM. *Medicine and Science in Sports and Exercise*, 48(5 Suppl 1), p. 428.

Pringle, A., Zwolinsky, S. and McKenna, J. (2013). Health improvement and professional football: Players on the same-side? *Journal of Policy Research in Tourism, Leisure and Events*, 5(2), pp. 207–212. DOI:10.1080/19407963.2013.798159.

Pringle, A., Zwolinsky, S., McKenna, J., Smith, A., Robertson, S. and White, A. (2013a) Effect of a national programme of men's health delivered in English Premier League Football Clubs. *Public Health*, 127(1), pp. 18–25.

Pringle, A., Zwolinsky, S., McKenna, J., Smith, A., Robertson, S. and White, A. (2013b) Delivering men's health interventions in English Premier League football clubs: Key design characteristics. *Public Health*, 127, pp. 716–726.

Pringle, A., Zwolinsky, S., McKenna, J., Smith, A., Robertson, S. and White, A. (2014) Men's health improvement for men/Hard-to-engage men delivered in English Premier League Football Clubs. *Health Education Research*, 29(3), pp. 503–520.

Robertson, S. and Baker, P. (2016) Men and health promotion in the United Kingdom: 20 years further forward? *Health Education Journal*, 76(1), pp. 102–113.

Robertson, S., Woodall, J., Henry, H., Hanna, E., Rowlands, S., Horrocks, J., Livesley, J. and Long, T. (2016) Evaluating a community-led project for improving fathers' and children's wellbeing in England. *Health Promotion International*, p.daw090.

Scriven, M. (1999) In Centers for Disease Control and Prevention. Framework for program evaluation in public health. Morbidity and Mortality Weekly Report, 48(No. RR-11).

Simmons, V., N., Klasko, L., Fleming, K., Koskan, A., Jackson, N., T., Noel-Thomas, Luque, J., Vadaparampil, S., Lee, J., Quinn, G., Britt, L., Waddell, R., Meade, C., Gwede, C. and Tampa Bay Community Cancer Network Community Partners (2015) Participatory evaluation of a community-academic partnership to inform capacity-building and sustainability. *Evaluation and Program Planning*, 52, pp. 19–26.

Sinclair, A. and Alexander, H. (2012) Using outreach to involve the hard-to-reach in a health check: What difference does it make? *Public Health*, 126, pp. 87–95.

South J. and Phillips G. (2014) Evaluating community engagement as part of the public health system. *Journal of Epidemiology and Community Health*, DOI:10.1136/jech-2013-203742.

South, J. and Tilford, S. (2000) Perceptions of research and evaluation in health promotion practice and influences on activity. *Health Education Research*, 15(6), pp. 729–741.

Sowden, S. and Raine, R. (2008) Running along parallel lines: How political reality impedes the evaluation of public health interventions: A case study of exercise-referral scheme. *Journal of Epidemiology and Community Health*, 62, pp. 835–841.

Sport England (2006) *Learning from LEAP*. London, Sport England.

White, A., de Sousa, B., de Visser, R., Hogston, R., Madsen, SA., Makara, P., McKee, M., Raine, G., Richardson, N., Clarke, N. and Zato ski, W. (2011) Men's health in Europe. *Journal of Men's Health*, 8, pp. 192–201.

White, A., Zwolinsky, S., Pringle, A., McKenna, J., Daly-Smith, A., Robertson, S. and Berry, R. (2012) Premier League Health: A National Programme of Men's Health Promotion Delivered in/by Professional Football Clubs, Final Report 2012. Centre for Men's Health & Centre for Active Lifestyles, Leeds Metropolitan University.

Whitehead, M. (2009) Designing and evaluating policy effectively. House of Commons Health Inequalities – Health Committee, London, HMSO.

Wholey, J., Hatry, H. and Newcomer, K. (2004) *Handbook of practical program evaluation*. 2nd Edition. San Francisco, Jossey-Bass.

Wilson, M., Basta, T., Bynum, B., DeJoy, D., Vandenberg, R. and Dishman, RK. (2010) Do intervention fidelity and dose influence outcomes? Results from the move to improve worksite physical activity program. *Health Education Research*, 25(2), pp. 294–305. DOI: 10.1093/her/cyn065. Epub 2009.

Wozniak, L. A., Soprovich, A., Rees, S., Johnson, S. T., Majumdar, S. R. and Johnson, J. A. (2016) A qualitative study examining healthcare managers and providers' perspectives on participating in primary care implementation research. *BMC Health Services Research*, 16(1), p. 316.

Zwolinsky, S. and McKenna, J. (2015) Leeds Let's Get Active: Final Report, August 2015. Centre for Active Lifestyles, Leeds Beckett University.

Zwolinsky, S. and McKenna, J. (2016). Leeds Let's Get Active: Lifestyle Behaviours Report, July 2016. Centre for Active Lifestyles, Leeds Beckett University.

Zwolinsky, S., McKenna, J. and Pringle, A. (2016) How can the health system benefit from increasing participation in sport, exercise and physical activity? In D. Conrad and A. White (Ed.), *Sports-based health interventions*. New York, Springer, pp. 29–52.

Zwolinsky, S., McKenna, J., Pringle, A., Daly-Smith, A., Robertson, S. and White, A. (2016a) Supporting lifestyle risk reduction: Promoting men's health through professional football. *Soccer & Society*, 17(2), pp. 183–195.

Zwolinsky, S., McKenna, J., Pringle, A., Widdop, P., Griffiths, C., Mellis, M., Rutherford, Z. and Collins, P. (2016b) Physical activity and sedentary behavior clustering: Segmentation to optimize active lifestyles. *Journal of Physical Activity and Health*, 13(9), pp. 921–928.

31

MODELLING THE COST EFFECTIVENESS OF PHYSICAL ACTIVITY INTERVENTIONS

The case of GP based interventions

Nana Kwame Anokye

Introduction

Global health policy documents (e.g. WHO 2016, 2009) highlight the need to implement programmes that work and to ensure that limited resources are used efficiently. This requires the application of economic evaluation methods to assess the relative efficiency of alternative programmes to achieve health outcomes. To date, most economic evaluation studies have focussed on clinical interventions although there is growing interest in evaluating the cost effectiveness of a broader range of healthcare programmes, including public health interventions (NICE 2014). The rationale for this is clear: public health interventions consume health (and in some case other public sector) resources and as such are associated with an opportunity cost. That is, the money spent on public health interventions could be used for other healthcare activities, and it is important to determine whether public health interventions offer value for money.

Modelling of the long-term costs and effects are more important where benefits and costs extend beyond the end of a trial, as in the case with disease prevention and health promotion programmes. It is of particular relevance to physical activity interventions, where the costs are mostly borne at the beginning (e.g. with expenditure on GP time) but benefits are not only experienced immediately but well in to the future too (as resource savings from reduced disease and therefore benefits in terms of increased quality of life). The methods of economic modelling in healthcare are based on a medical paradigm (Weatherly et al. 2009), that assumes that there is high quality evidence on their effectiveness, typically derived from randomised controlled trials conducted prior to widespread uptake in the health service. Those familiar with public health interventions will recognise that these methods may have limitations when applied to interventions such as health promotion. Limitations of the methods of economic evaluation when used in public health have been identified (Weatherly et al. 2009; Kelly et al. 2005). Particular concerns include the absence of robust evidence on effectiveness from randomised controlled trials which typifies many public health interventions; the fact that impacts of public health interventions may include both health and non-health effects and the applicability of standard outcomes (e.g. Quality Adjusted Life Year – QALY) to public health stakeholders. These limitations have been recognised by The National Institute for Health and Clinical Excellence (NICE) in the development of national public health guidance (Kelly et al. 2010).

This chapter will describe the application of economic evaluation technique to evaluate physical activity interventions using worked examples of GP based physical activity interventions, highlighting the associated challenges and how they have been addressed to date. In this chapter, GP based physical activity interventions are specified as exercise referral schemes (ERS), and brief advice for physical activity in primary care (BA). In line with the approach by Pavey et al. (2011), ERS is defined as a structured form of exercise programme at a leisure centre. This programme commences with an individual presenting themselves to a primary care professional who then refers to them to the exercise scheme. BA involves verbal advice, discussion, negotiation or encouragement, with or without written or other support or follow up (Campbell et al. 2015).

The chapter is structured in two main parts. First, an overview of the evidence base on the cost effectiveness of ERS and BA is provided. This is followed by a demonstration of the modelling of ERS and BA in the UK.

Overview of the cost effectiveness of GP based physical activity interventions

There is little economic evidence to inform resource allocation on whether brief advice should be used to promote physical activity and the local infrastructure and systems support to cost-effective delivery of brief advice on physical activity in primary care. This conclusion is corroborated by the findings of similar previous systematic reviews (e.g. Matrix 2006a).

A recent rapid systematic review of economic evidence on brief advice for adults in primary care (Anokye et al. 2014) found limited evidence (of moderate quality) from three studies: one model-based (Matrix 2006b), one trial-based (Pringle et al. 2010) and one audit-based analysis (Boëhler et al. 2011) suggest that brief advice on physical activity in primary care is more cost effective than usual care. The evidence should, however, be interpreted with caution as the three studies were based on a weak effectiveness base and did not fully explore uncertainty. For example, there is only evidence that the type of people delivering the intervention affects costs, but there is no evidence of any difference in impact. There is also only very limited and poor quality evidence that more costly screening with disease registers accesses people more likely to change behavior. The studies that do exist suggest brief advice, given by either GPs or other health workers and with or without written material is cost-effective, although the paucity of the evidence on effectiveness and concerns about its rigor coupled with inadequate exploration of uncertainty points to the need for further evaluation.

Systematic reviews of ERS have rather not yielded clear consensus on its cost effectiveness (Pavey et al. 2011, Matrix 2006b, Sorensen et al. 2006, and Williams et al. 2007). For example, Matrix (2006a) found that the economic case for ERS was unclear with one study reporting that intervention was less costly and more effective (i.e. a dominant strategy) than the comparator, three studies reporting it to be more costly and more effective and one study reporting it to be more costly and equally effective. On balance the authors indicate that the economic case for brief interventions is largely positive although the authors highlight concerns about the applicability of some of the evidence considered to the NHS. Pavey et al. (2011) identified only four primary economic evaluations that assessed the cost-effectiveness of ERS – three trial based economic evaluations and a model-based analysis commissioned by NICE as part of the development of guidance on the promotion of physical activity in primary care. On the whole, the studies suggested that ERS is cost effective.

Broadly, the evidence base suggests that GP based interventions are cost effective methods to improving physical activity levels in inactive but otherwise healthy populations. This is consistent with more recent similar but broader review, Vijay et al. (2015), who examined the economic evidence on the brief interventions promoting physical activity in primary care and the community. They concluded that brief interventions (compared with usual care) could lead to an additional cost of moving an inactive person to an active state was between £96 and £986, with the cost per quality-adjusted life year ranging from £57 to £14,002.

There is, however, significant uncertainty around the estimates of cost effectiveness in the long-term particularly due to the paucity of evidence on the long-term effectiveness of interventions. Whilst economic modelling could address this gap in knowledge (Vijay et al. 2015), ultimately these issues can only be resolved through better evidence of effectiveness derived from randomised controlled trials or other well-designed observational studies. For example, whilst there is evidence that physical activity levels change over time, economic models to date have not accounted for the varying behaviour patterns sufficiently due to data unavailability. The implication of this is decisional as the cost effectiveness of physical activity interventions is positively related to the onset of health benefits (e.g. reduced risks for long-term conditions such as stroke, CVD and diabetes) as a result of improved activity. As such, any criticism of the economic evidence should be considered in light of the evidence on short and long-term effectiveness that is available at the time of the analysis.

Modelling approach

This section demonstrates the modelling of GP based interventions in the UK. Any economic evaluation described in a standardised framework has a number of benefits, including comparability, generalisability and transferability. I adapt the NICE PH Methods Guide Reference Case (NICE 2014) as this framework (see Table 31.1).

One model of the cost-effectiveness of physical activity interventions in England has evolved over time, has had particular prominence in supporting policy advice in this area. The cost effectiveness analysis of exercise referral schemes (Campbell et al. 2015, Pavey et al. 2011, Anokye et al. 2011) and of brief advice (Anokye et al. 2014) have been used by NICE to update national guidance on GP based physical activity interventions (PH44 on brief interventions, PH2 on ERS guidance). The NICE ROI on physical activity is based on this model (Matrix 2014).

Figure 31.1 illustrates the model structure. A Markov model follows a cohort of physically inactive but healthy adults in annual cycles over their remaining life time. The initial age of the cohort is chosen to reflect the average age of participants in trials of interventions – 33 years for brief advice, and 50 years for exercise referral schemes. In the first year the cohort (100,000) is exposed to a GP based PA intervention or no active. At the end of the first year of the model, the cohort is either 'active' (i.e. minimum of 150 minutes of at least MVPA per week) or 'inactive'. The cohort could have one of three events (non-fatal CHD, non-fatal stroke, type 2 diabetes), remain event free (i.e. without CHD, stroke or diabetes) or die either from CVD or non-CVD causes. The 'inactive' individuals from the first year accrue a one-off short-term psychological benefit associated with achieving the recommended level of PA. This short-term psychological benefit was estimated by regressing all EQ-5D data collected in this on meeting the recommended level of MVPA using the methods set out in Anokye et al. (2014).

Table 31.1 Features of the economic evaluation

Aspects	Exemplified using GP based physical activity interventions
Decision problem/objective of the study	To evaluate the cost-effectiveness of GP based physical activity interventions
Policy context	To inform policy makers and practitioners of whether these interventions are value for money
Type of economic evaluation	Cost utility analysis
Perspective	NHS
Target population	Healthy but physically inactive individuals in the UK
Health outcomes	Physical activity, CHD, stroke, type 2 diabetes and short term psychological benefit, QALYs
Strategies	ERS and BA
Comparator	Usual care
Resources/costs	Cost of PA interventions, costs of treatment of disease conditions (CHD, stroke, type 2 diabetes and mental health)
Time horizon	Lifetime

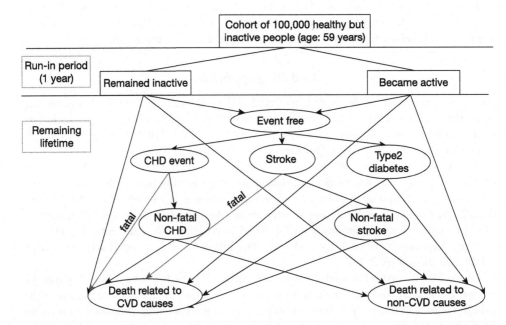

Figure 31.1 Illustration of pathways within the Markov model

Source: Anokye et al. 2014, Campbell et al. 2015

The 'active' state is associated with improved life expectancy and quality of life, as a result of a reduced risk of developing either coronary heart disease (CHD) (both non-fatal and fatal events), or stroke (both non-fatal and fatal events), or type 2 diabetes. The changes in the PA levels of the cohort overtime are accounted through the use of the relative risk (RR) of developing the disease conditions. These RR come from cohort studies, which assessed baseline PA (exposure) of their cohort and related this to subsequent onset of CHD, stroke or diabetes (outcomes) over a defined follow-up period. As these studies (Hu et al. 2003, 2005, 2007) followed up on the set of individuals (either active or inactive at baseline) for a number of years, during which some of the inactive people might have become active or vice versa, it indicates that irrespective of activity levels during the follow up years, once active (or inactive) at baseline, the relevant RR applies. The case-controls of these studies are only different in terms of baseline activity levels. Similarly, in the Markov model, as far as people are active or inactive at baseline i.e. Year 1 (irrespective of trial arm), the RR estimates are applicable regardless of activity levels in the subsequent years (equivalent to the follow-up years of the cohort studies).[1]

Beyond a period equivalent to the follow-up period in the cohort studies, a 100 per cent decay rate of physical activity is assumed and both active and inactive individuals are given the same risk of developing the disease conditions. Therefore, after the run-in period of the intervention (Year 0), we do not assume that physical activity levels as result of brief advice or usual care are sustainable. We recognise that this is a conservative approach and hence test its impact on the cost-effectiveness of brief advice in a sensitivity analysis.

Two separate models were run for ERS (Campbell et al. 2015) and brief advice (Anokye et al. 2014). Each model was run twice, once to estimate cost and health effects with the cohort offered intervention (the intervention arm), and once following usual-care with no active intervention (the control arm). Costs and outcomes of the cohort exposed (in the first one year cycle only) to GP based PA intervention are compared with the cohort not exposed to it (i.e. usual care). Health outcomes (from reduced disease) are expressed in terms of QALYs. Costs were assessed from a UK National Health Services perspective and costs and health outcomes were discounted. Table 31.2 sets out the details of the data used to populate the model.

Estimates of modelling

Table 31.3 presents the incremental cost-effectiveness ratio (ICER) for the GP based interventions based on a 100,000 cohort as estimated by Anokye et al. (2014) and Campbell et al. (2015). The ICER is the ratio of the difference (between an intervention and usual care) in costs and QALYs (cost per QALY). Total costs and outcomes are divided by the cohort size (100,000) to derive per person estimates of costs and benefits.

Compared with usual care, Anokye et al. (2015) found brief advice to be more costly, generating additional costs of £8 per person (in 2011 prices), but it is also more effective (leading to QALY gain of 0.0047 per person). The ICER for brief advice compared with usual care was £1,730 per QALY gained. Campbell et al. (2015) found ERS (compared with usual care) was relatively more expensive (£226 per person – in 2013 prices) and more effective (0.003 QALY gain per person). The ICER for ERS was £76,059 per QALY gained. The usual cost effectiveness threshold for England ranges from £20,000–£30,000 per QALY. Based on this threshold, brief advice can be seen as cost effective but ERS not.

The results for both interventions were found to be highly sensitive to the impact of the interventions on the likelihood of individuals meeting the recommended level of physical activity, maintenance of that level of activity (reflected via the duration of protective health effects) and the short-term psychological benefit. For example, Campbell et al. (2015) found that a slight improvement in the probability of ERS participants becoming physical active (from 1.12 to 1.31) resulted in ERS becoming cost effective with an ICER below the £30,000 threshold. Univariate analysis that increased the maintenance of physical activity levels and hence the duration of protective health benefits to lifetime improved the cost

Table 31.2 Data used to populate the model

Parameter	Value	Source of data
Relative risks of:		
Becoming active (at year 1):		
Brief advice vs usual care	1.42	Campbell et al. (2012)
ERS vs usual care	1.12	Campbell et al. (2015)
Disease (active vs inactive)		
CHD	0.90	Hu et al. (2007)
Stroke	0.86	Hu et al. (2005)
Diabetes	0.67	Hu et al. (2003)
Non-CVD mortality after:		
Non-fatal CHD	1.71	Brønnum-Hansen et al. (2001)
Non-fatal Stroke	1.71	
Diabetes	1.49	Preis et al. (2009)
CVD mortality after:		
Non-fatal CHD	3.89	Brønnum-Hansen et al. (2001)
Non-fatal Stroke	3.89	
Diabetes	2.61	Preis et al. (2009)
Fatality cases:		
CHD		
59–64	11.55%	Ward et al. (2005)
65–74	21.07%	
75+	14.76%	
Stroke		
55–64	23.28%	Ward et al. (2005)
65–74	23.47%	
75+	23.42%	
Incidence rates for:		
CHD		
59–64	0.63%	Ward et al. (2005); NCGC (2011)
65–74	0.97%	
75+	0.97%	
Stroke		
59–64	0.29%	
65–74	0.69%	
75+	1.43%	
Diabetes		
59	0.06%	Gonzalez et al. (2009)
60–69	0.10%	
70–79	0.11%	
80+	0.11%	
Quality of life		
Age specific quality of life		
59–64	0.82	National Centre for Social Research (2008)
65–74	0.78	
75+	0.72	

Parameter	Value	Source of data
Health state utility weight		
Healthy	1.00	Ward et al. (2005); NCGC (2011)
CHD 1st event	0.80	
post CHD 1st event	0.92	
Stroke 1st event	0.63	
Post stroke 1st event	0.65	
Diabetes	0.90	
Short-term psychological benefit of achieving 150 mins of MVPA per week	0.72	Pavey et al. (2011)
Annual cost		
Brief advice	£9.50	Campbell et al. (2012, 2015)
Exercise Referral Scheme	£229	
CHD 1st event	£4,248	NCGC (2011)
Post CHD 1st event	£485	
Stroke 1st event	£10,968	
Post stroke 1st event	£2,409	
Diabetes	£979	

Table 31.3 Cost-effectiveness results for brief advice (Anokye et al. 2014) and ERS (Campbell et al. 2015), compared with usual care

Physical activity intervention	Mean cost	Mean QALY	Incremental cost	Incremental QALY	ICER
Brief advice*	£1550	18.28	£8.06	0.0047	£1,730
Exercise referral scheme**	£4572	18.14	£225	0.003	£76,059

Notes: *discount rate=3.5%; ** discount rate=1.5%

effectiveness of the ERS from £76,059 to £33,056. On the other hand, the exclusion of the short-term psychological benefits resulted in higher ICERs, for example, an ICER of £27,000 per QALY gained (which is borderline cost-effectiveness) for brief advice.

Implications for practice and research

The illustrated approach for modelling the cost effectiveness of GP based physical activity interventions have used previous models in this field as a point of departure, and improved on the literature through using time-based model to account for the habitual changes in physical activity overtime and meta-analysed effectiveness data. The evidence suggests that the delivery of GP based physical activity interventions offer good value for money particularly for BA in primary care. The US Preventive Services Task Force (PSTF 2012) and NICE (NICE 2013) recommends BA in primary care as an effective programme for improving physical activity among adults. This view is supported by the European Union's guidelines on physical activity that encourage GPs to encourage patients to participate in physical activity (EU 2008). The implementation of these recommendations in practice is, however, challenged by provider related barriers that need addressing including inadequate time resources, conflicting priorities and lack of training (Campbell et al. 2012).

The modelling approach used in this chapter has a number of limitations that are worth mentioning. For example, a complete reflection of the variations of physical activity levels overtime was not captured with a 100 per cent decay rate of physical activity assumed for the whole cohort after year 10 of the time horizon in the model. This is a very conservative assumption, and the sensitivity analysis shows it is decisional. Further research could explore this through: (a) populating models with longitudinal data estimates on physical activity participation; (b) conducting physical activity trials with longer term follow up period; (c) using RR estimates on the impact of physical activity on disease conditions, which were based on follow up period that are equivalent to the time horizon in the economic models. In addressing this limitation, the methods ought to account for characteristics that influence the uptake and sustainability of physical activity (e.g. age, sex, health status). As individuals can opt in or out of interventions easily, it is important to reflect both the diversity in a population to maximise the efficiency accruable from interventions designed to increase physical activity.

Another limitation of the current modelling approach is that the inclusion of the long-term impact of PA on a few morbidities could have underestimated the cost effectiveness of the interventions. Related to this is the exclusion of the secondary transitions between the selected morbidities in the model, and this might have underestimated the protective health effects of physical activity. On the other hand, the model precluded adverse events associated with physical activity participation, for example, musculoskeletal injuries. Adverse effects could act as barriers in individual decision making to engage in physical activity and thereby the effectiveness and efficiency of interventions.

These highlight the urgent need for more robust evidence to populate the cost effectiveness of physical activity models: particularly on the long-term effectiveness of physical activity interventions, maintenance of physical activity levels overtime, long-term health benefits and costs of physical activity. This will enhance the provision of more reliable estimates for decision makers (including international, national and local commissioners) to allocate resources efficiently.

Note

1   The cohort studies controlled for other potential confounders, including: BMI, other types of physical activity, smoking and other morbidities. Given that such RR estimates already accounted for changes in physical activity that occurred during the cohort follow up periods, any further adjustment for changes in physical activity (e.g. decay rates) in the model would amount to double counting because any existing changes associated with PA during the follow-up is already incorporated in the RR estimate.

References

Anokye NK, Lord J, Fox-Rushby J. Is brief advice in primary care a cost-effective way to promote physical activity? *British Journal of Sports Medicine* 2014; **48**(3): 202–6.

Anokye NK, Trueman P, Green C, Pavey TG, Hillsdon M, Taylor RS. The cost-effectiveness of exercise referral schemes. *BMC Public Health* 2011; **11**:954 doi:10.1186/1471-2458-11-954.

Boëhler CEH, Milton KE, Bull FC, *et al.* The cost of changing physical activity behaviour: evidence from a 'physical activity pathway' in the primary care setting. *BMC Public Health* 2011, **11**:370. doi:10.1186/1471-2458-11-370.

Brønnum-Hansen H, Davidsen M, Thorvaldsen P. Long-term survival and causes of death after stroke. *Stroke* 2001; **32**(9): 2131–6.

Campbell F, Blank L, Messina J, *et al. National Institute for Health and Clinical Excellence (NICE) Public Health Intervention Guidance physical activity: BA for adults in primary care. Review of effectiveness, barriers and facilitators evidence.* London: NICE, 2012.

Campbell F, Holmes M, Everson-Hock E *et al.* A systematic review and economic evaluation of exercise referral schemes in primary care: A short report. *Health Technology Assessment*2015; **19**(60): 1–110.

European Union Working Group 'Sport & Health'. *European Union physical activity guidelines: Recommended policy actions in support of health-enhancing physical activity.* Brussels: EU, 2008.

Gonzalez ELM, Johansson S, Wallander MA, *et al.* Trends in the prevalence and incidence of diabetes in the UK, 1996–2005. *Journal of Epidemiology and Community Health* 2009; **63**(4):332–6.

Hu G, Jousilahti P, Borodulin K, *et al.* Occupational, commuting and leisure-time physical activity in relation to coronary heart disease among middle-aged Finnish men and women. *Atherosclerosis* 2007; **194**:490–7.

Hu G, Qiao Q, Silventoinen K, *et al.* Occupational, commuting, and leisure-time physical activity in relation to risk for type 2 diabetes in middle-aged Finnish men and women. *Diabetologia* 2003; **46**:322–29.

Hu G, Sarti C, Jousilahti P, *et al.* Leisure time, occupational, and commuting physical activity and the risk of stroke. *Stroke* 2005; **36**(9):1994–9.

Kelly M, McDaid D, Ludbrook A, *et al. Economic appraisal of public health interventions.*London: London Health Development Agency, National Health System, 2005.

Kelly MP, Morgan A, Ellis S, *et al.* Evidence based public health: A review of the experience of the National Institute of Health and Clinical Excellence (NICE) of developing public health guidance in England. *Social Science and Medicine* 2010; **71**(6):1056–62.

Matrix. *Rapid review of the economic evidence of physical activity interventions.* London: Matrix Knowledge, 2006a.

Matrix. *Modelling the cost-effectiveness of physical activity interventions.* London: Matrix Knowledge, 2006b.

Matrix. *Estimating Return on Investment for interventions and strategies to increase physical activity.* London: Matrix Knowledge, 2014.

National Centre for Social Research, University College London – Department of Epidemiology and Public Health. *Health Survey for England, 2008* [computer file]. *3rd Edition.* Colchester, Essex: UK Data Archive [distributor], July 2011. SN: 6397.

National Clinical Guideline Centre. Hypertension: The clinical management of primary hypertension in adults. Clinical guideline: Methods, evidence and recommendations. London: National Institute for Health and Clinical Excellence, 2011. Ref Type: Report.

National Institute for Health and Care Excellence. Physical activity: Brief advice for adults in primary care. NICE guidelines [PH44]. London: NICE, 2013.

National Institute for Health and Care Excellence (NICE). *Developing NICE guidelines: The manual.* London: NICE, 2014.

Pavey T, Anokye N, Taylor A, *et al.* The effectiveness and cost-effectiveness of exercise referral schemes: A systematic review and economic evaluation. Health Technology Assessment 2011; **15**(44):1–254.

Preis SR, Hwang SJ, Coady S, *et al.* Trends in all-cause and cardiovascular disease mortality among women and men with and without diabetes mellitus in the Framingham Heart Study, 1950 to 2005. *Circulation* 2009; **119**:1728–35.

Preventive Services Task Force. *Behavioural counselling interventions to promote a healthful diet and physical activity for cardiovascular disease prevention in adults: U.S. Preventive Services Task Force Recommendation Statement.* AHRQ Publication No. 11-05149-EF-2. 2012.

Pringle A, Marsh K, Gilson N, *et al.* Cost-effectiveness of interventions to improve moderate physical activity: A study in nine UK sites. *Health Education Journal* 2010; **69**:211–22.

Sorensen JB, Skovgaard T, Puggaard L. Exercise on prescription in general practice: A systematic review. *Scandinavian Journal of Primary Health Care* 2006; **24**(2):69–74.

Vijay GC, Wilson ECF, Suhrcke M, *et al.* Are brief interventions to increase physical activity cost-effective? A systematic review. *British Journal of Sports Medicine* 2015; **50**(7). doi:10.1136/bjsports-2015-094655.

Ward S, Jones ML, Pandor A, *et al. Statins for the prevention of coronary events.* London. National Institute for Clinical Excellence, 2005.

Weatherly H, Drummond H, Claxton K, *et al. Assessing the challenges of applying standard methods of economic evaluation to public health interventions.* York: Centre for Health Economics, 2009.

Williams NH, Hendry M, France B, Lewis R, Wilkinson C. Effectiveness of exercise-referral schemes to promote physical activity in adults: Systematic review. *British Journal of General Practice* 2007; **57**(545):979–86.

World Health Organization. *Interventions on diet and physical activity: What works.* Geneva: World Health Organization, 2009.

World Health Organization. *Physical activity strategy for WHO European Region 2016–2025.* Conpenhagen: World Health Organization, 2016.

32

CYCLING

A path to physical activity through transportation, sport and leisure

Richard J. Buning and Heather J. Gibson

Introduction

"When people ride bikes, great things happen"

Tim Blumenthal
President, PeopleForBikes

Cycling as one of the most popular outdoor recreation activities worldwide is an exemplar of lifetime physical activity enabling individuals to participate for sport, leisure, and/or transportation. A substantive body of knowledge confirms that cycling is a healthy activity that positively influences the regularity of physical activity, decreases obesity rates, improves cardiovascular health, and overall life expectancy and that these benefits far outweigh the risks from injury due to motor vehicle traffic (e.g., Bassett et al., 2008; Fishman, Schepers, & Kamphuis, 2015; Gordon-Larsen et al., 2009; Matthews et al., 2007; Shephard, 2008). Cycling advocates argue cycling participation alleviates the "physical activity crisis" by engaging individuals through competitive sport, recreational activity, and as a form of sustainable and efficient transportation (Birk, 2010; Blue, 2013; Mapes, 2009). This three pronged approach reaches the lifetime physical activity needs of a wide range of individuals and works toward addressing the general lack of physical activity during both leisure and transportation time, which are two of the most problematic areas for public health in the United States (Brownson, Boehmer, & Luke, 2005) and much of the western world (World Health Organization, 2015). Compounding this issue, racial/ethnic minorities and individuals from lower socioeconomic backgrounds historically are the least likely to engage in leisure-time physical activity (Crespo et al., 2000) despite being some of the most frequent bike riders for both recreation and transportation purposes (Breakaway Research Group, 2015). Moreover, class-based social disadvantage is also manifested in the lack of safe bicycling infrastructure such as dedicated bike lanes or bike paths, the presence of which tend to be significantly lower in communities with high proportions of racial minorities and families with lower socioeconomic status (Powell, Slater, & Chaloupka, 2004).

Cycling advocates also argue bicycling can save economies and develop communities by improving overall well-being and public health while decreasing transportation costs and pollution (Birk, 2010; Blue, 2013). Although cycling is an activity that poses valid safety

451

concerns especially with regards to the sharing of roadways with motor vehicles, evidence suggests cycling is a safer alternative to car driving when considering the related health benefits (De Hartog, et al., 2010) and cycling safety improves as cycling participation rises (Jacobsen, 2003). The benefits from cycling also extend outside of physical activity through the economic and social impacts from events and sport tourism and as a sustainable and green alterative to automotive transportation. Cycling provides individuals with important social benefits as individuals are able to bond and create community through a common interest across age groups and levels of involvement especially in regards to events (Buning & Gibson, 2015; Filo, Spence, & Sparvero, 2013; Gibson & Chang, 2012). Further, longitudinal evidence suggests that cycling to work is positively linked with psychological well-being (Martin, Goryakin, & Suhrcke, 2014). The benefits of cycling also extend to environmental impacts as cycling is a pollution free and an environmentally sustainable form of transportation. Indeed, cycling displaces carbon dioxide emissions from motor vehicles, conserves public space, reduces the need to build/service automobiles, and most importantly reduces the use of fossil fuels and the associated pollution (Komanoff et al., 1993). Lastly, cycling positively contributes to economies by reducing automobile transportation costs (Kenworthy & Laube, 1999), reducing oil consumption and carbon emissions (Higgins & Higgins, 2005), reducing health care costs (Rashad, 2007), the economic benefits accruing from cycling facilities (Krizek, 2006), and through sustainable tourism development (Meschik, 2012). However, cycling is not without its drawbacks as poor infrastructure, equipment costs, confrontations with other road users, and a rather homogenous participant demographic (in many countries) potentially inhibit its growth. This chapter will document cycling's connection to physical activity and other related economic, social, and cultural outcomes. Before a discussion of policy issues can be undertaken a wider understanding of cycling participation patterns is needed. Thus, the chapter will first provide background into cycling as leisure, as a competitive sport, and as a form of transportation and discuss the socio-demographic background of cyclists.

Cycling as leisure

The modern bicycle can be traced back to the early 1800s when farmers in southern Germany had difficulty feeding their horses due to a failed harvest creating a necessity that drove the invention of the first "horse replacement vehicle" by a German engineer and inventor (Vivanco, 2013, p. 27). In 1817, The Baron Karl von Drais of Karlsruhe revealed his invention known as the *draisienne* and later called the *velocipede*, or a hobby horse which was a crude form of the modern bicycle. This early machine had no pedals or brakes and required users to run with their legs and earned the nickname "boneshaker" due to the rough ride (Ritichie, 1975; Vivanco, 2013). The next 40 years was full of amateur mechanics attempting to improve the Baron's design, which led to the addition of pedals and the creation of the high wheeler in the late 1860s. The term "bicycle" also entered our vocabulary during this time as the word "velocipeiding" became more ambiguous as increasingly two wheeled designs were described using the words "bicycle" and "bicycling" (Ritchie, 1975). Due to safety concerns, the high wheelers were ultimately replaced by the modern *safety bicycle* in 1885, which featured two equal size wheels, brakes, and eventually pneumatic tires in 1888. As a result the first bicycle boom occurred during the 1890s in the US, France, Britain, and Germany as millions of safety bicycles were manufactured due to industrial advances and demand from the upper and middle classes (Vivanco, 2013).

It was during this time that the first cycle clubs were formed and cycle touring as a recreational activity became a popular pursuit of the more affluent classes. The unique aspect of these clubs was that cycling was a co-ed activity with men and women participating together unchaperoned. Cycling is often credited as providing freedom for women in a number of ways including freedom from social structures, increased geographical mobility, and in the wearing of less restrictive clothing (Ritchie, 1975). The long skirts of the day made it difficult to ride a bicycle and so some women chose to wear bloomers which were regarded as quite shocking in these quite staid Victorian times, although even Queen Victoria herself had a tricycle. The significance of cycling for women during this era is summed up by Susan B. Anthony who said:

> Let me tell you what I think of bicycling. I think it has done more to emancipate women than anything else in the world. It gives women a feeling of freedom and self-reliance. I stand and rejoice every time I see a woman ride by on a wheel . . . the picture of free, untrammelled womanhood.
>
> *Bly, 2014*

Today, cycling for leisure and recreation seems to be gaining popularity once more. A recent report commissioned by Sky and British Cycling suggests that in the UK cycling participation is increasing and cites the expansion of the National Cycle Network, heath concerns, and the success of British elite level cyclists in various world level events as inspiring this surge in the number of people regularly cycling (Grous, 2011). The report lists an estimated 3.7 million cyclists in the UK of which 1.7 million cycle for recreation, 654,000 cycle with their family for leisure and a further 550,000 are avid cyclists listing cycling as a passion. The popularity of the Sky Ride mass participation cycle events is cited as a way of bringing lapsed cyclists back into the sport and educating riders about opportunities in their community to take part in weekly organized rides in their local communities. In the US, the Rails to Trails Conservancy has been active in promoting the development of disused railways into a national network of cycling trails, many of which are used for leisure and tourism. In both the UK and the US, dedicated cycle trails, particularly in scenic areas such as the New Forest in the UK and coastal routes in Florida, encourage recreationists and tourists alike. The Adventure Cycling Association in the US works with state tourism agencies to develop cycling tourism as a viable part of their tourist attractions. Indeed, many states organize annual one week cycling tours that may draw 1,000 riders (e.g., Bike Florida), to the oldest and largest bike tour, the Registers Annual Great Bicycle Ride Across Iowa which was started in 1973 and is capped at 8,500 weeklong riders and has capacity for a further 1,500 day riders (RAGBRAI, 2015). Many of these rides attract participants of all ages and form a bicycle community that convenes year to year with a core of regular participants (Gibson & Chang, 2012). Over the past decade there has also been a proliferation of charity rides where recreational cycling is paired with raising money for various charities. Some of these are short events that range from a few hours to a day, whereas others are multi-day events (Pedaling.com, 2015). Web sites such as Pedaling.com are just one of many world-wide resources for the growing number of cyclists wishing to take part in events, independent, and guided cycle tours.

Cycling as sport

In addition to recreational cycling, competitive participation in the form of bicycle races also grew in popularity during the early years of bicycles. The exact date of the first competitive bike race is open to debate, however, many believe it occurred in Paris in 1868 on a velocipede (Sarig, 1997; Ritchie, 2011). With the invention of pneumatic tires and safety frames largely replacing early high wheeled bikes classic racing events started to flourish. Well-known long standing events including Paris-Brest-Paris and the Paris-Roubaix started in the 1890s and the first modern Olympics games in 1896 included six different cycling events (IOC, 2015; Ritchie, 2011). Many of these early events were overseen by the sport's first international governing body, the International Cycling Association (ICA), which eventually developed into the current international governing body the Union Cycliste Internationale (UCI) in 1900 (UCI, 2015). Now the UCI oversees eight different cycling disciplines and the related world championship events including: road, track, mountain bike, cyclo-cross, bmx, trials, indoor, and para-cycling (UCI, 2015). Cycling as a competitive sport is quite popular in the US and Europe. For example, the US national governing body, USA Cycling, sanctions more than 3,000 events, 2,000 clubs, and has 62,000 licensed members (2013), while their UK counterpart, British Cycling, reported having more than 100,000 members in 2014. Modern elite competitive events such as the Tour de France and the Tour Down Under draw spectators and TV viewers from all over the world.

Cycling as transportation

The invention and development of the bicycle was ultimately driven from the desire to be independent through transportation which led to the creation of the horseless carriage in the 1600s and has evolved through tricycles, high wheelers, and other similar inventions (Ritchie, 1975). The quest to make the activity safer in the late 1800s ultimately led to the creation of the modern triangle frame design still popular today (Ritchie, 1975). Cycling then became a primary and popular method of transportation until motor vehicles became available to the masses in the 1920s, which caused cycling to sharply decline. In developed counties with an emphasis on automobiles, trips by bike comprise a very small portion of overall transportation, whereas countries organized around cycling have vast ridership. For instance, approximately 1.0 per cent of trips are made by bike in the US and 2 per cent in the U.K whereas 26 per cent of trips are made by bike in the Netherlands (Pucher, Buehler, & Seinen, 2011; Ministry of Transport, Public Works and Water Management, 2009). However, cycling as a form of transportation in North America is on the rise and has been described as experiencing a "bicycling renaissance" as more and more people are using bikes as a utilitarian vehicle (Pucher et al., 2011). Based on data from national transportation and travel surveys the total number of bike trips in the US has tripled between 1977 and 2009 (Pucher et al., 2011). Cycling in Canada has also witnessed an increase in popularity as the number of bike commuters has increased by 42 per cent between 1996 and 2006. In some cities the rise of bike commuting has grown rapidly in recent years. For example, cycling as a mode of transportation in Portland, Oregon, an often cited model city for cycling, rose from 1.1 per cent to 5.8 from 1990 to 2008 and now has the highest rate of cycling among all large North American cities (Pucher et al., 2011). However, individuals partake in cycling as transportation disproportionately based on gender and age (Pucher et al., 2011). Thus, the following section will explore the socio-demographic background of cyclists related to transportation, sport, and leisure.

Socio-demographic background of cyclists

Despite the pervasive participation in cycling among all sectors of the population in the early 20th century, today in the low cycling participation countries such as the US, Canada, and the UK there are unequal participation patterns based on gender, age, income, and ethnicity. Although in the early days, cycling initiated a "cosmic shift in women's private and public lives" (Macy, 2011, p. 78), today the vast majority of trips by bike in these countries are made by men. The US Census Bureau reports that more than twice as many males commute to work via bicycle compared to females (McKenzie, 2014). Based on data from the National Household Travel Survey, men take 1.6 per cent of all trips by bike whereas women only take 0.5 per cent of all trips by bike in the US (Pucher et al., 2011). Further, the percentage of people who rode a bike within the last 12 months for both recreation and transportation was higher for men in the US (Breakaway Research Group, 2015). The UK is quite similar as males make three times as many cycle trips as women and ride four times as many miles according to the National Travel Survey (UK Department for Transport, 2014a). Competitive cycling is also largely dominated by male participants with women constituting 14 per cent of competitive cyclists in the US and 15 per cent in the UK (British Cycling, 2014; Larson, 2013). However, as noted by Heinen, Van Wee, & Maat (2010), while this gender imbalance may be present in countries with overall low cycling rates, in countries with overall high cycling levels (e.g., Netherlands), cycling participation by gender is more equal (Garrard, Rose, & Lo, 2008). These differential participation rates among men and women are likely due in part to perceived and actual cyclist safety (Garrard et al., 2008; Pucher et al., 2011). Certainly, in an analysis of six western US cities Emond, Tang, and Handy (2009) note that gender differences and cycling use are related to perceptions of bicycling safety combined with the type of bicycle infrastructure being used. The authors conclude by explaining "the high rates of bicycling for women in other countries suggest much room for improvement in the United States" (Emond et al., 2009, p. 23). Another possible reason for these unequal participation patterns in cycling by gender relates back to general sport participation patterns where women and girls generally are less physically active than their male counterparts, a pattern that may also extend over into a physically active pursuit such as cycling (Azevedo et al., 2007).

Regarding age, the general trend is a slight decline in cycling participation with age (e.g., Moudon et al., 2005; Pucher, Komanoff, & Schimek, 1999). US transportation estimates suggest those aged 5–15 years take the highest proportion of bike trips, and individuals aged 65 and older take the fewest bike trips (Pucher et al., 2011). However, Pucher et al. (2011) note the largest growth in cycling from 2001 to 2009 was amongst the 40–64 age group, which more than doubled its proportion of all bike trips. Some older adults due to health limitations may be sometimes unable to operate a bicycle and they generally consider their age as a reason not to cycle (Lohmann & Rölle, 2005). Certainly, the relatively low impact of cycling provides an opportunity from all ages and abilities to participate.

Cycling and income have a mixed relationship as conflicting studies suggest that the connection between income and cycling rates are either positive, negative or non-significant (Heinen et al., 2010). According to Pucher et al. (2011), in 2001 almost no differences were present between income groups based on cycling ridership, where in 2009 those with the lowest annual income reported the highest cycling level. Foreseeably those that have lower incomes and do not have access to a motor vehicle are more dependent on cycling as transportation, while those that have higher incomes are able to spend more on their health and leisure enabling them to purchase and maintain a bicycle. Evidence generally suggests that lower income individuals predominately cycle for transportation, while higher income groups cycle more for recreation, exercise, and competition (Heinen et al., 2010; Smart, 2010). Still, those that have higher incomes likely spend more on transportation and thus own and maintain a motor vehicle (Witlox & Tindemans, 2004). Evidence suggests that decreasing car ownership leads to increased bicycle ridership (e.g., Pucher & Buehler, 2008; Pucher et al., 2011; Stinson & Bhat, 2005), which creates an impediment to cycling for transportation as those with higher income are less motivated to cycle by necessity.

Conflicting evidence on ethnicity and cycling rates is also reported based on the study and type of cycling activity being investigated. Pucher et al. (2011) note that non-Hispanic whites have the highest share of bike trips, which account for 77 per cent of all bike trips in the US. Other US based evidence suggest that Hispanics are the most likely to have ridden a bicycle in the past year for both recreation and transportation (Breakaway Research Group, 2015).

Facilitators and barriers

There are a number of factors that can be identified that either facilitate or present barriers to cycling participation, however, these must also be contextualized within the wider social and political processes related to cycling in a region or country. The general assumption behind policies to increase participation in cycling as a form of transportation is a "build it and they will come" approach. As described by the former City of Portland Bicycle Program Manager, Mia Birk, "people will not drive in the river where no bridge exists, wait by the side of the road for a nonexistent bus, or walk on streets lacking sidewalks . . . similarly, few people will bike where no bikeways exist" (Birk, 2010, p. 25). Namely, by increasing opportunities and spaces for bicycle travel individuals will more likely participate. For cycling to become a viable and attractive form of transportation for residents of countries with lower cycling participation rates such as the US and the UK a multifaceted approach that integrates and creates cycling facilities, traffic control, education, promotion, policies, and programs is required (Pucher & Buehler, 2008). Similarly, by creating and maintaining cycling infrastructure, programs, and interventions while reducing barriers individuals will be more likely and willing to cycle for sport and leisure as well (e.g., Freeman & Thomlinson, 2014; Lamont & Buultjens, 2011). Thus, the next section will outline the various facilitators and barriers to cycling participation.

Cycling infrastructure

By far the primary approach to encourage cycling is through the construction and maintenance of cycling infrastructure such as bike lanes and paths. Numerous studies support the idea that a positive correlation exists between the presence of bike paths and lanes and cycling usage even when controlling for factors such as climate, income, and automobile ownership (e.g., Dill & Carr, 2003; Moudon et al., 2005; Nelson & Allen, 1997; Parkin, Warman, & Page, 2008; Pucher et al., 2010). For instance, individuals that live under a half a mile away from a bike path are at least 20 per cent more likely to ride a bicycle than individuals that live more than one to one and half miles away (Moudon et al., 2005). Further, evidence suggests that by building cycling infrastructure cyclist safety increases which leads to increased overall ridership (Elvik, 2009; Jacobsen, 2003). Bicycle infrastructure designed to encourage cycling with published support of their effectiveness includes the following (adapted from Pucher et al. (2010):

- *On-road bicycle lanes*: stripes on the margin of roads, some are coloured.
- *Contraflow bike lanes*: bidirectional travel on one-way streets allowing cyclists to ride in a protected lane against one-way traffic.
- *Cycle tracks*: similar to bike lanes, but include a physical barrier between lanes with curbs, vehicle parking, etc.
- *Off-street paths*: often labelled as a trail, are shared use, separate from motor vehicle traffic, and are bidirectional.
- *Signed bicycle routes*: shared roadways that adorn signage for preferred cycling routes.
- *Sharrows*: arrows painted on roads indicating the road is shared by cyclists and motorists.

- *Bicycle traffic signals*: specially timed traffic lights allowing cyclists to gain a head start through intersections.
- *Bike boxes*: painted areas in front of motor vehicle lanes at signalled intersections that allow for cyclists' visibility.
- *Bicycle boulevards*: signed bicycle routes on streets with low traffic and often encompassing traffic calming features to slow vehicular traffic.
- *Traffic calming*: physical changes to streets that are intended to slow motor vehicle traffic examples include speed bumps, slow speed limits, traffic circles, trees, benches, etc.
- *Car-free zones*: often referred to as *ciclovía*, a section of street or neighbourhood temporary closed to motor vehicle traffic. Also, constructed as permanent pedestrian malls and car-free neighbourhoods.
- *Public transit integration*: racks on buses, bike parking at transit stations (bus and rail), bike storage on ferries and rail cars, and short term bike rental.
- *End-of-trip facilities*: bike parking (general, guarded, lockers, and sheltered bike racks) shower facilities at workplaces, bicycle stations offering repair, storage, rentals, and showers often located near transit stations or in urban commercial areas.

Compounding the need for increased cycling infrastructure, research into the characteristics of cyclist and non-cyclists demonstrate that cyclists are more likely to engage in physical activity and exercise at home and report a higher level of perceived health (Moudon et al., 2005). Evidence from the Netherlands also suggests that many individuals are able to meet recommended levels of physical activity simply by cycling to work (Engbers & Hendriksen, 2010). The need for improved infrastructure is critical as 46 per cent of adults in the US would be more likely to cycle if they were physically separated from vehicles, while only 31 per cent are satisfied with the current bike lanes, paths, and trails available (Breakaway Research Group, 2015). Improving cycling infrastructure is critical to attracting new individuals to cycling as inexperienced individuals are far more concerned with paths that provide a physical separation from automobile traffic than more experienced cyclists (Stinson & Bhat, 2005). Studies also demonstrate that building cycling infrastructure is important for tourism as tourists are willing to increase their travel time by 100 per cent in order to cycle on a path completely segregated from motor vehicle traffic and by 40–50 per cent to cycle in a bike lane (Deenihan & Caulfield, 2015). Further, research suggests some cycling infrastructure does not accomplish its intended goals as a US study found that "Share the Road" signs do not increase driver comprehension or perceptions of safety for cyclists (Hess & Peterson, 2015). Thus, not only is cycling infrastructure needed, the overall effectiveness of current infrastructure programs should be critically assessed.

Cycling interventions

Many communities and advocacy groups have supplemented the construction of cycling specific infrastructure with programs and legal assistance aimed at promoting cycling participation. As outlined by Pucher et al. (2010), interventions exist as general travel programs, bicycling specific programs, bicycle access programs, and legal interventions. The most common strategy seems to be general travel awareness programs created to reduce motor vehicle traffic and increase public transit, walking, and bicycling (Pucher et al., 2010). These programs typically are implemented by local municipalities or community groups. Similar interventions include employer based trip-reduction programs and safe routes to school programs. The safe routes to school program provides infrastructure, education, and reinforcement to increase walking and cycling to school and has been quite effective at increasing walking, but seems to have only marginally increased cycling trips in the US (Safe Routes, 2015). Still, the US program reports over a six year period ending in 2013 that parents believed their child's school supported walking and bicycling at a rate of 24.8 per cent to 38 per cent. Other interventions that are bicycle specific include bike-to-work days, promotional programs, and educational programs. For instance, the US based organization The League of American Bicyclists (LAB) creates educational programs and certifies trainers to teach kids and adults the skills necessary to safely operate a bicycle. Promotional programs are wide ranging, from the People for Bikes' National Bike Challenge, a nationwide event encouraging cyclists to ride and record their miles ridden, to the LAB's bicycle friendly community program aimed at recognizing communities that integrate cycling through engineering, education, encouragement, enforcement, and evaluation/planning.

Interventions are also aimed at increasing access and providing legal support. To increase access, many communities have installed public bicycle sharing programs that offer low cost short-term bike rentals that can be picked and returned to docking stations throughout urban areas. Beginning in the 1960s in Amsterdam as a free service, modern systems use technology to track and provide secure access to the bikes. A recent study by Fuller et al. (2013) suggests the implementation of a public bicycling share program leads to a significant increase in cycling among people living in the installed area when controlling for weather, environment, and other individual variables. Other interventions to increase cycling have focused on legal issues such as helmet laws and reducing the speed limits to vehicular traffic. Overall, the most effective programs to increase cycling are those that integrate complementary interventions that include infrastructure, promotional bicycle programs, land use planning support, and car use restrictions (Pucher et al., 2010).

Barriers to cycling

Although infrastructure and interventions have been created to increase cycling participation a number of barriers exist that prevent individuals from partaking in the activity. From a study of cyclists and non-cyclists in the Netherlands the primary barriers for biking to work identified by non-cyclists included perspiration when arriving at work, weather, and travel time (Engbers & Hendriksen, 2010). Based on Australian evidence, a study by Lamont and Buultjens (2011) identified three primary impediments for the development of cycling tourism as consisting of cyclist perception of road safety, inadequate physical infrastructure/support, and difficulty transporting bicycles on public transit. Road safety concerns were manifested as cyclists' statutory rights (i.e., shared use of roadways) and the power imbalance between motorists and cyclists which creates a culture of disrespect towards cyclists. The infrastructure/support impediment consisted of five factors: physical infrastructure (e.g., trails, road shoulder widths), amenities (e.g., water, bathroom access), cycling services (e.g., storage facilities, rentals facilities), motorist attitudes, and information services (e.g., cycling websites, guided tours). Indeed, access to land for cycle paths and trails for recreation and tourism is a commonly raised, for all types of cycling especially for mountain biking, which often has to compete with government officials and private landowners for land access (International Mountain Bike Association, 2012). The final impediment discussed by Lamont and Buultjens (2011) and is one that is rather unique to cycling tourism is the carriage of bikes on air, bus, and rail services. Air services provide the biggest challenge as airlines often are inconsistent with the administration of excess baggage fees for bikes. The fees and related polices vary based on the different airlines and the decision to charge an excess baggage fee will often be based on the individual staff member checking the baggage, which is a serious obstacle as airlines charge between $100 to $300 each way (Elliot, 2014). The highest priority items for the cyclists surveyed by Lamont and Buultjens (2011) were the creation of dedicated bike paths/lanes, education of motorists, and wide/sealed/consistent road shoulders.

Road user conflict

A commonly cited barrier to all cyclists using shared roadways is conflict with the drivers of motor vehicles. Most cyclists at one point or another have had a run in with an angry or distracted motorist as Elly Blue explains an incident while riding: "'Get off the road' - "at least, I think that's what the woman yelled at me . . . I've heard those words before, though, or their more profane variations" (Blue, 2013, p.76). In some cases, this conflict has led to disastrous results, with cyclists being injured or killed due to motorists' purposeful or reckless driving. Often cyclists have little recourse if struck by a vehicle even if the driver was cited for a traffic violation. A landmark case that received considerable national and international coverage occurred when a California physician purposely used his car to attack a group of cyclists on two different occasions, with the final incident leading to severe injuries for two of the cyclists as they collided with his car (Pelkey, 2010). The driver was ultimately convicted of six felonies and a misdemeanour for the incidents, but many cyclists were outraged by the incidents and the lenient sentence imposed.

Road user conflicts are all too common as over 700 bicyclists were killed in the US in 2013 by motor vehicle crashes according to the Governors Highway Safety Association (Williams, 2014). Cyclist deaths and injuries from car crashes are not uniquely a problem for the USA, as the UK Department for Transport (2014b) reports that 109 cyclists were killed and 19,438 cyclists were injured in car accidents in 2013. Unfortunately, cyclists face an elevated risk of injury when involved in a crash with a motor vehicle, while motorists are not; thus cyclists are often classified as *vulnerable road users*. Generally, the association between cyclist fatalities and ridership is negative as the proportion of trips made by bike increases the safer cycling becomes, suggesting "safety is in the numbers" (Elvik, 2009; Jacobsen, 2003; Pucher et al., 2011). Thus, this relationship can be considered bidirectional by increasing cycling safety more individuals are encouraged to ride and by having more cyclists on the road overall cycling safety improves. Further, vast evidence confirms that perceived and actual danger imposed by motor vehicle traffic discourages individuals from cycling (Jacobsen, Racioppi, & Rutter, 2009). Indeed, bicycling on cycle tracks is less risky than cycling on roads shared with motor vehicles (Lusk et al., 2011). Risk aversion varies by gender though as women more than men are concerned with risk aversion and more strongly prefer cycling routes with maximum separation from motor vehicle traffic (Garrard et al., 2008; Lamont & Buultjens, 2011). Thus, improving cycling infrastructure and driver education is not only important for cyclist safety, but for increasing overall ridership especially among population groups where cycling participation is historically low.

Another issue that has manifested itself in the conflict between cyclists and motor vehicle users is the myth that cyclists do not pay to use the roads (Blue, 2013). Motor vehicle users commonly pay various road taxes including tax on their vehicles and fuel tax. This perceived inequity in the payment of taxes by the two user groups is a commonly cited argument by motorists as to why they should have priority in road usage over cyclists. In fact, in Gainesville, Florida a local government official proposed adding a usage fee/license for cyclists to use the roads (Curry & Alcantara, 2014). Yet many who use this argument fail to recognize that cyclists are also motorists, but they choose to sometimes use their bikes instead of their cars.

Implications for future physical activity policy and practice

In reviewing cycling participation patterns across different countries, it appears all is not equal. As noted previously, there are countries such as the Netherlands where cycling is integrated into everyday life. Dedicated cycling paths criss-cross the major cities and pedestrians and cyclists are urged to share the space. Mass cycling racks are located outside of public buildings and transportation hubs such as train stations. Thus, the obvious direction for policy should be to use these bicycle intensive countries as role models. But this is a simplistic approach as advocated by Pucher & Buehler (2008). Certainly much can be learned from these high cycle participation countries, but role modelling and policy change along will only go so far. The biggest barrier appears to be a cultural shift from one that views motorized transportation, namely the car, as the preferred mode for not only getting around, but in many regions of the US is regarded as having priority usage over the roads. For example, in Gainesville, Florida, a university town of about 125,000 people and roads that average between 25 and 45 miles per hour, various attempts have been made to make the city more cycle friendly and to entice the populace to ride their bikes both for transportation and leisure. However, in reading the local newspaper on any week, you will see letters to the editor admonishing the local government for spending money on bicycle lanes or restructuring roads so that bikes have priority. Eventually, most of these cycle friendly experiments in Gainesville have been abandoned and the roads have been turned back over to the cars. In the UK, 50 years ago a majority of the population, young and old, cycled to work, to school and for recreation. Yet, while the UK has witnessed an increase in recreational cycling over the past ten years (Dirs, 2014), the country has also seen a decline in cycling for transport and a rise in car ownership (Fisher, 2012). Thus, while policy can encourage the development of cycling infrastructure and engage in public health campaigns to encourage more people to cycle, the biggest challenge appears to be a cultural shift to one where the bicycle is an everyday choice for transportation and leisure and car drivers willingly share the road.

References

Azevedo, M. R., Araujo, C. L. P., Reichert, F. F., Siqueira, F. V., da Silva, M. C., & Hallal, P. C. (2007) Gender differences in leisure-time physical activity. *International Journal of Public Health*, *52*(1), 8–15.

Bassett, D., Pucher, J., Buehler, R., Thompson, D., & Crouter, S. (2008) Walking, cycling, and obesity rates in Europe, North America, and Australia. *Journal of Physical Activity Health*, *5*(6), 795–814.

Birk, M. (2010) *Joyride: Pedalling toward a healthier planet.* Portland, OR: Cadence Press.

Blue, E. (2013) *Bikenomics: How bicycling can save the economy.* Portland, OR: Microcosm Publishing.

Bly, N. (2014) Champion of her sex: Miss Susan B. Anthony. In Lutes, J. (ed.). *Around the World in Seventy-Two Days and Other Writings.* New York, NY: Penguin Group.

Breakaway Research Group (2015) U.S. bicycling participation benchmarking study report. www. peopleforbikes.org /pages/u.s.-bicycling-participation-benchmarking-report [Accessed 29 August 2017].

British Cycling. (2014) *British Cycling annual report 2014.* www.british cycling.org.uk/zuvvi/media/ bc_files/corporate/BC_ANNUAL_REPORT_2014_FINAL_DIGITAL.pdf [Accessed: 1 October 2015].

Brownson, R. C., Boehmer, T. K., & Luke, D. A. (2005) Declining rates of physical activity in the United States: What are the contributors? *Annual Review of Public Health*, *26*, 421–443.

Buning, R., & Gibson, H. (2015) The evolution of active-sport-event travel careers. *Journal of Sport Management*, *29*(5), 555–569.

Crespo, C. J., Smit, E., Andersen, R. E., Carter-Pokras, O., & Ainsworth, B. E. (2000) Race/ethnicity, social class and their relation to physical inactivity during leisure time: results from the third national health and nutrition examination survey, 1988–1994. *American Journal of Preventive Medicine*, *18*(1), 46–53.

Curry, C. & Alcantara, C. (2014) Hinson-Rawls thinks city should require bike licenses. *Gainesville Sun* April 8, 2014. www.gainesville.com/article/20140408/ ARTICLES/140409657/0/search [Accessed: 26 October 2015].

Deenihan, G., & Caulfield, B. (2015) Do tourists value different levels of cycling infrastructure? *Tourism Management*, *46*, 92–101.

De Hartog, J. J., Boogaard, H., Nijland, H., & Hoek, G. (2010) Do the health benefits of cycling outweigh the risks? *Environmental Health Perspectives*, *118*(8), 1109–1116.

Dill, J. and Carr, T. (2003) Bicycle commuting and facilities in major U.S. cities: If you build them, commuters will use them. *Transportation Research: Part B*, *1828*, 116–123.

Dirs, B. (2014) Is the newly 'cool' sport of cycling really the new golf? www.bbc.com/sport/0/golf/30422698 [Accessed: 29 October 2015].

Elliot, C. (2014) Airlines change gears on passengers flying with bikes. *The Washington Post*. 12 June. www.washingtonpost.com/lifestyle/travel /airlines-change-gears-on-passengers-flying-with-bikes/2014/06/12/a4d2af42-edc3-11e3-b84b-3393a45b80f1_story.html [Accessed: 20 October 2015].

Elvik, R. (2009) The non-linearity of risk and the promotion of environmentally sustainable transport. *Accident Analysis and Prevention*, *41*(4), 849–855.

Emond, C. R., Tang, W., & Handy, S. L. (2009) Explaining gender difference in bicycling behaviour. *Transportation Research Record*, *2125*, 16–25.

Engbers, L. H., & Hendriksen, I. J. (2010) Characteristics of a population of commuter cyclists in the Netherlands: Perceived barriers and facilitators in the personal, social and physical environment. *International Journal of Behavioral Nutrition and Physical Activity*, *7*, 1–5.

Filo, K., Spence, K., & Sparvero, E. (2013) Exploring the properties of community among charity sport event participants. *Managing Leisure*, *18*(3), 194–212.

Fisher, M. (2012) It's official: Western Europeans have more cars than Americans. www.theatlantic.com/international/archive/2012/08/its-official-western-europeans-have-more-cars-per-person-than-americans/261108/ [Accessed: 29 October 2015].

Fishman, E., Schepers, P., & Kamphuis, C. B. (2015) Dutch cycling: Quantifying the health and related economic benefits. *American Journal of Public Health*, *105*(8), 13–15.

Freeman, R., & Thomlinson, E. (2014) Mountain bike tourism and community development in British Columbia: Critical success factors for the future. *Tourism Review International*, *18*(1), 9–22.

Fuller, D., Gauvin, L. F., Kestens, Y. F., Daniel, M. F., Fournier, M. F., Morency, P. F., & Drouin, L. (2013) Impact evaluation of a public bicycle share program on cycling: A case example of BIXI in Montreal, Quebec. *American Journal of Public Health*, *103*(3), 85–92.

Garrard, J., Rose, G., & Lo, S. K. (2008) Promoting transportation cycling for women: The role of bicycle infrastructure. *Preventive Medicine*, *46*(1), 55–59.

Gibson, H. J., & Chang, S. (2012) Cycling in mid and later life: Involvement and benefits sought from a bicycle tour. *Journal of Leisure Research*, *44*(1), 23–51.

Gordon-Larsen, P., Boone-Heinonen, J., Sidney, S., Sternfeld, B., Jacobs, D., & Lewis, C. (2009) Active commuting and cardiovascular disease risk: The CARDIA study. *Archives of Internal Medicine*, *169*(13), 1216–1223.

Grous, A. (2011) *The British cycling economy: 'Gross cycling product' report.* www.britishcycling.org.uk/zuvvi/media/bc_files/corporate/The_British_Cycling_Economy_18Aug.pdf [Accessed: 26 October 2015].

Heinen, E., Van Wee, B., & Maat, K. (2010) Commuting by bicycle: An overview of the literature. *Transport Reviews*, *30*(1), 59–96.

Hess G., & Peterson M. N. (2015) "Bicycles may use full lane" signage communicates U.S. roadway rules and increases perception of safety. *PLoS ONE*, *10*(8), 1–16.

Higgins, P, & Higgins, M. (2005) A healthy reduction in oil consumption and carbon emissions. *Energy Policy*, *33*(1), 1–4.

International Mountain Bike Association. (2012) Bicycle leadership conference report an update in IMBA's public lands initiative for the bicycle industry. http://issuu.com/imbapublications/docs/2012_blc_reportprintable [Accessed: 10 October 2015].

International Olympic Committee (IOC). (2015) *Athens 1896: Cycling.* http:// www.olympic.org/content/news/all-news-groups/athens-1896/ [Accessed: 15 September 2015].

Jacobsen, J. L., Racioppi, F., & Rutter, H. (2009). Who owns the road? How motorised traffic discourages walking and bicycling. *Injury Prevention*, *15*(6), 369–373.

Jacobsen, P. (2003) Safety in numbers: More walkers and bicyclists, safer walking and bicycling. *Injury Prevention, 9*(3), 205–209.

Kenworthy, J. R., & Laube, F. B. (1999) Patterns of automobile dependence in cities: An international overview of key physical and economic dimensions with some implications for urban policy. *Transportation Research Part A, 33*(7–8), 691–723.

Komanoff, C., Roelofs, C., Orcutt, J., & Ketcham, B. (1993) Environmental benefits of bicycling and walking in the United States. *Transportation Research Record, 1405*, 7–12.

Krizek, K. J. (2006) Two approaches to valuing some of bicycle facilities' presumed benefits. *Journal of the American Planning Association, 72*(3), 309–320.

Lamont, M., & Buultjens, J. (2011) Putting the brakes on: Impediments to the development of independent cycle tourism in Australia. *Current Issues in Tourism, 14*(1), 57–78.

Larson, D. (2013) *USA Cycling membership survey and analysis.* https://s3.amazonaws.com/USACWeb/forms/encyc/2013-USAC-Membership-Survey-Report.pdf [Accessed: 15 September 2015].

Lohmann, G., & Rölle, D. (2005) "I would ride a bicycle, but . . .!" Changes in transport use in from the background of the ipsative theory of behavior. *Umweltpsychologi [Ecopsychology], 9*(1), 46–61.

Lusk, A. C., Furth, P. G., Morency, P., Miranda-Moreno, L. F., Willett, W. C., & Dennerlein, J. T. (2011) Risk of injury for bicycling on cycle tracks versus in the street. *Injury Prevention, 17*(2), 131–135.

Macy, S. (2011) *Wheels of change: How women road the bicycle to freedom.* Washington, D.C.: National Geographic Society.

Mapes, J. (2009) *Pedalling revolution: How cyclists are changing American cities.* Corvallis, OR: Oregon State University Press.

Martin, A., Goryakin, Y., & Suhrcke, M. (2014) Does active commuting improve psychological well-being? Longitudinal evidence from eighteen waves of the British Household Panel Survey. *Preventive Medicine, 69*, 296–303.

Matthews, C., Jurj, A., Shu, X., Hong-Lan, L., Yang, G., Li, Q., Yu-Tang, G., & Zheng, W. (2007) Influence of exercise, walking, cycling, and overall nonexercise physical activity on mortality in Chinese women. *American Journal of Epidemiology, 165*(12), 1343–1350.

McKenzie, B. (2014) *Modes less travelled – Bicycling and walking to work in the United States: 2008–2012.* www.census.gov/prod/2014 pubs/acs25.pdf [Accessed: 1 September 2015].

Meschik, M. (2012) Sustainable cycle tourism along the Danube cycle route in Austria. *Tourism Planning & Development, 9*(1), 41–56.

Ministry of Transport, Public Works and Water Management. (2009) *Cycling in the Netherlands.* www.fietsberaad.nl/library/repository/bestanden/ CyclingintheNetherlands2009.pdf [Accessed: 20 October 2015].

Moudon, A., Lee, C., Cheadle, A., Collier, C., Johnson, D., Scmid, T., & Weather, R. D. (2005) Cycling and the built environment, a US perspective. *Transportation Research Part D, 10*(3), 245–261.

Nelson, A., & Allen, D. (1997) If you build them, commuters will use them. *Transportation Research Record, 1578*, 79–83.

Parkin, J., Wardman, M., & Page, M. (2008) Estimation of the determinants of bicycle mode share for the journey to work using census data. *Transportation, 35*(1), 93–109.

Pedaling.com. (2015) *Bike routes and rides, cycling tours and events, cycling resources.* www.pedaling.com/ [Accessed: 26 October 2015].

Pelkey, C. (2010, January) L.A. road rage doctor gets five years. *Velonews.* http://velonews.competitor.com/2010/01/news/l-a-road-rage-doctor-gets-five-years_102274 [Accessed: 15 September 2015].

Powell, L. M., Slater, S., & Chaloupka, F. J. (2004) Race/ethnicity, social class and their relation to physical inactivity during leisure time: Results from the third national health and nutrition examination survey, 1988–1994. *Evidence-Based Preventive Medicine, 1*(2), 135–144.

Pucher, J., & Buehler, R. (2008) Making cycling irresistible: Lessons from the Netherlands, Denmark and Germany. *Transport Reviews, 28*(4), 495–528.

Pucher, J., Buehler, R., Bassett, DR., & Dannenberg, AL. (2010). Walking and cycling to health: a comparative analysis of city, state, and international data, *American Journal of Public Health, 100*, 1986–1992.

Pucher, J., Buehler, R., & Seinen, M. (2011) Bicycling renaissance in North America? An update and re-appraisal of cycling trends and policies. *Transportation Research Part A, 45*(6), 451–475.

Pucher, J., Komanoff, C., & Schimek, P. (1999) Bicycling renaissance in North America? Recent trends and alternative policies to promote bicycling. *Transportation Research Part A, 33*(7/8), 625–654.

RAGBRAI. (2015) The Register's *Annual Great Bicycle Ride Across Iowa.* http://ragbrai.com/ [Accessed: 26 October 2015].

Rashad, I. (2007) *Cycling: An increasingly untouched source of physical and mental health.* National Bureau of Economic Research Working Paper no. 12929.

Ritchie, A. (1975) *King of the road: An illustrated history of cycling.* Berkley, CA: Ten Speed Press.

Ritchie, A. (2011) *Quest for speed: A history of early bicycle racing 1868–1903.* San Francisco, CA: Cycle Publishing.

Safe Routes. (2015) *Trends in walking and bicycling to school from 2007 to 2013.* http://saferoutesinfo.org/ sites /default/files/SurveyTrends_2007-13_final1.pdf [Accessed: 10 September 2015].

Sarig, R. (1997) *The everything bicycle book: A freewheeling collection of bike know-how-from buying and maintaining to exercising and touring.* Holbrook, MA: Adams Media Corporation.

Shephard, R. (2008) Is active commuting the answer to population health? *Sports Medicine, 39*(9), 751–758.

Smart, M. (2010) US Immigrants and bicycling: Two-wheeled in autopia. *Transport Policy, 17*(3), 153–159.

Stinson, M. A., & Bhat, C. R. (2005) A comparison of the route preferences of experienced and inexperienced bicycle commuters. Transportation Research Board 84th Annual Meeting, Washington D.C., January 2005.

UK Department for Transport. (2014a) *National Travel Survey* (Publication No. 0601 and 0605). www. gov.uk/government/statistical-data-sets/nts06-age-gender-and-modal-breakdown#table-nts0601 [Accessed: 10 September 2015].

UK Department for Transport. (2014b) *Reported road casualties in Great Britain: 2013 Annual Report Focus on Pedal Cyclists.* https://www.gov.uk/government/ uploads/system/uploads/attachment_data/ file/358042/rrcgb2013-02.pdf [Accessed: 10 September 2015].

Union Cycliste Internationale (UCI). (2015) *About: History.* www.uci.ch/inside-uci/about/history/ [Accessed: 1 September 2015].

Vivanco, L. A. (2013) *Reconsidering the bicycle: An anthropological perspective on a new old thing.* New York, NY: Routledge.

Williams, A. (2014) *Bicyclist safety.* www.ghsa.org/html/files/pubs/spotlights/bikes_2014.pdf [Accessed: 10 September 2015].

Witlox, F., & Tindemans, H. (2004) Evaluating bicycle-car transport mode competitiveness in an urban environment: An activity-based approach. *World Transport Policy and Practice, 10*(4), 32–42.

World Health Organization. (2015) *Physical activity fact sheet.* www.who.int/mediacentre/factsheets/ fs385/en/ [Accessed: 1 September 2015].

33

WILL TO WIN

The darker side of elite swimming

Jenny McMahon

Access to sport and physical activity is a fundamental human right. According to The United Nations Sport for Development and Peace (2011), sport is a culturally accepted activity that brings people together and unites families, communities and nations. It is no surprise that sport has been found to contribute to a variety of positive outcomes such as improved health, a sense of achievement, teamwork, social inclusion, improved self-esteem, social capital and fair play (Cronin & Armour, 2015; Eime et al., 2013; Kavanagh, 2014). From a socioeconomic perspective, sport participation has been shown to benefit the economy by reducing ill health associated costs (Bloom, Grant & Watt, 2005; Cameron, Craig & Beaulieu, 2000; Katzmarysk, Gledhill & Shephard, 2000).

In recent years, a large number of elite athletes have been presented as "faces" of healthy eating and physical activity as a means of fighting the obesity epidemic (i.e. Kobe Bryant [basketball]; Dwight Howard [basketball]; Stephanie Rice [swimming]; Sharon Miller [gymnastics]; Michael Phelps [swimming]). While elite athletes may be viewed as the ultimate figures of healthy eating and physical activity, what has been generally overlooked is the negative effects associated with sport participation, in particular how sport may come to impact upon participants' health, wellbeing and engagement in physical activity both in the short term and also long term. A growing number of recent studies have contributed to the evidence associating sport with various detrimental effects such as emotional and physical harm (McPherson et al., 2015); physical and sexual abuse (Brackenridge, 2006); long term injury (Barker-Ruchti & Tinning, 2010); disordered eating; body dissatisfaction; depression and fractured identities (McMahon & Barker-Ruchti, 2015; Walters et al., 2015; Kavanagh, 2014; McMahon, Penney & Dinan-Thompson, 2012; Lang, 2010; Anderson, 2010; David, 2005; Jones, Glintmeyer & McKenzie, 2005; Hoberman, 1992).

In the chapter that follows, the darker side of sport will be explored. Three key but interrelated aspects will form the basis of this chapter and in so doing, the chapter will be formatted according to these sections drawing on various relevant scholarly literature throughout. First, the "why" and "how" of dominant ideologies and practices prevalent in elite sporting contexts will be explored. Then, a number of studies will be drawn upon to highlight how ideologies and practices have come to affect athletes both in the short term and also long term. While a large section of this chapter is focussed on the sport of swimming and specifically the elite context, literature and practices occurring in other sporting contexts will also be drawn upon to highlight how sport more broadly can have negative consequences for athletes or sporting participants at all levels. This latter point is significant, particularly as it was revealed in the research of McMahon et al. (2012) that dominant ideologies and practices occurring in elite swimming were indeed permeating the amateur and community sport contexts with both short term and long term detrimental effects.

Dominant ideologies and practices in [elite] sport: Why and how

Vince Lombardi, a pro footballer's famous statement, "winning isn't everything, it is the only thing," encapsulates the meritocractic ideology, a notion that continues to pervade sporting contexts at all levels. Terms such as "moral victory," "personal victory" and "being robbed of victory" exemplify the importance of meritocracy in sport at a micro level. It is also exemplified in any sporting environment where sporting participants are rewarded for their ability to produce and perform. Such rewards may include (but are not limited to): social rewards; being chosen on teams because of their sporting talent or ability to score; financial incentives or through the distribution of medals and trophies. This is because winning/losing, knowing how to play the game or perfect the necessary skills needed to participate successfully in a particular activity have become a major focus of sport. The importance placed on meritocracy at a macro level is exemplified through government funding policies (i.e. Australia's Winning Edge: 2012–2022). Another such example was the massive cash injection that Olympic sports in the United Kingdom received in the lead up to 2012 Olympics when London won its bid to host the Games. UK Sport's funding was increased from £70 million for the 2004 Athens Games to £264 million in the lead up to London 2012 with the intention of winning a greater amount of medals. As a result of this extra £165m funding, an additional 17 more medals were achieved and Great Britain left the Summer Olympic Games with a total of 65 medals (29 gold, 17 silver and 19 bronze) finishing third in the medal table rankings (BBC Sports, 2012).

Meritocracy in sport is by no means a new revelation as it has been long argued that coaches, team managers and committees in various sporting programs from the elite to community youth sports place an emphasis on effort and achievement (McMahon & Dinan Thompson, 2008; Fine, 1987; Dubois, 1986; Bain, 1990; Coakley, 1995). Kyle (2015) explains that as a result of meritocracy, athletes have come to be judged on their athletic merit and in so doing, meritocracy has fuelled technocentric ideologies in sport where athletes' bodies are seen as valuable commodities in order to achieve meritocratic ideals (i.e. competitive performance).

The technocentric ideology in sport is when athletes are "viewed as instruments and objects for manipulation" (Bain, 1990, p. 29) in order to achieve competitive success. Bain (1990, p. 29) uses the analogy "of the coach or choreographer treating the athlete or dancer as an instrument with which to achieve the desired performance." As such, the athlete "learns to view his or her body as an instrument to be trained, manipulated and in some cases drugged for the sake of performance". More recently, the voice of Leisel Jones, an Australian swimmer who won nine Olympic medals, revealed one of her experiences with the technocentric ideology occurring in the Australian swimming culture.

> This is the first time that I have had to do altitude training. We have to train up here for a couple of weeks, and then when we return home, we will swim like gods. We will restore Australian swimming glory. We've been told altitude training will affect every physiological system in our bodies: cardiovascular, nervous, endocrine, the works. Even your mental state will be affected. Our coaches expect we'll all shed weight. Up to a kilo a day and we have to stand on the scales and see

how much weight has slipped off us in the night thanks to the wonders of altitude training. Jeremy [our gym coach] has also got us all walking 20 kilometres to some mountain while we are here. We are at the will of coaches.

Jones, 2015

The voice of Leisel Jones reveals how her swimmer body was "viewed as a human resource" (Bain, 1990, p. 29; McMahon et al., 2012), trained to be efficient and obedient for the sake of achieving competitive performance. While this is only one such example, a vast majority of sports have strived to develop an increasingly effective and efficient means whether it be coaching methods, policy, processes or measures which permeate various levels of sport and are promoted through the concepts of productivity, efficiency and enhancing competitive performance. As a result, discourses of performance and perfection were established and in so doing these discourses privileged the technological criteria of efficiency and effectiveness in producing measurable outcomes (Bain, 1990; Eisner, 1985), all in the name of competitive performance.

Performance discourse

The *performance* discourse in sport places importance on the productivity of athletes in sport. It relates to pedagogy or methods that focus on and serves to regulate and monitor the output of athletes, by honing in on the specialised skills necessary for the production of the specific outputs [competitive performance] (Evans, Rich & Holroyd, 2004). Ball (2004, p. 143) provides an additional definition, describing the performance discourse as:

A technology; a culture and a mode of regulation, or even a system of terror that employs judgements, comparisons and displays as a means of control, attrition and change. The performances of individual subjects or organisations serve as measures of productivity or output, or displays of "quality," or "moments" of promotion or inspection. They stand for, encapsulate or represent the worth, quality and value of an individual or organisation within a field of judgement.

As such, within the discourse of performance, conversations occurring in sporting contexts, training and practices are based around improving sporting performance. Tinning (1997) further explains how it is about methods of instruction, practices, conversations, ideas that serve to enhance the performance of athletes. The performance discourse is thus legitimated through training, measurements and tests which Vertinsky (1985, p. 85) describes as "values packaged in a scientific wrapping". Tinning (1997) says that such a discourse is usually primarily underpinned by science, specifically science relating to performance and the physiology of the body. Language within the performance discourse is based on "training, workloads, thresholds, selection and supports competition usually with the less fit or able being excluded" (Tinning, 1997, p. 102). Consequently, coaches are viewed as being the bearers of all knowledge because of their claims to expertise, experience, wisdom and resources (Johns and Johns, 2000). Below, the voice of an 11 year old swimmer is drawn upon to exemplify the performance discourse in action in the amateur context of swimming.

It is 6.30pm. The rest of the swimmers in my squad get out of the pool but I am not allowed as I have to repeat what we did earlier because I did not make the times that my coach asked of me. I don't know how I am going to do 34 seconds for each effort now at the end of an eight kilometre session when I couldn't make it earlier. My body feels so tired from the long day. My mother sits in the stand watching but does not say anything to my coach.

Young swimmer: "Why am I the only one that has to stay in?"

Coach: "You better get on with it otherwise we are going to be here all night. Champions don't complain. How are you going to be the best 12 year old in the country next year with an attitude like that? If you want to be the best, you need to do what I am asking of you properly the first time."

McMahon, 2010

A similar experience related to the performance discourse was revealed in the gymnastics culture by Barker-Ruchti and Tinning (2010, p. 242).

Phoebe climbs onto the beam and tries again. But she falls. "Your gymnastics makes me sick"! Dina (coach) shouts at the young gymnast. This is like level zero gymnastics – so basic. Go back to baby gymnastics if you behave like this! "Arrgh, this girl just needs to grow up. Be more patient – and focused. I definitely need to talk to her mother. We must find a way for Phoebe to become more determined and focused" says the coach.

These extracts are two examples of how in the amateur context of swimming and gymnastics, young girls were trained to be efficient and obedient for the sake of competitive performance. Some other examples of practices occurring in a variety of sports as a result of the discourse of performance have also been found to include: social isolation due to a lack of performance, extra training to make up for lack of performance, heart rate tests, strength tests, long training hours in the name of improvement (McMahon, 2010).

Perfection

The *perfection discourse* closely aligns with the performance discourse, however, pedagogy and social interactions are primarily based on the ideology that the body is flawed or imperfect and in need of being changed (Evans et al., 2004). The discourse of *perfection* is described as "structures of meaning defining what the body [in size, shape, predisposition and demeanour] is and ought to be; and how, for those who do not meet these ideals, there is treatment, repair and restoration" (Rich & Evans, 2007, p. 44). When applied to sporting contexts specifically, the athlete body would be viewed as unfinished with the intention of making or becoming better in the name of competitive performance. As a consequence, athlete bodies are managed, regulated, measured and compared against and thus their results are subject to a wider technology which judges (Rich & Evans, 2007) how their athlete body measures up these standards.

Leisel Jones, an Australian swimming female icon, recently revealed how Australian swimming coaches would label female athletes who they viewed as fat with the code number 6:1:20 representing the order of f.a.t. letters in the alphabet after public weigh-ins (Zaccardi, 2015). Jones also revealed how she was actively encouraged by coaches to skip meals. Meal-replacement shakes were also recommended in an effort to lose weight. As a teenager, Jones revealed how she often felt ridiculed in front of her peers at thrice weekly weigh ins (Geary, 2015). The revelations from Leisel Jones in relation to the perfection discourse are not only isolated to the elite context of swimming and have also been found to permeate the amateur context. Below, an 11 year old swimmer exemplifies practices that she was exposed to as a result of the perfection discourse.

I hear banging on the window and my name being called. I look at the clock beside my bed and it is 11pm. It is pitch black. The banging on the window continues. I realise that it is my coach.

Coach: "Get up Carly, you need to run off that ice-cream you ate today! Get your running shoes on; you haven't burnt it off yet!"

11 year old swimmer: "What do you mean? It is 11pm?"

Coach: "Get your running shoes on and get out here! You haven't burnt off that ice-cream yet! You've got 11 kilometres kiddo! Need to burn off that ice cream you ate."

McMahon et al., 2012

The sport of swimming is not the only sporting context that has been found to place an emphasis on achieving an ideal body shape through particular body practices. Other sporting cultures such as dancing, athletics, light weight rowing and gymnastics have also been found to be part of a wider cultural discourse within sport that aligns "thin body ideals" for both male and female athletes with certain practices to achieve such ideals (e.g., skin folds, disordered eating/food monitoring, over-exercising) in the name of improving competitive performance (Busanich, McGannon & Schinke, 2014; Cosh, Crabb, Kettler, LeCouteur & Tully, 2014; Papathomas & Lavallee, 2014). Some other examples of practices occurring as a result of the discourse of perfection in sport have been found to include: weigh-ins, skin fold measurements, punishment (extra running, extra training), conversations that are focused on body imperfections when the body is not seen as the ideal size, surveillance of food intake and social isolation (*ibid*). Acquiring the ideal shape for competitive performance is not just limited to the athletes and coaches and has also been found to be adopted by team managers and other social regulators including parents of athletes, media, physiologists, dieticians (McMahon, 2010) and the general public (McMahon & Barker-Ruchti, 2016).

Effects of dominant ideologies and practices in [elite] sport

In the section of the chapter that follows, a number of studies will be drawn upon to highlight how sport has come to have detrimental effects on participants in both the short term (at time of the participation) and also long term (after participants have left the sport). As Eitzen (2012) highlights, sport is something that can be both "healthy and destructive" and there is a growing understanding of the dangers of participation where there is an emphasis on "winning." Eitzen's (2012) findings were recently confirmed by McPherson et al. (2015), who found that although children's sport in Australia had positive benefits, there were also negative effects. Other studies, including the research of Alexander et al. (2011); Gervis and Dunn (2004); Leahy et al. (2008); and Rhind et al. (2014) revealed how abuse, particularly emotional abuse, was becoming relatively common in children's sport with Alexander et al. (2011) revealing that up to 75 per cent of children in their study experienced shouting, threats and humiliating behaviour from coaches or other adults while 24 per cent of participants experienced physical abuse, all in the name of athletic performance. Examples of abuse occurring were exemplified in specific language used and included degrading, bullying, teasing and threatening to enhance competitive performance as well as training while exhausted or injured (Alexander et al., 2011). Indeed, research conducted by McPherson et al. (2015) found that this abuse resulted in the onset of severe eating disorders, depression, self-harm and suicidal ideation for sporting participants.

The risks associated with sport were also revealed in the research conducted by McEwen and Young (2011) who investigated dance culture. In their study, it was revealed that the ballet culture became a 'culture of risk' as pain and injury were normalised by encouraging dancers to understand and talk about their pain in ways that both suppressed and trivialised it. In so doing, the pain-injury experience was found to have negative emotional effects on the dancers, such as feelings of crisis and loss, shame, guilt and anxiety. Further, dancers who became complicit in accepting the often unhealthy conventions of the dance culture were also found to have unhealthy approaches to eating and weight. The research of McEwen and Young (2011) reveals some short term effects of practices occurring in dance culture on dancers. Recently, in the sport of swimming, Leisel Jones (multiple Olympic Gold medallist) revealed how coaching practices impacted swimmers in the short term saying,

> Girls would often sob in the showers after they were "weighed, weighed and weighed again" as men "as old as our dads" would pass judgement, labelling some girls a "6:1:20" [f.a.t]
>
> *Zaccardi, 2015*

After a number of years as a member of the Australian swimming team, Jones further revealed how she had contemplated suicide. At an Australian team altitude training camp in Sierra Nevada, Spain, in 2011, Jones explained that due to the practices and expectations placed on her by coaches, she contemplated ending her life. Her voice reveals the pain and torment that she was feeling at the time:

> I sit down on the bathroom floor with sleeping tablets and plan how I will steal a paring knife from the hotel kitchen to try to kill myself. I will start with my legs, with the big veins in my thighs. Then I will slash at my arms, at my pale white wrists. I shake as I think about it. I imagine the knife and how I will run its blade gently over my skin, scrape it across the smooth skin of my wrist – then go further and do what I need to do. I was picturing myself in a body bag leaving Sierra Nevada.
>
> *Zaccardi, 2015*

While the revelations from Jones exemplify the effects of pressures that she was feeling in the elite context of swimming, detrimental effects were also found to impact upon junior or amateur swimmers during their time of participation. In a study conducted by McMahon et al. (2012), an 11 year old swimmer revealed how she wanted to self-harm as she was not meeting her coach's or parent's competitive expectations and felt she could no longer deal with the pressure. Her voice below.

> I am ashamed of the way I am swimming. I just don't want to go through it anymore.
>
> Maybe I can get out of it?
>
> My mind works overtime, thinking of ways that I can get out of swimming tonight. If I say I have the flu, it won't be enough, they will still make me swim.
>
> Then it suddenly dawns on me: If I break a bone, then I won't have to swim!
>
> I then think of ways that I could break a bone, making it look like an accident to get me out of competing for the rest of the competition. Collarbone would work! If I fall out of my bed, rolling the wrong way, I could fall and break my collarbone.
>
> I found it. I have the answer! I place my body on the very edge of the bed, readying myself to fall out.
>
> *McMahon, 2010*

While there has been an abundance of research attributing sporting participation with a variety of short term effects (as outlined above), little research has been done on how sport may come to impact sporting participants in the long term after they have left the sport. This is an important aspect to understand in terms of how sport may come to impact upon participants' self, wellbeing, engagement in physical activity and diet in the long term. Recent research into Australian swimming culture revealed that specific practices that adolescents were exposed to were found to affect the athletes not only at the time of their participation but alarmingly 10–30 years on after they had finished with the sport thus revealing the long term effects of sport (McMahon, 2010; McMahon et al., 2012). It was revealed that young swimmers learned behaviours in relation to the performance and perfection discourses which were still evident in the way that they treated their bodies as adults, up to 30 years after they had left the sport suggesting that their athlete bodies were impressed with the practices of the swimming culture (*ibid*). A specific example from this study revealed the durability of cultural practices on young swimmers who were punished during their adolescence when they were caught eating outside of meal times and consequently as adult women, eating remained a "corporeal [bodily] sin that filled them with anxiety thus dismantling it as a pleasurable experience" (Evans et al., 2004, p. 126; McMahon, 2010). For these swimmers, food resembled that of an 'eating toxin' and as adult women, they became overridden with guilt and toxic thoughts once food was consumed. Below are two extracts; the first is from an amateur swimmer during her adolescence while the second is from the same person, but reveals her voice as an adult woman some 20 years after she has left the sport. These two extracts exemplify how exposure and effect of a sporting culture may be inextricably linked.

Adolescent swimmer

Outside the shop we all eat our ice-creams. As we are eating it, the white team bus with the coach driving passes us. As it starts to disappear down the street, some of the boys who did not run hang out the bus window and yell.

"Busted!"

I hope my coach didn't see me otherwise I will cop it. The boys immediately start to tease me for eating the ice cream when I arrive at the pool. Their taunts panic me. I really hope my coach did not see me and I hope the boys don't tell him! As I approach the end of the pool, my coach's eyes connect with mine and he says,

Coach: "Did you enjoy your ice cream? I hope it was worth it? You have got 16 kilometres to run after the session. Losers eat ice-cream."

McMahon, 2010

Adult woman

There are five left. Need to eat them even though I know I shouldn't. I know they are unnecessary calories and I know they will make me fat, yet I wonder why I am having trouble resisting. Have to sneak them so nobody sees. I grab all five of them. I walk into the lounge room so my kids don't see me and I shove them into my mouth one by one, until the last one is eaten. The sweet sugary taste gives me a good feeling, but it is only momentarily. Then my voices start.

You are fat!

You are disgusting!

Some familiar words come back to me. They are my coach's words.
Winners aren't weak.
Winners aren't fat.
Losers eat biscuits.
But I am weak. Feel so terrible now for eating the biscuits.

McMahon, 2010

While this data highlights the effects on an amateur swimmer, similar effects were encountered by elite swimmers (i.e. continuing to purge food 30 years post elite sport).

The research of McMahon et al. (2012) is not the only research to reveal the impact of sport on the eating practices of athletes in the long term. A study conducted by Jones et al. (2005) provides us with further insight into the effects of a culture of slenderness also in the sport of swimming revealing how for their swimmer participant, her experiences in the sport of swimming led her to develop an eating disorder. Thus, the findings of McMahon et al. (2012) and Jones et al. (2005) reveal a connection between exposure and effect of swimming culture and that within the discourses of performance and perfection, a number of social and emotional issues are created which pervade the sport participants' lives in both the short term and long term. This in turn points to the "durability" (Lee & Macdonald, 2010) of dominant ideologies and practices on athletes, long after they have left the sport as they continue to permeate their adult lives. In this respect, their exposure and adoption of such practices has had a sustained lived effect on their lives and their health and wellbeing. Thus, it is essential to realise how sporting organisations may support or constrain the protection of athletes by determining the extent to which practices are accepted (McMahon, 2010; Gervis & Dunn, 2004; Lang, 2010; Papaefastathiou, Rhind & Brackenridge, 2013; Pinheiro et al., 2014).

Implications for future physical activity policy and practice.

As outlined in this chapter, sport has been found to have both short term and long term detrimental effects for athlete participants. Ideologies and practices relating to the performance and perfection discourses have not only been found to occur in elite sporting contexts but have also been found to occur in amateur and community sporting contexts.

While a large section of this chapter has been focussed on the sport of swimming, other research presented in this chapter has revealed that similar practices are occurring in a variety of other sporting contexts with subsequent detrimental effects for the participants. In so doing, sporting participants have come to experience negative effects physically, emotionally and mentally in both the short term and long term (Kalleberg, 2009; McMahon et al., 2012) as a result of their involvement in sport.

In terms of what can be learned from this chapter in regards to increasing levels of physical activity in populations in the long term, the studies of McMahon (2010), McMahon et al. (2012) and others reveal how sport has affected participants' experience of sport/physical activity as well as eating behaviours in both the short term and long term. Thus, sections of this chapter indeed highlight a link between sporting participation and ill health, specifically disordered eating and a lack of wanting to participate in any type of exercise or physical activity in the long term. We draw on a voice of an adult woman who was once an amateur swimmer to exemplify this lack of wanting to engage in physical activity post sport.

I have not exercised for seven years. Not so much of a throwing over of the arms in the pool or even a walk up to the shops. I even avoid walking up stairs if I can.

My husband often asks me if I want to go for a walk at the beach and I cannot be bothered to even leave the house, even though I can see that he wants to do something with me. I feel tired, unmotivated and exercise is the furtherest thing from my mind. If I can avoid doing it, I do. My experiences during my adolescence have scarred me and I just do not enjoy it nor want to do it.

McMahon, 2010

While the literature included in this chapter reveals evidence that there is a link between physical activity/sport and ill health, this does not mean that all sport has detrimental effects for all participants, with many studies highlighting the potential value of sport participation (i.e. Cronin & Armour, 2015; Eime et al., 2013; Kavanagh, 2014). What this chapter does highlight is that sporting cultures that place a large emphasis on meritocracy or winning have neglected to consider sporting participants' wellbeing in the long term, in particular their life after sport. The emphasis on meritocracy and performance has been long reflected at a federal level, in that, a large number of policies continue to financially support and reward those athletes who are performing at an elite level (i.e. Australia's Winning Edge 2012–2022; Olympic Athlete Program – Making Great Australians; Maintain the Momentum). While there are some other policies that have been implemented over the years to support athletes in other ways such as limiting the prevalence of binge drinking (see: Be the Influence) and racism (see: Racism: It stops with me), there is little government support for elite athletes post sport or during their transition into retirement. While sporting performance will always remain a key objective of elite sport, coaches and sporting organisations should be equally concerned with the health and wellbeing of their athletes both in the short term and also long term. This would mean a greater emphasis placed on developing each and every athlete physically, emotionally, mentally, spiritually and socially. It is important for those involved in sport to provide a nurturing and supported environment for athletes as well as acknowledging the detrimental effects associated with the performance and perfection discourses in sport. This in turn will limit the long term effects on athletes' physical activity levels and healthy lifestyles. In closing, it is important to acknowledge that while this chapter draws a number of studies to outline the darker side of sport, the contents of this chapter may not represent nor resonate with all those who have been involved with sport. Instead it is hoped that the contents of this chapter may evoke a sense of significance for some and prompt on-going reflection and discussion.

References

Alexander, K., Stafford, A., & Lewis R. 2011. *The experiences of children participating in organised sport in the UK*. London, UK: NSPCC.

Anderson, E. 2010. *Sport, theory and social problems: A critical introduction*. London: Routledge.

Bain, L. 1990. A critical analysis of the hidden curriculum in physical education. In D. Kirk & R. Tinning (eds), *Physical education, curriculum and culture: Critical issues in the contemporary crisis* (pp. 23–41). Hampshire, UK: Falmer Press.

Ball, S. 2004. Performativities and fabrications in the education economy: Toward the performative society. In S. Ball (ed), *The RoutledgeFalmer reader in sociology of education* (pp. 143–155). London, UK: RoutledgeFalmer.

Barker-Ruchti, N., & Tinning, R. 2010. Foucault in leotards: Corporeal discipline in women's artistic gymnastics. *Sociology of Sport Journal, 27*(3): 229–250.

BBC sports. 2012. Olympic Sport Funding. *BBC sports*. Retrieved from: www.bbc.com/sport/0/olympics/20780450.

Bloom, M., Grant, M., & Watt, D. 2005. *Strengthening Canada: The socio-economic benefits of sport participation in Canada*. Ottawa: The Conference Board of Canada.

Brackenridge, C. H. 2006. Youth sport re-focussed – A review essay on Paulo David's human rights in youth sport: A critical review of children's rights in competitive sports. *European Physical Education Review*, *12*(1): 119–125.

Busanich, R., McGannon, K. R., & Schinke, R. 2014. Comparing elite male and female distance runner's experiences of disordered eating through narrative analysis. *Psychology of Sport & Exercise*, *15*(6): 705–712.

Cameron, C., Craig, C. L., & Beaulieu, A. 2000. *Increasing physical activity: Creating effective communities.* Ottawa: Canadian Fitness and Lifestyle Research Institute.

Coakley, J., 1995. Ethics, deviance and sports: A critical look at crucial issues. In A. Tomlinson & and S. Fleming (eds), *Ethics, sport and leisure – Crisis and critiques* (pp. 3–24). Oxford: Meyer and Meyer Sport.

Cosh, S., Crabb, S., Kettler, L., LeCouteur, A., & Tully, P. J. 2014. The normalization of body regulation and monitoring practices in elite sport: A discursive analysis of news delivery sequences during skinfold testing. *Qualitative Research in Sport, Exercise and Health*, 7: 338–360.

Cronin, C., & Armour, K. 2015. Lived experience and community sport coaching: A phenomenological investigation. *Sport Education and Society*, *20*(8): 959–975.

David, P. 2005. *Human rights in youth sport.* London, UK: Routledge.

Dubois, P.E., (1986) The effect of participation in sport on the value orientations of young athletes. *Sociology of Sport Journal*, *3*: 29–42.

Eime, R., Young, J., Harvey, J., Charity, M., & Payne, W. 2013. A systematic review of psychological and social benefits of participation in sport for children and adolescents: Informing development of a conceptual model of health through sport. *International Journal of Behaviour Nutrition and Physical Activity*, *10*: 10–98.

Eisner, E. 1985. *The educational imagination.* New York: Macmillan.

Eitzen, D. S. 2012. *Fair and foul: Beyond the myths and paradoxes of sport.* Lanham, MD: Rowman & Littlefield.

Evans, J., Rich, E., & Holroyd, R. 2004. Disordered eating and disordered schooling: What schools do to middle class girls. *British Journal of Sociology of Education*, *25*(2): 123–142.

Fine, G. 1987. *Little league baseball and preadolescent culture.* Chicago: University of Chicago Press.

Geary, B. 2015. 'It nearly killed me': Olympic gold medallist Leisel Jones says teen years were plagued with obsessive dieting – as she reveals her battles with mental health issues. *Daily Mail.* Retrieved from www.dailymail.co.uk/news/article-3253729/It-nearly-killed-Olympic-gold-medallist-Leisel-Jones-says-teen-years-plagued-obsessive-dieting-including-banning-chocolate-year-reveals-mental-health-battles.html.

Gervis, M., & Dunn, N. 2004. The emotional abuse of elite child athletes by their coaches. *Child Abuse Review*, *13*(3): 215–223.

Hoberman, J., 1992. *Mortal engines: The science of performance and the dehumanization of sport.* New Jersey: The Blackburn Press.

Johns, D., & Johns, J. 2000. Surveillance, subjectivism and technologies of power. *International Review for the Sociology of Sport*, *35*(2): 219–234.

Jones, L. 2015. Olympic Swimmer Leisel Jones dive into depression. *Sydney Morning Herald.* Retrieved from www.smh.com.au/good-weekend/olympic-swimmer-leisel-joness-dive-into-depression-20150910-gjjkkq.html#ixzz3oxXZsgoZ.

Jones, R., Glintmeyer, N., & McKenzie, A. 2005. Slim bodies, eating disorders and the coach-athlete relationship: A tale of identity creation and disruption. *International Review for the Sociology of Sport*, *40*(3): 377–391.

Kalleberg, A. L. 2009. Precarious work, insecure workers: Employment relations in transition. *American Sociological Review*, *74*(1): 1–22.

Katzmarysk, P., Gledhill, N., & Shephard, R. 2000. The economic burden of physical inactivity in Canada. *Canadian Medical Association Journal*, *163*(11): 1435–1440.

Kavanagh, E. 2014. *The dark side of elite sport: Athlete narratives of maltreatment in high performance environments.* Unpublished PhD thesis, Bournemouth University.

Kyle, D. 2015. *Sport and spectacle in the ancient world.* Chichester, UK: John Wiley and Sons.

Lang, M. 2010. Surveillance and conformity in competitive youth swimming. *Sport, Education and Society Journal*, *15*(1): 19–38.

Leahy, T., Pretty, G., & Tenenbaum, G. 2008. A contextualized investigation of traumatic correlates of childhood sexual abuse in Australian athletes. *International Journal of Sport and Exercise Psychology*, *6*(4): 366–384.

Lee, J., & Macdonald, D. 2010. Are they just checking our obesity or what? The healthism discourse and rural young women. *Sport, Education and Society Journal*, *15*(2): 203–219.

McEwen, K., & Young, K. 2011. Ballet and pain: Reflections on a risk dance culture. *Qualitative Research in Sport, Exercise and Heath*, *3*(2): 152–173.

McMahon, J. 2010. *Exposure and effect: An investigation into a culture of body pedagogies*. Unpublished PhD thesis, University of Tasmania.

McMahon, J., & Barker-Ruchti, N. 2015. Assimilating to a boy's body shape for the sake of performance. *Sport Education and Society*. doi: 10.1080/13573322.2015.1013463.

McMahon, J., & Barker-Ruchti. 2016. The media's role in transmitting a cultural ideology and the effect on the general public. *Qualitative Research in Sport Exercise and Health*, *8*(2): 131–146. doi: 10.1080/2159676X.2015.1121912.

McMahon, J., & Dinan-Thompson, M. 2008. A malleable body – Revelations from an Australian elite swimmer. *Healthy Lifestyles Journal*, *55*(1): 23–28.

McMahon, J., Penney, D., & Dinan-Thompson, M. 2012. Body practices – Exposure and effect of a sporting culture? Stories from three Australian swimmers. *Sport, Education and Society*, *17*(2): 181–206.

McPherson, L., Long, M., Nicholson, M., Cameron, N., Atkins, P., & Morris, M. 2015. Children's experiences of sport in Australia. *International Review for the Sociology of Sport*. doi: 10.1177/1012690215608517.

Papaefstathiou, M., Rhind, D., & Brackenridge, C. 2013. Child protection in ballet: Experiences and views of teachers, administrators and ballet students. *Child Abuse Review*, *22*(2): 127–141.

Papathomas, A., & Lavallee, D. 2014. Self-starvation and the performance narrative in competitive sport. *Psychology of Sport and Exercise*, *15*(6): 688–695.

Pinheiro, M. C., Pimenta, N., Resende, R. et al. 2014. Gymnastics and child abuse: An analysis of former international Portuguese female artistic gymnasts. *Sport, Education and Society*, *19*(4): 435–450.

Rhind, D., McDermott, J., Lambert, E. et al., 2014. A review of safeguarding cases in sport. *Child Abuse Review*. doi: 10.1002/car.2306.

Rich, E., & Evans, J. 2007. Rereading voice: Young women, anorexia and performative education. *Junctures: The Journal for Thematic Dialogue*. Retrieved from: www.junctures.org/issues.php?issue=0 9&title=Voice&colour=rgb(176,153,0).

Tinning, R. 1997. Performance and participation discourses in human movement: Towards a socially critical physical education. In J. Fernandez-Balboa (ed), *Critical postmodernism in human movement, physical education and sport* (pp. 99–121). Albany, NY: State University of New York Press.

United Nations. 2011. United Nations Sport for Development and Peace. Retrieved from: www. un.org/wcm/content/site/sport/.

Vertinsky, P. 1985. Risk benefit analysis of health promotions: Opportunities and threats for physical education. *Quest*, *37*(1): 71–83.

Walters, S., Payne, D., Schluter, P., & Thompson, R. 2015. It just makes you feel invincible: A Foucauldian analysis of children's experiences of organised team sports. *Sport, Education and Society*, *20*(2): 241–257.

Zaccardi, N. 2015. Leisel Jones details depression in 'Body Lengths'. *NBC Sports*. Retrieved from: http://olympics.nbcsports.com/athlete/leisel-jones/.

PART III

International perspectives on physical activity policy and practice

THEME F INTRODUCTION
Physical activity policy and practice around the world

The final section of the Handbook presents a series of regional and country-specific case studies of physical activity policy and practice. Government departments around the world are formulating policy responses as a result of the escalating importance placed on physical activity. The chapters which follow explore historic and current policy initiatives, the pertinent political, economic and cultural priorities of the area which inform policy and a description of the dominant forms of physical activity in the area's occupations, leisure and education systems.

By analysing the agendas and discourses of policy makers around the world, we can understand more about how justifications for intervention are emerging, how policy decisions are made and how policies are implemented. This section also provides an opportunity to consider the gaps between policy rhetoric (discourse) and reality, and raises questions about the replicability of policy from one area or country to another. The case studies offered here are certainly not intended to represent idealistic best practice. Instead, they show the array of styles, structures and funding that currently exist and are themselves morphing over time.

First, Mahfoud Amara examines the Arab region, and in particular the countries of the Gulf Cooperation Council: Bahrain, Kuwait, Oman, Qatar, Saudi Arabia and the United Arab Emirates. Amara notes that data on physical activity and health in the Arab world are scarce, possibly explained by the low priority of physical activity as opposed to other more prevalent issues, including education, employment, development of infrastructures and (in)security. Nevertheless, obesity is becoming a major health concern for many of these countries, which is giving impetus for policy makers to give more import to sport and physical activity as health.

Next, Margaret Heffernan, Constantino Stavros, Kate Westberg, Angela Dobele and Aaron Smith examine a country which many people think of as one of the most physically active, sporting nations in the world – Australia. The authors reveal a paradox between high achievement in world sport and low population rates of physical activity. The authors then advocate for cultural and resource reprogramming from elite sport to a preventative health agenda through increasing participation in various types of physical activity.

In a chapter dedicated to Brazil, Thiago Hérick de Sá, Marco Antonio Bettine de Almeida and Danielle Keylla Alencar Cruz illuminate the enormous changes the country has experienced in recent years. The last two decades has seen enormous economic growth in Brazil, leading to social and distributive policies which have in turn reduced the historic income inequality. However, major challenges remain. The democratic process is described as fragile and urbanisation as precarious, with poor urban conditions in municipalities an on-going problem. Significant inequities in physical activity remain. The authors argue that increasing physical activity (along with other rights) will only be possible with the deepening of social participation and strengthening democratic institutions.

Mads de Wolff's chapter investigates how physical activity is conceived of at a supranational level – in the European Union. De Wolff examines how the discourse about health enhancing physical activity (HEPA) recently entered the EU agenda via the Council of Health Ministers, until the sport divisions within the EU took control of the issue. Similar to many other countries' approaches to physical activity, the EU's policy priorities with regard to physical activity have increasingly become focused on grassroots sport. By drawing on theory to explain the emergence of physical activity as an important issue, de Wolff captures how physical activity is becoming increasingly legitimate as a core policy concern.

Next, Aman Dhall explores India and its changing approach to physical activity policy. Soon to be the most populous nation on Earth, India, as the cliché suggests, is a land of contrast. There are enormous wealth disparities in India. These socio-economic obstacles severely limit the ability to partake in safe, fulfilling physical activity for many people. There also appears to be a general lack of support and facilities in which to be active. However, Dhall, notes that changes are occurring slowly. The central government and the private sector have attempted to develop a culture in which sport and physical activity is prioritised. Notwithstanding all these positive sentiments, India continues to struggle with rising levels of health problems and administration apathy.

Tracey L. Kolbe-Alexander and Estelle V. Lambert discuss the South African policy context in great detail. Typical of many low to medium income countries, the authors note low income contributes to many health disparities in South Africa, including discretionary physical activity. Both government and non-government initiatives and policies are examined. The authors conclude that despite South Africa having higher levels of total physical activity compared to more developed countries, there are lower levels of leisure time physical activity. Increasingly sedentary occupations and travel both further highlight the importance of policy interventions to promote health enhancing physical activity.

Emily Knox examines physical activity policy in the United Kingdom. The discussion focuses on the opportunities presented and the difficulties of achieving or maintaining sporting excellence and furthering physical activity on the public health agenda, in light of increasing devolution and conflicting regional priorities. A description of the dominant forms of physical activity in occupations, leisure and education is also provided.

Lastly, Sean Bulger, Emily Jones and Eloise Elliott discuss physical activity policy in the United States of America. The authors explain how the policy issue of physical activity in the USA is complex with multiple biological, social and environmental factors. Adopting an ecological perspective, the authors examine policy making at the national and state levels. These include policy interventions to use school, transport and facilities as spaces and places to increase population-wide physical activity rates.

34

THE ARAB REGION

Mahfoud Amara

Introduction

Obesity has reached an epidemic rate in Arab countries for both children and adults. Among adolescents aged 15–18 years, the proportions that were overweight and obese in seven Arab countries ranged from 25 per cent to 60 per cent (Museiger et al 2013). Seven out of 10 Saudis are suffering from obesity, and 37 per cent of Saudi women face problems related to overweight (Khan 2014). According to the Saudi Obesity Research Centre "based on the National Nutrition Survey of 2007, the prevalence of obesity in the KSA was 23.6% in women and 14% in men. The prevalence of overweight in the community was determined to be 30.7% for men as compared to 28.4% for the women" (Obesity Research Centre 2015). Despite differences in health system size, structure, and financing, evidence suggests that across the region particular sections of the population are disproportionately affected by barriers to accessing health care (Kronfol 2012). Kronfol explains these barriers as follows:

- transportation to reach health care particularly in rural areas and for people with disability;
- regional variations and rural-urban disparities;
- cultural barriers to access particularly in relation to gender related to access, rights for care;
- deficit in the "responsiveness" of health care services;
- financial barriers with regard to funding of the health sector, access to health care and medication.

To understand the overwhelming health issues in the Arab world, a region which is going through drastic changes (political, urban, and socio-economic), *The Lancet* medical journal devoted a special issue on health in the Arab world. In this issue, the Regional Officer of WHO for the Eastern Mediterranean explained the five priorities to strengthening health systems in Arab countries:

- Accelerating progress towards universal health coverage by reforming health systems;
- Communicable diseases, the region has the fastest rate of increase among WHO regions in the number of HIV infections and the lowest coverage with antiretroviral therapy;
- Maternal and child health; 899,000 children younger than 5 years and 39,000 mothers needlessly die each year in the region from avoidable causes;

– Non-communicable diseases, particularly cardiovascular diseases, cancers, and diabetes. Up to 40 per cent of those dying from non-communicable diseases are aged younger than 60 years;
– Emergency preparedness and response (Alwan 2014).

In the same special issue, Rahim et al. (2014: n.p) stated that

> the burden of non-communicable diseases (cardiovascular disease, cancer, chronic lung diseases, and diabetes) in the Arab world has increased, with variations between countries of different income levels. Behavioral risk factors, including tobacco use, unhealthy diets, and *physical inactivity* are prevalent, and obesity in adults and children has reached an alarming level. Despite epidemiological evidence, the policy response to non-communicable diseases has been weak. So far, Arab governments have not placed a sufficiently high priority on addressing the high prevalence of non-communicable diseases, with variations in policies between countries and overall weak implementation (highlight added by the author).

Data and policies on physical activities

Data on physical activity and health in the Arab world are scarce, possibly explained by the low priority of physical activity as opposed to other more prevalent issues, such as education, employment, development of infrastructures, and of course (in)security. The few available studies explain that the highest levels of insufficient physical activity are seen in Saudi Arabia and Kuwait, where over two thirds (60%) of adults are classified as insufficiently active (World Health Organization 2014). Furthermore, in most Arab countries, with the exception of Iraq and Lebanon, men are more active than women. Physical activity is defined here as less than 5 times 30 minutes of moderate activity per week, or less than 3 times 20 minutes of vigorous activity per week, or equivalent. Three countries (Bahrain, Iraq, and occupied Palestinian territory) have national non-communicable disease policy or strategic plans, which have an objective focusing on physical activity. Four countries (Morocco, Oman, Qatar, and Saudi Arabia) have a specific policy on the promotion of healthy lifestyles or a national strategy addressing both nutrition (diet) and physical activity. In terms of sport and health awareness, the study reported a number of initiatives including:

– The King Abdullah II Prize for Fitness is a physical fitness promotion program intended to complement the regular physical education curriculum for children aged 9–17 years
– Exercise is medicine, Kuwait. An initiative aiming to encouraging primary care physicians and other health care providers to integrate physical activity into standard care for patients
– Urban design to promote physical activity example of Wadi Hanifa development (a valley of over 100 km in length which runs through the capital city Riyadh)
– The Nizwa healthy lifestyles project in Oman, which is a community-based project for the primary prevention of non-communicable diseases and the promotion of healthy lifestyles

In his study on barriers to female participation in sport in the Gulf region in general and in Qatar in particular Harkness (2012: 2167) concluded that:

> Female athletes in the Gulf region encounter a sort of triple jeopardy vis-à-vis sports participation: the first being that encountered by all women in general; the second being that encountered by female athletes the world over and the third based upon the

especially patriarchal environment of the Gulf region. Women throughout the world are subjected to patriarchy in most facets of social and economic life. In the Gulf region, women who do not play sports are already subjugated to immense patriarchy; female athleticism only adds to this. Influenced by Islamic principles, these gender dynamics impact sports and female athletic participation in a variety of ways, including the realms of gender segregation and clothing regulation.

Harkness goes on to highlight other structural hindrance to sport participation such as family structure, Hijab, gender segregation. These factors explain low numbers of female members in sports federations estimated in 2012 at 7.3 per cent (of the total athletes registered).

In addition to socio-cultural factors the other significant variable to explain lack of physical activity in the Arab World and in the GCC is the rapid urbanization and sedentary life. Abdul-Rasoul (2012: n.p) explains obesity epidemic in the GCC by

> the rapid urbanization in everyday life, accompanied by decreased levels of physical activity and increased caloric intake of non-traditional food has become responsible for the emerging of obesity in children and adolescents as a major public health issue in these countries.

In their study about prevalence of overweight, obesity, and abdominal obesity among urban Saudi adolescents, conducted during 2009–2010 in three major cities in Saudi Arabia, Al-Hazaa et al. (2014) found that there is a higher prevalence of overweight and obesity in adolescents attending private schools compared to those attending public schools. They concluded that differences in lifestyle factors, including lack of physical activity, might have also influenced differences in the regional obesity rates.

> Total physical activity in METs-min per week as well as several eating habits, like intake of breakfast, milk, and sugar-sweetened drinks, were shown to be significantly different among adolescents living in the three regions [online].

In another study Al-Hazaa et al (2012) contended that overweight/obesity was associated with lower levels of physical activity. Similarly, a lack of exercise was a significant risk factor for obesity among adolescents from south-western Saudi Arabia. The region is considered among urban centres of the Kingdom, where according to Al-Hazaa Western calorie-dense fast foods are increasingly available and consumed by the young generation.

Having discussed the general context of health challenges and priorities in the Arab world, particularly non-communicable diseases associated with the lack of physical activity, the second part of the chapter is devoted to analysis of sport and health policies in two countries with an ambition to be a hub of global sport industry in the Middle East and North Africa, the UAE, and Qatar.

Sport and social change in the UAE and Qatar

Both countries are engaged in an international venture of using sport for urban regeneration, diversification of economy (decreasing dependency on non-renewable natural resources), and image making. Staging regional and international sports events is one of the pillars of their international strategy to develop infrastructures and other economic sectors such tourism, estate, and retail. Both countries emphasize human development and technology as their path toward modernization. Doha, the capital of Qatar, is branded as the capital of sport, while

Dubai in the UAE is branded as the capital of e-government. Both Qatar (since 2012), followed by the UAE, starting from 2015, have their National Day of Sport. According to Qatar National Olympic Committee:

> Celebrating the National Sports Day reveals the importance of sport as a significant factor to help domestic institutions achieving their goals by creating a healthy community at both physical and psychological levels.
>
> *Qatar National Olympic Committee Webpage*

The National Sport Day has a different significance in the UAE, a country that is a federation of seven emirates or federal-states. This is emphasized in the UAE newspaper, *The National*: "Organizers of the UAE National Sports Day believe that as well as promoting healthy living, sporting competition also helps create a harmonious society" (Alwasmi 2015).

The urban landscape of cities in the GCC is being shaped by sport at multiple levels. New development projects have been and are being built, specifically around sport themes. Sport is now at the core of the modern project of urbanization in the region. "Sport cities" and "urban zones" built around sport themes, combined with high tech, retail, and tourism, are emerging and offering the local population, both citizens and residents, the possibility of being part of the global sporting experience. Examples of these regional initiates include Dubai Sports City, Ferrari World in Abu Dhabi, and Dubai Motor City in the UAE, and Aspire Zone in Qatar. As described by Scharfenort, sport is at the heart of the neoliberal urbanization policies of coastal cities in the Gulf region, which combine "a confluence of strategies of consumerism, entertainment, and global tourism" (Scharfenort 2012: 211). In the same vein Thani and Heenan (2015: n.p) asserted that:

> With the amalgamation of sport, tourism, entertainment and business in these spaces, Dubai and Abu Dhabi have conformed to Walt Disney's concept of building theme parks with activates and facilities to cater for all comers. This "Disneyfication" signals UAE's goal of becoming a global tourism and business hub in the Arab world. Post 9/11 sport has been used to "Disneyfying" Dubai and Abu Dhabi for Westerners' consumption.

In 2010 Qatar National Olympic Committee launched Sport and Health Campaign urging all members of the Qatari community to walk on regular basis as walking for 20 minutes would mean losing 100 calories. In 2011 recognizing the effect of increasing sedentary lifestyles and lack of population's (particularly nationals) engagement with physical activity, guided also by the Qatar National Vision 2030 that calls for development of a healthy and competitive human capital, Qatar National Olympic Committee launched Qatar Active initiative. It is designed as one of the key projects of Qatar Sport Sector Strategy (2011–2016). The aims of Qatar Active as formulated by the government are:

- Increasing youth programs to encourage sport participation – this will include the implementation of a national sports curriculum; certification and on-going professional development for teachers; development of curriculum support materials, including specific guidelines on the encouragement of students with disabilities; and the development of a monitoring and evaluation system.
- Healthy lifestyle interventions – an in-depth sports participation survey will be conducted to develop promotional strategy;
- The Active Qatar Campaign will in turn educate and advocate the benefits of healthy lifestyle within the community.

Table 34.1 Qatar Active – physical activity in schools (adapted from The Peninsula 2014)

Physical activity	Aims
Physical Activity through Physical Education	to enhance the method of providing physical education to early years (grade 1–3) so that all students are given the opportunity to practice physical activity during the whole 55 minutes allocated for each physical education class.
Physical Activity inside the Classroom	to increase the level of students' physical activity inside classrooms by providing physically active breaks as well as offering physically active teaching methods.
Physical Activity outside the Classroom	to increase the physical activity in the early morning assembly, recess time, breaks, additional activity classes, as well as at the end of the school day while children are waiting for the school bus.

To implement Active Qatar a number of projects are underway, including Qatar Active School (QAS) which is a community-based program provided by Aspetar (Orthopedic and Sport Medicine Hospital) in cooperation with the Supreme Education Council, Aspire Academy, Aspire Active, and the Primary Health Care Corporation (PHCC). The intended targets of the project are illustrated in Table 34.1.

Aspire Academy and Aspetar are part of Aspire Zone, which is the country's centre of sport excellence. It is also the heart of Doha city and representing the sporting ambition of Qatar in terms of prestige, design, and architecture. When the weather is cooler it is the place to be for casual sport (e.g. five-a-side football and jogging) and for family picnics. Outdoor exercise machines are also available for the general public to use as well as cycling paths. Teachers and administrators are encouraged to implement the four QAS components, which are: healthy heart, healthy bones, healthy muscle, and healthy person. The goal is to achieve the 60 minutes requirement of physical activity per day. It is expected that by 2020, the physical activity of children in Qatar will increase by 20 per cent, and QAS will be integrated into 50 per cent of schools in Qatar.

Some of the requirements for health promotion are already being enforced by the High Council of Education in Qatar as illustrated in the following recommendation to parents by a British school (Compass International) in Doha:

> Children are asked to bring a healthy snack and lunch to school to encourage healthy living and maximize brain capacity for learning. Please do not include sweets, chocolates or fizzy drinks in your child's lunch and always try to include a piece of fruit or vegetable.

In December 2015 following a survey conducted among Independent school children aged six to 19 years which found that 16 to 22 per cent of Independent school children in Qatar are to be either obese or overweight, the Supreme Council of Health (SCH) has partnered with Qatar Olympic Committee, Aspetar, and Weill Cornell Medical College in Qatar to launch a joint initiative to fight obesity among kids. The program is promoted as to be "an extension of various health initiatives implemented in schools in the past years under the National Health Strategy 2011–2016" (The Peninsula 2015). As an attempt to shift the focus in sport development in Qatar from elite sport to community sport the newly established Ministry of Youth and Sports inaugurated (officially in December 13, 2015) Qatar Sports for

All Federation. One of the on-going studies of the federation is to map out the level and types of sport practice in the country and explore the trends in participation in sports and physical activities among Qatari nationals – adults and students, and define the number of nationals from different ages and genders who practice sports and physical activities. Furthermore, knowledge is sought about their preference for the type of sport, the timing and season to practice sports activities, as well as the best sports venues.

Aspire, which is one of the pillars of sport excellence in the country, is also engaged in sport and health agenda. The organization launched a new program, sponsored by RasGas (the national Gas company), called "Every Step Counts" with the ambition to:

– Improve physical activity among the population of Qatar
– Increase number of organizations adopting physical activity programs
– Create and enhance access to places where people can be physically active
– Fight rising obesity, diabetes, and heart diseases

The philosophy of the program is

> to promote the concept of holistic health change to the people of Qatar to engage in a self-managed lifelong program based on a moderate amount of daily physical activity, encouraging each person to walk 10,000 steps and more a day in competitive, recreational and social approach.

The tool used to measure the steps and calculated routes in various malls and parks is apple and android applications. Participants had to register online (www.stepintohealth.qa). Aspire Zone and under the supervision of Aspetar would provide free online assistance and feedback on progress.

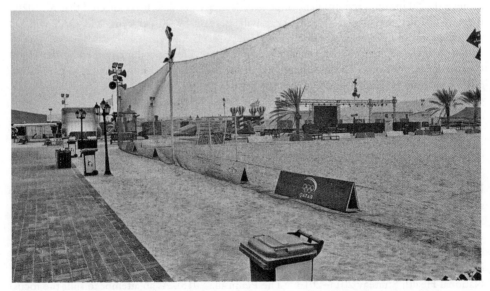

Figure 34.1 Olympic Park at Sealine Beach in Qatar, open to the public during the weekend.

Source: Taken by the author.

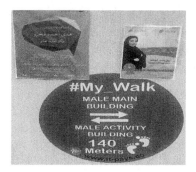

Figure 34.2 An initiative to promote walking among male students at Qatar University. A similar initiative was launched at the female side of the campus. With free WIFI inside the campus social media is becoming central for communication among the student population.

Source: Taken by the author.

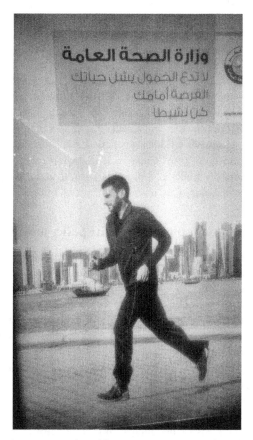

Figure 34.3 A poster by the Ministry of Health in Qatar promoting physical activity among general population designed around the motto "Do not let laziness disable your life. The opportunity is in front of you. Be active". The picture is depicting "male" with a full sport suit in daylight (more convenient in the winter) running in Doha Cornish which is seven kilometres [4.4 miles] long. It is lined with luxury hotels, government buildings, museums, and parks.

In the UAE a similar strategy is pursued of using Zayed Sport City in Abu Dhabi as a hub for health promotion and prevention from chronic diseases. Branded as *HealthPoint*, and financed by *Mubadala* "exchange", which is the Sovereign Investment Authority of the state of Abu Dhabi, it is approximately 1,000 square meters of physiotherapy and rehabilitation areas for men, women, and children, offering a range of orthopaedic, spine, and physiotherapy services. It also is the home of Abu Dhabi Knee and Sports Medicine Centre. The partner of *HealthPoint* is Etihad Airlines the sponsor of Manchester City. Manchester City launched a campaign "Exclusive Opportunity to Be a Mascot at a Manchester City Football Match" to promote the scheme. Pupils aged between 6–11 years of age were asked to submit 100 words on "what it takes to become a healthy child". According to Westerbeek and Smith (2015) the engagement of *Mubadala* and other corporations such Etihad Airways are to be seen as a way

> to rely on communities and their constituents to achieve economic prosperity and they have been slow to find ways of (re)connecting with these communities. One approach for corporations to reconnect, or indeed to attend to its corporate social responsibility, is through sport.

Considering the high level of obesity among children in the UAE, according to the 2010 Global School Health Survey, approximately 40 per cent of children in the UAE are overweight or obese; the country ranks the second highest in the world for the prevalence1 of diabetes, the Fat Truth Campaign was launched. It is a three-month awareness-raising initiative developed and implemented by UNICEF and multiple government and private-sector partners in order to sensitize children, adolescents, and parents to the risks of childhood obesity and the benefits of a healthy diet and regular physical exercise. Following the campaign in September 2010, the Ministry of Education passed a law banning the sale of unhealthy items such as chocolate and high-sugar drinks in school canteens. New health policies have also been developed requiring schools to shift focus from "education only" to include health promotion. Health education sessions are now a mandatory part of the new school curriculum.

Implications for physical activity policy and practice

To conclude, realizing the seriousness of health problems related to lack of physical activity a number of initiatives and programs are funded and implemented by governments and other public and private partners. Social media and other communication strategies such as digital phone applications are being utilized to sensitize the population about the health benefits of physical activity and the urgency to take actions against health related problems with low participation in sport and physical activity. There are, however, some major structural issues to consider:

–   In a car centred culture encouraged by low petrol prices, low interest bank loans, and large roads with no accommodated space for pedestrians or cyclists, the act of walking can be perceived as synonymous with unskilled low-paid jobs.
–   Visiting shopping malls seems to be a popular family activity to escape the outside high temperature. Shopping malls are designed around food courts, which start by McDonalds in the one side and finish with KFC or Burger King in the other. And in between Middle Eastern fast foods offering high calorie dishes.
–   Suitable period for outdoor activities are between the end of October to the end of March. This period can witness a sentiment of saturation and over promotion of sport activities and sport events centred around corporate branding and less on individuals.

- School time is between 7 am and 2 pm, which allows few opportunities for PE classes and other school sport activities.
- The recent budget cut due to the steady drop of oil price will have an impact in the short and medium terms on the access for public resources for sport for all initiatives and physical activity promotions.

To overcome some of these challenges more rigorous studies are needed to analyse the true impact of the lack of physical activity on general population's health (citizens and residents, male and female) as well as existing opportunities to access to sport facilities and to partake in community sport. Cities in the region are undergoing a massive transformation to cater for a growing population and for a changing economy. Sport and physical activity should be placed at the centre of the new urban design and economic development (outside the paradigm of Oil depending economy). At policy level there is a need to set and implement, at Gulf Cooperation Council (GCC) and individual states, a standard for a minimum sport practice per day and per week for the national population, including in work places and particularly in schools. More engagement from elite sport clubs, receiving a big share of state's funding, in developing community sport for local population as part of their social responsibilities is to be pushed for by sport and education authorities. Having said this, and based on my general observation since I moved to Doha, there are some signs of behavioural change. Shopping malls in Doha open early to allow for active walking. The Cornish is becoming a meeting point for runners in the evening. The large Aspire Zone area is expanding to include further open access to outdoor equipment. The alarming data on health issues related to lack of physical activity is here to remind us of the seriousness of the problem and hence the importance of a general mobilization of governments and non-government organizations, private and public entities, experts, civil society, and the media, to spark a new dynamic to allow for a cultural need for sport and physical activity among general population.

References

Abdul Rasoul, M.M. (2012) Obesity in children and adolescents in Gulf countries: Facts and solutions, *Avances en Diabetología*, 28, 3, 64–69.

Al-Hazaa et al. (2012) Lifestyle factors associated with overweight and obesity among Saudi adolescents, *BMC Public Health*, **12**, 354 [online]. Retrieved from www.ncbi.nlm.nih.gov/pmc/articles/PMC3433559/ [accessed 1 November 2015].

Al-Hazaa et al. (2014) Prevalence of overweight, obesity, and abdominal obesity among urban Saudi adolescents: Gender and regional variations, *Journal Health Population Nutrition*, 32, 4, 634–645.

Alwan, A. (2014) Responding to priority health challenges in the Arab world, *The Lancet, 383*, 9914, 284–286.

Alwasmi, N. (*The National*, 29 September 2015), National Sports Day to bring UAE together in friendly competition. Retrieved from www.thenational.ae/uae/government/national-sports-day-to-bring-uae-together-in-friendly-competition [accessed 29 September 2015].

Harkness, G. (2012) Out of bounds: Cultural barriers to female sports participation in Qatar, *The International Journal of the History of Sport*, 29, 15, 2162–2183.

Khan, F (*Arabnews*, 17 February 2014), 70% of Saudis are obese, says study. Retrieved from www.arabnews.com/news/527031 [accessed 1 October 2015].

Kronfol, N.M. (2012), Access and barriers to health care delivery in Arab countries: A review, Eastern Mediterranean Health Journal, 18 [online]. Retrieved from www.emro.who.int/emhj-volume-18-2012/issue-12/09.html [accessed 12 September 2015].

Museiger, A. et al. (2013) Perceived barriers to healthy eating and physical activity among adolescents in seven Arab countries: A cross-cultural study, *The Scientific World Journal*, 2013 [online]. Retrieved from www.hindawi.com/journals/tswj/2013/232164/ [accessed 14 September 2015].

Obesity Research Centre. (2015) Retrieved from www.obesitycenter.edu.sa [accessed 20 September 2015].

Rahim, H.F.A. et al. (2014) Non-communicable diseases in the Arab world, *The Lancet*, 383, 9914, 356–367.

Scharfenort, N. (2012) Urban development and social change in Qatar: The Qatar National Vision 2030 and the 2022 FIFA World Cup, *Journal of Arabian Studies: Arabia, the Gulf, and the Red Sea*, 2, 2, 209–230.

Thani, S. & Heenan, T., (2015) Sport and the 'Disneyfication' of the UAE. Retrieved from www. inter-disciplinary.net/probing-the-boundaries/wp-content/uploads/2015/08/Thani-sport4-dpaper.pdf [accessed 1 November 2015].

The Peninsula (12 December 2014) Qatar Active Campaign launched. Retrieved from http://thepeninsulaqatar.com/news/qatar/311257/qatar-active-campaign-launched [accessed 1 September 2015].

The Peninsula (08 December 2015), Qatar- Joint initiative to fight obesity among kids. Retrieved from www.menafn.com/qn_news_story_s.aspx?storyid=1094465917&title=Qatar-Joint-initiative-to-fight-obesity-among-kids&src=RSS [accessed 8 December 2015].

Westerbeek, H. & Smith, A. (2015) Corporate social responsibility and community health in the UAE the case of the Al Jazira Sport and Health Foundation, 1, 1 [online]. Retrieved from www.mejb.com/flash_content/Vol1_Issue1/Corporate-Social-Responsibility.htm [10 September 2015].

World Health Organization [Regional Office for the Eastern Mediterranean] (2014) Promoting physical activity in the Eastern Mediterranean Region through a life-course approach. Retrieved from http://applications.emro.who.int/dsaf/EMROPUB_2014_EN_1603.pdf [accessed 1 October 2015].

35

AUSTRALIA

Margaret Heffernan, Constantino Stavros,
Kate Westberg, Angela Dobele and Aaron Smith

Introduction

This chapter presents an overview of the practices and policies that have contributed to Australia's rich sporting reputation and social conundrum of dwindling physical activity. It chronicles the multi-disciplinary initiatives and policies undertaken by government and health organizations to motivate citizens to partake in physical activity, the paradox of policy and promotion for culturally diverse sectors, and how these factors have translated to current participation trends. Interventions and advocates are reviewed, particularly health perspectives and programs that have cast an urgent spotlight on the need to rethink approaches to influencing participation, particularly among vulnerable and disadvantaged groups in society. This chapter identifies the disconnect between Australia's image as an elite sporting nation and the reality of declining physical activity participation rates and the associated health concerns resulting from more sedentary lifestyles. Finally, the chapter reflects upon the issues associated with future policy alternatives and their implications for the practice of sport and its impact on physical activity.

As the Australian nation matures, the meaning and social significance of sport and its impact on physical activity demand a fresh perspective. This chapter will explore the need for this change, positing the requirement for a new approach to sport and physical activity to ensure that stereotypical representation of national identity and an over-emphasis on elite success does not undermine future health and wellbeing. The chapter argues that cultural and resource reprogramming is required to address the strategic direction of sports and physical activity by shifting the focus from elite sports to a preventative health agenda through increased participation.

Australia's population of 24 million will almost double over the next half-century (Australian Bureau of Statistics 2013a), bringing with it many complex challenges, including how to keep the burgeoning populace active and healthy. That an ostensibly sporting-fanatic nation such as Australia needs to be concerned with such a predicament might appear strange. The stereotypical Australian persona transmitted globally and reinforced by the national identity is that of an outgoing and natural sportsperson, incessantly surfing spectacular waves and jogging through pristine exotic nature.

While the "bronzed Aussie" image is largely the work of clever marketing, the reality is that Australians of all ages face unprecedented health and lifestyle risks. The nation, which has long prided itself on its sporting endeavours, has been subsumed by sedentary practices, poor diet and an ageing population. This new landscape is challenging governments at all levels to respond with policy that goes beyond the historic expectation that elite sporting success will filter down to stimulate grassroots participation in physical activity.

Sport policy and government cycles

Not only has Australia invested a large amount of emotional energy in its sporting practices, but its governments have also allocated extensive financial resources to the country's sporting infrastructure, which is now one of the most accessible and varied in the world. Historically, Local and State Government have been major providers of funds for facility construction. Local Government has been instrumental in building indoor sport centres, swimming pools and outdoor playing fields for their local communities, while State Governments have typically focused their funding contributions on larger scale venues more geared to spectator sports (Suter 2009; Richards 2016). The Commonwealth Government's role in sport funding and assistance is far more recent; indeed, for most of the twentieth century, it gave only limited assistance to sport. However, in the 1970s the Commonwealth Government became a major contributor to sport and is now the single most powerful influence on Australian sport and physical activity (Australian Institute of Sport 2015).

The institutional framework for Australian sport development is underpinned by a three-tier federalist system of government, established in 1901. Under this model, power is shared between the eight States and Territories and the Commonwealth, or Federal Government. The Constitution was structured to give the Commonwealth Government a number of specific and limited powers centred on defence, foreign relations and customs. Tax matters were initially left to the States. However, taxing powers were handed over to the Commonwealth Government during World War Two and since then it has taken over full responsibility for all major economic management, financial and revenue raising matters. The model is pivotal to understanding how public policy gains traction through the deployment of resources. For example, States were initially dependent on the Commonwealth Government for the funding of key services, but due to a broadening tax base, the balance has shifted over time with sport and physical activity currently the purview of Local, State and Commonwealth Governments (Hume 2016).

The other important institutional feature of Australian society is the clear division between the public and private sectors. The public sector comprises government, its agencies and infrastructure. The private sector comprises a variety of shareholder-based corporations, owner-operated businesses and non-profit entities like welfare organizations, community support groups, associations and clubs. Economic, cultural and recreational activity is generated and supported by both sectors. When the three tiers of government are combined with the private and not-for-profit sectors, a broad range of service and infrastructure delivery options become available. First, the Commonwealth Government, or a nationally based corporation, community agency or association, can deliver services and infrastructure centrally. Second, the services and infrastructure can be delivered at the local level by State Government, the local authority, business, association, community groups or commercial operators (Australian Government 2016a; Hume 2016).

Commonwealth Government sport policy is multi-dimensional, endeavouring to strike the elusive balance between elite sport development and community sport development and participation (Green & Houlihan 2005; Commonwealth of Australia 2010). Prior to the 1970s, the Australian Commonwealth Government took an ad hoc approach toward sport and recreation, partially driven by the political cycles of change in government ideologies. During the early 1970s, a newly elected Labor Government showed signs of a greater interest in sport and health policy. Although its initiatives were few, some policy changes survived into legacy. For example, the government viewed sport as an avenue to improve the overall welfare of the nation, and the future direction for sport in Australia was seriously considered through legislative frameworks. As a result, the Department of Tourism and Recreation was established, which subsequently commissioned a series of reports recommending more funding to professionalize elite sport, as well as the need for school and community-based programs to improve physical activity. The idea for a National Institute of Sport was first mooted at this time, but with another change of government in 1975 the initiative was abandoned along with other structural changes. However, Australia's poor performance in the 1976 Montreal Olympic Games became a major catalyst for change in Australian sport policy. Faced with criticism of its sporting system as being amateur, unstructured and poorly funded, coupled with public outrage and lobbying by sporting groups, the government was forced to re-think its perspective on elite sport. The government responded by pursuing sporting excellence on the world stage, most notably through the establishment of the Australian Institute of Sport (AIS) in 1981 in the nation's capital, Canberra, supported by a dramatic increase in Commonwealth sport funding (Hogan & Norton 2000; Eggins 2002; Green & Houlihan 2005; Jolly 2013).

The next decade saw the development of peak bodies designed to reshape the national sports agenda. In 1983, the Department of Sport, Recreation and Tourism was established followed by the Australian Sport Commission (ASC) in 1985, an independent statutory authority with a mandate of deploying public sport policy by allocating funding and overseeing strategic development programs. The ASC has been instrumental in directing the country's sporting success on the world stage, but has also proved a decisive advocate of sport participation and physical activity more broadly (Eggins 2002). One of the ASC's first projects in 1986 was to tackle the trend in declining youth physical activity. The result was the *Aussie Sport* program, which aimed to increase sport participation in schools by focusing on fun over competition, and within a decade had reached 96 per cent of Australian primary schools. Because the program modified sports and focused on values of achieving one's personal best, as opposed to winning, some critics suggested that it compromised opportunities for identifying talented athletes (Jolly 2013).

The paradox of Australian sport policies

The historical top-down approach to Australian sport policy is somewhat understandable due to its notable record of high-level sporting achievement, including winning world championships just this century in sports as diverse as cricket, pole-vaulting, surfing, field hockey and rugby. Australian cities have twice hosted the Olympic Games, Melbourne in 1956 and Sydney in 2000, and an Australian team has attended every Summer Olympics of the modern era, a feat shared by just four other nations, France, Great Britain, Greece and Switzerland. Coupled with a natural inclination to demonstrate global relevance through achievements on the sporting field, the confluence of government support and public enthusiasm has helped ensure that sporting achievement receives priority in the international arena. Politicians and policy makers assume that such success is important to Australians, irrespective of whether the benefits go further than medals and pride (Australian Government 2008).

The antecedents to the ingrained notion of sport's broader importance to the Australian psyche are difficult to pinpoint precisely. A strong British colonial heritage played a part, as has timing, given that many sporting teams were formed at the infancy of sport's professionalization.

Today, fans of elite sport are spoilt for choice. They can attend four codes of football (Australian Rules football, rugby league, rugby union and soccer), which are all played on a national level and receive significant media exposure. The championship match of Australian Rules football was the most watched television show in Australia in 2015, with a Rugby League match between two State teams in second place (Knox, 2016). National leagues also exist in other team sports including basketball and cricket, and positive gender policies are reflected in national competitions for women, including basketball, cricket, netball and soccer. On a participatory level for both groups and individuals, a wide variety of sport and recreation alternatives may be undertaken through accessible subsidized facilities, including beaches and swimming pools, indoor stadiums and well-resourced parks. Outdoor sports are popular due to a favourable climate, enabling participation in a myriad of activities, including surfing, swimming, golf, running, tennis and lawn bowls (Commonwealth of Australia 2010).

On a broader level a festival approach to sport consumption is increasingly common throughout Australia on the assumption that multi-faceted events can engage the wider community by attracting audiences and volunteers that might otherwise have not attended a pure sporting contest (Chalip & McGuirty 2004). Events and festivals tend to be facilitated and funded by State Governments, sometimes even legislating public holidays connected to sport. For example, in the state of Victoria two major sporting events have secured their own public holiday, one aligned with the Australian Rules football season, (the "Grand Final"), and the second linked to horse racing (The Melbourne Cup, "the race that stops a nation"). Government investments in these and many other designated major events are geared toward generating positive economic and social benefits for the community (Ruhanen & Whitford 2011). However, little evidence suggests that economic activity and entertainment deliver a commensurate improvement in sport participation, physical activity or health (Hajkowicz et al. 2013).

Investments in sport development have not come cheaply or easily. The last twenty years of policy implementation required more than AUS$1 billion of Commonwealth Government funding. Most of this investment was directed at elite sport and national sporting bodies, while at the same time State and Local Governments built a sporting infrastructure unparalleled on a per capita basis. With estimates that Olympic gold medals cost upwards of AUS$10 million each, policy makers have long insisted that the benefits of elite funding yield wider benefits in terms of national pride, economic stimulation, social capital and community participation (Australian Institute of Sport 2015).

At a community level, as described earlier, strong government-supported infrastructure gives the impression that sport and physical activity participation should come easily. It therefore constitutes somewhat of a paradox that despite their enthusiastic spectatorship, Australians are less inclined than ever before to join sport clubs. As we shall examine, participation rates in organized sport remain relatively disappointing. At best, informal physical activity is more likely to capture Australians' discretionary leisure time than structured, competitive sport. More alarmingly, there are few positive signs of improvement in the key physical health indicators of Australians whose increasingly sedentary lifestyles are fuelling metabolic conditions such as obesity and diabetes (Hills et al. 2014).

Australian sport policy and social capital

Sport development strategies have struggled to impact positively upon social capital. While there is limited evidence linking sport policy with lower levels of juvenile crime or dysfunctional social behaviour, connections have been shown between sporting cultures and binge-drinking, assaults, bullying incidents, racism and gender inequality. National sport policies have also failed to attenuate the risks of alienation and social dislocation that runs through many impoverished Australian communities. Much of Australian sport operates with little government interference. With the exception of the role the State and Local Governments play in funding the country's sport infrastructure, sport clubs, associations, leagues and governing bodies largely act autonomously. Self-reliant and resourceful, they mobilize interest in their sporting products, for both participation and entertainment (Nicholson & Hoye 2008).

The drivers of sport policy result from numerous political forces, with election policies at all tiers of government frequently forming the basis of inconsistent policy. Furthermore, policies are seldom sufficiently responsive to changing conditions and contexts, such as the growing obesity problem. Another source of policy development is the major stakeholder groups who may be seen as policy communities, at times with competing agendas. These groups comprise a diverse assemblage including the Australian Sports Commission, which is responsible for implementing Commonwealth Government policy as well as managing the AIS; the Australian Olympic Committee; the Commonwealth Games Association; major sport leagues; national and state sporting bodies; the Australian Sport Anti-doping Agency; the digital, electronic and print media; elite athletes; sport scientists and physicians; health and physical education professionals; and volunteer sport officials. Each prioritizes its own political agenda and consequent sporting ideology. Governments have an interest in fostering policy communities since they facilitate consultation, make the policy process more predictable, reduce policy conflict and provide the opportunity for non-government funding for sport. At the same time, all of these stakeholders and policy communities pull sport in different directions, more often towards commercial outcomes than health advantages.

Sport policy and health agendas

At the State and Local government levels, sport has intermittently been viewed as a conduit for improving social cohesion and health, particularly as a means of combating rising rates of obesity. Unfortunately, the latter outcome has not eventuated. Physical inactivity has been acknowledged as a growing problem in Australia and has been linked to more than 13,000 deaths. It has been estimated that an increase in physical activity by 15 per cent by 2018 would save up to AUS$434 million (Australian Sports Commission 2015a). However, governments have promoted exercise and activity through a steady stream of fragmented programs, most of which operate independently and on a trivial scale compared to those driving elite performance.

In 1996, the ASC launched *Active Australia – A National Participation Framework* designed to increase physical activity with the support of State Governments. The framework aimed to provide facilities, programs and services to boost physical activity of all Australians, but with a focus on schools and Local Government organizations. In 1999 a specially formed Sport 2000 Task Force produced a report entitled *Shaping Up: A Review of Commonwealth Involvement in Sport and Recreation in Australia*. It recommended that the government allocate more resources for sport, physical activity and participation programs, which previously had commanded 10 to 15 per cent of total Commonwealth Government spending. Despite the success of the *Aussie Sports* and the *Active Australia* programs, the sport participation rate increased only marginally between 1985 and the year 2000.

In 2001 the Commonwealth Government launched a new policy entitled *Backing Australia's Sporting Ability: A More Active Australia*, which was subsequently implemented by the ASC. The policy focussed on four primary goals: first, ensuring that athletes, including those with disabilities, continue to compete successfully at an international level; second, enhancing sport management structures and practices to increase the professionalism of Australia's national sporting system and to maintain and develop the elite sport feeder system; thirdly, creating a "drug free" and equitable sporting environment. The final goal was to significantly increase public participation in sport.

The Commonwealth Government allocated approximately AUS$132 million a year from 2001–05 to support the new goals, although the spending allocations revealed its real emphasis. The first policy goal related to elite sport and high performance development was allocated AUS$103 million in each of the four years. In contrast, the fourth policy goal, which aimed to increase public participation in sport, was allocated AUS$22 million for each of the four years. As a result, while elite sport continued to deliver medals, physical activity and sport participation continued to languish.

In June 2004, the Commonwealth Government introduced the initiative *Building a Healthy Active Australia*, which had a major emphasis on facilitating access to free, structured physical activity programs for children after school. In addition to improving physical activity, the program also addressed parental concerns related to children playing in unsupervised settings as well as time constraints in supporting extracurricular activities. The program received high levels of satisfaction from stakeholders and was supported from 2005 until 2015 when it was replaced by yet another initiative: the *Sporting Schools* program (Australian Sports Commission 2014). However, despite numerous programs developed by the Commonwealth Government to enhance sport at the elite and community levels, as well as initiatives to encourage physical activity, there is little evidence to suggest that these investments have led to improved health outcomes for the community. Sport policy that attempts to cater for both the elite and grassroots level does not deliver a healthier nation. As a result, on-going criticism of the government's prioritization of elite sport funding has gathered momentum (Jolly 2013).

Addressing the challenges

In 2008 the Commonwealth Government expressed concern at the increasing intensity of sport competition on the world stage, acknowledging that it was time for a much-needed reform of the sport system to enable it to meet future challenges. A report entitled *The Future of Sport in Australia*, also known as the *Crawford Report*, recognized the "complex, inefficient and cumbersome" system associated with Australian sport, the multiple portfolios related to sport and recreation, health and education, and also the proliferation of fragmented sporting organizations, universities and schools (Crawford 2009, p. 11). The report acknowledged the need for a single point of focus to provide leadership and an overarching policy. Further, it highlighted that community sport had been neglected and underfunded compared to the support provided for winning medals at the elite level. Criticism was levelled at all three tiers of government for their ad hoc approach toward community sport, and lack of impact on health. Finally, the report identified a need to cater for the changing profile of the Australian population, taking into account ageing, immigration and increased urbanization, factors that had been previously ignored.

The strategic response to the report resulted in *Australian Sport: The Pathway to Success*, which exposed a "critical junction" for sport. The report highlighted the impotency of prior approaches, and the desperate need for system-wide "collaboration, reform and investment" (Australian Government 2010, p. 1). Again, a significant financial commitment was made for

Australian sport (AUS$1.2 billion) to be deployed by the ASC over the forthcoming four years. Key priorities included increased funding for:

(i)   sport and education strategies focusing on increasing participation in schools;
(ii)   national sporting organizations to grow participation at the community level, including people from diverse backgrounds;
(iii) promoting women's participation and leadership in sport;
(iv)   support and training for coaches and officials involved in community level sport; and
(v)   support for high performance athletes.

The Crawford Report further argued the need for a more integrated commitment between the three tiers of government in aligning elite and community initiatives. As a result, the Sport and Recreation Ministers' Council established the first *National Sport and Active Recreation Policy Framework* in 2011 to help guide policy and resource allocation at all government levels. Key priorities focused on increased participation at the local level, strong national competitions, and success at international levels. Its overarching goal of improved public health, social inclusion and community development was a critical change to previous strategic priorities, which were targeted towards under-represented and under-active groups. To date, one of the key challenges in developing and implementing an effective physical activity strategy remains a lack of reliable information, not only about participation levels, but also about what kinds of intervention programs bolster activity and health outcomes. To address this, the ASC has committed to undertaking research to better understand participation trends, inform decision-making and enhance participation strategies (Australian Sports Commission 2015b).

Behavioural change through public campaigns

Various levels of Australian government have sought to promote physical activity through a range of promotional campaigns, but as the following examples illustrate, behavioural change has been difficult to attain. In fact, physical activity participation rates continue to decline, especially amongst those between the ages of 25 and 34 (Hills et al. 2014) . Whilst educational and promotional campaigns successfully raise awareness about health, diet and physical activity, behavioural change impacts are not easily identified (Cavill & Bauman 2007) with reliable data in short supply.

The introduction of one of the first health and physical activity campaigns, launched in the 1970s, was *Life. Be In It! (Be in it today, live more of your Life. Be. In. It.)*. This campaign proved "instrumental in changing Australians' attitudes to exercise and healthy eating" (Xu et al. 2014, n.p.). Its key cartoon character, Norm, represented a typical overweight, un-fit, sedentary middle-aged Australian man. Using various media, the messages cautioned the population on obesity (causes and health implications), diet and the need to participate in exercise (www.lifebeinit.org/).

Two decades later in 1997–8, the *Active Australia* campaign promoted the importance of regular, moderate-intensity exercise, targeting men and women aged 25–60, along with health, sport, recreation and fitness professionals. The campaign also aimed to maintain the physical activity motivation in people already sufficiently active. Other specific population groups have been targeted in subsequent campaigns. For example, the 2006 national *Get Moving* campaign was directed at children and parents in order to promote exercise and healthy weight ranges with the intention of ameliorating the alarming increase in childhood obesity stemming from physical inactivity and poor dietary practices. Similarly, the subsequent 2007–8 Victorian Government *Go For Your Life* campaign aimed to improve the socio-cultural, policy and physical environments in children's care and educational settings.

Several other large scale campaigns have encouraged adults to change their lifestyles and improve their overall health and wellbeing. Some examples include the *Measure Up Campaign* (and Phase 2 *Measure Up*) of 2008–13; the Western Australian program *Live Lighter*, which extended to Victoria and the Australian Capital Territory in 2012; *Get Set 4 Life – Habits for Healthy Kids*; *Healthy Spaces and Places*; *Learning from Successful Community Obesity Initiative*; *Healthy Weight Information and Resources* (Australian Government 2015). The most recent attempts to improve national health and wellbeing have been through two unique partnerships. First, in a response to the discussion paper *Australia: The Healthiest Country by 2020* (Commonwealth of Australia, 2008) the Australian Local Government Association, Heart Foundation and Planning Institute of Australia in 2008–16 created the *Healthy Spaces & Places* programme, a national guide that aimed to improve health and wellbeing through the development of healthy, built environments (Planning Institute of Australia 2009, 2016). Whilst the Heart Foundation continues to promote the program's fundamental principles, the short-termism of Government initiatives poses a major barrier to the sustainability of sound initiatives, and hence Australia being the "healthiest country".

A second policy framework, *An Australian Vision for Active Transport* was launched in 2010 through a national partnership with organizations from the health, transport and local government sectors. The framework sets out a nine point plan to boost participation in walking, cycling and public transport. It encourages the Australian government to make a major commitment to support strategic initiatives that enable delivery of physical activity policies; setting clear, realistic targets for active transport and physical activity outcomes; resourcing local government authorities to implement the policy; embracing the *Healthy Spaces and Places* planning principles; investing in infrastructure to encourage active domestic tourism; increasing safety measures for active transport participants; embed the principles through cycle training and pedestrian education in schools; and provide employer incentives to encourage employee to use more active forms of transport to get to work. Although the long term benefits are anticipated to enhance environmental and social-cohesion factors, the success of this initiative will require significant behavioural change from the general public and legislators. Many urban dwellers continue to use private transport to commute due to congested public transport systems, perceptions of unsafe walking environments prevail among females in particular and varying approaches related to the availability of cycling access on roads across the country (Bicycle Network 2016) suggests there is no universal government support for the *Active Transport* policy.

While Australians are aware of the need for regular physical activity as a means to promote health and assist in the prevention of non-communicable diseases, they are not translating that knowledge into action. A major challenge for health professionals revolves around how to motivate individuals and groups to adopt and maintain physical activity (Hills et al. 2014).

In order for physical activity promotion in Australia to improve its success, campaigns need to focus on five key factors. First, since the level of promotional media around lifestyle behaviours, from physical activity to nutrition, alcohol consumption and smoking, has increased, the corresponding noise in the informational marketplace has increased. In this crowded space is the potential for contradictory information, diversity of well-intentioned messages and conflicting agendas, which can lead to "uncertainty and ultimately intertia by stakeholders" (Hills et al. 2014, p. 31). Second, the pattern of physical activity tends to be higher in younger populations, which reveals a correspondingly small window of opportunity to engage and cultivate long-term physical activity rather than a lifetime of sedentary habits. This narrow window represents a pivotal point where interventions should be directed.

Third, public health communications tend to take a "shotgun" approach, presenting generic information without real relevance to specific groups or those between developmental stages (Hills et al. 2014, p. 32). Interventions and campaigns designed with heterogeneous consumer groups in mind will have a greater chance of success (Lee et al. 2012). Fourth, more evidence is being captured about activity levels before and after promotional campaigns (Brug et al. 2010; Estabrooks & Glasgow 2006; Glasgow et al. 2003). Decisions based on solid evidence offer an "improvement loop between evidence and practice" that could allow for the tailoring of messages to specific groups while accounting for social context and technology. Finally, campaigns need to create a supportive environment to better enable an individual to make healther decisions and choices (Hills et al. 2014, p. 32).

Despite the surfeit of policies and intervention campaigns, little evidence of a unified approach can be seen. In addition, further campaigns could be more focussed on the intention and planning stages of physical activity rather than just informing and educating. Previous research has shown that national mass-media campaigns involving a television advertising component can increase physical activity levels (for a summary see Craig et al. 2015). Perhaps the shortfall separating physical fitness awareness and action can be located between the environmental factors (where a campaign is informative and perhaps even inspiring) and the second stage of the health process where intention and planning fall short, or start off well but languish. Beyond the campaign, other environmental factors that impact behavioural decisions include peer or family pressure, community facilities and resources and even the weather (Xu et al. 2014). Also salient are a host of factors shown to be particularly relevant to physical participation in culturally diverse communities discussed shortly.

Active lifestyle trends

The active lifestyle previously embedded in Australia's culture and identity has been under threat for some time, as it has in many countries. In terms of the nature of physical activity, increased time pressure for much of the population has resulted in a shift from participation in organized sport toward more flexible and individual forms of exercise such as running, walking, aerobics and gym membership (Australian Sports Commission 2015a). Unfortunately this trend toward individual fitness pursuits may exclude lower socioeconomic groups that do not traditionally have high levels of access to these activities (Hajkowicz et al. 2013).

According to the Australian Bureau of Statistics (2015), of the Australian population aged 15 years and over, an estimated 60 per cent (11.1 million people), reported that they had participated in sport and physical recreation at least once during the twelve months in 2013–14, a 5 per cent decline from the previous two years. Walking as a form of exercise, fitness and gym are the most popular physical recreational activities, particularly among females. Males were more likely than females to play golf or participate in cycling and BMX cycle sport. Figure 35.1 indicates the ten most popular sports and activities in 2014 for children between the ages of 6–13, and well as teenagers and adults over the age of 14. For both groups, swimming had the most regular participation. With children, over two-thirds (77 per cent) spend their leisure time watching television, and only one third of children achieve the recommended levels of physical activity (Australian Sports Commission 2015b). Children living in areas of lower socioeconomic status are 9 per cent less likely to participate in organized

Rank	Sport	Percent Participation, age 6–13	Rank	Sport	Percent Participation, age 14+
1	Swimming	48.8	1	Swimming	10.1
2	Soccer	48.7	2	Cycling	7.3
3	Cycling	37.7	3	Hiking/Bushwalking	4.4
4	Athletics/Track and Field	31.7	4	Aerobics	3.2
5	Basketball	30.5	5	Soccer	3.1
6	Dancing	30.3	6	Dancing	2.9
7	Cricket	25.7	7	Tennis	2.4
8	Netball	20.5	8	Netball	1.8
9	Tennis	20.0	9	Basketball	1.7
10	Gymnastics	18.1	10	Cricket	1.2

Figure 35.1   Top 10 sports and activities by regular participation rate 2014

Source: Roy Morgan Research (2015)

sport, as compared with children who come from a "mid-range" socioeconomic status (Australian Bureau of Statistics 2012).

Australia is struggling with rising levels of metabolic diseases and obesity related to physical inactivity. As a nation, Australia's girth is expanding, contributing to the nation's health burden and to its reputation as "one of the fattest nations in the developed world" (Obesity in Australia 2015, n.p.). One in two Australian adults and one in four children are categorized as obese, the prevalence increasing by 7 per cent in the last 15 years, figures well above the OECD countries' average of 18 per cent adult obesity (Australian Bureau of Statistics 2012). Geography also contributes to this grim picture. Men and women who live in inner regional, outer regional and remote areas (predominantly an Indigenous population) of Australia show higher rates of obesity compared with their counterparts living in major cities (Australian Bureau of Statistics 2013b).

In 2008, the Commonwealth Government's national preventative health strategy, ambitiously titled *Australia: The Healthiest Country by 2020*, highlighted obesity, tobacco and excessive alcohol consumption as three areas of priority. With obesity the goal was to drive environmental change leading to increased physical activity, and reduce sedentary behaviour including prolonged sitting. In mid-2014 the Department of Health elevated its recommended amount of weekly physical activity from two and a half to five hours of moderate physical activity for adults between the ages of 18–64, or one and a quarter, to one and a half hours of vigorous physical activity. For children aged 5–17 years old, the aim should be one hour of moderate to vigorous physical activity per day with "screen time" occupying a maximum of two hours per day (Australian Government 2014). With regard to adults, in response to the sedentary patterns of 71 per cent of the Australian working population, workplace physical activity policies have been introduced at Federal and State levels of government. Whilst the implementation of these policies is voluntary, employers are encouraged to provide access to, or opportunities for, physical activity both at work and through active travel to and from work (Australian Government 2016b). Many new buildings in the Central Business Districts of major cities now eschew car parking in basements, preferring instead to provide secure bicycle parking and showering facilities to encourage workers to ride.

Australian migrants' participation in sport and physical activity

The multi-disciplinary initiatives and policies undertaken by government and health organizations as described have not addressed participation among the populations most in need. The focus on elite sport policy and an Anglo-Saxon focus in the promotion of sport participation and physical activity have contributed to women's social disadvantage in culturally and linguistically diverse (CALD) population groups. Even the best of intentions have contributed to some unintentionally discriminatory and inequitable practices that have undermined participation goals (Solar and Irwin 2010).

Australia is a culturally diverse nation with migrants from more than 200 countries comprising 28 per cent of its population (~ 6.6 million people) (Australian Bureau of Statistics 2013c). Most of these individuals arrive in Australia in good health as part of their eligibility for migration. This "healthy migrant effect" is not sustained with many first generation migrants gaining excess weight with change of diet as a result of acculturation, and increases in their sedentary lifestyle (Australian Bureau of Statistics 2013b).

Many of these migrants do not reflect the average Australian when it comes to rates of participation in sporting and physical recreation activities, including attendance at sporting events (Dassanayake et al. 2011). Significant sections of the population have unequal access and opportunities to participate, diminishing their prospects for social inclusion and good health (Sawrikar and Muir 2010). Whilst peak sporting bodies provide inclusive and culturally targeted initiatives such as the ASC *All Cultures* strategy through a supported and structured environment, migrant enthusiasm for sport is not necessarily translated into participation (Australian Sports Commission 2015a). Among migrant men, and increasingly for younger women, soccer has played an important role in their social inclusion and social capital (Civitillo 2014). These disparate participation trends in physical activity and sport are mirrored in children often through parental acculturation patterns. Noticeably lower participation in organized sport, such as swimming, outdoor soccer, football and netball outside school hours has been shown among children from families with low English literacy (Australian Bureau of Statistics 2009).

Many migrant groups are often unfamiliar with Australian cultural norms around sport and physical activity. For example, in Queensland the *CALD Physical Activity Mapping Project* found that despite most physical activity service providers assuming that their initiatives were inclusive, only 10 per cent of sports and physical activity initiatives specifically met the needs of CALD communities. A culturally proficient community-engagement approach to program development and community awareness may help overcome these barriers (Caperchione et al. 2013; Queensland Health 2010).

Barriers to access and participation in sport and recreation exist for many migrant women, and may be attributed to cultural differences, interpersonal, institutional and internalized attitudes, and a lack of awareness, knowledge and accessibility (Diabetes 2012). Direct inhibitors include institutional constraints that compromise cultural issues including: dress codes; language and communication barriers; personal issues around cultural traditions of family responsibilities and family expectations (being a common barrier across all population groups); adherence to religious codes which do not condone women's participation in sport; a lack of understanding of Australia's sporting culture; and discrimination.

Historically, women's participation in many sporting codes has been overlooked in general, which has impacted upon the integration of new social norms and health promoting behaviours within the broader community (Chau 2007). However, progress is being shown with the establishment of walking clubs, increasing access through "women only" swim and gym sessions across all states in Australia and culturally appropriate swimwear and sport clothing being manufactured, although inflexible dress codes prevail in some sports (McCue 2008).

The lack of women's sports participation nationally was of such concern that in 2006 the Commonwealth Government instigated a Senate Committee report, *"About Time!" Women in Sport and Recreation in Australia* (Commonwealth of Australia 2006). The report found CALD women's participation was constrained by the numerous cultural and social factors described above. It also reported that many sporting bodies were unable to deliver participation opportunities that met the cultural needs of CALD participants. The Queensland State Government through its *Start Playing Stay Playing* plan (MacDonald 2013) identified enablers designed to increase women and girls' participation through diversity policies across the three tiers of government. Examples include economic enablers like reducing costs and increasing access, culturally and gender inclusive attitudes and facilities, culturally targeted promotion, partnership and social support models with other community programs and media awareness about physical activity access.

Implications for future physical activity policy and practice

The Australian sports landscape is continually changing. In 2013, an ASC report *The Future of Australian Sport: Megatrends* identified six social, economic and environmental megatrends that were considered most likely to influence community, industry and government policy and investment choices in shaping Australia's sports and recreation sector to 2045 (Hajkowicz et al. 2013). The report highlighted the following trends:

(i)   personalized and socialized elements of sport for health and fitness across the broader population catering to individualized schedules (as currently shown with women) rather than organized sporting codes which will show a decrease in participation;
(ii) increased participation especially driven by younger sub-cultures and social media in lifestyle, adventure and alternative sports and recreational activities;
(iii) the increased alignment of government sporting policies to social capital through improved health and civil cohesion;
(iv) policies will be driven by societal demographic (especially an ageing population), general and cultural changes to maintain and sustain participation;
(v)   increased market competition for the sports sector due to the rise of Asia's economic growth and sports development; and finally,
(vi) market and economic pressures on elite athletes and new business models, impacting on the viability of grass-roots community sports associations and community participation.

The above trends foreshadow increasing complexity in the physical activity and sporting marketplace, and suggest that governments will have an even more difficult job in stimulating health behaviours. Transferring national objectives through national sporting organizations (NSOs), non-governmental organizations (NGOs) and sporting enterprises into positive physical activity or health related outcomes remains an enduring challenge because it leaves government with few viable methods for determining the effectiveness of its own policies other than via the judicious use of secondary, indirect performance measures.

In practice, the role of government is to set strategic direction by charting a national course, distributing funding for aligned initiatives, and hoping that the trickle-down effect gains momentum. This is usually accomplished by stating general rather than detailed policy. In the case of sport, it is the Australian Sports Commission as the agency of the Commonwealth Government, which is responsible for the delivery of the government's sports programs, providing funds to NSOs for a range of both elite and participatory purposes, and for determining the effectiveness of those programs. However, the ASC does not provide funding for State, regional and local sporting organizations or individuals. This is achieved through State Departments of Sport and Recreation as well as local municipalities. As a result, even the most vigorous of government policies aiming to bolster physical activity, health or a more functional sporting culture has little relevance to the non-elite Australian householder uninterested in organized competition.

In essence the challenge is clear at the government level: deliver the twin objectives of increasing the number of successful elite athletes and increasing the numbers of people playing sport. The latter task is devolved to the ASC, and to NSOs. The funding received from government may then, in whole or in part, be passed from the NSO to State sports organizations, to individual clubs, or NGOs charged with the stewardship of health or physical activity related programs. Where funding goes to State organizations or individual clubs, that funding may represent only a small portion of that organization's or club's overall income. By implication, national physical activity policies have never mustered sufficient potency to overcome the dilution of funding pools that trickle down the sporting system. Conversely, the hyper-commercial world of professional sport entertainment inexorably channels its resources into elite performance and its economic dividends.

Having determined some of the difficulties facing the Commonwealth Government, the ASC and NSOs, how then might these organizations proceed in order to improve physical activity and health outcomes for the Australian population? The process must start with the policy itself. Invariably, the focus of the outcome will be on the effect the government can have on the community, the economy or the national interest. Despite the political appeal of elite success, any serious improvements in physical activity must begin with a commitment prioritising national health. In turn, the agency tasked with implementing the government policy, the ASC, must determine the most appropriate organization to service their requirement. Unlike current arrangements that favour yearly initiatives, a superior approach would preference long-term agreements and programs in order to affect the growing culture of inactivity. It may be undertaken at the national, state or local level, or it may be accomplished by setting up ASC sponsored programs. Far more attention must also be allocated to ensuring that specific demographic groups in the community such as youth, older people, people with a disability and people with a CALD background are also likely to be recipients of program opportunities.

Conclusion

The last 30 years of Australian sport policy has transformed the Australian sporting landscape. It has largely abandoned its amateur values, ventured boldly into the corporate world and professionalized its management structures and systems. At the same time the Commonwealth Government has progressively increased its financial assistance to elite sport while leaving most of the programs associated with bolstering physical activity to the sport system and health authorities. Although local, club and State sport associations still underpin the sport system, they have fallen subservient to high performance sport institutes and high profile, commercialized professional sport league competitions. One outcome has been a radical escalation in performance standards allowing Australia and its athletes to remain amongst the world's elite. On the other hand, there are many serious health and wellbeing issues left unresolved, including fading community sport volunteerism and resourcing, declining participation rates, alarming increases in metabolic illness caused by inactivity and poor diet, chronic drinking encouraged through sport cultures, and all while marginalized groups, ethnicities and women remain disadvantaged.

While some social benefits from the high performance policy area have yielded returns in national pride, the outcomes from the mass participation policy have not. Informal and unstructured exercise options seem the only resilient areas of interest. Physical activity participation remains the great weakness of Commonwealth Government sport policy, although it should also be recognized that State and local governments have some direct responsibilities in this area. It is difficult to see how the current Commonwealth Government policy, which gives only moderate attention to broad participation, social integration, grassroots assistance and equity, can reverse the declining activity levels of Australian people. Few stakeholders dispute that sport is an integral part of the Commonwealth policy mix, and can generate a significant array of social benefits, but it is also clear that some of the benefits are seriously under-realized when it comes to health outcomes, access and equity.

When the last 30 years of Australian sport and physical activity policy are viewed in aggregate, a number of objectives are evident. First, and foremost, there are policies that aim to train elite athletes who can successfully compete internationally. Second, there are policies that aim to improve the management systems of national sport bodies. Third, there are policies that aim to leverage a variety of economic benefits from major sport events and the expertise residing in our sporting bodies. Fourth, there are policies that aim to extend and improve opportunities for community participation. Fifth, there are policies that aim to build social capital through the support of community sport clubs and associations. Finally there are policies that aim to create diversity and equity by changing the culture of sport organizations. However, as we have suggested, not all of these policy themes have been equally successful, or met the expectations that were set for them.

References

Australian Bureau of Statistics 2009, *Year Book Australia 2009–10*, cat.no. 1301.0. ABS Canberra.

Australian Bureau of Statistics 2012, *Australian Social Trends, June*, cat.no. 4102.0, ABS Canberra.

Australian Bureau of Statistics 2013a, *Population Projections, Australia, 2012 (base) to 2101*, cat no. 3222.0, ABS Canberra.

Australian Bureau of Statistics 2013b, *Profiles of Health Australia 2011–13. Overweight and Obesity*, cat. no. 4338.0, ABS Canberra.

Australian Bureau of Statistics 2013c, *Migration, Australia 2013–14*, cat.no. 3412.0, ABS Canberra.

Australian Bureau of Statistics 2015, *Participation in Sport and Recreation 2013–14*, cat.no. 4177.0, ABS Canberra.

Australian Government 2008, *Australian Sport: Emerging Challenges, New Directions*, viewed 12 May 2016, www.clearinghouseforsport.gov.au/__data/assets/pdf_file/0005/165839/Australian_Sport_Emerging_Challenges, _New_Directions.pdf.

Australian Government 2010, *Australia Sport: The Pathway to Success*, viewed 21 October 2015, www.health.gov.au/internet/main/publishing.nsf/Content/aust_sport_path_report_chapter.

Australian Government 2014, *Department of Health Physical Activity and Sedentary Behaviour Guidelines*, viewed 21 October 2015, www.health.gov.au/internet/main/publishing.nsf/content/health-pubhlth-strateg-phys-act-guidelines.

Australian Government 2015, *Department of Health: A Healthy and Active Australia*, viewed 20 October 2015, www.healthyactive.gov.au/internet/healthyactive/publishing.nsf/Content/home.

Australian Government 2016a, *How Government Works*, viewed 12 May 2016, www.australia.gov.au/about-government/how-government-works.

Australian Government 2016b. *What is a Healthy Workplace?* Australian Government Department of Health, viewed 30 March 2016, www.healthyworkers.gov.au/internet/hwi/publishing.nsf/Content/what.

Australian Government 2016c, *Healthy Workers Initiative*. Australian Government Department of Health, viewed 30 May 2016, www.healthyworkers.gov.au/internet/hwi/publishing.nsf/Content/movemore.

Australian Institute of Sport 2015, *Investment Announcement 2015–16,* viewed 12 May 2016, www.ausport.gov.au/supporting/investment_announcement_2015-16.

Australian Local Government Association, Bus Industry Confederation, Cycling Promotion Fund, National Heart Foundation of Australia, & International Association of Public Transport, *An Australian Vision for Active Transport 2010,* viewed 30 March 2016, www.beactive.wa.gov.au/index.php?id=1267.

Australian Sports Commission 2014, *Sporting Schools,* ASC & AIS, Australian Government, viewed 20 October 2015, www.ausport.gov.au/news/asc_news/story_585663_sporting_schools.

Australian Sports Commission 2015a. *Participating in Sport.* ASC & AIS, Australian Government, viewed 20 October 2015, http://www.ausport.gov.au/participating/resources/resources.

Australian Sports Commission 2015b. *Play. Sport. Australia. The Australian Sports Commission's Participation Game Plan. March.* ASC & AIS, Australian Government, viewed 20 October 2015, http://www.ausport.gov.au/participating/playsportaustralia.

Bicycle Network 2016, *Our Campaigns,* viewed 30 May 2016, www.bicyclenetwork.com.au/general/policy-and-campaigns/2552/.

Brug, J, van Dale, D, Lanting, L, Kremers, S, Veenhof, C, Leurs, M, van Yperen, T, & Kok, G 2010, 'Towards evidence-based, quality-controlled health promotion: The Dutch recognition system for health promotion interventions', *Health Education Research,* vol. 25, no. 6, pp. 1100–1106.

Caperchione CM, Kolt GS, & Mummery WK 2013, 'Examining physical activity service provision to Culturally and Linguistically Diverse (CALD) communities in Australia: A qualitative evaluation', *PLoS ONE,* vol. 8, no. 4, p. e62777.

Cavill, N & Bauman, A 2007, 'Changing the way people think about health-enhancing physical activity: Do mass meda campaigns have a role?' *Journal of Sports Sciences,* vol. 22, no. 8, pp. 771–790.

Chalip, L & McGuirty, J 2004, 'Bundling sport events with the host destination', *Journal of Sport & Tourism,* vol. 9, no. 3, pp. 267–282.

Chau, J 2007, *Physical Activity and Building Stronger Communities,* Premier's Council for Active Living, NSW Centre for Physical Activity and Health, report no. CPAH07-001.

Civitillo, J 2014, 'The role of soccer in the adjustment of immigrants to South Australia', *Australian Population & Migration Research Centre,* vol. 2, no. 4, pp. 1–5.

Commonwealth of Australia 2006, *About Time! Women in Sport and Recreation in Australia.* The Senate Parliament of Australia, 6 September, ISBN 0 642 71708 7.

Commonwealth of Australia 2008, *National Preventative Health Taskforce Australia: The Healthiest Country by 2020. A Discussion Paper.* P3–4510. Online ISBN: 1-74186-728-2.

Commonwealth of Australia 2010, *Australian Sport: The Pathway to Success.* Online ISBN: 978-1-74241-233-7, viewed 12 May 2016, www.health.gov.au/internet/main/publishing.nsf/Content/aust_sport_path_report_chapter/$file/aust_sport_path.pdf.

Craig, CL, Bauman, A, Latimer-Cheung, A, Rhodes, RE, Faulkner, G, Berry,TR, Tremblay, MS, & Spence, JC 2015, 'An evaluation of the My ParticipACTION campaign to increase self-efficacy for being more physically active', *Journal of Health Communication: International Perspectives,* vol. 20, no. 9, pp. 995–1003.

Crawford, D 2009, *The Future of Sport in Australia,* viewed 22 October 2015, http://apo.org.au/files/Resource/Crawford_Report.pdf.

Dassanayake, J, Dharmage, SC, Gurrin, L, Sundararajan, V, & Payne, WR 2011, 'Are Australian immigrants at a risk of being physically inactive?', *International Journal of Behavioral Nutrition and Physical Activity,* vol. 8, p. 53.

Diabetes 2012, *Immigrant & Refugee Women Factsheet 4 August,* Multicultural Centre For Women's Health, viewed 13 October 2015, www.mcwh.com.au/downloads/factsheets/MCWH%20FS%204%20Diabetes%202012.pdf.

Eggins, M 2002, *The AIS - An Icon for Excellence in Sport* from Excellence: The Australian Institute of Sport. Canberra, Australian Sports Commission. 1998 (updated Jan 2002), viewed 12 May 2016, www.ausport.gov.au/ais/about/history.

Estabrooks, PA & Glasgow, RE 2006, 'Translating effective clinic-based physical activity interventions into practice', *American Journal of Preventive Medicine,* vol. 31, no. 4, S45–56.

Glasgow, RE, Lichtenstein, E, & Marcus, AC 2003, 'Why don't we see more translation of health promotion research to practice? Rethinking the efficacy-to-effectiveness transition', *Journal of Public Health,* vol. 93, no. 8, pp. 1261–1267.

Green, M & Houlihan, B 2005, *Elite Sport Development: Policy Learning and Political Priorities.* Routledge, London, UK.

Hajkowicz, SA, Cook, H, Wilhelmseder, L, & Boughen, N 2013, *The Future of Australian Sport: Megatrends Shaping the Sports Sector over Coming Decades*. A Consultancy Report for the Australian Sports Commission. CSIRO, Australia.

Hills, AP, Street, SJ, & Harris, N 2014, 'Getting Australia more active: Challenges and opportunities for health promotion', *Health Promotion Journal of Australia*, vol. 25, no. 1, pp. 30–34.

Hogan, K & Norton, K 2000, 'The "Price" of Olympic gold', *Journal of Science and Medicine in Sport*, vol. 3, no. 2, pp. 203–218.

Hume, C 2016, *Structure of Australian Sport*, Australian Sports Commission, 09112-17, viewed 12 May 2016, www.clearinghouseforsport.gov.au/knowledge_base/organised_sport/sport_systems_structures_and_pathways/structure_of_australian_sport.

Jolly, R 2013, *Sports funding: Federal balancing act*, viewed 28 August 2015, www.aph.gov.au/About_Parliament/Parliamentary_Departments/Parliamentary_Library/pubs/BN/2012-2013/SportFunding.

Knox, D 2016 2015, *Ratings: The Final Word*, viewed 23 May 2016, www.tvtonight.com.au/2016/01/2015-ratings-the-final-word.html.

Lee, IM, Shiroma, EJ, Lobelo, F, Puska, P, Blair, SN, & Katzmarzyk, PT for *The Lancet* Physical Activity Series Working Group 2012, 'Effect of physical inactivity on major non-communicable diseases worldwide: An analysis of burden of disease and life expectancy', *The Lancet*, vol. 380, no. 9838, pp. 219–229.

MacDonald, D (Chair) 2013, *Start Playing Stay Playing: A Plan to Increase and Enhance Sport and ActiveRecreation Opportunities for Women and Girls*, Ministerial Advisory Committee on Women and Girls in Sport and Recreation. State of Queensland, Australia, viewed 28 August 2015, www.qld.gov.au/recreation/health/women-girls/.

McCue, H 2008, *The Civil and Social Participation of Muslim Women in Australian Community Life*, Department of Immigration and Citizenship (DIAC), Canberra, Australia.

Nicholson, M & Hoye, R 2008, *Sport and Social Capital*, Elsevier, Abingdon, UK.

Obesity in Australia 2015, *Obesity in Australia*, viewed 8 October 2015, www.modi.monash.edu.au/obesity-facts-figures/obesity-in-australia/.

Planning Institute of Australia 2009, 2016, *Healthy Spaces & Places: A National Guide to Designing Places for Healthy Living*, Australian Government Department of Health & Ageing, viewed 18 May 2016, www.healthyplaces.org.au/site/.

Queensland Health 2010, *Engaging culturally and linguistically diverse (CALD) Queenslanders in physical activity: Findings of the CALD Physical Activity Mapping Project*, Division of the Chief Health Officer, Queensland Health, Brisbane, Australia.

Richards, R 2016, *Sports Facility Planning and Use*, viewed 12 May 2016, www.clearinghouseforsport.gov.au/knowledge_base/organised_sport/sports_administration_and_management/sports_facility_planning_and_use.

Roy Morgan Research 2015, *The Top 20 Sports Played by Aussies Young and Old(er)*, viewed 9 October 2015, www.roymorgan.com/findings/6123-australian-sports-participation-rates-among-children-and-adults-december-2014-201503182151.

Ruhanen, L & Whitford, M 2011, 'Indigenous sporting events: More than just a game', *International Journal of Event Management Research*, vol. 6, no. 1, pp. 33–51.

Sawrikar, P & Muir, K 2010, 'The myth of a "fair go": Barriers to sport and recreational participation among Indian and other ethnic minority women in Australia', *Sport Management Review*, vol. 13, no. 4, pp. 355–367.

Solar, O & Irwin, A 2010, 'A conceptual framework for action on the social determinants of health', *Social Determinants of Health Discussion Paper*, no. 2, Policy and Practice, World Health Organization, Geneva, viewed 8 October 2015, www.who.int/sdhconference/resources/ConceptualframeworkforactiononSDH_eng.pdf.

Suter, S 2009, *Issues and Directions Paper for Local and Regional Sport and Recreation Facilities: 'A Time for Fundamental Change'*, viewed 12 May 2016, www.lga.sa.gov.au/webdata/resources/files/Rec_and_sport.pdf.

Xu, X, Millar, M, & Mellor, D 2014, 'Examining the structural validity of health motivation scale in physical activity', *Anthropology*, vol. 2, no. 3, pp. 126–129. doi: 10.4172/2332-0915.1000126.

36

BRAZIL

*Thiago Hérick de Sá, Marco Antonio Bettine
de Almeida and Danielle Keylla Alencar Cruz*

Introduction

The historical and interdisciplinary analysis of the Brazilian context regarding physical activity/ sport policies is necessary to critically assess the past and to better understand the current scenario. In view of the rapid and intense changes taking place in Brazil in recent decades, we aim to discuss the recent past and the contribution of different forces to the current situation of physical activity in the country, focusing on policies and programs from three sectors – Sports and Leisure, Health and Urban Development, as well as on intersectoral actions with impact on physical activity in Brazil.

Brazil: Brief historical context

Brazil is characterized by a federal political system and a market economy still based on agricultural commodities and raw materials exportation. Since the beginning of the Republic (1889), the country has a history of alternation between democratic and dictatorial periods, with the constant presence of clientelistic political systems, populist politicians (Bresser-Pereira 2014), a patrimonial and violent elite (Maricato 2006) and a significant proportion of the population deprived of minimum citizenship guarantees (Vasconcellos 2014). The last Constitution of Brazil, from 1988 (FC/88), established a democratic state of law, in force until the present day. The current version of the FC/88 also establishes important universal rights for the Brazilian people, such as the right to health, education, work, leisure, decent housing and to the city, which in turn directly influences the development of policies and practices for sport/physical activity in the country.

Over the past 15 years, Brazil's significant economic growth together with social and distributive policies contributed to reduce the historic income inequality in the country while intensified mass consumption and the process of precarious urbanization (UN-Habitat 2012). In the same period, there has been the stabilization of the Brazilian population and the consolidation of the epidemiological (Omran 1971) and nutritional (Popkin 1999) transitions. The beginning of the twenty-first century also confirms the assumption of a political ideology that emphasizes macroeconomic factors while building a social agreement to improve the basic living conditions of the poorest people without compromising privileges of a powerful minority that historically ruled the country (Singer 2009). As a result, the eradication of historical wounds, such as hunger and extreme poverty, occurs at the same time as the persistence of large Brazilian social problems, like urban violence, restricted access to education and health, poor urban condition of the metropolis and racial and gender issues. There is also a prominent accumulation of capital, which consolidated the conservative economic advancement and a huge concentration of power, despite the reduction of inequalities.

Without proper political education, the centrality of the interests of finance capital and consumption-driven citizen inclusion strengthened the prospect of a fatalistic and alienated 'modus vivendi' by establishing routines centred on hard work, limited periods of leisure time and consolidation of a collective conception of sport/physical activity as a product with limited opportunities to experience sport/physical activity as a social transformation tool, essential for the health and quality of life of the population. This political and economic environment had a strong influence on the development of public policies and governmental actions – including those related to sports/physical activity and leisure. It also indirectly influences the practice of physical activity in Brazil through other sectors policies (Gomez et al. 2015), as discussed below.

Sports and leisure

During the Brazilian military dictatorship, which took place between the years 1964 and 1985, sports policy was marked by a nationalist and vainglorious character (Athayde 2014). The focus on high performance sport, with athletes representing the country in international events, was characteristic of this period and led to stronger sense of hierarchy, centralization of decisions and low interdisciplinarity in sports policies (Bueno 2008).

This approach to sports policies applies to many other areas during the 60s and early 70s, when the possibility of social participation was vastly restricted. In the late 1970s, Brazil experienced various forms of organizations seeking to promote social participation in government decisions, which was especially manifested by the health reform movement (Paim et al. 2011). These experiences became popular with time and participatory democracy would receive status of a constitutional principle with the FC/88 having to concurrently occur with representative democracy. From the 1990s onwards, Brazil had a significant increase in the number and types of participatory arrangements (Martins 2013).

The democratization process was a milestone for challenging rules and paradigms of military dictatorship and brought important changes to various sectors of Brazilian public policies, including the sports sector. In addition, during the 1980s, the organization of an epistemic community resulted in strong advocacy for the creation of a chapter in FC/88, in which sports activity would be recognized in three dimensions: sports-education, sports-leisure/participation and sports-performance.

The FC/88 established, in its Article 217, that sport is a duty of the state and right of the population, determining that public resources should be channelled to promote educational sports and, in specific cases, to promote high performance sports. According to Carvalho (2013), it was left to the sub-constitutional laws to determine the levels of government responsible for promoting sport/physical activity in its different dimensions as well as their respective objectives. Public enterprises and the private sector have played an important role in the sponsorship of sports activities, although these actions still lack the regulatory and institutional framework and alignment with the National Sports Policy (the National Sports Policy will be discussed in more detail below).

The period following the FC/88 is marked by various regulatory and institutional frameworks that would influence the formation of the conception of sport as a prominent area in the public policies of the country. Some of the key moments can be seen in Table 36.1.

Although part of the country's political agenda for decades, it is only in 1995 that sports received ministerial status. In 2003, the Sports Ministry is created. Since then, four ministers have chaired the institution, none of them with substantial previous technical experience or major contributions to the area. The Sports Ministry has as its main goals:

i) Democratic and universal access to sport and leisure, with a view to improving the quality of life of Brazilian population;
ii) Promotion of the construction and strengthening of citizenship, ensuring access to sports and related scientific and technological knowledge;
iii) Decentralization of sports public policies management;
iv) Promotion of sports practices of educational and participatory nature for the entire population and strengthening of sports cultural identity through intersectoral policies and integrated actions; and
v) Encouragement of the development of sports talents and improvement of the performance of athletes and disabled athletes.

Based on this, the Ministry of Sports is currently divided into three national secretariats, one of them devoted only to football and football supporters' rights. Although there is a relative diversity on the ministry's programs, ranging from financial support to high performance athletes to the expansion of programs of sports infrastructure and the coordination of research and documentation centres, the Ministry has been focusing on high-performance sports to the detriment of other activities, including in the allocation of resources (Athayde et al. 2015). This prioritization is to a great extent related to the realization of the 2007 Pan American Games in Rio de Janeiro, the 2014 Men's Football World Cup and the 2016 Olympics in Rio de Janeiro.

Sport in schools has also been influenced by the priority given to high performance sport in recent years (Silva et al. 2015). Programs such as the 'Second Time', which aims to democratize access to sport among children and adolescents by offering activities after school, has lost power in favour of other initiatives, such as programs 'Discovery of Sports Talent' and 'Brazilian School Games', which function as actions to support high performance sport by identifying young sporting talents. In the case of physical education, under the responsibility of the Ministry of Education, there is a low coverage of physical education classes, despite the fact that the subject is mandatory in the curriculum until high school (Hallal et al. 2010). This scenario is particularly worrying, given that promotion of physical activity through the school has strong evidence of effectiveness in the Latin American context (Hoehner et al. 2013).

Despite all efforts to define sport/physical activity as a citizens' right in FC/88, to have an institutional control in this area, through the creation of the Ministry of Sport in 1995, and to create laws highlighted in the Table 36.1, the reorganization of the sports public policy framework failed to achieve the intended advances. Few intersectoral actions with education, health and culture have been implemented, which have consequences to the institutional organization of sports policies as illustrated by the lack of solid public budget structure and by the extensive dependence on incentive laws.

The National Sports Policy

On August 19, 2005, the ex-President of Brazil, Luiz Inácio Lula da Silva, launched the National Sports Policy. The president's speech markedly emphasized the need for the State

Table 36.1 Evolution of legislation and agencies responsible for sports public policies within the federal government

Institutional or normative landmark	Year	Characteristics
1988 Federal Constitution (FC/88)	1988	Sports established as state duty and citizens' right, including the statement that public resources should be devoted to sports promotion.
Law 8.672/93 (Zico Law)	1993	Defined sports practice as physical and intellectual activity and defined three dimensions: sports-education, sports-leisure/participation and sports-performance. Created the Superior Sports Council.
Creation of the Extraordinary Sports Ministry	1995	Created during the first mandate of President Fernando Henrique Cardoso with the future goal of creating a permanent sports ministry. In 1998, it joined the tourism sector turning into the Ministry of Sports and Tourism.
Law 9.615/98 (Pelé Law)	1998	Terminated the Higher Sports Council and the Department of Sport and created the National Institute of Sport Development. As the Zico Law, it prioritized football. It did not create important landmarks for the sports-education and sports-leisure/participation.
Law 9981/00 (Maguito Vilela Law)	2000	Apart from creating the Ministry of Sports and Tourism and strengthening the role and functions of the Brazilian Sports Development Council, it dealt with issues related to athletes in Brazil.
Law 10264/01 (Agnelo/Piva Law)	2001	Determined that 2% of gross revenues from federal lotteries should be given to Brazilian Olympic Committee (85%) and Brazilian Paralympic Committee (15%) and determined that these two entities should invest 10% of their revenues in school sports and 5% in university sports.
Creation of Ministry of Sports	2003	Composed by the National Sports Council and three departments, which were responsible for the following areas: leisure, education and high performance. At the time of its creation, the Ministry of Sports was responsible for establishing a national policy for the development of sports practices.
Creation of the National Educational Sport Secretariat	2003	It is aimed at democratizing access to sports practice, promoting development, citizenship, quality of life and reducing social vulnerability. It also has the responsibility to establish centres of educational sports in partnership with public and private entities.
Creation of the National Secretariat for Development of Sports and Leisure	2003	This Secretariat was created with the purpose of generating knowledge and access to the practice of recreational sport and leisure through sports, artistic, physical practices and leisure activities for all age groups. It also contemplates the establishment, renovation, expansion and modernization of sports infrastructure for the promotion of such activities.
Launch of National Sports Policy	2005	Results from the activities of the 1st National Sports Conference, the Policy established guidelines for the sport as a state's duty. Among its main themes are: universal access, health promotion, economic development, social control and decentralization.
Law 11.438/06 (Law of Sports Incentive)	2006	Created the possibility for companies and individuals to apply 1% and 6%, respectively, of income tax on sports projects approved by the Ministry of Sports.

Source: Based on data and information from Ministério do Esporte (2005), Silva (2015), Carvalho (2013) and Bueno (2008).

to take responsibilities for sport policies in Brazil, and the importance of professional sports, sports clubs on the national context and mega sports events. The speech at the official launch mirrored the priority given to issues regarding high performance sport and to the 'club-based' model over sport-education and sport-leisure approaches (Presidência da República 2005).

The National Policy of Sport was a milestone for the field of public policies for sport in Brazil. The policy is the result of a set of legal guidelines, including both constitutional and sub-constitutional laws. In the document, dramatic inequalities in Brazilian sports practices were recognized, sport was considered as a cultural manifestation and as a matter of state. Also, the need for a more concise diagnosis of Brazilian sport and clearer definitions of the roles of Federal government and segments of society in sport were emphasized. Another innovation was the emphasis on sports activities for people with disabilities (Ministério do Esporte 2005).

In the document, it was also recognized that state activities and important political decision making in Brazil were historically dominated by the elite. Even though social participation was still modestly approached in the law's text as can be illustrated by the limited discussion on democratic governance, social participation and social control when dealing with the need of strengthening institutional links (Ministério do Esporte 2005).

The issue of participation in sports public policies requires commitment to expand the communication and dialogue between government and society. However, there is no clear initiative regarding the creation, strengthening and expansion of participation means, except for the National Sports Council. The council is the main structure with an important role in the national sports political system (Ministério do Esporte 2005).

The National Sports Council is an independent and auxiliary entity to the government, linked to the Ministry of Sport as a collegiate organ. It has the capacity of deliberating and intervening with a number of decisions of state entities, representing the interests of the sports community towards the federal government (Ministério do Esporte 2005). The council also has responsibility for updates on regulatory rules against doping.

The national sports political system is comprised of the Ministry of Sports, National Sports Council, states sports systems, Federal District and municipalities, Brazilian Olympic and Paralympic committees, national and regional sports organizations, regional and national leagues and institutions of sports practice.

Mega-events

Despite the evidence that major events have failed to increase sports/physical activity practice or to result in other health gains (Mahtani et al. 2013), the country pursued these mega events aimed at obtaining international publicity that portrayed Brazil's economic growth and administrative capacity (Silva et al. 2015). Moreover, these major events served as mechanisms for the acceleration of capital accumulation, both for the media and entertainment industries and for their commercial, multinational partners in the fields of construction, real estate development, security, food and automobiles, through urban gentrification projects and the creation of consumer islands (Paula & Bartelt 2014; Dilger 2014; Capela & Tavares 2014; Comitê Popular Rio Copa e Olimpíadas 2013).

As observed in other countries hosting large sporting events (Paula & Bartelt 2014), the false argument of legacy was used to justify making exceptions concerning rules and legality (Paula & Bartelt 2014; Dilger 2014; Capela & Tavares 2014), which, for instance, allowed the highest profit in history for the *Fédération Internationale de Football Association* (FIFA) in the 2014 World Cup in Brazil (approximately R\$16 billion or US\$5 billion) (FIFA 2014), notably higher than the government investments to promote sport and leisure that year. This reinforces sports as a product in a business model in detriment to the democratization of sports inside and outside the school or the promotion of leisure-time physical activity. Although there is no national evidence of the number of high-performance athletes, it is possible to observe a significant reduction in the fraction of leisure-time Brazilian football participation precisely in the years before the World Cup in Brazil (from 9.1% in 2006 to 7.2% in 2012) (de Sá et al. 2014).

The environment of juridical and legal exception that took place for the organization of mega-events also allowed a series of injustices against the most vulnerable segments of the population (Paula & Bartelt 2014; Dilger 2014; Capela & Tavares 2014). In addition to job insecurity faced by mega events construction workers, many families were expelled from their homes to make way for construction of mega-events structures and urban projects of interest to the real estate market. It is estimated that, by 2013, at least 11,000 families have been removed only in Rio de Janeiro (approximately 40,000 people) (Comitê Popular Rio Copa e Olimpíadas 2013), and a significantly greater number have been forced to move to outermost regions on account of real estate valuation. This removal of job opportunities, education and health weakens the right to the city, reduces the free time of these families and encourages the use of individual motorized transport, with negative effects on physical activity in daily travel (Sa et al. 2013) and increased risk of road traffic injuries, particularly among motorcycle users and pedestrians (Reichenheim et al. 2011).

Health

In Brazil's history, several initiatives contributed to the understanding of health as part of government actions and to define the structure and goals of the health sector, especially at the beginning of the last century and during the creation of the Unified Health System (in the 80s). This organization of the sector has had an impact on the role of physical activity in the health system, as discussed below.

In the early twentieth century, infectious epidemics demanded health actions based on prevention and hygiene, which included mass vaccination, demolitions of unhealthy houses and removal of the population housed in slums to remote areas. The practice of physical activity, although not a core part of the actions of the health sector at the time, was indirectly influenced by the actions of that sector, as illustrated by the urban reform. In Rio de Janeiro, the most important city in Brazil during this time, the state-centred sanitary interventions in the city's central area contributed to the occupation of the hills by the poorest – now known as 'favelas'.

While sanitary actions regarding vaccination and prevention of communicable diseases were aimed at the entire population, other health actions, including health care, were a privilege of formal workers (who had signed a contract with guaranteed labour rights). They were the ones entitled to retirement and pensions that originated from financial contributions of the workers themselves and of enterprises that guaranteed pension to the worker in case of disability, to the family in case of death of the worker and health care/medicine access to the worker and family. Until very recently, the legal condition of the majority of Brazilian workers was 'non-formal' workers, those with a precarious or absent legal condition, such as street sellers, freelancers and housekeepers.

The Ministry of Health was only created in 1953, after the segregation of the then Ministry of Education and Health. In 1964, at the beginning of the military dictatorship, access to health via social security contributions was strengthened. Those who could not contribute to the social security system accessed health services through specific programs. Those who did not fit as beneficiaries of government specific health programs had to seek assistance in private philanthropic institutions (Giovanella 2008). During this period, the understanding that prevailed on health was focused on the doctor and on a clinical and hospital-centric perspective. At the time, physical activity was not considered part of health care by health services.

In the 1970s, still during the military period, the movement of the Health Reform took place, emphasizing health as a right of all citizens, resulting from social determinants (Paim 2008), and as achievable only through the institutional reorganization of the country towards democracy and social rights. The Health Reform, driven by employees, managers and the epistemic community of public health, was a milestone in the definition of health as a universal right and responsibility of the State (as well as sport and leisure, as seen previously), expressed in the FC/88. In 1990, the Unified Health System (SUS) was implemented, having among its principles universality, integrality and community participation (Brasil 1990). Primary care was placed at the core of the health system network (Ministério da Saúde 2010). Primary care is the closest level of community health care since it is organized in health areas where people live (Brasil 2012b). Therefore, most of the initiatives of physical activity promotion policies and programs in the health sector have been developed within the primary care setting.

The main primary care program involved in population-level physical activity promotion is the Family Health Strategy (*Estratégia de Saúde da Família*), which is also the central program in primary care. The Family Health Strategy is composed of professionals from the areas of nursing, medicine and dentistry, as well as community health workers, who form the basis of the Family Health team. These teams are responsible for covering an area that generally corresponds to 4,000 people. In addition to the Family Health team, there are the Centers of Support for Family Health (*Núcleos de Apoio à Saúde da Família*), responsible for supporting the Family Health team and providing multiprofessional care when needed. This program consists of several kinds of health professionals, including a Physical Education expert, recognized in Brazil as a health professional since 1997 (Conselho Nacional de Saúde 1997). Strategies to promote physical activity through Family Health teams and Centers of Support for Family Health in recent years have proved effective in empowering health professionals for advice on physical activity as part of care (Florindo et al. 2014).

Incentives to encourage and practice physical activity in primary care as part of the SUS have occurred since 2002, with the implementation of *Hiperdia* Program, aimed at the registration and monitoring of individuals with hypertension or diabetes (Benedetti 2014). In this program, in addition to access to medicines, users participate in walking groups monitored by professionals of the Family Health team. Another program developed in primary care since 2007 is the School Health Program, which links Family Health teams to the public schools with the aim of developing actions to promote health and disease prevention among schoolchildren. Among the actions of the School Health Program, we highlight the anthropometric measurements and the promotion of healthy lifestyles, all developed by Family Health teams in partnership with school professionals and the Centers of Support for Family Health (Presidência da República 2007). In 2015, the School Health Program covered 4,878 municipalities (86%) and 18 million students (41%).

Addressing non-communicable chronic diseases

In Brazil, as in other countries, the impact of chronic diseases in morbidity and mortality of the population demanded broad actions to reduce the incidence of these diseases. Since the publication of the Global Strategy on Diet and Physical Activity in 2003 by the World Health Organization (Organização Mundial da Saúde 2004), Brazil has carried out national initiatives to promote physical activity practice. In 2005, the Ministry of Health allocated financial resources to the states and large municipalities to develop programs and projects related to the themes of the Global Strategy.

In 2006, the National Policy for Health Promotion was launched with seven priority themes, among them physical activity and body practices (Ministério da Saúde 2006). In the same year, the National Policy for Integrative and Complementary Practices of SUS was launched, which placed traditional Chinese medicine as part of health care practices, including body practices (e.g. tai chi chuan, lian gong and yoga). Between 2005 and 2010, financial resources were given to over 1,000 municipalities to develop health promotion actions within the perspective of the National Policy for Health Promotion. However, this corresponds to only 27 per cent of Brazilian municipalities contrasting with the SUS principle of universality.

In 2006, the Ministry of Health started a telephone survey for the surveillance of risk and protective factors for chronic non-communicable diseases, which annually monitors the trend of these factors in adults over 18 years living in the 27 Brazilian state capitals. Physical activity is monitored in four domains: leisure time, occupation, transportation and domestic activities. In 2014, 35.3 per cent of Brazilian adults (41.6% of men and 30.0% of women) practiced at least 150 minutes of moderate physical activity per week. Although total physical activity practice presents an upward trend since 2006, there are important differences in temporal variation by domain and sex (Ministério da Saúde 2015).

In 2011, the Health Academy Program was launched with the aim of contributing to health promotion through the implementation of centres with the required infrastructure and skilled professionals (Ministério da Saúde 2013). This Program unified health promotion actions from the National Policy for Health Promotion and included health education (Malta et al. 2012). To implement the Health Academy program, it is required that financial resources are transferred from the federal government to the municipalities for the construction of physical space where the actions and services are developed (known as 'centres'). These centres are considered primary care structures that support health care and contribute to the Health Care Networks.

The Health Academy Program implementation is on-going in 3,132 (56%) municipalities in all regions of the country. Monitoring of the target population coverage is continuous and occurs through the Primary Care Information System. The centres encompass health promotion activities beyond physical activity/body practices, as, for example, health education activities and healthy eating promotion, community mobilization and artistic/ cultural practices (Ministério da Saúde 2013). Brazil's option for focusing on NCDs prevention and health promotion within the primary care and to promote multiple actions beyond physical activity is relevant to the cultural diversity of the country, economic and social inequalities in the regions, complexity of the problem and need of strengthening health actions within local territories. These require long term intersectoral and multidisciplinary initiatives.

The experience of Brazil to promote physical activity in the health sector, integrated with health services – especially the primary care – and strongly supported by the multidisciplinary expertise, represents a major advance compared with the period prior to the FC/88. It should also be emphasized the important insertion of the Physical Education professional in SUS, as well as the understanding of health care beyond medicalization, which strengthens physical activity and body practices as health care components.

Urban development

Until mid-twentieth century, Brazil was a predominantly rural country, a situation that changed with the rapid and disorganized urbanization faced by its major cities, similar to that observed in other Latin American countries (UN-Habitat 2012). As an example, between 1940 and 1980, the population of Greater São Paulo expanded from 1.6 to 12.6 million. The result of this urban growth – influenced both by external factors, such as increasing globalization, as by internal factors, such as inter-regional migration – brought important repercussions for the population's health and quality of life, as well as for physical activity (Gomez et al. 2015).

Policies for transport, housing and urban planning of this time were designed based on a project for 'middle-class cities' (Vasconcellos 1999; Vasconcellos 2014), extensively favouring private modes of transport at the expense of mass transit and active modes (walking and cycling), the development of a poverty belt around the richer centre, where most of the employment and education opportunities are concentrated, and the unequal distribution of leisure spaces such as squares, parks and public facilities for physical activity (Vasconcellos 1999; Vasconcellos 2014). All these factors have contributed to greater leisure time physical activity among the richest and greater practice in other domains among the poorest in several Brazilian cities (Gomez et al. 2015).

Given this precarious urban condition and the recognition of the need for urban reform, the City Statute was promulgated in 2001 (Oliveira 2001), a law that regulates the chapter on urban policy in the FC/88 and establishes the universal right to the city, making Brazil the first country in the world to feature this right in its federal constitution. The City Statute also requires municipalities to establish and regularly review their master plans, with the right to the city and environmental sustainability as guiding principles. In 2003, the Ministry of Cities was created, which meant a breakthrough for the development and implementation of development and urban mobility policies. Finally, in 2007, the National Policy on Urban Mobility was promulgated (Brasil 2012a), with the general objective of establishing principles, guidelines and tools to enable municipalities to perform their urban mobility plans to ensure universal access to cities and their opportunities, contributing to sustainable urban development. The National Urban Mobility Policy recognized the importance of active forms of commuting, and prioritized active travel and public transport instead of private modes (car and motorcycle), new renewable and cleaner energy matrix in mobility, democratization of public space, the promotion of the right to the city and accessibility for people with disabilities. These were followed by a series of actions by municipalities aimed at solving the urban crisis, in favour of more dense, diverse, safe and sustainable cities. All these urban development measures seem to have had a positive impact on the quality of public transport, cycling and pedestrian infrastructure, land use and spatial segregation between rich and poor, although the number of initiatives rigorously evaluated has been very small.

However, more recently, federal programs and policies to warm up the internal consumption in face of the latest global financial crisis contributed to reinforce a spatially segregated city model, dependent on private transport modes. Tax incentives for the purchase of vehicles contributed to a significant increase in the number of cars and motorcycles across the country (Presidência da República 2010). The housing program 'Minha Casa, Minha Vida' (My House, My Life) focused on the poorest, prioritized the construction of new housing in low-cost land, which are even more peripheral and away from the city centre (Amore et al. 2015). In addition, efforts to democratize access to green areas appear to have been insufficient.

As a consequence, inequities in physical activity and maintenance of poor urban condition in municipalities are perpetuated (Gomez et al. 2015). The combination of the current structure of cities and the real gain in purchasing power of the poorest led to greater increases in motor-ization rates in this population subgroup, since cars and motorcycles are cost-effective options to overcome the large and complex commuting in metropolises. In São Paulo, for example, where the average accumulated commuting time is around an hour and a half (Sá et al. 2015a), there appears to be an inverse trend of increasing bicycle use among the wealthiest in parallel to a reduction among the poorest (Companhia do Metropolitano de São Paulo 2013). In addition, there was an acceleration of the reduction in walking and cycling practice when commuting to school between the years 2007 and 2012 compared to the period between 1997 and 2007 (Companhia do Metropolitano de São Paulo 2013; Sá et al. 2015b).

Changes in urban development are mandatory for improving quality of life, increasing physical activity and reducing inequities in physical activity practice. There is evidence that only the combination of the reduction of distances and a travel pattern that favours public transport and active commuting could improve physical activity without necessarily increasing the total time of daily commuting (Sá et al. 2015a). To what extent the recent policies and programs to improve urban conditions in Brazilian cities will be able to promote these changes is a question yet to be answered.

Implications for future physical activity policy and practice in Brazil

Despite the difficulties outlined above, such as the priority given to high performance sport and the lack of integration of sport/physical activity with key areas, it is undeniable that sports and physical activity gained greater prominence and investment on the political agenda in past two decades. Significant advances are embodied in national policies that directly or indirectly deal with the subject, such as the National Sport Policy, the National Policy for Health Promotion and the City Statute.

The main challenge for increasing participation of citizens in the different manifestations of sport and the promotion of culturally integrated physical activity is the effective imple-mentation, assessment and continuous review of these policies. Moreover, another major challenge is to create institutional arrangements that promote the integration of these policies and other actions related to sport/physical activity at the different levels of government. One option could be the creation of intersectoral governance bodies at every level – federal, state and municipal – as well as the elaboration of a federal pact, as already happens in key sectors of the country, such as health and education.

These challenges become even greater given the fragility of Brazilian democracy, the social and cultural heritage of secular processes (such as slavery and precarious urbanization) and the pressure exerted by the interests of finance capital, with negative consequences to different aspects of life. The guarantee of constitutionally provided rights that are intimately related with sport/physical activity practice, among which is the right to health, leisure and the city, will only be possible with the deepening of social participation and strengthening democratic institutions in the country.

References

Amore, C. S., Shimbo, L. C. Z. & Rufino, M. B. C. 2015. *Minha Casa . . . E a cidade? Avaliação do Programa Minha Casa Minha Vida em seis estados brasileiros*, Rio de Janeiro: Letra Capital.

Athayde, P. F. A. 2014. *O ornitorrinco de chuteiras: determinantes econômicos da política de esporte do governo Lula e suas implicações sociais*. Doctorate, Universidade de Brasília.

Athayde, P., Mascarenhas, F. & Salvador, E. 2015. Primeiras aproximações de uma análise do financiamento da política nacional de esporte e lazer no Governo Lula. *Revista Brasileira de Ciências do Esporte*, 37(1), pp 2–10.

Benedetti, T. E. A. 2014. *A formação do profissional de Educação Física para o setor saúde*, Florianópolis: Postmix.

Brasil. 1990. *Lei n. 8.080, de 19 de Setembro de 1990. Dispõe sobre as condições para a promoção, proteção e recuperação da saúde, a organização e o funcionamento dos serviços correspondentes e dá outras providências.* Presidência da República. Brasília: Diário Oficial da União.

Brasil. 2012a. *Lei No. 12.587, de 3 de janeiro de 2012. Institui as diretrizes da Política Nacional de Mobilidade Urbana e dá outras providências.* Presidência da República (ed.) 3. Brasília: Diário Oficial da União.

Brasil. 2012b. *Política Nacional de Atenção Básica*, Brasil.

Bresser-Pereira, L. C. 2014. *A Construção Política do Brasil: Sociedade, Economia e Estado desde a Independência*, São Paulo: Editora 34.

Bueno, L. 2008. *Políticas públicas do esporte no Brasil: razões para o predomínio do alto rendimento*. Doctorate, Fundação Getúlio Vargas.

Capela, P. & Tavares, E. 2014. *Os megaeventos esportivos: suas consequências, impactos e legados para a América Latina*, Florianópolis: Editora Insular.

Carvalho, C. M. 2013. *Esporte como política pública: um estudo sobre o processo de formulação da política de esporte no Brasil*. Masters, Universidade Federal de Campinas.

Comitê Popular Rio Copa e Olimpíadas. 2013. *Megaeventos e violações dos direitos humanos no Rio de Janeiro* (Rio de Janeiro).

Companhia do Metropolitano de São Paulo. 2013. *Pesquisa de Mobilidade da Região Metropolitana de São Paulo: Principais Resultados da Pesquisa Domiciliar* (São Paulo).

Conselho Nacional de Saúde. 1997. *Resolução n. 218, de 6 de março de 1997. Reconhece as categorias profissionais como da saúde*, Conselho Nacional de Saúde.

Dilger, G. 2014. *Resistências no país do futebol – A Copa em contexto*, São Paulo: Fundação Rosa Luxemburgo.

Fédération Internationale de Football Association (FIFA). 2014. *FIFA financial report 2014*. [Online]. Available at: www.fifa.com/about-fifa/news/y=2015/m=3/news=fifa-financial-report-2014-frequently-asked-questions-2568090.html.

Florindo, A. A., Costa, E. F., Sa, T. H., dos Santos, T. I., Velardi, M. & Andrade, D. R. 2014. Physical activity promotion in primary health care in Brazil: A counseling model applied to community health workers. *Journal of Physical Activity and Health*, 11(8), pp 1531–1539.

Giovanella, L. E. A. O. 2008. *Políticas e Sistemas de Saúde no Brasil*, Rio de Janeiro: Editora FIOCRUZ.

Gomez, L. F., Sarmiento, R., Ordoñez, M. F., Pardo, C. F., de Sá, T. H., Mallarino, C. H., Miranda, J. J., Mosquera, J., Parra, D. C., Reis, R. & Quistberg, D. A. 2015. Urban environment interventions linked to the promotion of physical activity: a mixed methods study applied to the urban context of Latin America. *Social Science & Medicine*, 131, pp 18–30.

Hallal, P. C., Knuth, A. G., Alencar Cruz, D. K., Mendes, M. I. & Malta, D. C. 2010. Physical activity practice among Brazilian adolescents. *Ciência & Saude Coletiva*, 15, pp 3035–3042.

Hoehner, C. M., Ribeiro, I. C., Parra, D. C., Reis, R. S., Azevedo, M. R., Hino, A. A., Soares, J., Hallal, P. C., Simoes, E. J. & Brownson, R. C. 2013. Physical activity interventions in Latin America: Expanding and classifying the evidence. *American Journal of Preventive Medicine*, 44(3), pp e31–e40.

Mahtani, K. R., Protheroe, J., Slight, S. P., Piva Demarzo, M. M., Blakeman, T., Barton, C. A., Brijnath, B. & Roberts, N. 2013. Can the London 2012 Olympics 'inspire a generation' to do more physical or sporting activities? An overview of systematic reviews. *BMJ Open*, 3(1), pp. e002058.

Malta, D. C., Silva, S. A., Oliveira, P. P. V., Iser, B. P. M., Bernal, R. T. I., Sardinha, L. M. V. & Moura, L. 2012. Resultados do monitoramento dos Fatores de risco e Proteção para Doenças Crônicas Não Transmissíveis nas capitais brasileiras por inquérito telefônico, 2008. *Revista Brasileira de Epidemiologia*, 15(3), pp 639–650.

Maricato, E. 2006. O Ministério das Cidades e a política nacional de desenvolvimento urbano. *Políticas Sociais: Acompanhamento e Análise*, 12, pp 211–220.

Martins, S. H. Z. 2013. *Mobilização e mudança social: experiências de participação política na sociedade contemporânea*, São Paulo.

Ministério da Saúde. 2006. Portaria n. 687 MS/GM, de 30 de março de 2006. *Política Nacional de Promoção da Saúde*, Ministério da Saúde (Brasília).

Ministério da Saúde. 2010. *Portaria n. 4.279, de 30 de dezembro de 2010. Estabelece diretrizes para organização da Rede de Atenção à Saúde no âmbito do Sistema Único de Saúde (SUS)* [Online]. Available at: http://conselho.saude.gov.br/ultimas_noticias/2011/img/07_jan_portaria4279_301210.pdf.

Ministério da Saúde. 2013. *Portaria n. 2.681, de 7 de novembro de 2013. Redefine o Programa Academia da Saúde no âmbito do Sistema Único de Saúde*, Ministério da Saúde.

Ministério da Saúde. 2015. *Vigitel Brasil 2014 Saúde Suplementar: vigilância de fatores de risco e proteção para doenças crônicas por inquérito telefônico*, Ministério da Saúde (Brasília).

Ministério do Esporte. 2005. *Política Nacional do Esporte* [Online]. Available at: www2.esporte.gov.br/arquivos/conselhoEsporte/polNacEsp.pdf.

Oliveira, I. C. E. 2001. *Estatuto da Cidade: para compreender*. Rio de Janeiro: Ibam/Duma, 64.

Omran, A. R. 1971. The epidemiologic transition. A theory of the epidemiology of population change. *Milbank Memorial Fund Quartely*, 49(4), pp 509–538.

Organização Mundial da Saúde. 2004. *Estratégia Global em Alimentação Saudável, Atividade Física e Saúde* [Online]. Available at: www.who.int/dietphysicalactivity/publications/releases/pr84/en/.

Paim, J. 2008. *Reforma sanitária brasileira: contribuição para a compreensão e crítica*, Salvador/ EDUFBA Rio de Janeiro/Editora Fiocurz.

Paim, J., Travassos, C., Almeida, C., Bahia, L. & Macinko, J. 2011. Health in Brazil 1 The Brazilian health system: History, advances, and challenges. *The Lancet*, 377(9779), pp 1778–1797.

Paula, M. & Bartelt, D. D. 2014. *Copa para quem e para quê? Um olhar sobre os legados dos mundiais de futebol no Brasil, África do Sul e Alemanha.*, Rio de Janeiro: Fundação Heinrich Böll.

Popkin, B. M. 1999. Urbanization, lifestyle changes and the nutrition transition. *World Development*, 27(11), pp 1905–1916.

Presidência da República. 2005. *Discurso do Presidente da República, Luiz Inácio Lula da Silva, na cerimônia de lançamento da Política Nacional do Esporte*, Presidência da República (São Paulo).

Presidência da República. 2007. *Decreto n. 6.286, de 5 de dezembro de 2007. Institui o Programa Saúde na Escola - PSE, e dá outras providências*, Presidência da República.

Presidência da República. 2010. *Decreto n. 7.222, de 29 de Junho de 2010. Altera a Tabela de Incidência de Imposto sobre Produtos Industrializados-TIPI, aprovada pelo Decreto n. 6006, de 20 de dezembro de 2006*, Presidência da República.

Reichenheim, M. E., de Souza, E. R., Moraes, C. L., Jorge, M., da Silva, C. & Minayo, M. C. D. 2011. Health in Brazil 5 Violence and injuries in Brazil: The effect, progress made, and challenges ahead. *The Lancet*, 377(9781), pp 1962–1975.

Sá, T. H., Salvador, E. P. & Florindo, A. A. 2013. Factors associated with physical inactivity in transportation in brazilian adults living in a low socioeconomic area. *Journal of Physical Activity & Health*, 10(6), pp 856–862.

Sá, T. H., Garcia, L. M. & Claro, R. M. 2014. Frequency, distribution and time trends of types of leisure-time physical activity in Brazil, 2006–2012. *International Journal of Public Health*, 59(6), pp 975–982.

Sá, T. H., Parra, D. C. & Monteiro, C. A. 2015a. Impact of travel mode shift and trip distance on active and non-active transportation in the São Paulo Metropolitan Area in Brazil. *Preventive Medicine Reports*, 2, pp 183–188.

Sá, T. H., Garcia, L. M. T., Mielke, G. I., Rabacow, F. M. & Rezende, L. F. M. 2015b. Changes in travel to school patterns among children and adolescents in the São Paulo Metropolitan Area, Brazil, 1997–2007. *Journal of Transport & Health*, 2(2), pp 143–150.

Silva, D. S., Borges, C. N. F. & Amaral, S. C. F. 2015. Gestão das políticas públicas do Ministério do Esporte do Brasil. *Revista Brasileira de Educação Física e Esporte*, 29, pp 65–79.

Singer, A. 2009. Raízes sociais e ideológicas do lulismo. *Novos estudos – CEBRAP*, (85), pp 83–102.

UN-Habitat 2012. *Estado de las Ciudads de América Latina y el Caribe – rumbo a una nueva transición urbana*: UN-Habitat.

Vasconcellos, E. A. 1999. *Circular é preciso, viver não é preciso: a história do trânsito na cidade de São Paulo*, São Paulo: Annablume.

Vasconcellos, E. A. 2014. *Urban transport environment and equity: The case for developing countries*, New York: Taylor & Francis.

37

THE EUROPEAN UNION

Mads de Wolff

With the coming into force of the Lisbon Treaty in 2009 the European Union (EU) has been awarded a supporting competence in sport with Article 165 of the Treaty on the Functioning of the European Union (TFEU). While excluding harmonisation, Article 165 TFEU allows for the creation of soft monitoring mechanisms through recommendations of the Council of the European Union (Council), thereby providing a structured if voluntary tool for stimulating policy convergence across the EU's Member States. On 26 November 2013 the Council adopted its first recommendation in the field of sport on promoting health-enhancing physical activity (HEPA). Accordingly, for the first time EU governments will be subject to monitoring of how EU sport policy is implemented.

Thus far, most scholarship on EU sport policy has sought to explore *how* sport became a competence of the EU. The EU's entrance into the field of sport has thus been described as reactive and indirect, an instance of gradual task expansion due to the accumulation of legal rulings from the 1970s and onwards where various rules adopted by the governing bodies of sport have been challenged by stakeholders and brought before the European Commission and the European courts (García and Meier 2012; Meier 2009; Tokarski *et al.* 2004). The infamous 1995 *Bosman* ruling, in which a football player succeeded in contesting the power of football governing bodies to restrict player mobility, pushed sport to the top of the EU agenda (García 2007). The rise of EU sport policy has been described as a struggle of two competing definitions of sport: one, principally adopted by the European Courts, framing sport in economic terms and hence falling under regulation related to the Single European Market; and two, the countering socio-cultural definition invoked by sport bodies and their alternating EU-level supporters, emphasising the social-cultural "specificity" of sport (e.g. Parrish 2003a; Parrish 2003b). Following years of negotiations with the sports movement and the Commission, the EU Member States included an article on sport in the Lisbon Treaty and Article 165 TFEU then represents the current compromise between these two definitions of sport (García and Weatherill 2012).

Thus, the question of how sport came to be included in the Lisbon Treaty has been subject to great deal of scrutiny. However, less work has addressed what has transpired following the coming into force of the Article 165 TFEU or how particular issues become part of the EU's sport agenda (see, however: Kornbeck 2015).

To remedy these gaps, this chapter analyses the rise of promoting physical activity on the EU agenda. As this chapter will show, the EU's priorities in sport have increasingly become focused on grassroots sport and, in particular, the promotion of health-enhancing physical activity. The chapter analyses how HEPA entered the EU agenda via the Council of Health Ministers, before the sport venues within the EU eventually managed to claim authority for this issue. The analysis relies on written sources and semi-structured interviews with policy-makers. As for the former, the article uses official EU documents. The interviews informing this research comprise a total of 28 semi-structured interviews with key actors, mainly from Member State governments (n=16), the European Commission (n=5) and stakeholders (n=7).

This chapter draws on agenda-setting theory in order to analyse HEPA's rise on the EU agenda (Princen 2007; Princen 2011). As argued, HEPA represents an example of the "low politics route" agenda route of initiation, specification, expansion and entrance (Princen and Rhinard 2006). Accordingly, the chapter is structured in five sections. First, the chapter explores how HEPA came onto the EU agenda, *initiation*. The second examines the low-political and technical work undertaken to *specify* the European dimension of promoting physical activity. The third section looks at the key stage of *issue expansion* when, between 2012 and 2013, the European Commission and the Council of Ministers were negotiating how, and to what extent, to move forward with the promotion of physical activity at the EU level. The fourth section examines the negotiations on the final recommendation, i.e. *issue entrance*. Finally, the concluding section teases out the key findings of the chapter and considers what this case illuminates about the international dimension of developing physical activity policy.

Initiation

Around the turn of the millennium, the issue of promoting physical activity started gathering momentum, especially within the World Health Organization (WHO). In 2000 WHO released a report called "Obesity: preventing and managing the global epidemic" (World Health Organization 2000), which prescribed better diets and increased physical activity to solve the "epidemic" of obesity. In 2002, a WHO resolution called for the development of a "global strategy on diet, physical activity and health" (World Health Organization 2002). Accordingly, a "Global Strategy on Diet, Physical Activity and Health" was developed in consultation with scientists and stakeholders which was endorsed on May 2004, which again identified diet and increasing physical activity as the key factors in avoiding noncommunicable diseases (World Health Organization 2004).

The EU, in particular its health venues, took an active part in this wider international process. On the one hand, the EU's Council of Health Ministers started taking an interest in managing obesity though diet and physical activity in the same period as the WHO (e.g. Council 2003) and the EU Member States supported the adoption of WHO's Global Strategy (Council 2005).

Furthermore, the promotion of HEPA grew in visibility on the EU agenda during these years. In 2005 the European Commission's Directorate General for Health and Food Safety set up the EU Platform on Diet, Physical Activity and Health (European Commission 2005) as a forum where organisations voluntarily commit to "tackling current trends in diet and physical activity" (European Commission 2015). Further, when the European Parliament and the Council designated 2004 the European Year of Education Through Sport, they also acknowledged how "exercise improves psychological and physical health" (European

Parliament & Council 2003: article 1:9). At the request of the Commission's Directorate General for Health and Food Safety, the first special Eurobarometer survey on physical activity was commissioned (European Commission 2003).

Thus, there had emerged a global network of scientists, stakeholders and governments sharing a common set of beliefs on physical activity, in particular that physical activity can be a tool to managing public health problems such as obesity. That is to say, the issue *initiated* out "of professional concerns in epistemic communities" (Princen and Rhinard 2006: 1122). Specifically, physical activity commanded much visibility in the EU's health communities *circa* 2004. The development of a HEPA policy within the EU should be seen as part of what Piggin and Bairner (2016) have described as rise of the "global physical inactivity pandemic". In short, physical activity framed as *health-enhancing* had entered a period of "internationalization", i.e. reached a moment where this national collective problem could become international and/or EU problem (Stephenson 2012: 799).

As pointed out by Piggin and Bairner (2016), framing a problem as a "pandemic" – urgently requiring action – has consequences, as actors will seek to affect issue-definition so as to shape proposed targets and the distribution of resources. Thus, actors within the EU sport policy sought actively to stake a claim in solving this "pandemic".

As noted in the introduction, sport had not yet become of competence of the EU at this stage. However, as recalled by a Commission official, senior ranking officials within the European Commission's Sport Unit were aware of the issue's high visibility around 2004: "[m]y head of unit at that time had realised that there was much talk about 'couch potatoes' and a decrease in daily physical activity among young people" (Interview with Commission official, 16 July 2014). Accordingly, the Commission's Sports Unit took an interest in this issue which was floating around on the wider EU agenda, in particular by commissioning four studies on HEPA. One of these studies argued that the rise in obesity was not only related to people eating less healthily, but that European people also lead more sedentary lives, wherefore it suggested re-introducing more physical activity into people's lives to "restore the balance" (Brettschneider and Naul 2004: 146). This study gathered much attention amongst the EU's ministers of sport:

> [T]his one has had the far greater impact than any of the three others, and that's the sort of thing you don't know when you launch the study because the budget for the studies was practically the same, and the technical description were fairly similar [. . .] The final report was a result of a structured review of then available academic knowledge around physical activity and increase in obesity. It was a comparative structured review of what was then the 25 Member States, and some of the data was frankly 10 years old, but nobody had done this exercise before.
>
> *Interview, Commission official, 16 July 2014*

Thus, the Commission's Sport Unit picked up on a problem with a high degree of visibility in the EU's adjacent health agenda – "couch potatoes", i.e. sedentary behaviour – and sought to carve out a role for EU sport policy. Thus, a new set of strong indicators – or indicators *perceived* to be strong (Kingdon 1995: 93ff) – fixed the attention of the EU ministers of sport. One particularly study commanded a lot of attention not only because it diagnosed a problem, obesity, but also offered a solution (Princen 2007), namely increased physical activity, a message easily "sold" to the concerns of the sport ministers.

Lastly, it is important to recognise that HEPA emerged at a particular point in time in which the Commission and the EU Member States had started exploring "what" EU sport policy was supposed to look like, where HEPA was an especially appealing subject to the EU sport ministers:

> Because [the study] was just about information sharing, at that moment in time when some Member States were still very reluctant to accept any formal structures for sport, it was actually quite welcome because they could pick it and use for their own purposes [. . .] And then very importantly the UK – who at that point thought sport should not be in the Treaty – used its Presidency in 2005 to put a proposal on the table at an informal ministerial meeting in Liverpool, to set up the first informal EU working group – which was the EU working group Sport & Health – to see how Member States could cooperate on the knowledge gained through this study.
>
> *Interview, Commission official, 16 July 2014*

Indeed, the EU Sports Ministers in 2005 decided to set up a Sport & Health Working Group, with a remit to exchange information and good practice, and, through this, develop new models (European Commission 2007a: 126).

Thus, the rise of HEPA on the EU agenda must be understood as an outcome of two interlinked processes: the increasing internationalisation of promoting physical activity and the gradual development of EU sport policy. However, the EU's specific approach to promoting HEPA had not yet been specified.

Specification

Around 2004, promoting physical activity had become an increasingly visible issue on the EU agenda, especially within the EU's health and sport communities, who had both shown an interest in HEPA. However, at this stage, it was still unclear which venues had the remit to specify the European dimension HEPA – or, rather, who would claim this authority.

Crucially, during the Finnish Presidency of the Council in 2006, the Sport & Health Working Group received a mandate by the EU sport ministers to start preparing a set of "Physical Activity Guidelines". This process was completed in 2008 when the Sport & Health Working Group adopted the final set of Guidelines, which were later informally confirmed by EU Sport Ministers at a meeting November 2008 (EU Working Group Sport & Health 2008). In other words: the EU dimension of HEPA was further *specified*, with the EU's sport venues being the key drivers in facilitating this.

In the lead-up to the ratification of the Lisbon Treaty, the Commission furthermore gave HEPA special attention, with HEPA being the first presented agenda item in the White Paper on Sport (European Commission 2007c: 3–4). The Commission released the White Paper as its first step to define an approach towards a coherent EU sport policy under the Lisbon Treaty. The White Paper defines EU sport policy around three thematic sections: (1) the societal role of sport, (2) its economic dimension and (3) its organisation. In the White Paper, HEPA was defined under the social dimension, with the Commission pledging that it "will make health-enhancing physical activity a cornerstone of its sport-related activities" (European Commission 2007c: 4).

For each dimension a series of Preparatory Actions were outlined, which were supported by a limited funding scheme through 2009–2013 (see European Commission 2012). As promised, the European Commission gave HEPA special priority, ultimately financing nine (out of 42) Preparatory Actions between 2009–2011 on the topic HEPA, more than any other issue (European Commission 2012). Thus, HEPA had become the most developed area in EU sport policy. The issue aroused the most interest amongst sporting stakeholders. As noted by a Commission official:

> The field that was most developed was this one. It was the one, we saw, I mean we funded certain projects, 9, 10, 11, and the ones on sport and health were the ones soliciting the most interest – by far the highest number of applications.
>
> *Interview, European Commission official, 10 May 2014*

Once Article 165 TFEU came into force at the end of 2009, Directorate Generale Education and Culture (DG EAC) under the Commission re-emphasised HEPA as its flagship initiative in sport. This is directly reflected in a Communication released by the Commission in 2011 which announced that it would "consider proposing a Council Recommendation in this field" (European Commission 2011: 7). Notably, this was the only place such a measure was proposed:

> [HEPA] picked up with the communication. After the Lisbon Treaty we did a communication in 2011, in order to, shall we say, pronounce ourselves on what this means for us now. Ok, so we now have a Treaty article, how are we gonna translate this into something more concrete?
>
> *Interview, Commission official, 12 May 2014*

The first Special Eurobarometer on physical activity (European Commission 2003) had been commissioned by DG Health and Food Safety, who later bundled questions concerning physical activity with questions on diet, health and weight in a survey on "health and food" (European Commission 2006). After the ratification of the Lisbon Treaty, DG EAC was allowed to take charge of the commissioning of surveys on physical activity (European Commission 2010; European Commission 2014), now with an exclusive focus on physical activity.

During the same period the Commission also released White Papers on Health (European Commission 2007d) and Obesity (European Commission 2007b), which included HEPA-related proposals. While HEPA also commanding interest within the EU's health venues, there was seemingly little institutional competition within Commission compartments on who should lead initiatives related to the *promotion* of HEPA. When asked whether a HEPA recommendation could have been dealt with by another DG, an official from DG EAC replied:

> It could have been, yes, except that there is a difference in approach. If our colleagues in [Health and Food Safety] work on it, they will not start first by thinking about sport and physical activity input but would look at it from a public health perspective.
>
> *Interview 38*

Thus, the DG's seem to have peacefully divided responsibilities, with DG EAC in charge of the promotion of physical activity – the "input" side, framed in terms of promoting activity – whilst DG Health and Food Safety would focus on clinical "public health" (e.g. diet, consumer protection, etc.).

Thus, since 2004, an EU dimension of HEPA had been initiated and specified by the Commission and Sport Ministers through low-political and technical work (Princen and Rhinard 2006), resulting in the development of European guidelines on physical activity. Crucially, in these years physical activity in EU sport policy venues became "divorced" from diet and consumer protection; the framing of HEPA became focused on promoting physical activity. This reflects the institutional bias (Baumgartner and Jones 1993) of the venue which showed HEPA the most sustained interest and who set expert networks to develop technical proposals for promoting HEPA, specifically the Commission's sport unit and the EU sport ministers.

Furthermore, HEPA emerged as DG EAC's flagship initiative in sport, an area in which it had claimed authority within the Commission, and where this claim to authority was not internally contested. However, it is important to recognise that HEPA was not just any issue on the EU's sport agenda; it commanded the most visibility in the sport policy subsystem. Next, it is explored how the European Guidelines on Physical Activity – the specified European dimension of HEPA – began its conflict expansion.

Conflict expansion

The Commission had floated the idea of a HEPA recommendation to the Member States just after the ratification of the Lisbon Treaty (Interview, Member State representative, 5 May 2014). Indeed, early drafts of the Council's 2011–2014 Work Plan had proposed explicitly setting the adoption of a HEPA recommendation as a target (Council 2011a).

However, the Member States were not quite ready to explicitly endorse a Council recommendation on HEPA at this point in time. Nonetheless, the Council's 2011–2014 Work Plan on Sport did establish a new expert group on "Sport, Health and Participation" which was instructed to explore "ways to promote health enhancing physical activity and participation in grassroot sport" by mid-2013 (Council 2011b: 4). The first planned deliverable was "Input for the Commission's proposal for a Council Recommendation in the field of HEPA building on [the EU Guidelines on Physical Activity]" (XG SHP 2011: 3).

The Commission had commissioned a study to develop a monitoring framework on HEPA, focused on possible "indicators" to be used. These indicators were discussed in the expert group (XG SHP 2012b: 3) before it adopted its first deliverable on "Input for an EU initiative to promote HEPA" (XG SHP 2012a). The release of this deliverable meant that the EU sport ministers had some idea of the Commission's concrete plans on HEPA, hence allowing the Member States to make an informed decision as far as how to go forward with HEPA; that is, whether to support or constrain conflict expansion.

In the Council, there was awareness that if a recommendation of HEPA was to be achieved, the Commission would need the explicit support of the Council:

> The Commission needs an input from the Member States in order to be able to initiate a recommendation, so in the Working Parties, during the Cypriot Presidency, we had conclusions on HEPA, where we [. . .] invited the Commission to propose the Council Recommendation. This was very needed. On that basis, the Commission could start the work internally, which I know is also very complicated; they have to prove that this initiative is really necessary, "without it this and that would happen". And the current atmosphere is not really supportive to any new initiatives, so I think that we are quite lucky, and the Sport Unit and the sport colleagues in the Commission did very well.
>
> *Interview, Member State representative, 21 May 2014*

However, there was not universal support among the Member States for moving forward with a HEPA recommendation. This became obvious when, on 27 June 2012, the Cypriot Presidency released a set of draft Council conclusions on "promoting health enhancing physical activity" (Council 2012c).

During the negotiations on this set of Council conclusions – which are not legally binding but serve to more a political function in terms of starting the legislative process – there was resistance to two parts of the texts as initially drafted by the Cypriot Presidency (Council 2012c):

> The first issue we had was with the Nordic countries because they didn't want – there was an item in the Council conclusions that the Commission should prepare this Council convention on HEPA. So the Nordic countries were not in favour that this should happen, so we had a kind of conflict there [. . .] The other one was for the establishment of the European Week of Sport, because some Member States already have national or local initiatives, very successful one, and they thought that this campaign would replace these initiatives and should do something new.
>
> *Interview, Member State representative, 2 May 2014*

Thus, the conflict revolved around (i) whether the Commission should be explicitly invited to propose a HEPA recommendation to the Council and (ii) concerns about encouraging the Commission to move forward with the launch of a "European Week of Sport". That these were the disagreements is supported by documentary analysis (Council 2012b; Council 2012c; Council 2012d; Council 2012e; Council 2012f; Council 2012g). However, only Sweden lodged formal reservations against the text, which were ultimately released following a minor rewording regarding the particulars regarding the European Week of Sport (Council 2012a; Council 2012b; Council 2012g). As explained by a Swedish representative, if Sweden was sceptical as regards to the HEPA recommendation and the European Week of Sport, the majority of Member States were very enthusiastic:

> It's always difficult to be against these things in a way. You can be against [the recommendation] in maybe you can argue that "is this really EU competence, should we be dealing with it?" [. . .] More or less all Member States thought that it's good to raise these issues and emphasise the importance of sport for public health and so on. At the same time, from the Swedish perspective, we were kind of doubtful about the efficiency when it comes to this [EWoS] because we believe maybe this is work which needs to be done during the whole year [. . .] it's always a weight of preferences. If someone is very, very keen on having it, yeah, then it goes through [. . .] As I said before, it's about public health and blablabla, and it's always strange when you are totally against these things. "Don't you find it important? Sweden is the most sporting people in the world!"
>
> *Interview, Member State representative, 14 May 2014*

Evident here is how it can be socially and politically hard to say "no" to certain things in EU sport policy, especially something as "irresistible" as HEPA ("it's always difficult to be against these things"), with Sweden's subsidiarity concerns not accepted at this stage.

With Sweden releasing its reservations, the Council adopted conclusions on "promoting health-enhancing physical activity" (Council 2012a). The conclusions take note of the HEPA Guidelines, the work of WHO in the field, and the scientific consensus that "[p]hysical activity is one of the most effective ways to prevent non-communicable diseases and combat obesity" (Council 2012a: 22). Member States and the Commission are called on to promote HEPA in various ways, for instance by urging the inclusion of physical activity in the European Statistical Programme for 2013–2017. The conclusions further invited the Commission to "make a proposal for a Council Recommendation on HEPA, and consider including a light monitoring framework" (Council 2012c: 23).

Thus, after many years low-political work had led to a large majority of Member States supporting the adoption of a HEPA recommendation, resulting in conflict expansion with the Council conclusions calling on the Commission to initiate further work. However, for this to happen, certain institutional constraints had to be negotiated, especially within the Commission itself.

Issue entrance

The Commission had commissioned a study to help develop the indicators for the monitoring framework. This study was finalised October 2012 (European Commission 2013a: 8). DG EAC's Sport Unit had gone through internal consultations and procedures since July 2011, ultimately submitting an impact assessment to the Impact Assessment Board on 7 November 2012, which gave the measure a positive assessment (European Commission 2013a: 7).

With the support of the Sport Council and the Commission's internal Impact Assessment Board, this would suggest the road was paved for the Commission to release a recommendation. However, interviews suggest a lot of "in-house" Commission resistance against going forward with the HEPA recommendation, as illustrated below:

> Some parts of the house was not too keen on us going out with a recommendation on HEPA because you have to appreciate that in this period increased criticism on the EU, any interventions perceived as being in the field of lifestyle, are not favoured by many people – at the political level in Council, but also the Commission [. . .] It was about whether or not to do it entirely. Once you decided you are going to do this, I don't think there was much controversy about the actual document. In fact there was hardly any, it was very smooth, but pressing the 'yes button' was the problem, right from the beginning. And you have to see this in the broader political context of increasing pressure on the EU, the rise of the far right, everywhere in Europe, the pressure on [European Commission President] Barroso, also from the European Council, right? [. . .] at the Heads of State there was a political climate that was not conducive to this level of initiatives, you know? It's a Council recommendation, right? And I think at that time the Commission was not in favour of doing more recommendations, because recommendations are of questionable value, shall we say, because: you throw it out there, it attracts bad press because the far right's growing everywhere and stuff, and the press will feed on anything.
>
> *Interview, Commission official, 12 May 2014*

Hence, the political climate was not felt as conducive to proposing further recommendations, not least in something dealing with "lifestyle". This represents the point at which "low politics" intersect with "high politics" (Princen and Rhinard 2006: 1129); how bureaucratic, expert processes on HEPA eventually confronted agenda dynamics "from above", namely the "broader political context of increasing pressure on the EU". That is to say: while actors within EU sport policy recognised the promotion of HEPA as an important and credible issue, this was not necessarily so beyond the EU's sport venues. Accordingly, the issue of HEPA had to be re-framed.

Thus, in order to mobilise further support within the Commission, DG EAC argued that HEPA was not "micro-management" but that it rather had "significant macro-level implications, you know in the economy for example. And we had to make that argument" (Interview, Commission official, 12 May 2014). It was further argued that the sharing of best practices and pooling of resources would provide a European added value and, ultimately, that HEPA promotion is conducive to the reaching the Europe 2020 goals (Interviews with Commission officials, 12 and 16 May 2014). Hence, overcoming internal blockades required emphasising the HEPA's economic dimension, a point prominently made in the Commission's explanatory memorandum of its draft recommendation:

> While evidence demonstrates vast discrepancies between individual Member States, most countries have not achieved the principal policy objective, namely to increase the proportion of citizens who reach the HEPA levels recommended by the WHO and reiterated in the EU Physical Activity Guidelines. For the Union as a whole, the HEPA promotion policies of Member States have not been effective. This situation runs not only counter to the Europe 2020 Strategy, which acknowledges the need to fight health inequalities as a prerequisite for growth and competitiveness, but is also incompatible with the Union's stated policy ambitions in the fields of sport and health. Research indeed confirms the "evidence-policy gap for action" in addressing physical inactivity and has led to urgent calls for policy action on physical activity as a standalone public health priority.
>
> *European Commission 2013b: 3–4*

Evident here is the framing of HEPA in terms of the Europe 2020 strategy, as well as how EU HEPA policy is part of a broader international movement (e.g. WHO). Further, the research cited by the Commission on the "evidence-policy gap for action" draws on an article (Lee *et al.* 2012), part of the *The Lancet* Physical Activity Series which, as argued by Piggin and Bairner (2016), reflects how the "obesity epidemic" is slowly morphing into "the physical inactivity pandemic". In this sense, this is reflected here since the European Commission proposes moving towards physical activity as "a standalone public health priority".

Ultimately, DG EAC was able to overcome internal resistance and on 28 October 2013 the Commission released its "Proposal for a Council Recommendation on promoting health-enhancing physical activity across sectors" (European Commission 2013b). The incumbent Lithuanian Presidency of the Council quickly set aside meetings to deal with the dossier. All interviewees, regardless of institutional affiliation, provided analogous accounts of Council negotiations on this dossier. Negotiations were largely consensual and positive, with the vast majority of Member States in favour of the initiative. The main discussions concerned specific indicators to be used, with the Netherlands declaring early on that it would resist the recommendation. The negotiations are here summarised by a Member State representative:

> The Netherlands took a reservation against the whole document because of – and they said that at the very beginning – because they had a political decision at the highest level, not just in sport but in general, in all the spheres – they see the value of the EU only when it's really added value for the national, or something like that. And yeah, they didn't see, they thought it's just the competence of the Member

State, and they said they won't participate in this at all. Britain was also like doubting at first, but then at the end they took their reservation back. But mainly – what did I want to say – we didn't need the full majority, so that was ok. We were not scared, you know, only one Member State, Netherlands, and other Member States were surprisingly very much in favour. France, even Sweden – they always object to everything [laughing] but somehow they were like "mmm, ok", they were just . . . As I said, the main discussion was about the indicators. What to measure.

Interview 20

This narrative is supported documentary process tracing of earlier drafts (Council 2013b; Council 2013c; Council 2013d; Council 2013e; Council 2013f) until the adopted Council recommendation (Council 2013a). While the indicators may have been heavily discussed, only few alterations were made, and the indicators proposed by the Commission, heavily work-shopped via expert groups and informal meetings, were essentially adopted. The documents further reveal the UK entering a parliamentary scrutiny and the Netherlands entering a general reservation (Council 2013f). However, Council recommendations are adopted by the qualified majority voting procedure, meaning that the adoption of the recommendation was never in real danger.

This brings us full circle in our analysis of how HEPA rose to the top of the EU agenda on sport, ultimately becoming the EU's first recommendation in the field of sport. The importance of this process is profound. First, Member States will henceforth be subject to light monitoring on HEPA, which would allow for stimulating voluntary policy coordination and sharing of best practices across the EU on HEPA (Kornbeck 2015). Second, the effect on EU sport policy has been strong since, as noted by the European Commission, the "majority of activities in the field of sport now focus on implementing the Council's Recommendation to promote health-enhancing physical activity" (European Commission 2016b). This is evident in how, from 2013 and onwards, the majority of funding earmarked for sport through the Erasmus+ programme has been devoted to HEPA and related priorities like the European Week of Sport (see: European Commission 2016a).

Conclusions

This chapter has analysed how HEPA became the first issue in which the EU has adopted a Council recommendation in the field of sport. The rise of HEPA has followed the "low politics route" of issue initiation, specification, expansion and entrance (Princen and Rhinard 2006), ultimately reaching the highest possible level of political decision allowed under Article 165 TFEU. From an early stage physical activity was framed as health-enhancing. *Initiating* in wider international trends in the WHO and spurred on by new sets of indicators, DG EAC and the Council of Sport Ministers started a period of technical *specification* in the years prior to Article 165 TFEU coming into force, resulting in the development of EU Physical Activity Guidelines. From then on, there was a sustained, gradual build-up in developing these technical guidelines, with the Commission earmarking HEPA as the first possible recommendation in the field of sport. The Sport Council eventually encouraged the Commission to propose a HEPA recommendation during the Cypriot Presidency in 2012. Finally, HEPA managed to gain agenda *entrance* as the Commission overcame in-house resistance to the initiative and the Council finally adopted the Commission's proposal for a HEPA recommendation.

Thus, one key to HEPA's upward agenda expansion, affecting framing and hence conflict expansion (Princen 2007), has been the strong *perception* of working on a solid evidence-base.

As shown in this chapter, the framing of physical activity as health-enhancing has been consistent, with the rise of this issue on the global public health agenda creating a "window of opportunity" (Kingdon 1995) for the EU's sporting venues to stake a claim. That is to say, actors within EU sport policy have used developments in other international fora, in particular the WHO, to serve their own goals, a common strategy in agenda-setting (Princen 2011).

Crucially, the proposals on HEPA were backed by a perceived authority "that appear to external policymakers to be 'scientifically objective' and susceptible to truth tests and also appear to benefit the international community as a whole" (Drake and Nicolaïdis 1992: 39). Hence, the evidence and recommendations supporting actions promoting the framing of physical activity as health-enhancing seem universally accepted in the policy subsystem – poor health the problem, physical activity the solution. As expected, the validity of HEPA was only questioned once the issue expanded beyond sporting venues, requiring a framing towards the macroeconomic contribution of HEPA to overcome institutional constraints in the Commission. In conceptualising the "low politics" agenda-setting route, Princen and Rhinard (2006: 1121) draw on Haas (1989) and argue that that "epistemic communities" play a crucial part in the initiation and specification phases; in developing consensus. The findings of this chapter certainly underline the importance of experts in developing policy consensus. However, when mobilising supporters, different types of evidence may be required in order to frame an issue persuasively. That is to say, while the legitimacy of HEPA was so strong within the EU sport policy subsystem that it was almost "difficult to be against", mobilising support beyond the sport system required deliberately framing the issue in more economic growth oriented terms.

Importantly, DG EAC and the Sport Council managed claim authority with regards to the *promotion of* HEPA compared to the competing EU venues. This has had two consequences. First, DG EAC and the Sport Council, who have used HEPA to assert and mainstream sport policy within the EU system, have arguably been key to bringing visibility to HEPA on the EU agenda. Indeed, it is unlikely that a recommendation of HEPA would have been initiated by the EU's health ministers, who have not devoted the issue as much attention. Second, this has allowed EU policy and funding initiatives to be framed more in terms of promoting physical activity and sport rather than the more traditional clinical projects which had been the key focus thus far (Kornbeck 2015).

The findings of this chapter are also important for students of EU sport policy. Despite the ratification of Article 165 TFEU, most research remains focused on the EU's role in the regulation and governance of professional sport and the EU's relationship with the governing bodies of sport (García and Meier 2012; Geeraert and Drieskens 2015; Meier and García 2013; Parrish 2011). While these questions remain intriguing and important, this chapter has shown how such issues no longer remain at the core of EU's work in the field of sport, not least in terms of funding. Thus, more attention to the "social" dimension of EU sport policy is needed if we are to achieve a more nuanced understanding of the dynamics governing this particular policy area.

Finally, this chapter's findings reveal some broader implications for practitioners involved in the promotion of sport and physical activity. First, that framing HEPA as a vehicle for economic growth can be a useful strategy when mobilising support and, ultimately, funding. At the same time, given the centrality of the internal market to the EU's supranational remit, such an "economised approach" (Princen 2011: 937) to agenda-setting may not be equally successful in other settings, given how national sport policy tends to operate under a different logic (e.g. Grix and Carmichael 2012). Nonetheless, evidence in this chapter suggests that highlighting the European sport sector's documented growth potential and labour intensiveness

(SportsEconAustria 2012) may be a fruitful strategy also in national and local spheres of public policy in the low-growth, austerity dominated Europe.

Second, and related, the fact that the promotion of HEPA has become the EU's main priority within the field of sport means that there is now a plethora of new funding possibilities for projects that serve to promote HEPA. This includes the Erasmus+ programme but also EU Cohesion policy through its Structural Funds (European Commission 2016c). Indeed, as EU sport policy becomes ever more mainstreamed within the EU system, funding opportunities for HEPA promotion should only increase, and practitioners involved in the promotion of sport, health and physical activity should take advantage. Moreover, the increasing amounts of cross-national HEPA data and the best practices developed through multinational projects means actors involved in the promotion of physical activity will have access to an increasing amount of evidence when developing policy, programmes and activities.

References

Baumgartner, F. R. and Jones, B. D. (1993) *Agendas and Instability in American Politics*, Chicago: University of Chicago Press.

Brettschneider, W.-D. and Naul, R. (2004) *Study on young people's lifestyles and sedentariness and the role of sport in the context of education and as a means of restoring the balance. Final report*, Paderborn, available at http://eose.org/wp-content/uploads/2014/03/Study-on-young-people-lifestyles_20041.pdf (accessed 10 January 2016).

Council (2003) 'Council conclusions of 2 December 2002 on obestiy', *Official Journal C 11/02*, 17 January, Brussels.

Council (2005) 'Council conclusions on obesity, nutrition and physical activity – Outcome of proceedings', *Council Document 9803/05*, 6 June, Brussels.

Council (2011a) 'Draft Resolution of the Council and of the Representatives of the Governments of the Member States, meeting within the Council, on a European Union Work Plan for Sport', *Council Document 7880/11*, 24 March, Brussels.

Council (2011b) 'Resolution of the Council and of the Representatives of the Governments of the Member States, meeting within the Council, on a European Union Work Plan for Sport for 2011–2014', *Official Journal C 162/01*, 1 June, Brussels.

Council (2012a) 'Conclusions of the Council and of the Representatives of the Governments of the Member States, meeting within the Council, of 27 November 2012 on promoting health-enhancing physical activity (HEPA)', *Official Journal C 393/22*, 19 December, Brussels.

Council (2012b) 'Conclusions of the Council and of the Representatives of the Governments of the Member States, meeting within the Council, on promoting health-enhancing physical activity (HEPA) – Adoption', *Council Document 15871/12*, 14 November, Brussels.

Council (2012c) 'Draft conclusions of the Council and of the Representatives of the Governments of the Member States, meeting within the Council, on promoting health-enhancing physical activity (HEPA)', *Council Document 11334/12*, 27 June, Brussels.

Council (2012d) 'Draft conclusions of the Council and of the Representatives of the Governments of the Member States, meeting within the Council, on promoting health-enhancing physical activity (HEPA)', *Council Document 14160/12*, 28 September, Brussels.

Council (2012e) 'Draft conclusions of the Council and of the Representatives of the Governments of the Member States, meeting within the Council, on promoting health-enhancing physical activity (HEPA)', *Council Document 13519/12*, 14 September, Brussels.

Council (2012f) 'Draft conclusions of the Council and of the Representatives of the Governments of the Member States, meeting within the Council, on promoting health-enhancing physical activity (HEPA)', *Council Document 12229/12*, 13 July, Brussels.

Council (2012g) 'Draft Conclusions of the Council and of the Representatives of the Governments of the Member States, meeting within the Council, on promoting health-enhancing physical activity (HEPA) – Adoption', *Council Document 15664/12*, 6 November, Brussels.

Council (2013a) 'Council Recommendation of 26 November 2013 on promoting health-enhancing physical activity across sectors', *Official Journal C 354/01*, 4 December, Brussels.

Council (2013b) 'Proposal for a Council Recommendation on promoting health-enhancing physical activity across sectors', *Council Document 14434/13*, 17 October, Brussels.

Council (2013c) 'Proposal for a Council Recommendation on promoting health-enhancing physical activity across sectors', *Council Document 15107/13*, 25 October, Brussels.

Council (2013d) 'Proposal for a Council Recommendation on promoting health-enhancing physical activity across sectors', *Council Document 15300/13*, 31 October, Brussels.

Council (2013e) 'Proposal for a Council Recommendation on promoting health-enhancing physical activity across sectors', *Council Document 14188/13*, 7 October, Brussels.

Council (2013f) 'Proposal for a Council Recommendation on promoting health-enhancing physical activity across sectors – Adoption', *Council Document 15755/13*, 14 November, Brussels.

Drake, W. J. and Nicolaïdis, K. (1992) 'Ideas, interests, and institutionalization: "trade in services" and the Uruguay Round', *International Organization* 46(1): 37–100.

EU Working Group Sport & Health (2008) 'EU physical activity guidelines: Recommended Policy Actions in Support of Health-Enhancing Physical Activity', *Approved by the EU Working Group 'Sport & Health' at its meeting on 25 September 2008, Confirmed by EU Member State Sport Ministers at their meeting in Biarritz on 27–28 November 2008*, 10 October, Brussels, available at http://ec.europa.eu/sport/library/policy_documents/eu-physical-activity-guidelines-2008_en.pdf (accessed 10 January 2016).

European Commission (2003) 'Special Eurobarometer: Physical Activity', *Special Eurobarometer 183–186,* available at http://ec.europa.eu/health/ph_determinants/life_style/nutrition/documents/ebs_183_6_en.pdf (accessed 10 January 2016).

European Commission (2005) 'Mandate Working Groups: Diet, Physical Activity and Health – A European Platform for Action', *Rev1 – 25/05/2005,* 25 May, Brussels, available at http://ec.europa.eu/health/ph_determinants/life_style/nutrition/platform/docs/ev20050525_md_en.pdf (accessed 12 January 2016).

European Commission (2006) 'Eurobarometer 64.3: Health and food', *Special Eurobarometer 246,* available at http://ec.europa.eu/health/ph_publication/eb_food_en.pdf (accessed 10 January 2016).

European Commission (2007a) 'Commission staff working document: The EU and Sport: Background and Context. Accompanying document to the White Paper on Sport', *SEC(2007) 935,* 11 July, Brussels.

European Commission (2007b) 'White Paper on a Strategy for Europe on Nutrition, Overweight and Obesity related health issues', *COM(2007) 279 final,* 30 May, Brussels.

European Commission (2007c) 'White Paper on Sport', *COM(2007) 391 final,* 11 July, Brussels.

European Commission (2007d) 'White paper: Together for Health: A Strategic Approach for the EU 2008–2013', *COM(2007) 630 final,* 23 October, Brussels.

European Commission (2010) 'Eurobarometer 72.3: Sport and Physical Activity', *Special Eurobarometer 334,* Brussels, available at http://eose.org/wp-content/uploads/2014/03/european-barometer-survey_334_en_20101.pdf (accessed 10 January 2016).

European Commission (2011) 'Communication from the Commission to the European Parliament, the Council, the European Economic and Social Committee and the Committee of the Regions: Developing the European Dimension in Sport', *COM(2011) 12 final,* 18 January, Brussels.

European Commission (2012) *Towards an EU Funding Stream for Sport: Preparatory Actions and Special Events 2009–2011*, Luxembourg: Publications Office of the European Union, available at http://bookshop.europa.eu/en/towards-an-eu-funding-stream-for-sport-pbNC3212200/ (accessed 10 January 2016).

European Commission (2013a) 'Impact assessment Accompanying the document Proposal for a Council Recommendation on promoting health-enhancing physical activity across sectors', *SWD(2013) 311 final,* 28 August, Brussels.

European Commission (2013b) 'Proposal for a Council Recommendation on promoting health-enhancing physical activity across sectors', *COM(2013) 603 final,* 28 August, Brussels.

European Commission (2014) 'Special Eurobarometer 412: Sport and physical activity. Report', *Special Eurobarometer 412,* Brussels, available at http://ec.europa.eu/health/nutrition_physical_activity/docs/ebs_412_en.pdf (accessed 10 January 2016).

European Commission (2015) 'EU Platform on Diet, Physical Activity and Health', *ec.europa.eu,* available at http://ec.europa.eu/health/nutrition_physical_activity/platform/index_en.htm (accessed 22 May 2015).

European Commission (2016a) 'Erasmus+: Selection results', *https://eacea.ec.europa.eu,* available at https://eacea.ec.europa.eu/erasmus-plus/selection-results_en (accessed 24 October 2016).

European Commission (2016b) 'Health and Participation', *http://ec.europa.eu*, available at http://ec.europa.eu/sport/policy/societal_role/health_participation_en.htm (accessed 24 October 2016).

European Commission (2016c) 'Study on the contribution of sport to regional development through the Structural Funds published', *http://ec.europa.eu*, available at http://ec.europa.eu/sport/news/2016/1018_regional-development-structural-funds_en.htm (accessed 24 October 2016).

European Parliament & Council (2003) 'Decision No 291/2003/EC of the European Parliament and of the Council of 6 February 2003 establishing the European Year of Education through Sport 2004', *Official Journal L 43/1*, 18 February, Brussels.

García, B. (2007) 'From regulation to governance and representation: agenda-setting and the EU's involvement in sport', *Entertainment and Sports Law Journal* 5(1), available at http://www2.warwick.ac.uk/fac/soc/law/elj/eslj/issues/volume5/number1/garcia/ (accessed 16 January 2016).

García, B. and Meier, H. E. (2012) 'Limits of interest empowerment in the European Union: The case of football', *Journal of European Integration* 34(4): 359–378.

García, B. and Weatherill, S. (2012) 'Engaging with the EU in order to minimize its impact: sport and the negotiation of the Treaty of Lisbon', *Journal of European Public Policy* 19(2): 238–256.

Geeraert, A. and Drieskens, E. (2015) 'The EU controls FIFA and UEFA: a principal–agent perspective', *Journal of European Public Policy* 22(10): 1448–1466.

Grix, J. and Carmichael, F. (2012) 'Why do governments invest in elite sport? A polemic', *International Journal of Sport Policy and Politics* 4(1): 73–90.

Haas, P. M. (1989) 'Do regimes matter? Epistemic communities and Mediterranean pollution control', *International Organization* 43(3): 377–403.

Kingdon, J. W. (1995) *Agendas, Alternatives, and Public Policies*, 2nd Ed., New York: Harper Collins Publishers.

Kornbeck, J. (2015) 'Lisbonisation without regulation: engaging with sport policy to maximise its health impact?', *The International Sports Law Journal* 15(1–2): 112–122.

Lee, I. M. et al. (2012) 'Effect of physical inactivity on major non-communicable diseases worldwide: An analysis of burden of disease and life expectancy', *The Lancet* 380: 219–229.

Meier, H. E. (2009) 'Emergence, dynamics and impact of European sport policy – Perspectives from political science', in S. Gardiner, R. Parrish, and R. C. R. Siekmann (eds). *EU, Sport, Law and Policy: Regulation, Re-regulation and Representation*. The Hague: T.M.C. Asser Press, pp. 7–34.

Meier, H. E. and García, B. (2013) 'Abandoning hopes for veto power: institutional options for sport governing bodies in the European Union', *International Journal of Sport Policy and Politics* 5(3): 421–443.

Parrish, R. (2003a) *Sports Law and Policy in the European Union*, Manchester: Manchester University Press.

Parrish, R. (2003b) 'The politics of sports regulation in the European Union', *Journal of European Public Policy* 10(2): 246–262.

Parrish, R. (2011) 'Social dialogue in European professional football', *European Law Journal* 17(2): 213–229.

Piggin, J. and Bairner, A. (2016) 'The global physical inactivity pandemic: An analysis of knowledge production', *Sport, Education and Society* 21(2): 131–147.

Princen, S. (2007) 'Agenda-setting in the European Union: A theoretical exploration and agenda for research', *Journal of European Public Policy* 14(1): 21–38.

Princen, S. (2011) 'Agenda-setting strategies in EU policy processes', *Journal of European Public Policy* 18(7): 927–943.

Princen, S. and Rhinard, M. (2006) 'Crashing and creeping: Agenda-setting dynamics in the European Union', *Journal of European Public Policy* 13(7): 1119–1132.

SportsEconAustria (2012) *Study on the Contribution of Sport to Economic Growth and Employment in the EU*, Final report, commissioned by the European Commission, Directorate-General Education and Culture, available at http://ec.europa.eu/sport/library/studies/study-contribution-spors-economic-growth-final-rpt.pdf (accessed 16 January 2016).

Stephenson, P. J. (2012) 'Image and venue as factors mediating latent spillover pressure for agenda-setting change', *Journal of European Public Policy* 19(6): 796–816.

Tokarski, W., Steinbach, D., Petry, K. and B. Jesse (2004) *Two players one goal? Sport in the European Union*, Oxford: Meyer and Meyer Sport.

World Health Organization (2000) 'Obesity: preventing and managing the global epidemic', *WHO Technical Report Series 894*, Geneva: World Health Organization, available at www.who.int/nutrition/publications/obesity/WHO_TRS_894/en/ (accessed 10 January 2016).

World Health Organization (2002) 'Diet, physical activity and health', *WHA55.23,* 18 May, available at http://apps.who.int/gb/archive/pdf_files/WHA55/ewha5523.pdf (accessed 10 January 2016).

World Health Organization (2004) 'Global strategy on diet, physical activity and health', *WHA57.17,* May, available at www.who.int/dietphysicalactivity/strategy/eb11344/strategy_english_web.pdf (accessed 16 January 2016).

XG SHP (2011) 'Expert group "sport, health and participation": Report from the 1st meeting (27 September 2011)', *ec.europa.eu,* October, available at http://ec.europa.eu/sport/library/documents/expert-groups/shp_en.pdf (accessed 16 January 2016).

XG SHP (2012a) 'Deliverable 1: "Input for an EU initiative to promote HEPA" – A monitoring framework on the implementation of the EU Physical Activity Guidelines (EU PA GL)', *ec.europa.eu,* June, available at http://ec.europa.eu/sport/library/documents/expert-groups/shp_en.pdf (accessed 16 January 2016).

XG SHP (2012b) 'Expert group "sport, health and participation": Report from the 3rd meeting (27 June 2012)', *ec.europa.eu,* July, available at http://ec.europa.eu/sport/library/documents/expert-groups/anti-doping_en.pdf (accessed 16 January 2016).

38

INDIA

Aman Dhall

India has a population of 1.25 billion people (second in terms of population) and ranks third in terms of recent economic growth. However, when it comes to sports and physical activity statistics, India does not fare so well in many respects. For a country with such a large population and landmass, India ranked 55th in the 2012 London Olympics, and 67th in Rio four years later. Even as India has taken big strides in almost every field in the last few decades, its achievements in sports do not match the kind of presence it wields among other countries of the world in different spheres. A nation's failure to produce sporting talents is often attributed to the physical activity rate of its people.

Economic development and urbanization in India have brought about many changes in individual behaviour, especially among the affluent classes, which is conducive to an increased problem of obesity (TNN, 2017). These changes have driven people more towards a sedentary lifestyle with an increased level of television and computer use, a rising availability of energy-dense processed foods and the growing tendency of replacing previously laborious household chores with electronic appliances. All these result in a significant reduction in the amount of physical exertion needed for day-to-day life. According to the World Health Organization, "[t]he trend toward physical inactivity is increasing in many economically developing countries, such as India, partly due to the unhealthy environments and behaviours that rapid urbanization and globalization promote" (WHO 2010). This is quite alarming, as physical inactivity has been identified as the fourth leading risk factor for global mortality, accounting for 9 per cent of deaths worldwide.

A study by the Global Physical Activity Observatory shows that the physical activity rate among Indian youth is moderately high. The prevalence of physical activity among girls (aged above 18 years) and that among boys (above 18 years) in India are 84 per cent and 89 per cent respectively. However, the rate of physical activity decreases with age, and this is evident from the rising prevalence of obesity and diabetes in India. In the fight against physical inactivity, an increase in diabetes, obesity and other health related issues, the government has recognized the importance of promoting physical activity and sport at the grassroots among young people. With the growing tendency of sedentary lifestyles in India, this is an enormous challenge at the time of growing social media intrusion into young people's lives, despite a heightened understanding about health and fitness in urban youth.

When it comes to physical activity, many youth in India find it more exciting and engaging to play games online rather than going out to play with friends. With the growing number of gaming applications available on smart phones and the ease of access of smart phones to middle class young people, there are dangers to physical activity rates in the future. However, technology might also be motivational for young people who wish to engage in physical activity, and for those who young people in urban cities who regularly attend the gym.

Physical activity culture and practices in India

Like many others, India is a country of contrast. In major cities there are pockets of enormous wealth, contrasting starkly with large populations that live in poverty. Urban areas which have become increasingly "westernised", can be juxtaposed with rural communities, which maintain traditional habits and customs. The differences in physical activity levels and types varies enormously within and between urban and rural spaces. Rural communities often maintain traditional habits and customs, including work practices which rely heavily on manual labour. Many of the large city areas (including some of the largest in the world) are also witnessing the negative effects of sedentary lifestyles which often correlate with most urban landscapes and technological advances.

Still, physical activity remains a core part of Indian culture from traditional dancing to the practice of yoga for physical wellbeing and meditation, to the passion amongst many Indians for the sport of cricket. It should be mentioned that it would be cliché to state that cricket is the only sport that Indians play and watch – hockey and wrestling are also popular, and in recent years football has risen dramatically in popularity. For many adults, walking and jogging are popular in cities, while gyms tend to be the domain of only those who can afford the membership fees, in cities which have significant wealth gaps. Large cities in India do have numerous public parks for physical activities to take place – walking and yoga are popular here for adults and older adults alike. Cycling is very common, particularly as a means of commuting for those in poorer income brackets. With regard to employment, while many occupations in large cities are as sedentary as those in other parts of the world, employment in more rural areas is often heavily reliant on manual labour. Jobs which could (and perhaps should) be done by machines are done by humans. This raises interesting questions about the value of technologies – while they are often blamed for increasing sedentary lifestyles, it could be argued that technological advances would be enormously helpful overall for people working in rural communities. One more interesting aspect of activity in India, similar to many other countries is the tradition of squatting, a practice which is commonplace at meal times in parts of the countries and for ablutions.

Given that urbanization and economic development have a strong correlation, and with the trend of an increasing urban population in India as compared to the rural population, it has been suggested that India could focus on developing at least 25–30 world-class mega cities in the future. Physical activity opportunities would need to be high on the agenda to contribute to the health of people who live there. At the same time, India, like other developing countries, is struggling to deliver sufficiently on poverty eradication, infrastructure development for basic housing, water supply and electricity.

The sport and physical activity industry

Very few Indian parents encourage their children to take up sports as a career. It is mostly perceived more as a hobby or fitness regime than as a prospective career option. Reasons behind this are many. A career in sports and physical activity does not seem financially lucrative. Moreover, in India, the cultural dominance of cricket means that many other sports can be perceived as less important. No other sport receives as much importance as cricket. Cricketers are celebrities in India and hence, people associate cricket with glamour. As a result, other sports receive neither encouragement nor much financial support.

Even Indian schools never paid much heed towards cultivating the habit of sports and physical activity among students. Though physical activity and sports have always been part of the co-curricular activity of the Schools in India, there has been always a gap in the training provided to students. The outlook towards sports amongst Indian families has certainly improved over the years but it has not achieved the kind of importance and focus that it receives in other nations. Aspiring urban class families of the 21st century are generally supportive in providing an opening to their children in sports. However, when these children graduate to the top level, they are hit hard by the wide gap between themselves and counterparts from other countries. Lack of professional scientific coaching, missing grassroots structure and sustainable funding support are generally attributed as reasons.

1991 proved the turning point for India's fortunes when the then Finance Minister Manmohan Singh, who later served two terms as the Prime Minister, liberalized the economy and India has never looked back. The abolition of the Licence Raj not only brought about huge changes to the economy of the country but also paved the way for the globalization of sports in India. The arrival of private sports channels like Prime Sports and ESPN Star Sports helped change people's attitude towards sports. Programmes like badminton, tennis, golf, "Formula One" motorsports, basketball and even baseball matches were aired by Prime Sports, which made people interested in world sports. Football also received a global outlook from Indian sports enthusiasts.

The ministry of Youth Affairs and Sports has revealed the budget proposal for the year 2016–17 in which Rs. 900Cr (plan) and Rs. 96Cr (non-plan) are allocated for all sports altogether. The Sports Department of India had 21 schemes which, from 2016, have been merged under three umbrella schemes namely 1) *Sports Institutions and Schemes*, 2) *Encouragement and Awards to Sportspersons* and 3) *Khelo India National Programme*.

In the current financial year, an amount of more than Rs 900 crore was allocated for sports. It pales in comparison to what some other countries but even this amount is not utilized properly. Like the TOP (Target Olympic Podium) scheme for the 2016 Rio Olympics received a lot of criticism for the way the selection of athletes was made and delay over payments.

A large problem in India is the way sports in India are managed. Most sports associations are government funded and managed by administrators, mostly politicians, who do not have the expertise or vision to see India grow as a sporting superpower. The suspension of the Indian Olympic Association in 2012 for not following the Olympic charter in election of its officials was a black day and this dented the image of sport governance in India. Boxing, in which India was emerging as top competitors in international events, has also suffered from infighting over the official body and as a result, Indian boxers are troubled to fight under the national flag, a matter of pride and motivation.

The National Sports Development Bill, floated by the previous United Progressive Alliance regime, to bring in changes in the working of these associations was not allowed to have the kind of teeth it was projected to have. Corruption, nepotism and indifference towards sports are rampant and the athletes are often not supported as much as they could be. How the dominance in India's national game hockey was allowed to fade away over the years is a perfect example of general apathy and indifference towards sports.

Government and policies

The government has traditionally been a driver of sport and physical activity in India. It has been a chief engineer of the promotion of Olympic sports with a larger overview to achieve broader social goals. The role has been further divided between the centre and the states, the Indian Olympic Association, the Sport Authority of India (SAI) and the National Sports Federations and its affiliates (Mukherjee, Goswami, Goyal & Satija, 2010).

It is observed over the years that children who regularly participate in sports and other physical activities tend to perform academically better in schools. Studies have shown that regular physical activities help to improve memory and concentration among children. The role of physical activity, therefore, is considered crucial for the cognitive development of children. Besides, regular participation in sports and physical activities allows children and youth to develop necessary social and emotional skills by providing them with opportunities to socialize and interact with their peers in a healthy sporting environment. Hence, in order to promote sports and physical activity among children, the Government of India has implemented many schemes like *Rajiv Gandhi Khel Abhiyan* (RGKA) and *Khelo India National Programme*. Though the Government has also implemented schemes for the development and maintenance of infrastructure for various sports with the help of MoRD (Ministry of Rural Development) and MUD (Ministry of Urban development), there are opportunities in the future for private organizations to be incentivized for setting up playgrounds and for providing sports facilities to schools, colleges and community areas.

Ministry of Youth Affairs & Sports (MoYAS)

The ministry was established by the government of India when it hosted the Asian Games in 1982. In 2000 this department was granted a status of the ministry. The role of ministry is to build sports infrastructure and develop sport at the grassroots level by working with multiple autonomous agencies such as Sport Authority of India, the Indian Olympic Association and sports developmental institutions.

State governments

State governments are in charge for the development of physical activity and sport in their respective provinces. Apart from their own allocation of funds, the state governments receive finances from the MoYAS under the government's five-year plans.

National Sports Federations

These organizations work in conjunction with the IOA and prepare athletes for participation at the international sporting meets. It's generally on the recommendation of the NSFs that IOA select and train athletes. Apart from the above duties, NSFs are also responsible for organizing national and international tournaments in India.

Sports Authority of India (SAI)

After the 1982 Asian Games in New Delhi the government set up the Sports Authority of India (SAI), as part of its efforts to boost sports and attract youth with the objective of promotion of sports and games. It was entrusted with maintaining and utilizing infrastructure facilities for athletes, on behalf of Ministry of Youth Affairs and Sports. The sports development institutions – the Lakshmibai National College of Physical Education and the Netaji Subhash National Institute of Sports – are the educational wings of the SAI.

Among the policies, the Sports Promotional Schemes of SAI was developed to boost development and promotion of sports in the country at grassroots level to attain excellence at National and International level through scouting sports calibre and further developing talented athletes by inducting them in SAI Sports Promotional Schemes. Currently among the other notable schemes for the promotion of sports in the country include National Sports Talent Contest Scheme (NSTC) and the Army Boys Sports Company Scheme (ABSC). While the former scheme was launched during 1985 for spotting talented young children in the age group of 8–14 years from schools and nurturing them by providing scientific training, the latter was developed with the objective of achieving excellence at international level by making use of good infrastructure and efficient administrative and disciplined environment of the Army.

Sports received a tremendous increase in budget allocation during the year 2015–16. The Ministry of Youth Affairs and Sports received an extra Rs 384 crore. The scheme for the Benefit of North Eastern Area and Sikkim was given Rs 151.23 crore this year as compared to just Rs 81.95 crore last year. The acknowledgement that north-eastern states of India have an abundance of youth whose sports talent needs to be optimized was well received.

However, lack of transparency when it comes to implementation and lackadaisical attitude of bureaucracy has somewhat negatively affected the public's enthusiasm on a regular basis and slowed down India's progress as a sporting nation. The country needs to further visualize and implement both long-term and short-term policies that can impact sports development.

Infrastructure in India

Lack of adequate sports infrastructure and effective utilization of existing spaces has been a major hindrance to promote sports and physical activity amongst young people in India. Sports complexes are either located in big cities far out of reach of communities in smaller towns and villages out. At many activity sites, the infrastructure is in such deplorable condition that it limits sports training. Sportspeople have to compromise with deteriorating training machines.

Infrastructure is a key element for sports development in India and the government plays an important role in this not only in granting money for building of infrastructure but by auditing, monitoring and maintaining it at periodic intervals. Huge sports complexes were constructed for the Asian Games in 1982 and 28 years later in 2010 it was the Commonwealth Games raising hopes that there would be a boost in sports participation in the country. However, after the events, these sports facilities and the Games Villages were used for purposes other than for which they were constructed. The Asian Games Village was handed over for government residential quarters while the Commonwealth Games Village remained deserted. Most of the stadia are used more often for political meetings with an occasional sporting event thrown in between. The lackadaisical attitude of the government towards sports and the use of the stadia for purposes other than for which they were constructed also contribute to a lack of importance placed on a wide variety of sports. It is clear that the nation needs to become realistic about the budget allocation on the maintenance of sports and physical activity infrastructure. This situation is made worse by what is perceived as ineffective utilization of existing sports infrastructure. Playgrounds, indoor halls in schools and sports complexes around the country are not being utilized to their maximum potential. They are often underutilized and stay empty for a number of hours on weekdays. For large stadiums and small local village facilities alike, there is space to develop a vision and put in a long-term roadmap to create sustainable sports infrastructure across the country. Rather than hosting specific events, an importance focus should be larger goals of youth development and healthy society.

Not many would disagree that India has never been a sporting nation. And after nearly seventy years of independence, it still aspires to be one despite producing world beaters like Major Dhyanchand (hockey), Sachin Tendulkar (cricket), Sania Mirza and Leander Paes (tennis), Vishwanathan Anand (chess) and Saina Nehwal (badminton) among others. Notable achievements in sports, sporadic and few, fuel aspirations among fans to see India emerge as a sporting superpower but then the idea has come time and again and died an untimely death.

Influence of sport events

Since independence, India has hosted several major sporting events with many of them more than once such as the Cricket World Cup, World Table Tennis Championship, the Asian Games twice in 1951 and 1982 and the Commonwealth Games in 2010. In 2017 India hosted the FIFA U-17 World Cup in 2017, the first time India would be organizing a football tournament of such scale. The launching of the Indian Premier League Cricket in 2008, after winning the inaugural T20 World Cup in South Africa, cemented the popularity of the sport. It was hoped the Commonwealth Games in 2010 would leave a positive legacy and add to the popularity of many sports, but the tournament was beset with a variety of organizational problems which meant goodwill and spectatorship at the event was limited.

The recent development of the professional football league and the Kabbadi league (associated with the glamorous Bollywood) have captured the interest of many people in India. However, it is yet to be clear if these leagues really motivate and inspire the youth to take up the sports or they just create more TV-glued watchers who watch for the charm of Bollywood and regional sentimentality.

The hosting of sporting events has had both a positive and negative impact on the nation's politics and economy. The 1982 Asian Games hosted by India in New Delhi did boost the image of the then Prime Minister Indira Gandhi as it saw the capital attaining several world class stadia with the centre piece being the Jawaharlal Nehru Stadium where the opening and closing ceremonies of the Games were held. But, after the event, this stadium virtually lay unused except for an occasional international sports meet or a football match but mostly school sports being held there. The stadium became the office of the Sports Authority of India (SAI) while two other indoor stadia too were largely used for political activity while another stadium which was renovated for football saw the holding of wrestling matches and public meetings.

Though the 2010 Commonwealth Games was successful attracting a large number of spectators, the lead up proved politically costly for the Delhi Government of the then Chief Minister Mrs Shiela Dikshit and the Chairman of the Organizing Committee of the Games Suresh Kalmadi who was jailed for corrupt practices. The capital got a facelift worth Rs 66,550 crore for the Commonwealth Games, with taxpayers picking up a major part of the tab. Delhi's beautification made up for the bulk of the total expenses on the Games – Rs 70,608 crore. This was far above the estimated original price tag of the Games, and more than what the government spends on the National Rural Health Mission every year. This caused further embarrassment to the Sheila Dikshit government, which had been on a taxation spree on the pretext of the Games.

According to Majumdar (2010), "[s]uch an escalation is unheard of in the history of world sport. These figures aren't polemic, but empirically based on facts". Of the total Games-related spending on improving Delhi's infrastructure, Rs 5,700 crore was allocated for flyovers and bridges alone, Rs 650 crore for stadia, Rs 16,887 crore for the Delhi Metro expansion and Rs 35,000 crore for new power plants. Intriguingly, none of these sums figure in the data submitted in Parliament by successive sports ministers or in the internal records of the Games organising committee (OC).

India was the third developing country to host this multi-sports mega-event after Jamaica in 1966 and Malaysia in 1998 and the objective was to leave behind a "lasting legacy" with an overhaul of the existing city infrastructure and sporting infrastructure. The benefits that did accrue to the Indian capital were that it got a world class public transport system in Metro Rail and broad roads though the construction of these roads left much to be desired for the rains in the post-Games period saw most of them becoming virtually impossible to drive on as they were full of potholes.

The Games went off smoothly showcasing Indian culture which was indeed appreciated. India gave its best ever performance in the Commonwealth Games with a record haul of 101 medals, the highest ever in an international sporting event of this nature. Not many would disagree that India has never been a sporting nation. Ganguly (2013) observes that the short-term outlook that "prevails within the sporting set up is another spanner in the works of the Indian sports machine". Most Indian "sports fans" are mere enthusiasts and limit themselves to watching an occasional cricket match and viewing EPL football matches on TV. And after nearly seventy years of independence from colonial rule, it still aspires to be one. Notable achievements in sports, sporadic and few, fuel aspirations among fans to see India emerge as a sporting superpower.

An important issue in context of developing countries is not the "conduct" of the mega-event. Rather it is the potential for mega-events to contribute to sustainability, including socio-economic development and long-term environmentally sound practices that is most important. At the India-Brazil-South Africa (IBSA) Dialogue Forum Fourth Summit, the Heads of States of the three countries recognized that hosting of mega-events reflected the positive momentum of developing countries and could potentially act as a tool for their social and economic development (Konrad Adenauer Stiftung, 2011). The Games did not produce the tangible benefits for the tourism industry that were expected. The CWG did create a number of jobs and livelihoods during the Games but most of these were temporary and concentrated in the informal sector. Moreover, a number of jobs were lost due to eviction and displacement related to the games. For Delhi, the 2010 Commonwealth Games accelerated infrastructure, especially in the transportation sector at the local (city) level which has the potential to benefit the expanding urban area around Delhi. Transportation-linked infrastructure projects as well as small projects linked to increasing supplies of energy and water can be considered a beneficial legacy. Apart from awareness-raising initiatives, it is not clear what the environmental legacy of the Games will be in the long run.

Implications for physical activity policy and practice

Physical inactivity is a global problem and is one of the reasons behind the growing numbers of lifestyle disorders and non-communicable diseases. However, it is observed that middle-income countries often show a higher rate of physical inactivity. And India is no exception to this. This calls for the immediate implementation of various policies to encourage more physical activity among children and adolescents. Here are some considerations for policies that might help Indians live more physically active lives.

The mere inclusion of sports in school curricula is not enough. Since sport is a state subject, primary responsibility for development and promotion of sports in schools is that of the State Governments. However, there is a need to involve all the States and Union territories. In 1998, the Government instituted the National Sports Development Fund (NSDF) with a view to mobilizing resources from the Government as well as non-governmental sources including the private and corporate sector and non-resident Indians.

There appears to be a lack of collaboration between the two tiers of government (Central and State) and the private-public sector to provide equitable access to basic physical activity and sporting facilities programmes. However, in recent years, government and the private sector have made an attempt to engender a culture in which sports is prioritized. Notwithstanding these positive sentiments, India continues to struggle with rising levels of health problems, administration apathy and lack of a sustainable sport development program that could improve activity levels.

The Ministry of Youth Affairs and Sports receives contributions from a host of public sector units, private companies and sporting bodies (2015). These include the Board of Control for Cricket in India (BCCI), Steel Authority of India Limited (SAIL), Oil & Natural Gas Commission (ONGC), Jindal Steel and Power Ltd, Oriental Bank of Commerce, Videocon International Ltd, Powergrid Corporation of India, State Bank of India, Jaypee Sports International Limited, India Infrastructure Finance Company Limited (IIFCL). This was part of the effort by the government to bring in the Corporate Sector, both public and private, to promote and develop sports in the country.

According to the current Minister for Sports and Youth Affairs, training to promote rural sports, nationally recognized sports, paralympic sports and Olympic sports have been included in the Companies Act, which would allow companies to spend on development of sports from the funds earmarked for Corporate Social Responsibility (CSR) related activities. The move to include sports in the CSR activities was done as it was felt that this would give a boost to the promotion and development of sports in the country and the much needed funds from companies, both in the public and private sector, will flow to the sports sector. However, there are question marks raised over whether supporting these sports projects is more an obligation to abide by the rules or being taken up as a true responsibility for carrying out sustainable efforts for sport development at the grassroots.

It is rather unfortunate that the centre and most states have not worked with a holistic approach for a system geared to promote physical activity and sports in a comprehensive manner. The objective of evolving into a healthy and active nation requires concerted effort to secure free access to good facilities for the youth. A unified national structure must work in a mission-mode – with central and state governments functioning in close co-ordination with the Sports Authority of India (SAI), the Indian Olympic Association (IOA) and the National Sports Federations (NSFs). There is a need for sustained supply of funds and resources to develop and maintain facilities and stadia as also skills in technical and managerial aspects for the development of physical activity in India. India needs more youngsters to take up coaching and sport science related careers.

The foundation of a physically active nation is the grassroots level itself. Education and training should begin at the grassroots level. There is space for every village and every town to promote physical activity more. Physical activity for all and sports-for-all is what India needs.

References

Ganguly, A. (2013). What ails Indian Sport?. [online] Sportskeeda. Available at: http://www. sportskeeda.com/general-sports/what-ails-indian-sport

Konrad Adenauer Stiftung. (2011). *Sustainable mega events in developing countries.* [online] Johannesburg: Konrad Adenauer Stiftung. Available at: www.kas.de/wf/doc/kas_29583-1522-1-30.pdf

Majumdar, B. (2010) In Games makeover is a Rs 66,550 cr bomb. Available at: http://indiatoday. intoday.in/story/games-makeover-is-a-rs-66550-cr-bomb/1/110410.html Accessed 8 September 2017.

Ministry of Youth Affairs & Sports (2015). *Annual report 2014–15.* [online] New Delhi: Ministry of Youth Affairs & Sports. Available at: http://yas.nic.in/sites/default/files/Annual%20Report%20 2015%20English.pdf

Mukherjee, A., Goswami R., Goyal, T. and Satija, D. (2010). *Sports retailing in India: Opportunities, constraints and way forward.* [online] India: Indian Council for Research on International Economic Relations. Available at: http://icrier.org/pdf/Working_Paper_250.pdf

TNN. (2017). India has second highest number of obese children in world: Study. *The Times of India.* [online]. Available at: http://timesofindia.indiatimes.com/india/india-has-second-highest-number-of-obese-children-in-world-study/articleshow/59135548.cms

WHO (2010) *Global Recommendations on Physical Activity for Health.* Geneva, Switzerland: WHO.

39

SOUTH AFRICA

Tracy L. Kolbe-Alexander and Estelle V. Lambert

Introduction

With a population of more than 50 million people and 11 official languages, South Africa is culturally diverse. Seventy-five per cent of South Africans are literate, contrasted against a 21 per cent rate of unemployment. Children under the age of 15 make up one-third of the population, while adults over 65 constitute approximately 5 per cent of the total population (Statistics South Africa, 2012). Rapidly urbanizing South Africa has one of the highest GINI coefficients in the world, 0.67, indicating a wide gap between rich and poor. Against this demographic backdrop, nearly 1 in every 5 to 6 adults is estimated to be HIV-positive, while approximately 40 per cent of adult mortality may be attributable to 4 chronic conditions, including: cardiovascular disease, diabetes, chronic lung disease and certain cancers (Levitt, Steyn, Dave & Bradshaw, 2011). Moreover, 1 in 5 children under the age of 5 years is stunted, with nearly an equal number considered to be overweight or obese (Shisana, Labadarios, Rehle et al., 2014). More than two-thirds of South African women are overweight or obese, while more than half of all South Africans are reportedly inactive or doing insufficient physical activity for health benefit (Norman, Bradshaw, Schneider et al., 2007).

Physical activity is well-established as one of the four major risk factors for non-communicable disease (Lee, Shiroma, Lobelo et al., 2012). It has been estimated that 30 per cent of ischaemic heart disease, 27 per cent of colon cancer and 20 per cent of diabetes in South Africa may be attributed to physical inactivity (Joubert, Norman, Lambert et al., 2007). This translated to more than 17,000 deaths (3.3% of all deaths), and 176,000 DALYs (1.1% of all DALYs) in 2000 (Joubert, Norman, Lambert et al., 2007).

Only 36 per cent of South African men and 24 per cent of women report sufficient levels of daily health-enhancing physical activity (Guthold, Ono, Strong, Chatterji, & Morabia 2008). Furthermore, the South African Youth Risk Behaviour Survey found that nearly half of all school children did not meet the recommended levels of physical activity, with more than 36 per cent of the boys and 46 per cent of the girls reportedly inactive (Reddy, James, Sewpaul et al., 2010). There were concerning increasing trends for inactivity from 2002–2008, suggesting that South African adolescents are becoming less physically active, with 30 per cent spending 3 or more hours per day in front of the television (Reddy, James, Sewpaul et al., 2010). Thus, there is a major health imperative to promote physical activity and reduce levels of inactivity in the general South African population.

In lower and middle-income countries such as South Africa, where there are often large income disparities, there is typically an inverse association between occupation- and transport-related physical activities and time spent in recreational physical activity (Guthold, Louazani, Riley et al., 2011), reflecting socio-economic and education gradients. For example, a study reporting the prevalence of leisure time physical activity showed that people in developing nations were less active than those in developed countries (Haase, Steptoe, Sallis & Wardle, 2004). While active travel and non-motorized transport have been shown to contribute significantly to total daily physical activity in some settings, in South Africa, the National Household Travel Survey showed a trend for a decline in active travel from 2003–2013, from just over 23 per cent to 20 per cent (Statistics South Africa, 2014). Furthermore, there is an inverse association between car ownership and daily physical activity in both developed and developing countries (Shoham, Dugas, Bovet et al., 2015).

Therefore, with the decline in occupational- and transport-related activities, leisure time physical activity has become increasingly important as a target for changing levels of habitual physical activity. It is the role of government along with civil society to address the declining levels of physical activity through policies and programmes aimed at promoting physical activity and sport. The aim of this narrative review is to highlight government and non-government initiatives and policies, past, current or pending, that may have impacted or have the potential to impact on population levels of physical activity.

A historical context for physical activity-related policies and programmes in South Africa

The following is a brief overview of policies and programmes that relate to physical activity (and sport) that have been promulgated in South Africa over the past two decades. Figure 39.1 highlights some of the policy development and national level evaluation and monitoring activities from the early 1990s to 2015. South Africa has made significant progress, including the development of many new policies since the abolition of Apartheid in the early 1990s. (*Apartheid was a political and societal system that enforced segregation between indigenous [African, Indian and Coloured people] and Caucasian people. Although segregation occurred for many years, Apartheid was legalized by the National Party of South Africa in 1948. This system enforced segregation by the Caucasian minority and systematically disadvantaged and denied other racial groups basic human rights. Loosely translated, Apartheid is "being apart".*) Much of the focus in new polices has been aimed at addressing past injustices by improving equity, access and opportunity for participation in physical activity and sport for all citizens.

This period was characterized by an emergence of non-governmental organizations, which emphasized physical activity and "sport for good" or "sports for development" in under-resourced communities and settings. The first democratic South African government released a White Paper on Sport and Recreation in 1994, aiming to ensure increased access and equity to sport and recreational opportunities for all South Africans. Physical activity was therefore highlighted in this report and mass participation was encouraged through the "Siyadlala Mass Participation Campaign" in 2004. Siyadlala is the Xhosa phrase for "we are playing". The main objective of the initiative was to increase the number of sports and recreation clubs in the country, especially in rural and remote areas, and to provide access to a wide variety of activities to impoverished communities, identified as "hubs". Although Siyadlala has had a greater focus on organized sports such as athletics and gymnastics, it also promoted indigenous games and dance. Examples of indigenous games includes "Dibeke or skun
unu" and "drie stokkies (3 sticks)". Dibeke/skununu is a running game played by two teams of six players

each. Attacking players try to kick a ball down the length of a field without being tagged by a defender. If an attacking player is tagged, they are "out" the game. The defenders are allowed to use their hands and feet, while attackers can only use their feet to move the ball. In "drie stokkies", three sticks are placed parallel to each other, one metre apart. Players take turns to run and one step between the sticks without touching them. The last player that jumps aims to leap as far forward after the 3rd stick, which is then moved to where his heel (foot) landed, thus increasing the distance between the sticks with each round of jumping. Local implementers, mainly unemployed youth, were recruited and trained as coaches/administrators to implement at community centres and schools. Hub Coordinators are responsible for managing the delivery/implementation of sporting codes at community level.

Over this same time period, physical activity for health was receiving widespread attention, globally. In 2002, the World Health Organization (WHO) World Health Day in 2002 focused on Move for Health, and the main event was celebrated in Sao Paulo, Brazil, with the "Agita Sao Paulo and Agita Brazil" campaigns to promote physical activity. These campaigns eventually led to the global social movement for physical activity promotion, Agita Mundo. Subsequently, the World Health Assembly's Resolution on Diet, Physical Activity and Health advocated that WHO member states celebrate Move for Health day and to use it as a vehicle to encourage and promote regular physical activity for well-being and as part of a healthy lifestyle.

Global surveillance instruments such as the International Physical Activity Questionnaire (IPAQ) and the Global Physical Activity Questionnaire (GPAQ) were developed over this time and validated both internationally and locally (Bull, Maslin & Armstrong, 2009; Craig, Marshall, Sjostrom et al., 2003). Monitoring and evaluation of physical activity initiatives and harmonization of global prevalence data were made possible using these instruments. The first prevalence measures for physical in/activity surveillance as part of the National Demographic and Health Survey were made in South Africa in 2003. At this time, more than 50 per cent of South Africans were insufficiently active. Fitness levels were assessed in the more recent South African National Health and Nutrition Survey (SANHANES) in 2013, and showed that 62 per cent of the men and 42 per cent of the women participating in the survey were physically fit (Shisana, Labadarios, Rehle et al., 2014).

The international focus on non-communicable disease and associated risk factors culminated in the UN High Level Meeting on Non-Communicable Disease in September 2011. This meeting, along with national surveillance, and secular trends, served as an important catalyst in underscoring the importance of population-based strategies to promote physical activity for health.

As a direct result of these global and other local developments, strategies for the promotion of physical activity have been recognized and articulated in policies and white papers from the Departments of Health, Basic Education, Sport and Recreation, and Transport. These strategies are also highlighted in the National Development Plan 2030, which recognizes that physical activity and a physically active lifestyle have the potential to positively impact on the economy, the environment and the development of social capital in children and youth.

The next section of this chapter provides examples of current physical activity-related policies in South Africa. Perhaps what is most notable about these strategies, plans and policies is the degree of alignment, the articulation of the need for inter-sectorial cooperation and the emphasis on social and environmental justice, access and redress. Moreover, there is a clear, settings-based approach. What remains to be determined is the extent to which these plans will be implemented successfully, as well as the plans for monitoring and evaluation of implementation within and across sectors and settings.

Physical activity within South Africa's National Development Plan (NDP) 2030

The key challenges for the promotion of physical activity in South Africa relate to competing priorities, for example: poverty alleviation and unemployment; the provision of housing and basic services, crime and personal violence; education; reducing the burden of HIV and TB, as well as under-nutrition in children. South Africa's main political, cultural and economic priorities have been clearly articulated in The National Development Plan 2030.

The National Planning Commission (NPC) was comprised of 25 independent commissioners appointed by the South African president in 2010. The mandate of the commission was to take a broad, cross-cutting, independent and critical view, to help define an aspirational South Africa. Then, looking ahead to 20 years' time, the commission was tasked with developing a national plan designed to map out a path to achieve these aspirations (National Planning Commission, 2011).

The NDP includes 5 long-term nation-building objectives, one of which is to "promote social cohesion across society". Sport and physical activity play an important role in promoting wellness and social cohesion, and therefore, the plan treats sport and physical activity, as a cross-cutting issue, with related proposals in the chapters on education, health and nation building. The Department of Basic Education and the Department of Sports and Recreation have taken important steps to reintroduce sport in schools. The NDP proposes that this initiative should be expanded so that all schools develop and maintain infrastructure for at least two sports. Some of the popular sports in South Africa, dependent on region and demographics, include: soccer, netball, rugby, cricket and athletics.

Further, the NDP recommends that all communities should have access to sports and recreational facilities and that local authorities promote physical activity by ensuring that urban roads have adequate sidewalks, developing cycle lanes and installing traffic-calming measures. Finally, the NDP proposes an initiative to encourage South Africans to walk, run, cycle or play team games on the second Saturday of every month, mobilizing the extensive network of formal and informal sporting clubs to organize these events.

National Department of Sport and Recreation Strategic Plan 2015–2020

The tag line for Sport Recreation South Africa's (SRSA) Strategic Plan 2015–2020 is "For the Active You" (Department of Sport and Recreation, 2014). This comprehensive plan has two main strategic objectives including "an active nation" and a "winning nation". The strategic goal under "an active nation" is that citizens will have access to sport and recreation activities to help achieve the goal of a 10 per cent increase in participation in selected sport and recreation activities by 2019/20.

Within this plan, and under this strategic objective, there are several sub-programmes including Active Recreation, Community Sport and School Sport. Active Recreation offers mass participation opportunities to "improve the health and well-being of the nation", and aims to deliver "at least 25 active recreation campaigns or programmes with a specific focus on designated groups". Activities such as the Big Walk – a mass participation event with more than 30,000 participants – the Golden Games for seniors, the Move for Health social mobilization campaign and national youth camps form some of the baseline events already convened under this sub-programme. However, the plan articulates the need to upscale these activities, and that this will require resources and planning.

Under the Community Sports sub-programme, the goal is to promote "lifelong physical activity by providing at least 10 structured sport promotion programmes to community members". Typically, the focus under this sub-programme is sport-for-development, and expanding reach into disadvantaged communities.

Finally, the School Sports programme focuses on increasing access, and its primary objective is to "increase learners' access to sport at schools by supporting 8 national school sport championships for learners". The underlying rationale in the policy is that schools sports lead to active youth and an active nation. SRSA and the Department of Education are working together to reintroduce sport in schools as they both acknowledge that both sport and physical education contributes to children's development and health.

SRSA's Strategic Plan 2015–2020 builds on the National Development Plan and includes the following proposals related to school-based physical activity such as ensuring that physical education classes are mandatory at all schools and led by a qualified physical education teacher. In addition, schools and the local community should have facilities and equipment required for physical education and sport. The plan aims to encourage organized sports events from local to national level competitions. Lastly, they aim to encourage healthy lifestyles among school employees and have suggested that this could be promoted using incentives (Department of Sport and Recreation, 2014).

Another important activity of SRSA highlighted in their Sport and Recreation South Africa Strategic Plan 2015–2020 is their role in revising the International Charter of UNESCO on Physical Education, Physical Activity and Sport. Furthermore, South Africa has been selected as a pilot country for UNESCO's physical education programme, promoting physical activity in schools, using UNESCO's new guidelines for Quality Physical Education. These guidelines seek to halt the steady decline in physical education globally over the past few years (McLennan & Thompson, 2015).

Strategic Plan for the Prevention and Control of Non-Communicable Diseases: 2013–2017

In response to the UN High Level Meeting on Chronic, Non-Communicable Diseases in 2011, the South African Department of Health released the Strategic Plan for the Prevention and Control of Non-Communicable Diseases 2013–2017 (Department of Health, 2013). Prior to the UN meeting, the South African National Department of Health hosted a "National Summit", which included delegates from government, non-governmental organizations, professional organizations and representatives from tertiary institutions. The South African Declaration for Prevention and Control of Non-Communicable Diseases was adopted at this meeting. The declaration was comprised of 10 goals and targets for 2020, including: "to increase the prevalence of physical activity (defined as 150 of moderate-intensity physical activity per week or equivalent) by 10%".

The four strategies put forward to promote greater population levels of physical activity include:

a) Increasing knowledge and awareness on the benefits of physical activity;
b) Encouraging inter-sectoral collaboration thereby increasing access and opportunities to increase physical activity;
c) Implementing physical activity intervention programmes;
d) Disseminating examples of evidenced-based physical activity interventions and policies (Department of Health, 2013).

Progress on the targets will be monitored via national surveys like the South African National Health and Nutrition Examination Survey (SANHANES) and the Demographic Health Survey in 2016.

National Department of Education: Physical education and physical activity policies in South African schools

Physical education was previously a stand-alone subject in all schools. However, it now forms part (1/4) of the "Life Skills" subject area in schools from kindergarten (Grade R) through Grade 12. In the Curriculum and Assessment Policy Statements (CAPS) document presented in 2011, for implementation in 2012, schools were expected to deliver 2 hours of physical education per week in grades 1–5. From grades 6–12, Life Skills as a subject area is only allocated 2 hours in total per week, and thus physical education formed a much smaller component of the curriculum. Despite the fact that physical education is scheduled in the curriculum, studies in South Africa show that in urban primary schools more than one-third of learners did not participate in weekly physical education (Katzmarzyk, Barreira, Broyles et al., 2015) and in a rural sample, less than two-thirds of children participated in weekly physical education (Micklesfield, Pedro, Kahn et al., 2014). Clearly, there is a need for better monitoring and strategies to overcome the policy-implementation gap.

In November 2011, the Departments of Basic Education and Sports and Recreation South Africa put forward a Memorandum of Understanding, to promote an Integrated School Sport Framework (Departments of Basic Education, 2011). Under this MOU, Section 1.2, it is stated that:

> The integration of physical education and sports participation into the school day will make sport accessible to all children who attend school (regardless of their physical ability, gender, socio-economic or ethno-cultural backgrounds). This integration can build on children's early experiences by:
>
> a) ensuring that children develop their physical and motor capacities to lead active, healthy lives – a major factor in preventing non-communicable disease;
> b) providing children with opportunities to have fun and be active, reinforcing their desire to make physical activity a lifelong habit;
> c) helping children understand and overcome barriers to physical activity;
> d) informing, equipping and motivating children to make healthy lifestyle choices by integrating sport and physical activity with health education programmes.

Under Section 1.1, the MOU states that "ensuring optimal conditions for a child's participation in sport and recreation is one of the best investments the government can make", suggesting that the South African government demonstrates the political will to promote physical activity in a variety of sectors.

National Department of Transport: Policies that impact on physical activity

In 2008, a policy document was prepared by the National Department of Transport detailing the plan for Integrated and Non-Motorised Transport (NMT) in South Africa (Department of Transport, 2008). This policy was followed by numerous provincial and local municipal plans for NMT. Within this policy document there is recognition that non-motorized transport should be made widely accessible and that most forms of NMT are healthy, non-polluting, versatile and reliable. The policy emphasized a shift away from private car use to NMT and an integrated public transport system. The underlying rationale was to utilize the existing road network more efficiently, providing not only economic and environmental benefits, but individual health and lifestyle benefits and the potential for greater social cohesion within communities (Department of Transport, 2008).

One of the key thrusts of the Department of Transport, in the policy document for plans from 2007–2020, is the development of Integrated Rapid Public Transport Networks (IRPTS). In the draft policy, it was envisaged that the IRPTS Networks will "form a viable, car-competitive mobility option and hence enable stricter penalties and incentives to get car users to switch to these networks". There are plans to implement measures to lower car dependency, particularly during peak traffic hours, through financial disincentives for parking and private vehicle use, and tax incentives for employers and individuals utilizing the networks. In addition, there is the stated intention to implement these networks in conjunction with NMT options (Department of Transport, 2008).

The Bus Rapid Transit (BRT) systems are being rolled out in 6 metropolitan areas in South Africa, including the Rea Vaya system in Johannesburg and MyCiTi in Cape Town. Preliminary evidence from intercept interviews on the MyCiTi system (Bartels, Lambert, Kolbe-Alexander & Behrens, 2015) suggests that those people using the BRT accumulate 30 min of PA per day when walking to and from transit stations.

Inter-sectorial Strategy for the Prevention and Control of Obesity in South Africa: 2015–2020

Perhaps one of the most innovative and potentially far-reaching policy initiatives comes in the form of the Strategy for the Prevention and Control of Obesity in South Africa: 2015–2020. The over-arching mission of the strategy is to "empower the population of South Africa to make healthy choices by creating an environment that enables and promotes healthy eating and physically active lifestyles for the prevention and control of overweight and obesity" (Department of Health, 2014). What sets this policy initiative apart is the expressed intent for an inter-sectorial platform of implementation. The strategy itself was prefaced by a statement of commitment and/or support from the Ministers for Basic Education, Sport and Recreation, Transport, Cooperative Governance and Traditional Affairs, Trade and Industry, as well as Public Service and Administration, to work with the private sector and academia to reduce the prevalence of overweight and obesity by 10 per cent in 2020.

Increasing the prevalence of physically active South Africans has been identified as one of the 6 goals of this strategy. This goal has 4 main objectives:

a) Improve access to recreational facilities for all people, with a focus on equity; key actions under this objective include:

Increase equitable access to and maintenance of recreational and physical activity facilities in communities, strengthen partnerships between communities and local schools to access school grounds for physical activities, ensure that all urban planning and new developments are required to consider strategies to optimize PA opportunities and create walkable communities (zoning laws, bicycle lanes), establish community-based physical activity groups and strengthen the programme for mass participation.

b) Promote equitable access and increased use of active transportation;
c) Increase physical activity in the schools, both as part of the curriculum and improving the school environment;
d) Increase physical activity in workplaces by incorporating it as part of obesity management and other wellness programmes, and creating activity-"permissive" worksites.

In addition, there is a focus on increasing physical activity levels in early childhood, and importantly, creating a demand-side "push" or social mobilization for community-based physical activity programmes, facilities and campaigns. The aim is to support environmental changes that facilitate increased levels of physical activity; partner with and support evidence-based interventions that encourage healthy lifestyle behaviours, including physical activity; support research, evaluation and monitoring or surveillance, and lastly to align with the "National Strategic Plan on Non-Communicable Diseases". It is envisaged that this strategy adopt a phased approach, and it is notable that to date, there is no country which has effectively "rolled back" the obesity epidemic. The targets are bold, and the outcomes of this innovative strategy have yet to be evaluated, but it has proposed useful indicators for process and outcome evaluation. This may yet be the "call to action" that positions physical activity, along with appropriate dietary and fiscal strategies, firmly on the national agenda.

"Failure to launch": Department of Health's National Physical Activity Plan

The National Department of Health, under the Health Promotion Directorate, was approached by a lead tertiary, academic institution and subsequently requested work to begin drafting a National Physical Activity Plan in 2011, as physical activity is a "proven, scalable, population-based, multi-sectoral and culturally-relevant intervention that has health, social and economic benefits".

The National Physical Activity Plan aimed to provide a framework to achieve the global target of increasing the prevalence of physical activity by 5 per cent by 2020. Work on this plan preceded the National Strategy for the Prevention and Control of Non-Communicable Diseases, and was undertaken well before the promulgation of the national obesity strategy. The vision of the National Physical Activity Plan was to improve the health status and quality of life of all South Africans by increasing (participation in) physical activity, as an accessible and integrated part of one's daily life.

The plan articulated 5 over-arching strategies, within a settings-based approach:

a) Create knowledge and awareness of the importance of regular, moderate physical activity for health and wellbeing, for the prevention and management of disease and for the promotion of human and social capital.
b) Develop and support the implementation of policies to effect the necessary infra-structural, environmental and programmatic adjustments to enable access to routine physical activity for all South Africans.
c) Increase and promote inter-sectorial collaboration towards increased opportunities to be physically active.
d) Disseminate examples of evidence-based interventions and programmes and policies to promote physical activity.
e) Facilitate the development of programmes and interventions to promote physical activity; to monitor and evaluate the reach, effectiveness and impact of these programmes and interventions.

These strategies may be reflected by actions within different sectors that will form part of the planning framework going forward. Furthermore, the plan was situated within sectors and against strategies which have proven to be effective globally (Global Advocacy for Physical Activity and the Advocacy Council of the International Society for Physical Activity and Health, 2012).

These settings, strategies, and sectors include:

a) Primary health care

For example, in this setting, it has been proposed that physical activity be integrated into the primary health care setting. The tactics that have been identified include: developing and implementing a rapid assessment for PA as a monitoring tool for patients with NCDs/risk factors for NCDs; and to provide client PA education and appropriate supportive activities into waiting areas, club and counselling rooms; as well as integrating physical activity into community support groups, and providing training and support materials for members of the primary health care team concerning physical activity and health recommendations and exercise prescription for NCDs.

b) Education

For example, in the education sector, the following tactics have been identified: prioritizing and providing adequate pre-service and in-service training and support for implementing School Physical Education Curriculum (new life skills, CAPS); supporting the development of safe walking and cycling routes to and from school ("walking school bus"), traffic calming, zebra crossings and monitors); ensuring that there are gender- and ability-appropriate programs in schools for after school sport and physical activity for all learners through funding, programme development, training and partnerships; and promoting physical activity during break times by providing affordable and appropriate resources such as playground markings, exercise circuits, equipment (tyres, climbing frames) playing fields (sport-specific) and adult supervision or leadership.

c) Work places

In the worksite setting, there were many potential opportunities for intervention, including: providing tax and/or SETA-related incentives for worksites with NCD-related worksite health promotion programmes (WHPP); implement physical activity intervention programmes as part of WHPP; and provide shower and change room facilities, dedicated space and/or time for physical activity and incentives for employees to participate. Ultimately, the goal would be to develop a framework policy and guidelines for physical activity-permissive worksites.

d) Sports and recreation

Perhaps the most important tactic identified under this setting was to support and grow the mass participation programme, Siyadlala, by training community leaders, and to monitor and evaluate its impact and reach.

e) Mass media

Tactics proposed under mass media include: sequencing, planning and providing guidelines for dissemination of community-wide campaigns for physical activity, in a prospective, coordinated manner; promoting the "Move for health" Day and implementing on-going activities in the schools, worksites, health care and community settings, using the brand, messages and dissemination platform developed previously.

f) NGOs, FBOs, community-based organizations
Within the NPO, Community and Sports for Development settings, the strategies included: prioritizing and incorporating physical activity into existing community-based programmes, as well as promoting physical activity and health within existing community-based sport for development programmes, and partnering with national government on the Move for Health campaign.

g) Roads and transport, land use, urban planning and community development
With respect to active transport and urban design, the following tactics were recommended: developing and implementing standards for community design that incorporates land use, transportation, parks and trails and economic development planning which provides for increased opportunities for physical activity; consider safety, street connectivity, access to public transport, aesthetics, local destinations (retail, business and community facilities such as schools, places of worship, etc.).

The first draft, with input from tertiary academic institutions, and intra-departmental comment, was completed in 2012. This was circulated to a small group of stakeholders for comment and input, including representatives from the Department of Education and the Department of Cultural Affairs and Sport, as well as representatives from other tertiary institutions. The plan was updated and a national workshop was planned, where a wider range of stakeholders were to be given the opportunity to contribute to the development of the plan. Once the final version had been drafted, it was to be presented to the South African National Parliament.

However, the plan was never presented to the national government for adoption, and much of this plan has been subsumed in the Strategy for the Prevention and Control of Obesity 2015–2020, and the National Strategy for the Prevention and Control of Non-communicable Diseases 2013–2020. The question remains as to why the National Plan for Physical Activity had a "failure to launch" compared to the subsequent strategies. This may have been due, in part, to the political environment at the time, the lead government directorate which was Health Promotion or the lack of visibility of this initiative within government, or the lack of visibility of physical inactivity as a risk factor. It also highlights that in countries where there are competing demands, positioning physical activity/inactivity plans and policies within other "more pressing" strategies may be one way to increase priority and drive action.

Major physical activity initiatives

Access, opportunity and benefits of leisure time physical activity should be promoted, however, there are some unique challenges to implementing or promoting leisure-time physical activity in South Africa, which might include rapid urban change, low socioeconomic status, unequal access to health care, limited resources and civil and political instability. Despite these challenges, there are many examples of programmes and initiatives encouraging increased levels of physical activity that have been implemented over the past few years. The following section of this chapter provides examples of physical activity intervention programmes at the national level in various settings including schools, worksites, older adults and community settings.

The National Departments of Health, Education and Sport and Recreation South Africa, have worked together in the "Vuka South Africa – Move for your Health Campaign", are stakeholders in the National Plan for Physical Activity and Health. In addition, the

Departments of Health and Education are collaborating in schools, in programmes like the Health Promoting Schools campaign.

"Vuka South Africa" Move for your Health

Based on the burden of non-communicable diseases among South Africans, and also in response to the WHA's Resolution on Diet and Physical Activity, the National Department of Health's launched its "Healthy Lifestyle Campaign" in 2004. Promoting physical activity is one of the main components of this campaign which is advocated in each of the 9 provinces. This campaign, together with South Africa's involvement in the Move for Health Day in 2002, led to the development and launch of "Vuka South Africa – Move for your Health", which is based on the Agita Mundo initiative (Kolbe-Alexander, Bull & Lambert, 2012). Subsequent to the launch in 2005 and the workshop in 2007, there has been continued implementation of programs and events linked to Vuka SA. However, these have been sporadic, and limited data is available on the number of initiatives and participants.

Siyadlala: Sport and Recreation South Africa (SRSA)

The Ministry of Sport and Recreation South Africa's programme, "Siyadlala", a Zulu term meaning "let's play", was launched in 1994. This programme aimed at facilitating mass participation in sport and recreation activities, particularly during leisure time. Siyadlala's activities included handball, soccer, basketball, aerobics, gymnastics, fun walks, netball, rugby, cricket, volleyball and "learn to swim" and indigenous games. The Siyadlala campaign included the "30 minutes of physical activity on at least 5 days of the week" message at these community-based interventions, thereby promoting the physical activity guidelines to the broader South African community.

This programme is responsible for the organization and delivery of the "Golden games", a sports event for older adults (>60 years); Indigenous Games and other Siyadlala programmes across SA with a focus on marginalized groups including women, children, youth, elderly, persons with a disability and people living in rural areas. In addition, conditional grants have been awarded to each of South Africa's provinces (or states), to promote activities within communities and schools related to the FIFA World Cup legacy, mass participation hubs under Siyadlala and school sport.

Monitoring and evaluation reports for Siyadlala suggest that this mass participation programme is now reaping rewards, with increase in capacity and participation (38 hubs, 9,537 participants per week, 122 activity coordinators and more than 740 practice sessions per week, typically involving an average of 25 participants per session) (Burnett & Hollander, 2006).

Annual Recreation Day

In December 2014, the South African parliament announced that South Africa would celebrate an Annual Recreation Day on the first Friday of October every year. All South Africans will be encouraged to participate in recreational activities, including physical activity that can play a role in improving their health status. A National Steering Committee was established to promote and organize the Annual Recreation Day. Events for this day will link with other established initiatives such as TAFISA's World Walking Day (Department of Sport and Recreation, 2014).

School-based interventions

The South African Youth Risk Behaviour Survey found that 38 per cent of school children participated in less than the recommended levels of physical activity (Reddy, James, Sewpaul et al., 2010). Therefore schools have been identified as an important setting to promote leisure time physical activity. Interventions targeting schools include those that provide resources such as lesson plans for teachers, together with worksheets for learners. The aims of the lesson plans are to provide learners with physical activity experiences and also with the knowledge of the benefits of regular physical activity. The effectiveness of these interventions is still being measured, however, anecdotal reports suggest an increase in moderate intensity physical activity among the youth.

Community Health Intervention Programmes (CHIPS)

Physical activity interventions targeting older adults have also achieved significant improvements in functional ability and health status. An example of one such programme is the Community Health Intervention Programmes (CHIPS) based in South Africa. CHIPs is a community-based physical activity programme where the older adults meet twice per week for low intensity seated exercises. The older adults participating in the exercise sessions improved dynamic balance and lower body muscle strength after only 20 weeks of exercising (Kolbe-Alexander, Lambert & Charlton, 2006). There were significant improvements in blood pressure. The Yale Physical Activity Survey for older adults was used for self-reported physical activity in various domains. Weekly energy expenditure related to exercise increased in the intervention group, however there was no change in total energy expenditure (Kolbe-Alexander, Lambert & Charlton, 2006). Thus the older adults could have decreased physical activity in the other domains due to their increased leisure time exercise sessions.

Private sector: Health insurance initiatives

Several private national health insurers recognized and prioritized the importance of physical activity in the prevention and management of non-communicable diseases. Subsidized gym membership and also rewards for regular participation in leisure time physical activity are offered to their members. Clients receive points for going to the gym, or participating in running, cycling and golf-related events, and also for having their fitness assessed. The effect of habitual physical activity on health care expenditure was recently evaluated. This study showed a monotonic decrease in hospitalization costs and admission rates per member from the inactive to the high active categories (Patel, Lambert, da Silva et al., 2011).

There are also published results from the implementation of an incentivized health promotion programme, from South Africa's largest private health insurer, Discovery Health, with over 2.5 million beneficiaries. Wellness activities of the program include health risk assessments (HRA), subsidized gym memberships and smoking cessation or weight loss programmes. This incentive-based programme has shown a significant relationship between levels of participation in fitness-related activities, with lower medical claims and hospital admissions (Lambert, da Silva, Fatti et al., 2009). A retrospective longitudinal analysis demonstrated that participation in fitness-related activities increased over 3 years, and that these changes were associated with a significantly lower probability of hospital admissions and in-patient claims in the subsequent two years (Patel, Lambert, da Silva et al., 2011). Taken together, these studies highlight the use of physical activity and financial incentives for health promotion in the worksite or private health care setting, as a means of reducing health care expenditure.

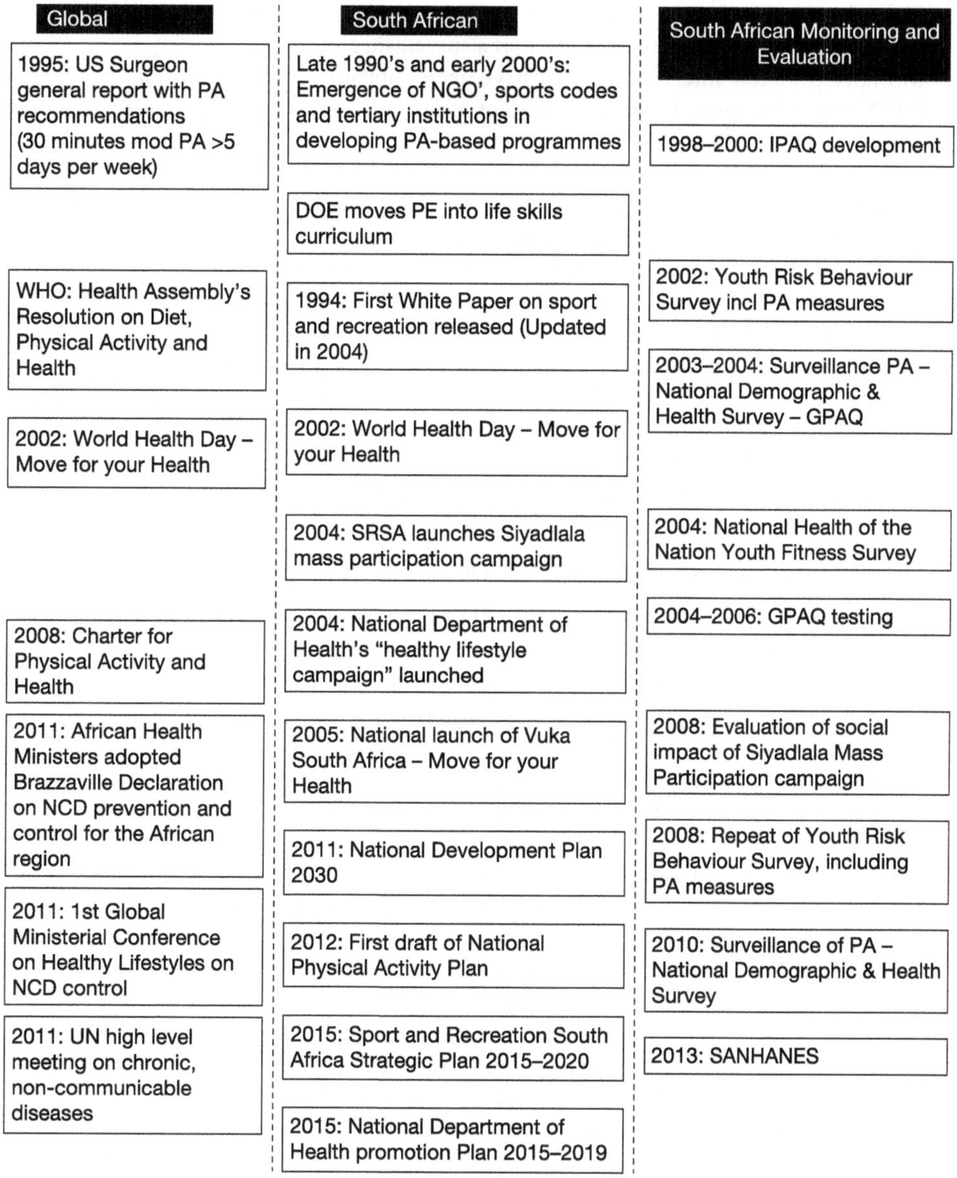

Global	South African	South African Monitoring and Evaluation
1995: US Surgeon general report with PA recommendations (30 minutes mod PA >5 days per week)	Late 1990's and early 2000's: Emergence of NGO', sports codes and tertiary institutions in developing PA-based programmes	1998–2000: IPAQ development
	DOE moves PE into life skills curriculum	
WHO: Health Assembly's Resolution on Diet, Physical Activity and Health	1994: First White Paper on sport and recreation released (Updated in 2004)	2002: Youth Risk Behaviour Survey incl PA measures
		2003–2004: Surveillance PA – National Demographic & Health Survey – GPAQ
2002: World Health Day – Move for your Health	2002: World Health Day – Move for your Health	
	2004: SRSA launches Siyadlala mass participation campaign	2004: National Health of the Nation Youth Fitness Survey
2008: Charter for Physical Activity and Health	2004: National Department of Health's "healthy lifestyle campaign" launched	2004–2006: GPAQ testing
2011: African Health Ministers adopted Brazzaville Declaration on NCD prevention and control for the African region	2005: National launch of Vuka South Africa – Move for your Health	2008: Evaluation of social impact of Siyadlala Mass Participation campaign
	2011: National Development Plan 2030	2008: Repeat of Youth Risk Behaviour Survey, including PA measures
2011: 1st Global Ministerial Conference on Healthy Lifestyles on NCD control	2012: First draft of National Physical Activity Plan	2010: Surveillance of PA – National Demographic & Health Survey
2011: UN high level meeting on chronic, non-communicable diseases	2015: Sport and Recreation South Africa Strategic Plan 2015–2020	2013: SANHANES
	2015: National Department of Health promotion Plan 2015–2019	

Figure 39.1 Overview of a selection of global and South African policy initiatives since 1990s

Source: Adapted from Kolbe-Alexander et al., 2012

Surveillance, monitoring and evaluation: Physical activity prevalence, reach and impact of programmes and policies

There have been some important milestones with respect to institutionalized surveillance of physical activity prevalence, within the National Demographic and Health Survey (2003) and in the South African National Health and Nutrition Survey (SANHANES) in 2012 and planned for 2016. On the other hand, the South African Youth Risk Behaviour Survey, conducted in 2002 and again in 2008, was largely funded by international research support, and as such, has not been institutionalized as a surveillance tool.

Moreover, the few interventions that have been implemented across school community or NPO settings have yielded little by way of evaluation and monitoring, and there is also very little information concerning scaling up these interventions, or on ensuring sustainability within the South African setting.

The Healthy Active Kids South Africa Report Card, now bi-annual expert consultation, and evaluation exercise provides some guidance and a bench-mark exercise for certain key indicators for physical activity in children, including physical education, active play, active transport, organized sport and sedentary behaviour, as well as the correlates and determinants of these indicators. However, as much of the monitoring and evaluation serves as advocacy tools, the impetus comes from the private sector, NPOs or tertiary academic partnerships, and are generally inadequately funded.

There is a need to change the culture of partnerships, and interventions, and to "begin with the end in mind" in establishing the evaluation matrix and measures for a pilot, for an efficacy trial, for a dissemination trial and for practice-based evidence.

Implications for future physical activity policy and practice

African countries are faced with an increasing burden of non-communicable diseases, which in part, can be prevented by leading a physically active lifestyle. However, despite higher levels of total physical activity compared to more developed countries, there are lower levels of leisure time physical activity. This, together with reduced energy expenditure in occupation and transport-related activity, underscore the importance of physical activity and sport-based intervention programs in Africa.

With regards to policy promoting sport and physical activity, there is room for improvement in this area within the African region. However, there is a noticeable gap between policy and implementation, and increased policy on the role of sport and physical activity in the promotion of health may not necessarily lead to improved implementation of sport and physical activity programmes.

The examples of good practice presented in this chapter align with policy and other high level recommendations from the United Nations and African Union, however they do not seem to have been driven by policy. Rather, it would appear that these programmes have been developed and implemented in response to the health and development needs in Africa, where creative and active methods have been sought to address these needs.

The challenge remains, however, to conduct widespread and rigorous evaluation of these types of programs so that practice-based evidence can be disseminated and evidence-based practice promoted. If evidence of effectiveness can be shown and communicated, the quality of other sport and physical activity interventions could be improved, and these interventions could reach a wider population. Ultimately, this could result in the increased promotion of health and prevention of disease on the African continent.

References

Bartels, C., Lambert, E.V., Kolbe-Alexander, T. & Behrens, R. (2015). The siketha ukuba nempilo (we choose to be healthy) project: Can taking public transport lead to a healthier lifestyle? *Journal of Transport and Health, 2.2*(S15).

Bull, F. C., Maslin, T. S. & Armstrong, T. (2009). Global physical activity questionnaire (gpaq): Nine country reliability and validity study. *Journal of Physical Activity and Health, 6*(6), 790–804.

Burnett, C. & Hollander, W. (2006). Mid-impact report of the mass participation project of sport and recreation South Africa 2004/2005 Johannesburg, South Africa: Sport and Recreation South Africa and University of Johannesburg.

Craig, C. L., Marshall, A. L., Sjostrom, M., Bauman, A. E., Booth, M. L., Ainsworth, B. E., Pratt M., Ekelund U., Yngve A., Sallis J. F. & Oja, P. (2003). International physical activity questionnaire: 12-country reliability and validity. *Medicine and Science in Sports and Exercise, 35*(8), 1381–1395. doi: 10.1249/01.mss.0000078924.61453.fb.

Department of Basic Education & Department of Sport and Recreation, Republic of South Africa. (2011). *Memorandum of understanding: An integrated school sport framework.* Pretoria, South Africa: South African Governement Retrieved from http://www.srsa.gov.za/pebble.asp?relid=1228.

Department of Health, Republic of South Africa. (2013). *Strategic plan for the prevention and control of non-communicable diseases 2013–2017.* South Africa: South African Government Retrieved from www.health-e.org.za/2013/09/19/strategic-plan-prevention-control-non-communicable-diseases-2013-17/.

Department of Health, Republic of South Africa. (2014). *Strategy for the prevention and control of obesity in South Africa 2015–2020.* Pretoria, South Africa: Department of Health Retrieved from www.sancda.org.za/wp-content/uploads/2015/09/National-Strategy-for-prevention-and-Control-of-Obesity-4-August-latest.pdf.

Department of Sport and Recreation, Republic of South Africa. (2014). *Sport and recreation South Africa: Strategic plan 2015–2020.* Pretoria, South Africa: South African Government Retrieved from www. srsa.gov.za/pebble.asp?relid=1024.

Department of Transport, Republic of South Africa. (2008). *Draft national non-motorised transport policy.* Pretoria, South Africa: Republic of South Africa Retrieved from http://unpan1.un.org/intradoc/groups/public/documents/cpsi/unpan037583.pdf.

Global Advocacy for Physical Activity (GAPA) the Advocacy Council of the International Society for Physical Activity and Health (ISPAPH). (2012). NCD prevention: Investments [corrected] that work for physical activity. *British Journal of Sports Medicine, 46*(10), 709–712. doi: 10.1136/bjsm.2012.091485.

Guthold, R., Louazani, S. A., Riley, L. M., Cowan, M. J., Bovet, P., Damasceno, A., Sambo, B. H., Tesfaye, F. & Armstrong, T. P. (2011). Physical activity in 22 african countries: Results from the world health organization stepwise approach to chronic disease risk factor surveillance. *American Journal of Preventive Medicine, 41*(1), 52–60. doi: 10.1016/j.amepre.2011.03.008.

Guthold, R., Ono, T., Strong, K. L., Chatterji, S., & Morabia, A. (2008). Worldwide variability in physical inactivity: A 51-country survey. *American Journal of Preventive Medicine, 34*(6), 486–494. doi: 10.1016/j.amepre.2008.02.013.

Haase, A., Steptoe, A., Sallis, J. F., & Wardle, J. (2004). Leisure-time physical activity in university students from 23 countries: Associations with health beliefs, risk awareness, and national economic development. *Preventive Medicine, 39*(1), 182–190. doi: 10.1016/j.ypmed.2004.01.028.

Joubert, J., Norman, R., Lambert, E. V., Groenewald, P., Schneider, M., Bull, F., & Bradshaw, D. (2007). Estimating the burden of disease attributable to physical inactivity in South Africa in 2000. *South African Medical Journal, 97*(8 Pt 2), 725–731.

Katzmarzyk, P. T., Barreira, T. V., Broyles, S. T., Champagne, C. M., Chaput, J. P., Fogelholm, M., Hu G.,Johnson W. D.,Kuriyan R., Kurpad A., Lambert E.V , Maher C., Maia J., Matsudo V., Olds T., Onywera V., Sarmiento O. L., Standage M., Tremblay M. S., Tudor-Locke C., Zhao P. & Church, T. S. (2015). Physical activity, sedentary time, and obesity in an international sample of children. *Medicine and Science in Sports and Exercise, 47*(10), 2062–2069. doi: 10.1249/mss.0000000000000649.

Kolbe-Alexander, T., Bull, F.& Lambert, EV. (2012). Physical activity advocacy and promotion: The South African experience. *South African Journal Sports Medicine, 24*(4), 6.

Kolbe-Alexander, T. L., Lambert, E. V. & Charlton, K. E. (2006). Effectiveness of a community based low intensity exercise program for older adults. *The Journal of Nutrition, Health and Aging, 10*(1), 21–29.

Lambert, E. V., da Silva, R., Fatti, L., Patel, D., Kolbe-Alexander, T., Derman, W., . . . Gaziano, T. (2009). Fitness-related activities and medical claims related to hospital admissions – South Africa, 2006. *Preventing Chronic Disease, 6*(4), A120.

Lee, I. M., Shiroma, E. J., Lobelo, F., Puska, P., Blair, S. N. & Katzmarzyk, P. T. (2012). Effect of physical inactivity on major non-communicable diseases worldwide: An analysis of burden of disease and life expectancy. *The Lancet, 380*(9838), 219–229. doi: 10.1016/s0140-6736(12)61031-9.

Levitt, N. S., Steyn, K., Dave, J. & Bradshaw, D. (2011). Chronic noncommunicable diseases and hiv-aids on a collision course: Relevance for health care delivery, particularly in low-resource settings – insights from South Africa. *The American Journal of Clinical Nutrition, 94*(6), 1690S–1696S. doi: 10.3945/ajcn.111.019075.

McLennan, N. & Thompson, J. (2015). Quality physical education (qpe) (S. a. H. S. Sector, Trans.) (pp. 88). United Kingdom: United Nations Educational, Scientific and Cultural Organisation.

Micklesfield, L. K., Pedro, T. M., Kahn, K., Kinsman, J., Pettifor, J. M., Tollman, S. & Norris, S. A. (2014). Physical activity and sedentary behavior among adolescents in rural South Africa: Levels, patterns and correlates. *BMC Public Health, 14*, 40. doi: 10.1186/1471-2458-14-40.

National Planning Commission, South Africa. (2011). *National development plan*. South Africa: Retrieved from www.gov.za/issues/national-development-plan-2030.

Norman, R., Bradshaw, D., Schneider, M., Joubert, J., Groenewald, P., Lewin, S., Steyn K., Vos T., Laubscher R., Nannan N., Nojilana B., & Pieterse, D. (2007). A comparative risk assessment for South Africa in 2000: Towards promoting health and preventing disease. *South African Medical Journal, 97*(8 Pt 2), 637–641.

Patel, D., Lambert, E. V., da Silva, R., Greyling, M., Kolbe-Alexander, T., Noach, A., Conradie, J., Nossel, C., Borresen, J. & Gaziano, T. (2011). Participation in fitness-related activities of an incentive-based health promotion program and hospital costs: A retrospective longitudinal study. *American Journal of Health Promotion, 25*(5), 341–348. doi: 10.4278/ajhp.100603-QUAN-172.

Reddy, S. P., James, S., Sewpaul, R., Koopman, F., Funani, N. I., Sifunda, S., Josie, J., Masuka, P., Kambaran, N. S., Omardien, R. G. (2010). *Umthente uhlaba usamila: The South African youth risk behaviour survey 2008*. Cape Town, South Africa: South African Medical Research Council.

Shisana, O., Labadarios, D., Rehle, T., Simbayi, L., Zuma, K., Dhansay, A., Reddy, P., Parker, W., Hoosain, E., Naidoo, P., Hongoro, C., Mchiza, Z., Steyn, N.P., Dwane, N., Makoae, M., Maluleke, T., Ramlagan, S., Zungu, N.; Evans, M.G., Jacobs, L.; Faber, M., & the SANHANES-1 Team. (2014). *The South African national health and nutrition examination survey, 2012: Sanhanes-1: The health and nutritional status of the nation* (Second Edition). Cape Town, South Africa: Human Sciences Research Council and Medical Research Council.

Shoham, D. A., Dugas, L. R., Bovet, P., Forrester, T. E., Lambert, E. V., Plange-Rhule, J., Schoeller, D. A., Brage, S., Ekelund, U., Durazo-Arvizu, R. A., Cooper, R. & Luke, A. (2015). Association of car ownership and physical activity across the spectrum of human development: Modeling the epidemiologic transition study (mets). *BMC Public Health, 15*, 173. doi: 10.1186/s12889-015-1435-9.

Statistics South Africa. (2012). *Census 2011 statistical release (revised)* po301.4 (pp. 88). Pretoria, South Africa: Statistics South Africa.

Statistics South Africa. (2014). National houshold travel survey 2013 *Statistical Release PO320*. Pretoria, South Africa: Statistics South Africa.

40

THE UNITED KINGDOM

Emily Knox

Introduction

The passage of policy in Westminster

The Department of Health and the Department for Digital, Culture, Media and Sport are mainly responsible for policy relating to physical activity and sport respectively in the UK, whilst the Department for Education leads on school sport. They propose policies which are debated in the House of Commons with a number of stakeholders, including opposition parties, the public and non-governmental organisations. Once enough support is secured for a policy to be finalised, a White Paper is produced alongside a detailed policy plan. Policy on a key issue is dictated by the vision and goals of the ruling party. On 7 May 2015 results of the UK general election saw a Conservative party majority government replace a Conservative-Liberal coalition, with a vision to support school sport, build on the Olympic and Paralympic legacy, and boost sport in the community (Conservatives 2015).

The evolution of UK physical activity policy

Physical activity has gained momentum on the public health policy agenda over recent years, largely stemming from efforts to tackle obesity. Obesity has been on the policy agenda since the early 1990s but it was not until the early 2000s when physical activity was thrown into the mix as an important element of tackling obesity and other health conditions. Physical activity was becoming increasingly recognised by policymakers as personal choices heavily influenced, sometimes even determined, by the environment in which they occur, with public health policies being needed to address the numerous behavioural, sociocultural and environmental factors which often make the healthful choice the most difficult choice to make (Musingarimi 2009). Further, lobbying groups such as the Richmond Group of Charities who champion better use of health and care resources, exert increasing influence. 'Prevention, early diagnosis and intervention' is one of five key themes promoted by the coalition of which physical activity plays an important part. During this period, sport lobbyists were also becoming savvier to the potential benefits of sport by positioning it alongside physical activity as a tool for improved public health.

Prior to 1997 the government position was that it should have minimal involvement in the running of sport. Factors such as the Carter and Select Committee reports suggested that there were market inefficiencies and inequalities to resolve requiring a major change in government involvement. Between 2000 and 2002 the UK Government released *A Sporting Future for All* (DCMS 2000) and *Game Plan* (DCMS/Strategy Unit 2002), the former laying out sport policy and the latter detailing the strategy to deliver. The key objectives from *A Sporting Future for All* were:

- bolster participation by delivering a minimum of two hours per week statutory quality PE and sport in schools
- establish Centres of Vocational Excellence in sport and related activities
- use sport development for social inclusion by brokering sports partnerships with further education institutions
- encourage the necessary support structures for key partners to replicate successful models for healthy living
- establish new national coaching qualifications and enable wide access to them
- support improved elite sport by establishing a scholarship network and seeking additional resources.

Whilst *Game Plan* did not change any of the policies introduced in 2000, a focus in the rhetoric on the benefit of *sport participation* for health and *sport performance* for elite success notably emerges: 'increasing participation in sport and physical activity and developing sustainable improvement in success in international competition'. Sport participation and performance remained as the main hinges of sport policy when the government changed in 2010. *2010 to 2015 government policy: elite sports performance* stated the four main aims of:

- funding elite athletes to train full time for each Olympic cycle
- keeping drugs out of UK elite sport
- improving the governance structures of sport in the UK
- bringing major sporting events to the UK.

2010 to 2015 government policy: sports participation stated the main aims of:

- funding Sport England (discussed later in the chapter) to help more people have a sporting habit for life
- run the School Games as a way of motivating and inspiring young people to take part in more competitive sport
- help primary schools improve the quality of their PE and sport activities through the PE and sport premium.

In placing sport and physical activity more firmly on the public health agenda, the attention of policymakers has turned towards public health policy which can directly address the wider contextual environment. According to popular policy rhetoric, this will require a more 'joined up whole-systems approach'. This has played a part in the UK Government's decision to release a new broad strategy for sport (HM Government 2015b). The main change in the strategy is an added focus on achieving gains in physical and mental wellbeing, and social and community development through sport. This is principally seen through the emphasis on measuring impact and the inclusion of measures designed to identify mobilisation i.e. previously, physical activity has been measured in terms of minutes spent active. This meant that participation levels could increase without a single inactive individual becoming active if active individuals became more active. With the new strategy, progress will be measured against the proportion of the population engaging in physical activity and sport rather than the total number of minutes being undertaken. This is an encouraging change with regards to potential gains in public health. Sport England followed up this release with the funding strategy to support *Sporting Future* (Sport England 2016b). Whilst much of the rhetoric mirrored that seen previously, a determination to ensure greater diversification of sporting opportunities and accountability of funding recipients to demonstrate success against *Sporting Future* objectives emerges.

Finally, the hosting of mega-events, most notably the Olympic and Paralympic Games held in London in 2012 and the Commonwealth Games held in Glasgow in 2014, has also had an influence on policy in recent years. Just as it has been for previous mega-events, 'legacy' was consistently referred to in the build-up and aftermath of both Games (Weed et al. 2012). Strategies to un-tap the potential of the Games beyond sport, to influence adult engagement in physical activity and improve communities were also presented (Coaffee 2012). Both bid campaigns promised to ensure that through hosting the respective event they would create an abundance of benefits which would positively impact the hosting community and the wider country. This led to a series of 'Inspired by 2012' policy documents (HM Government, 2015a; DCMS, 2015a; HM Government, 2014a; HM Government, 2014b) and a Commonwealth Legacy policy document being released by UK and Scottish Government's respectively (The Scottish Government 2009). The success of the London Olympic bid in particular has been largely attributed to its distinctive bid focused on young people, regeneration and the future (HM Government 2015a). Policy following the Olympic Games and the Commonwealth Games has been largely focused on young people as a result of efforts to deliver on legacy promises made leading up to the events. This will be discussed in more detail towards the end of this chapter. Both the English and Scottish legacy approaches share common ground by aiming for elite success, mass participation and school sport but with a subtle difference in tone. For instance, then First Minister of Scotland Alex Salmond commented: 'We have high hopes for Scotland and for winning medals in 2014. But from the outset we have been clear the Games are about much more than this.' For Scotland, a successful Commonwealth Games was perhaps just as crucial for highlighting Scotland's position on the map as it was for sporting gains.

The devolution of UK government

Devolution in the UK refers to the transfer of power from central government which sits in Westminster in England, to the national authorities of the relevant home countries. Devolution first became a major political issue in the UK during the early 1970s. At present, Scotland, Wales and Northern Ireland all have their own national authorities with control over aspects such as education and health. While the four home countries are still ultimately ruled under one central government, increasing devolution means that regional priorities dictate new policy to a greater extent than ever before. Sport policy is a devolved matter which presents a number of opportunities and challenges.

The challenges and promises of devolution regarding health policy

At a time where concern over the balance of power and resources between Westminster and the rest of the UK is high, the 'Devolution Revolution' offers a number of advantages:

1) It is a growing concern that more and more of the wealth in the UK is moving to London and the South East of England at the expense of Scotland, Wales, Northern Ireland and other regions of England. Devolving powers out to the other regional areas of the UK may enable local areas to protect against the increasing funnelling of wealth to London and reduce fears over the existing unbalanced economic policy of Westminster. Some areas, such as Greater Manchester, have already secured greater self-determination (Greater Manchester Combined Authority 2015).

2) There is no 'one size fits all' solution to dwindling levels of physical activity. Greater regional autonomy could benefit grassroots sport by allowing more effective adaptation to local circumstances and building on the model of County Sports Partnerships (CSPs) to increase the number of people taking part at local level. Further, certain regions within England may share fewer similarities with Westminster than they do with regions in the other home countries. Likewise, certain regions in Scotland, Wales or Northern Ireland may be more similar to regions in England than they are to other regions within their own country. Devolution may encourage a greater testing of context-specific approaches which may be a more effective and efficient means of identifying policies and approaches to tackling inactivity through shared learnings (DCMS 2015c).

3) If all of the devolved regions have a physical activity strategy in place this could lead to a more concerted and less 'piecemeal' effort to promote physical activity. In recent years, Northern Ireland has operated under less devolved power than the other UK regions. This is slowly changing and the move is welcomed by local politicians and policy-makers (Department of Health Social Services and Public Safety 2014).

On the other hand, devolution presents a number of challenges:

1) Any overhaul in political systems, especially on the scale of that occurring in Northern Ireland will inevitably face difficulties as councillors used to being commentators on major political issues instead become decision-makers. Policymakers interviewed in 2010 (N=58) stated that government policies were not joined up (Hallsworth et al. 2011). It takes time for new systems to achieve the type of joined-up working required for successful public health policy to be developed.

2) As a result of moving responsibility for formulating and enacting public health policies to the various devolved regions, differences in regional priorities are increasingly significant (Smith & Babbington 2006). Adopting the CSP model (discussed above) would result in loss of strategic oversight, scale and consistency which could dissipate the impact of policies tackling public health related issues (DCMS 2015c). One example illustrating the convolution of policies as a result of devolution are the regionally set standards for physical education in schools (which have occurred at different times), while interventions to promote physical activity guidelines have taken place at the UK level.

3) Physical activity interventions with the greatest chance of success will likely require profound societal and environmental changes (Heath et al. 2012) taking decades to bring

about measureable change. Public health campaigners already have to battle to convince politicians facing pressing short-term political contests to back long-term interventions, the effects of which will be realised during a different political cycle when a rival party could be in office. With devolution comes another layer of bureaucracy and competing interests to slow the passage of legislation. Further, devolution has hardened the reluctance of government to adopt interventions which could be viewed as impinging on individuals' freedom of choice. Concerns around being derided as a 'nanny state' and debates around the appropriate role of a central government in public health delivery have made government more cautious in implementing directive public health policies. Lang and Rayner (2007) have described the result as a 'policy cacophony drowning out the symphony of effort'.

4) As previously discussed sport/physical activity policies broadly aim to boost participation or performance. In the case of sport *participation*, the process is relatively simple. Each region develops their own strategy and initiative (some of which will be discussed later in this chapter) to boost participation in their area. National surveys such as the Health Survey for England, Active People Survey, Scottish Health Survey, Welsh Health Survey and Northern Ireland Sport and Physical Activity Survey, and other evidence can then be collected to support the continuation or modification of such strategies and policies. However, where sport participation comes through the grassroots sport *performance* pathway, the processes of administering and measuring impact of initiatives is murkier.

5) A lack of clarity over the powers and remit of local governments still pervades which weakens their ability to pass local policy. In a radio interview, Welsh constitutional affairs expert Jocelyn Davies stated: 'nobody knows what we can do, [the Welsh Assembly] spend time getting legal opinion about what is possible and what would bring us into conflict with Westminster' (BBC 2001). Calls to clarify devolved powers and systematise them across the four home nations have failed to simplify the process (BBC Wales 2015).

England

Central government is responsible for the overall development of sports policy in England as is laid out in *Towards an Active Nation* (Sport England 2016b) – the Government's national strategy for sport. *Towards an Active Nation* and the previously discussed *Government policy for elite sports performance* and *sports participation* will not be further explored here.

Sport England is the Council responsible for delivering government policy for sport across England. Unlike the other home country sports councils Sport England has no high performance targets and focuses exclusively on increasing the proportion of people (particularly 14–25 year olds) regularly playing sport (DCMS 2012). It has a planning policy to protect playing fields and influence provision of facilities. Sport England also has duties (Government Equalities Office 2010) to ensure adequate provision of opportunities amongst groups with protected characteristics. A triennial review of Sport England was published in 2015 (DCMS 2015c). As described in this review, Sport England currently channels the bulk of their resources towards 14–25 year olds and individuals who are most likely to engage in sport once a week. This is likely attributable to two main factors. The first is that participation has been shown to drop most sharply in this age group. The second is that current measurement of progress towards Sport England targets is based on minutes spent in sport and so does not incentivise them to increase the total number of people participating in sport or to engage the inactive.

Scotland

Since Scottish Parliament was re-established in 1999, the issue of Independence of Scotland from rule in Westminster has been high on Scotland's political agenda. Scotland have been vociferously moving to increase its limited devolved powers to create 'a more democratic Scotland, a more prosperous country and a fairer society' (The Scottish Government 2013). In September 2014, the Scottish people voted in a historic referendum to decide whether Scotland would become truly independent. While the outcome saw Scotland remain under central UK government, its charge for more self-determination regarding economic policy, international relations, defence spending and defence priorities, social security benefits, taxation and public spending gained more weight.

The Scottish Executive provides a lead on policy and direction for the Scottish national strategy for physical activity and sport. Following advice laid out in the 1999 White Paper *Towards a Healthier Scotland* (The Scottish Government 1999), Scotland released a strategy for physical activity in Scotland in 2003 entitled *Let's Make Scotland More Active* (Physical Activity Task Force 2003). This has been followed up with the subsequent strategy documents *Reaching Higher* (Scottish Executive 2007) and *On Your Marks* (The Scottish Government 2009). Scottish priorities for physical activity include using it as a vehicle to increase the visibility of Scotland as a nation for the benefit of business and the wider economy and Scotland's national identity.

Wales

In May 2007 the Government of Wales Act (National Assembly for Wales 2006) took effect which increased the law making powers of the Welsh National Assembly. Further law making powers were secured for the Welsh National Assembly following a referendum in 2011 enabling it to pass laws in the 20 Welsh regions without agreement from UK government.

The Welsh Assembly Government is responsible for physical activity related policy and has disseminated an increasing number of policies and strategies since their national review of health and social care in 2003 (Welsh Assembly Government 2003a). This review urged for a greater focus on long-term over short-term health and social care plans in Wales. Subsequent plans have therefore focused on children and young people (Welsh Assembly Government 2004; Welsh Assembly Government 2006a; Welsh Assembly Government 2006b; Welsh Government 2013a; Welsh Government 2013b), healthy ageing (Welsh Assembly Government 2005b; Welsh Assembly Government 2005a; Welsh Government 2008; Welsh Government 2013b) and a healthy workforce (Welsh Assembly Government 2010). In terms of strategy for children and young people, these documents set out seven core aims for children and young people including that all should have access to a range of play, leisure, sporting and cultural activities. Physical activity is listed as a priority for achieving public health targets and ensuring children have a good start in life. With regards to Welsh strategy for older adults, the most recent *Strategy for Older People 2013–2023* is grounded in ageing as a positive concept and has been praised internationally as the 'most coherent long term commitment to improving the position of older people of any administration in the UK in the last decade' (McCormick et al. 2009). Since 2007 Age Cymru has delivered The Healthy Ageing Programme, funded by Welsh Government, which is aimed at addressing the health needs of older people. The individual components of the programme are *Ageing Well Physical Activity Initiatives*, and *Gwanwyn. Ageing Well* is a peer health mentor model, whereby people aged 50 and over are trained to act as Ageing

Well volunteers to deliver key health improvement messages to their peers. The *Ageing Well* work is underpinned by national campaigns delivered by Age Cymru around topics such as Sexual Health, Falls Prevention and Keep Well This Winter. The key aim of the *Workforce Development Plan* is to improve the physical activity knowledge of professionals through an expert working group including bodies such as SkillsActive, Skills for Health and the Sports Council for Wales.

Northern Ireland

Of the four home nations, Northern Ireland has the most complicated political history. The political struggles experienced by Northern Ireland are beyond the scope of this chapter but it is important to note that the region has seen significant political unrest which has often manifested in Anglo-Irish tensions and violence. Northern Ireland was ruled by a devolved Parliament between 1921 and 1972. Due to an intensification of the Troubles in Northern Ireland, the British government lost faith in the devolved institutions abilities to deal with the growing crisis and brought Northern Ireland back under direct rule from Westminster. Devolution then occurred again in 1998 when the Northern Ireland Assembly was established as a result of the Belfast Agreement (Northern Ireland Assembly 1998) and the Northern Ireland Act (HM Government 1998). The Northern Ireland Assembly currently has full legislative and executive authority for all matters that are the responsibility of the Northern Ireland Government Departments. Political turmoil led to the suspension of the Northern Ireland Assembly and the devolved institutions in 2002 and their subsequent dissolution in April 2003. The Assembly was restored to a state of suspension in November 2003 following government elections which saw a change in the balance of power. The devolved institutions were not fully restored until 2007 following the Northern Ireland Act (St Andrews Agreement; HM Government 2006). The Northern Ireland Executive is responsible for taking decisions on behalf of the Northern Ireland Assembly on the significant issues put forward for new legislation.

As a region emerging from decades of turmoil and political unrest, physical activity has not been prominent on the policy agenda in Northern Ireland. Northern Ireland has identified seven priority areas for investment. These areas are: improved transport networks, skill development for young people such as through access to higher education and youth services, better health services, better social services such as social housing and enterprises, improved water and waste management, greater productivity and more efficient justice systems (Northern Ireland Executive 2011). Policies pertaining to physical activity could play a role in a number of these areas. The current Northern Ireland strategy for preventing and addressing overweight and obesity, *A Fitter Future for All* (Department of Health Social Services and Public Safety 2011), calls for cross-departmental action to tackle the 'obesogenic' environment, including policies to support physical activity choices.

Public health policy targets

In 2011, the Chief Medical Officers for the four home countries released *Start Active, Stay Active* (Department of Health Physical Activity Health Improvement and Protection 2011), which provided the first UK-wide guidelines for physical activity at four life stages.

Early years (under 5s): Minimise sedentary time and engage in 180 minutes of physical activity every day once the child can walk unaided.

Children and young people (5–18 years): At least 60 minutes of moderate-to-vigorous physical activity every day.

Adults (19–64 years): At least 150 minutes of moderate-to-vigorous physical activity every week.

Older adults (65+ years): At least 150 minutes of moderate physical activity every week.

It has been a popular practice in recent years to set targets in public health policy which relate to these physical activity guidelines. England's target of 70 per cent of adults meeting physical activity guidelines by 2020 is the most ambitious (Department of Health 2005). Scotland has set the target of 50 per cent of adults to meet recommendations by 2022 (Physical Activity Task Force 2003). In 1996, Northern Ireland set the target of 35 per cent of men and 25 per cent of women meeting physical activity recommendations by 2002 (Health Promotion Agency for Northern Ireland 2002). In 2009, this target became to collect suitable data to measure physical activity levels in 2011 and to then increase adult participation by 3 per cent by 2019 (Department of Culture, Arts and Leisure 2009). Wales set a somewhat different target in 2002, to increase the proportion of adults engaged in the minimum recommended level of physical activity by one percentage point per year for the following 20 years (The Welsh Assembly Government 2004). The differences between these targets demonstrate the diverging influence of devolution on physical activity-related policy. These differences appear to reflect differences in strategy.

Rigorous evaluation of policy and their related actions is needed to assess the impact of existing measures and support or refute the introduction of new measures. Monitoring and evaluation in the devolved regions is currently poor (Hallsworth et al. 2011) and this delays learning from policy. Northern Ireland and Wales are especially poor at surveying. For instance, there is little evidence that an evaluation of either the Northern Irish 1996 physical activity targets or the Welsh 2002 targets has occurred to determine whether targets were met and to inform next steps. The lack of available reliable surveillance data on which progress against targets can be measured represents another difference between regional targets which will have important further policy implications. In December 2015, the Global Observatory for Physical Activity published individual cards summarising physical activity and public health for 131 countries, including the four home nations (Global Observatory for Physical Activity 2015). These could provide a benchmark against which to measure targets going forward.

Strategies supporting physical activity policy of the home nations

Previous initiatives at the individual level have had only modest effects, with maintained changes in physical activity behaviour being difficult to achieve. There is a need to move towards broader population interventions that provide a supportive social and built environment. In order to facilitate this shift, physical activity should be integrated into cross-departmental policies. This means that physical activity policy needs to be considered by the Department for Education, the Department for Business, Innovation and Skill, the Department for Communities and Local Government and the Department for Environment, Food and Rural Affairs, amongst others (DCMS 2015b).

The National Institute for Health and Care Excellence (NICE) provides guidance and advice to providers and commissioners about health and social care issues such as physical activity. NICE is sponsored by the Government but is statutorily independent. Officially, its remit is England-only but the devolved administrations of Wales, Scotland and Northern Ireland often apply NICE guidance. Following the UK Foresight report (Department of Health 2007), UK government commissioned reviews to identify recommendations for policy, transport, urban planning and architecture, which could facilitate the incorporation of physical activity into activities of daily living (National Institute for Health and Clinical Excellence 2008). NICE has developed a pathway for physical activity strategy, policy and commissioning to facilitate the incorporation of physical activity into daily living. Three of the key recommendations were: national campaigns, active travel and exercise referral schemes.

National campaigns

Mass media campaigns can reach large sections of the population giving them the potential to influence on a grand scale (Richman et al. 1999). Further, policy actions concerning mass media and marketing strategies are recommended by the European Union to support health-enhancing physical activity (EU Expert Working Group 'Sport & Health' 2008). The National Health Service (NHS) of each home country (also called Health and Social Care in Northern Ireland [HSCNI] in Northern Ireland) is responsible for producing and disseminating health information. Its largest informational campaign to date is *Change4Life* which runs across England and Wales. Since 2009, upwards of £89 million have been spent encouraging different sub-populations, such as families with young children, adults and young people, to improve their health. In Northern Ireland *Get a Life, Get Active* has been running since 1999 targeting all adults, primarily those aged 30–35 (www.getalifegetactive. com/). In 2014, Scotland published its first ever national Physical Activity Implementation Plan, *A More Active Scotland – Building a Legacy from the Commonwealth Games* (The Scottish Government 2014) but has not launched a campaign of the same magnitude and gravitas as in its neighbouring nations. Most recently, the *This Girl Can* campaign, launched in October 2014, has garnered recognition for its media approach targeting inactive and typically non-sporty women (Sport England 2016a).

Unfortunately these campaigns have not been well evaluated. Despite having run for more than a decade, *Get a Life, Get Active* has not been evaluated at all and yet its perceived success has instrumentally influenced the Northern Ireland physical activity action plan (Department of Health Social Services and Public Safety 2011). A number of government reports on *Change4Life* have suggested that *Change4Life* messages have raised awareness amongst large segments of the target audience but fail to measure behaviour (Department of Health 2010; Department of Health 2011). Alternatively, independent reports on aspects of the campaign have suggested problems with its implementation (Piggin 2012) and disappointing outcomes (Croker et al. 2012). All of the home nations must make strides in evaluating national campaigns to increase the impetus for an active society. This is recognised by NICE (National Institute for Health and Clinical Excellence 2008) which has urged for the policies of research councils and funders to prioritise funding for the evaluation of effectiveness of environmental interventions on physical activity.

Active travel

The key role of walking and cycling as the main modes of transport for short trips, especially to local facilities such as shops, schools, etc. and in providing access to public transport for longer journeys is emphasised in the Government's *Guidance on Full Local Transport Plans* (Department of Transport 2009) and in *Transport 2010 – The 10 Year Plan* (Department of Transport 2010). A NICE policy goal is to ensure that government funding supports physically active modes of travel for instance through urban regeneration and improving walkability of the physical environment (National Institute for Health and Care Excellence 2015). A number of the devolved regions now have strategies for promoting sustainable, environmentally friendly means of travel for commuting e.g. *Walking and Cycling Strategy* (Welsh Assembly Government 2003c); *Walking Northern Ireland* (Department for Regional Development 2003). The Connswater Community Greenway project in Belfast (www.communitygreenway.co.uk) has resulted in major urban regeneration of a 9 km linear park, including the provision of new cycle paths and walkways. In addition to the environmental improvements, this complex intervention involves a number of programmes to promote physical activity in the regenerated area. The Connswater Community Greenway provides a significant opportunity to achieve long-term, population level behaviour change, and to investigate the public health impact of urban regeneration. Another example comes from the Sustrans Connect2 cycling networks which strive to create active environments by adapting existing infrastructure in ways which encourage physical activity (Sustrans 2007). For example, the initiative has built new bridges and crossings to increase pedestrian safety when crossing busy roads, rivers and railways and to link routes to walking and cycle paths (Goodman et al. 2014).

Exercise referral

Exercise referral is a specific and formalised programme whereby a medical professional refers a patient to a fitness programme often based within the community with which there is an existing formal agreement. In the UK, exercise referral (called exercise on prescription in Northern Ireland) is operated through the NHS and local councils. NICE has produced guidance for the delivery of exercise referral schemes (National Institute for Health and Care Excellence 2014) as has the NHS through the National Quality Assurance Framework (National Health Service 2001). Exercise referral schemes have been increasing steadily since they began in 1990 but reviews suggest that long-term outcomes are largely unknown (Northern Ireland Assembly 2010; Dugdill et al. 2005). A positive example comes from the Active Health Team in Camden, London which provides green gyms, sports groups, yoga and Pilates to referred adults free of charge for eight weeks (Northern Ireland Assembly 2010).

Priority groups

The 2010 Equality Act (Government Equalities Office 2010) states that there is a responsibility to consider vulnerable groups for instance, by ensuring equal access to amenities, conducting robust monitoring of identified groups and ensuring staff are trained to work with all types of individuals. Following this, in 2014 Public Health England released the document *Everybody Active, Every Day* (Public Health England 2014) which foregrounded common inequalities in access to physical activity and presented strategies to improve access for those living in less prosperous areas, those living in North West England, older adults, disabled individuals, ethnic minority groups, females and homosexual and transgender individuals.

Children and young people

The Youth Sport Trust is an independent charity which, since 1995, has worked to ensure high quality physical education and sport opportunities are available to all young people. Its influence on school-based youth sports development policies through its delivery of a clear message that school sport can improve social inclusion, educational attainment and community cohesion, and reduce crime has been discussed in detail elsewhere (Houlihan & Green 2006). Major policy documents concerning children and young people include *A Sporting Future for all* (DCMS 2000) launched in 2000 and the Physical Education and Sport Strategy *PE, School Sport and Club Links* (OfSTED 2005), which was launched in 2002 and extended in 2008 (DCSF & DCMS 2008). The plans aim to increase the percentage of school children participating in two hours a week of high quality physical education and sport through a network of School Sport Partnerships and School Sports Colleges created from *A Sporting Future for All.*

The School Sports Colleges policy was intended to:

- improve participation and achievement in physical education amongst students of all abilities,
- raise standards of teaching in schools,
- provide a structure through which students can progress to careers in sport and physical education,
- promote the development of young talented athletes through links with other schools, agencies, clubs and the regional centres of the UK Sports Institute.

Subsequent structures and strategies have therefore occurred at curricular and extracurricular level.

It is important to note that the recommended two hours a week of statutory PE is voluntary and is determined by individual schools. The quality of physical education in England and Wales is evaluated by Ofsted who report back to a range of stakeholders with a view to improving provision. Ofsted inspections have been suggested as a good example of a physical education scheme for policymakers by the United Nations Educational, Scientific and Cultural Organization (UNESCO 2015). While Scotland does not have Ofsted inspection its own new Curriculum for Excellence has drawn similar praise (UNESCO 2015). The Curriculum is part of Scotland's legacy plans and aims to ensure that every child receives two hours of quality physical education in primary school and two lessons in secondary school. Further, local authorities are adopting its *Better Movers and Thinkers* initiative to improve physical literacy. In Wales, the *PE and School Sport Initiative* aims to improve the range and quality of opportunities for physical activity available to school pupils. Local development centres have been established in partnership with the Sports Council for Wales and local authorities to connect primary and secondary schools with local partners to share expertise and facilities. This has proven particularly effective in bolstering the teaching of gymnastics, dance and health-related exercise (Welsh Assembly Government 2006a). In 2006, Northern Ireland introduced an extended school policy with a view to supporting after-school youth, sport and leisure activities particularly in disadvantaged areas (OFMDFM 2006).

Policy around school physical activity has become increasingly performance oriented in recent years with an increased focus on extracurricular competition. For instance, in England, *Sportivate* provides young people with six to eight weeks of coaching with a view to identifying talent for development (Sport England 2014). Further, in 2010 a revised policy was announced which reduced central funding for school sports in favour of encouraging local funding for School Sports Partnerships (HM Government 2010). The plan aimed to 'build a framework of competitions as part of the New School Games'. The School Games is delivered through partnerships at national and local level with policy leadership being provided by the Department for Digital, Culture, Media and Sport.

The aim of the Games is to motivate and inspire young people to take part in more competitive school sport across various levels of activity:

- competition in schools,
- competition between schools,
- competition at a country/area level.

Currently, regional School Games competitions which occur within and between schools are focused only on schools in England, but Scotland, Wales and Northern Ireland do compete at a country level.

School-based approaches focus on sport in favour of physical activity. Approaches geared towards increasing the physical activity levels of young people include creating environments which encourage children and young people to access opportunities for physical activity in their neighbourhoods. This might be achieved by changing the physical landscape or by providing/highlighting opportunities which fit with the existing landscape. The Welsh Assembly report released in 2006 (Welsh Assembly Government 2006a) states that 'a number of initiatives stemming from Welsh Government strategies have already begun to create an environment which is encouraging children and young people to utilise opportunities for physical activity across Wales'. *Climbing Higher* (Welsh Assembly Government 2009a) and *Food and Wellbeing* (Welsh Assembly Government 2007) are the main strategies reportedly behind these initiatives. A number of initiatives are also in place to encourage more walking to school e.g. England's *Travelling to School* action plan outlines a number of measures at national and local level for schools to promote more walking, cycling and use of public transport to and from school (Department of Transport and Department for Education and Skills 2003).

A final target of policies regarding physical activity amongst children is to support play. These policies are founded in the United Nations Convention on the Rights of the Child, which was ratified by the UK Government in December 1991 (HM Government 2011), and which recognises the importance of play and leisure activities for the child. Wales released its first policy on play in 2002, though the implementation plan for this never followed until 2006 (Welsh Assembly Government 2006b). Northern Ireland released a play policy in 2010 (NICMA 2010) and the strategy *Families Matter* coincided to assist families in capitalising on play opportunities for their children. The intention of the play and leisure policy for Northern Ireland is to ensure that the importance of play and leisure in children's lives is understood and given appropriate consideration in the context of increasingly restricted public spending and competing agendas. This is not the responsibility of a single service agency or provider. Whilst the Office of the First Minister and Deputy First Minister has taken the lead in coordinating policy on play and leisure, all government departments are committed to contributing to the development of the policy and to future action plans.

Older adults

By 2031 all four home countries are projected to have more than 21 per cent of the population above the state pension age threshold and there will be more pensioners than children (McCormick et al. 2009). The need to ensure healthy ageing has never been greater. As shown in *Building a Society for All Ages* (HM Government 2009), policymakers now recognise that active living can be used as a vehicle to prevent the cycle of loneliness and declining wellbeing associated with old age. The *Active at 60* programme has assisted communities to provide opportunities for older adults to stay or become more active and positively engaged with society (Hatamian et al. 2012).

The Welsh approach to physical activity policy for older adults has drawn praise from the Institute of Public Policy Research which stated:

> The Welsh approach seems to be the most coherent long term commitment to improving the position of older people of any administration in the UK in the last decade ... the Welsh Strategy appears the most likely of any to ensure a continuing high profile for older people's issues across many policy areas and at a local level.

The Welsh Government launched its first strategy for older people in 2003 (Welsh Assembly Government 2003b). It called for a joined-up approach to policy development which considered issues such as health alongside those of local government, life-long learning, housing and benefits. This was followed by Wales' first systematic strategy for older adults, named a *Healthy Ageing Action Plan* (Welsh Assembly Government 2005b). Since then, the Welsh Government have funded initiatives such as the Age Cymru delivered *Healthy Ageing Programme* which trains people aged 50 and over to act as Ageing Well volunteers to deliver key health improvement messages to their peers and delivers initiatives such as Nordic Walking groups and Low Impact Functional Training. Most recently, Wales released a ten year strategy (Welsh Government 2013b) for ensuring that older adults have access to opportunities for physical activity and can overcome the challenges they face to an active lifestyle. The 2013 strategy is an extension of the 2003 strategy but urges for a better integration of health and social services through pooling budgets and increased flexibility. The strategy highlighted some of the successes of the previous plan. Two of them are likely to have had a positive direct or indirect effect on physical activity, these are free swimming and bus passes. Further, it claims the main success of the strategy to be the establishment of mechanisms and structures at local and national level that allow older people to be involved in the decision-making process.

Women in sport

Women engage in less physical activity and sport than men and are underrepresented on National Boards and in the media (DCMS 2014). In 2013, the Government established a 'Women in Sport Advisory Board' to raise the profile of women's sport and come up with strategies to further the Women in Sport agenda. The Advisory Board informs the Governments work programme on women and sport. This programme deals with five specific areas: increasing women's participation in sport, improving the media profile of women's sport, increasing commercial investment in women's sport, improving women's representation in leadership and the work force and encouraging greater recognition of women's sporting achievements. The Board has also been tasked to work closely with Sport England to address barriers to women's participation in sport.

In January 2015, Sport England launched *This Girl Can*, a national campaign which aims to create more positive social norms around physical activity and sport for females, particularly those aged between 14 and 40. While this campaign is only running across England, Sport Northern Ireland, Sport Scotland and Sport Wales all have a remit for increasing female participation within those nations. Sport Wales launched the *What Moves You?* campaign to unpick the reasons why Welsh women do not engage in sport and identify what would attract them to become involved. Similarly to *This Girl Can*, the campaign links up with local partners who provide a variety of appealing opportunities within their local communities. Sport Scotland also focuses on barriers to participation amongst teenage girls and may provide the best examples so far of initiatives targeting leadership. For instance, the *Active Girls* and *Females Achieving Brilliance* programmes provide opportunities and inspiration to young women who are looking to become involved or are already involved in sport.

Income inequality

Within the UK, half of the population owns just 9.9 per cent of the wealth, while the richest 10 per cent own 43.8 per cent of the wealth (Office for National Statistics 2012). Income inequality in the UK is amongst the highest in the developed world and the country has some of the biggest regional differences in GDP per head than any EU nation (OECD 2011). This has translated into health disparities, with gaps in health and wellbeing increasing since the early 1990s (Welsh Assembly Government 2011). Of the four nations Wales demonstrate the greatest health inequality, with a level that is slightly worse than the average amongst OECD countries (UNICEF 2010). Gaps in health and wellbeing are even apparent from a very early age, with babies showing lower birth weight across gradients of socio-economic deprivation (Welsh Assembly Government 2011). In recognition, Wales have released a string of policy documents since the late 1990s namely, *Better Health, Better Wales* (Welsh Assembly Government 1998), *Targeting Poor Health* (Gordon 2004), *Review of Health and Social Care in Wales* (Welsh Assembly Government 2003a) and culminating with *Our Healthy Future* (Welsh Assembly Government 2009b). *Our Healthy Future* represents a step change in tackling health disparities by changing the focus from health inequalities (i.e. do different groups have different health outcomes) to health inequities (i.e. where can disparities be avoided, where are disparities unfair or immoral). This, the report states, is driven by the 'vision and principles reflecting our country [Wales]'. In this respect, Wales has taken a slightly different approach to the other regions of the United Kingdom, for instance, Scotland's *Equally Well* (The Scottish Government 2008) and England's *Fairer Society, Fairer Lives* (Strategic Review of Health Inequalities in England Post 2010 2010) maintain a focus on inequality. In Scotland the *Agenda for Change* urges for sport to be made more accessible, desirable and enjoyable and to adopt a policy of inclusive membership regardless of ability (Scottish Executive 2007). It aims to achieve this by linking with the European Foundation for Quality Management Excellence Model and existing policies from other areas to improve monitoring and evaluation of progress and enable continuous improvement of sporting strategies (Scottish Executive 2007).

Of course, in some cases responsibility for policies which impact on health inequities is not within the power of the devolved Executives. For instance, macro-economic policy, social security policy, policy relating to aspects of employment, taxation, benefits and pensions are determined by UK government in Westminster and need to work synergistically with regional public health approaches. Action by the UK government and even the European Union can either support or undermine efforts of the devolved UK regions to tackle health inequalities and inequities.

Implications for future physical activity policy and practice

While it is evident that policymakers still use sport as a vehicle for global recognition and furthering industry there is a steadily increasing awakening that sport can also be used as a vehicle for public health, social inclusion and other wider outcomes. As has been discussed in this chapter, UK policy around physical activity and sport has sought to boost participation and improve performance. In the consultation paper for the Government's new strategy for sport, current thinking around participation has been stated as being 'too simplistic' (DCMS 2015b) as it fails to recognise that supporting more inactive people to become active will likely bring more benefits to wider governmental aims than supporting (slightly active) people to become more active. The Minster for Sport, Tourism and Heritage writes that:

> As part of the funding process, should we ascribe more value to getting someone who was previously inactive to participate than someone who is already sporty doing a bit extra? We need to start thinking of participation as a means to an end and not necessarily the end result.
>
> *DCMS 2015b*

Thus, the future may see Government policy moving away from 'quick and easy' targets which result in lean keen runner beans also playing more football, towards more difficult challenges which might result in couch potatoes engaging in some physical activity. Policymakers are recognising that sport is only a part of that picture and that encouraging inactive people to take up physical activity in any form is hugely beneficial. Rather than moving away from sport, the definition of sport is expanding (and will continue to do so) to incorporate more types of activity. This is important for catering to a wider variety of needs within the population and for encouraging wider cross-departmental working. Further, future policy will need to cater to the needs of an aging population and sport as it is traditionally considered may not be an appropriate catalyst of more healthful behaviour within this population.

As the devolved Executives get to grips with the remit of their powers and more adeptly navigate the red tape involved, it is likely that policies will evolve to support more localised delivery of sport and physical activity and that practices will begin to target more specific local needs. Whether this will result in public health gains for any or all of the home nations remains to be seen.

References

BBC, 2001. Devolution. Available at: http://news.bbc.co.uk/news/vote2001/hi/english/main_issues/sections/facts/newsid_1220000/1220730.stm [Accessed August 29, 2017].

BBC Wales, 2015. Devolution should not be weakened, warns Carwyn Jones. Available at: www.bbc.co.uk/news/uk-wales-politics-34335248 [Accessed August 29, 2017].

Coaffee, J., 2012. Policy transfer, regeneration legacy and the summer Olympic Games: Lessons for London 2012 and beyond. *International Journal of Sport Policy and Politics*, 5(2), pp.295–311.

Conservatives, 2015. *The Conservative Party manifesto 2015*, London.

Croker, H., Lucas, R. & Wardle, J., 2012. Cluster-randomised trial to evaluate the 'Change for Life' mass media/social marketing campaign in the UK. *BMC Public Health*, 12(1), pp.404–429. Available at: www.ncbi.nlm.nih.gov/pubmed/22672587 [Accessed August 21, 2012].

DCMS/Strategy Unit, 2002. *Game plan: A strategy for delivering government's sport and physical activity objectives*, London.

DCSF & DCMS, 2008. *PE and Sport Strategy for young people*, DCSF & DCMS.

DCMS, 2000. *A sporting future for all*, DCMS, pp.1–20.

DCMS, 2012. *Creating a sporting habit for life: A new youth sport strategy*, London. Available at: www.cabdirect.org/abstracts/20123185861.html.

DCMS, 2014. *Interim report of the Government's Women and Sport Advisory Board*, DCMS.

DCMS, 2015a. *A living legacy: 2010–2015 sport policy and investment*, London.

DCMS, 2015b. *A new strategy for sport: Consultation paper*, London, UK.

DCMS, 2015c. *Triennial review of UK Sport and Sport England: Report*, DCMS.

Department for Regional Development, 2003. *Walking Northern Ireland: An action plan*, Belfast. Available at: www.roadsni.gov.uk.

Department of Transport and Department for Education and Skills, 2003. *Travelling to school: An action plan*, Available at: www.dft.gov.uk/pgr/sustainable/schooltravel/travelling/travellingtoschool anactionplan.

Department of Culture, Arts and Leisure, 2009. *Sport matters: A culture of lifelong enjoyment and success in sport*, Belfast.

Department of Health, 2005. *Choosing activity: A physical activity action plan*, London.

Department of Health, 2007. *Tackling obesities: Foresight: Future choices*, Department of Health.

Department of Health, 2010. *Change4Life one year on*, Department of Health.

Department of Health, 2011. *Change4Life three year social marketing strategy*, Department of Health.

Department of Health Physical Activity Health Improvement and Protection, 2011. *Start active, stay active: A report on physical activity for health from the four home countries' Chief Medical Officers*, London: Department of Health.

Department of Health Social Services and Public Safety, 2011. *A fitter future for all: Framework for preventing and addressing overweight and obesity in Northern Ireland 2012–2022*, Department of Health Social Services and Public Safety.

Department of Health Social Services and Public Safety, 2014. *Making life better. A whole system strategic framework for public health 2013–2023*, Belfast. Available at: www.dhsspsni.gov.uk/articles/ making-life-better-strategic-framework-public-health.

Department of Transport, 2009. *Guidance on local transport plans*, London.

Department of Transport, 2010. *Transport 2010 – The 10 Year Plan*, London.

Dugdill, L., Graham, R.C. & McNair, F., 2005. Exercise referral: The public health panacea for physical activity promotion? A critical perspective of exercise referral schemes; their development and evaluation. *Ergonomics*, 48(11–14), pp.1390–410. Available at: www.ncbi.nlm.nih.gov/pubmed/ 16338708 [Accessed June 10, 2013].

EU Expert Working Group 'Sport & Health,' 2008. *EU physical activity guidelines: Recommended policy actions in support of health-enhancing physical activity*, Brussels.

Global Observatory for Physical Activity, 2015. Country Cards. Available at: www.globalphysicalactivityobservatory.com/country-cards/.

Goodman, A., Sahlqvist, S. & Ogilvie, D., 2014. New walking and cycling routes and increased physical activity: One- and 2-year findings from the UK iConnect study. *American Journal of Public Health*, 104(9), pp.38–46.

Gordon, D., 2004. *Targeting poor health: Review of rural and urban factors affecting the costs of health services and other implementation issues*, Cardiff: National Assembly of Wales.

Government Equalities Office, 2010. *Equality Act 2010*, London. Available at: www.legislation.gov. uk/ukpga/2010/15/pdfs/ukpga_20100015_en.pdf.

Greater Manchester Combined Authority, 2015. *Greater Manchester Agreement: Devolution to the GMCA and transition to a directly elected mayor*, Greater Manchester Combined Authority.

Hallsworth, M., Parker, S. & Rutter, J., 2011. *Policy making in the real world: Evidence and analysis*, London. Available at: http://onlinelibrary.wiley.com/doi/10.1111/j.2041-9066.2011.00051.x/full.

Hatamian, A., Pearmain, D. & Golden, S., 2012. *Outcomes of the Active at 60 Community Agent Programme*, Sheffield: Department for Work and Pensions.

Health Promotion Agency for Northern Ireland, 2002. *Physical activity an investment in public health: The Northern Ireland Action Plan 1998–2002*, Belfast.

Heath, G.W. et al., 2012. Evidence-based intervention in physical activity: Lessons from around the world. *The Lancet*, 380, pp.272–281. Available at: www.ncbi.nlm.nih.gov/pubmed/22818939 [Accessed August 12, 2013].

HM Government, 1998. *Northern Ireland Act 1998*, HM Government.

HM Government, 2009. *Building a society for all ages*, Surrey.

HM Government, 2006. *Northern Ireland (St Andrews Agreement) Act 2006*, HM Government.

HM Government, 2010. *New approach for school sports: Decentralising power, incentivising competition, trusting teachers*, HM Government.

HM Government, 2011. *UK initial report on the UN convention on the rights of persons with disabilities*, London.

HM Government, 2014a. *Moving more, living more: The physical activity Olympic and Paralympic legacy for the nation*, London.

HM Government, 2014b. *The long term vision for the legacy of the London 2012 Olympic & Paralympic Games*, London.

HM Government, 2015a. *Inspired by 2012: The legacy from the London 2012 Olympic and Paralympic Games*, London.

HM Government, 2015b. *Sporting future: A new strategy for an active nation*, London. Available at: www. gov.uk/government/uploads/system/uploads/attachment_data/file/486622/Sporting_Future_ACCESSIBLE.pdf.

Houlihan, B. & Green, M., 2006. The changing status of school sport and physical education: Explaining policy change. *Sport, Education and Society*, 9(3), pp.73–92.

Lang, T. & Rayner, G., 2007. Overcoming policy cacophony on obesity: An ecological public health framework for policymakers. *Obesity Reviews*, 8(Suppl. 1), pp.165–181.

McCormick, J., McDowell, E. & Harris, A., 2009. *Policies for peace of mind? Devolution and older age in the UK*, London: The Progressive Policy Think Tank.

Musingarimi, P., 2009. Obesity in the UK: A review and comparative analysis of policies within the devolved administrations. *Health Policy*, 91(1), pp.10–16.

National Assembly for Wales, 2006. *Government of Wales Act 2006*, National Assembly for Wales.

National Health Service, 2001. *Exercise referral systems: A national quality assurance framework*, National Health Service.

National Institute for Health and Clinical Excellence, 2008. Physical activity and the environment. *NICE Public Health Guidance*, (8), p.56. Available at: http://guidance.nice.org.uk/PH8.

National Institute for Health and Care Excellence, 2014. *Exercise referral schemes to promote physical activity*, National Institute for Health and Care Excellence.

National Institute for Health and Care Excellence, 2015. *Physical activity strategy, policy and commissioning - NICE Pathways*, Available at: http://pathways.nice.org.uk/pathways/physical-activity#path= view%3A/pathways/physical-activity/physical-activity-strategy-policy-and-commissioning.xml &content=view-node%3Anodes-national-campaign-for-children-and-young-people.

NICMA, 2010. Play and resources. Available at: https://nicma.org/For-Childminders/Resources-(1). aspx [Accessed August 29, 2017].

Northern Ireland Assembly, 1998. *The Belfast Agreement*, Available at: http://archive.niassembly.gov. uk/io/agreement.htm.

Northern Ireland Assembly, 2010. *GP Exercise Referral schemes/Exercise on Prescription*, Northern Ireland Assembly.

Northern Ireland Executive, 2011. *Economic strategy: Priorities for sustainable growth and prosperity*, Northern Ireland Executive.

OECD, 2011. *An overview of growing income inequalities in OECD countries: Main findings*, Available at: www.i-red.eu/resources/publications-files/oecd-divided-we-stand.pdf\nhttp://egov.formez.it/ sites/all/files/OCSE - An Overview of Growing Income Inequalities in OECD Countries.pdf.pdf.

Office for National Statistics, 2012. *South East has biggest share of the wealthiest households*, London.

OFMDFM, 2006. *Our children and young people – Our pledge: A ten year strategy for children and young people in Northern Ireland 2006–2016*, Belfast.

OfSTED, 2005. *The physical education, school sport and club links strategy*, OfSTED.

Physical Activity Task Force, 2003. *Let's make Scotland more active: A strategy for physical activity*, Edinburgh: Crown.

Piggin, J., 2012. Turning health research into health promotion: A study of causality and 'critical insights' in a United Kingdom health campaign. *Health Policy*, 107(2–3), pp.296–303. Available at: www.ncbi.nlm.nih.gov/pubmed/22771080 [Accessed July 12, 2012].

Public Health England, 2014. *Everybody active, every day: An evidence-based approach to physical activity*, London.

Richman, W.L. et al., 1999. A meta-analytic study of social desirability distortion in computer-administered questionnaires, traditional questionnaires, and interviews. *Journal of Applied Psychology*, 84(5), pp.754–775.

Scottish Executive, 2007. *Reaching higher: Building on the success of Sport 21*, Edinburgh. Available at: http://scholar.google.com/scholar?hl=en&btnG=Search&q=intitle:Reaching+Higher:+Building+ on+the+Success+of+Sport+21#0.

Smith, T. & Babbington, E., 2006. Devolution: A map of divergence in the NHS. British Medical Association. Available at: www.bma.org.uk/ap.nsf/Content/hprsummer06~Devolution.

Sport England, 2014. *Sport England – Annual report and financial statements 2013–14*, Sport England.

Sport England, 2016a. *This Girl Can: Inspiring millions to exercise*, London.

Sport England, 2016b. *Towards an active nation: Strategy 2016–2021*, London.

Strategic Review of Health Inequalities in England Post 2010, 2010. *Fair society, healthy lives. Marmot Review: Executive summary*, London.

Sustrans, 2007. *The Connect2 Project*, Sustrans.

The Scottish Government, 1999. *Towards a healthier Scotland*, The Scottish Government.

The Scottish Government, 2008. *Equally well: Report of the ministerial task force on health inequalities*, Edinburgh.

The Scottish Government, 2009. *On your marks . . . A Games legacy for Scotland*, Edinburgh.

The Scottish Government, 2013. *Scotland's Future*,

The Scottish Government, 2014. *A more active Scotland: Building a legacy from the Commonwealth Games*, Edinburgh.

The Welsh Assembly Government, 2004. *Health gain targets*, Available at: http://gov.wales/splash?orig=/topics/health/ocmo/research/health-gain/.

UNESCO, 2015. *Quality physical education: Guidelines for policy-makers*, Paris: United Nations Educational, Scientific and Cultural Organization.

UNICEF, 2010. *The children left behind: A league table of inequality in child well-being in the world's rich countries*, Florence.

Weed, M. et al., 2012. Developing a physical activity legacy from the London 2012 Olympic and Paralympic Games: A policy-led systematic review. *Perspectives in Public Health*, 132(2), pp.75–80.

Welsh Assembly Government, 1998. *Better health better Wales*, Cardiff.

Welsh Assembly Government, 2003a. *The review of health and social care in Wales: Summary*, Cardiff.

Welsh Assembly Government, 2003b. *The strategy for older people in Wales*, Cardiff. Available at: http://wales.gov.uk/topics/olderpeople/publications/strategy2008-2013/;jsessionid=5176446FAB0976C594F2F9782F18439F?status=closed&lang=en.

Welsh Assembly Government, 2003c. Walking and cycling strategy, (August). Welsh Assembly Government.

Welsh Assembly Government, 2004. *National Strategy Framework for children, young people & maternity services*, Cardiff. Available at: www.wales.nhs.uk/sites3/Documents/441/EnglishNSF_amended_final.pdf.

Welsh Assembly Government, 2005a. *Draft National Service Framework for older people in Wales*, Cardiff.

Welsh Assembly Government, 2005b. *Healthy ageing action plan for Wales: A response to Health Challenge Wales*, Cardiff. Available at: http://wales.gov.uk/topics/olderpeople/publications/healthyageingactionplan;jsessionid=5176446FAB0976C594F2F9782F18439F?status=closed&lang=en.

Welsh Assembly Government, 2006a. *Food and fitness – promoting healthy eating and physical activity for children and young people in Wales*, Cardiff.

Welsh Assembly Government, 2006b. Play in Wales: The Assembly Government's Play policy implementation plan, (February), Welsh Assembly Government, pp.2–6.

Welsh Assembly Government, 2007. *Food and well being: Reducing inequalities through a nutrition strategy for Wales a mid-term review*, Welsh Assembly Government.

Welsh Assembly Government, 2009a. Climbing higher: Creating an Active Wales - a 5 year strategic action plan consultation document, Welsh Assembly Government.

Welsh Assembly Government, 2009b. *Our healthy future*, Cardiff. Available at: http://wales.gov.uk/docs/phhs/publications/100521healthyfutureen.pdf.

Welsh Assembly Government, 2010. *A workforce development plan*, Cardiff.

Welsh Assembly Government, 2011. *Fairer health outcomes for all*, Cardiff.

Welsh Government, 2013a. *Building a brighter future: Early years and childcare plan*, Cardiff.

Welsh Government, 2013b. *The strategy for older people in Wales 2013–2023*, Cardiff. Available at: http://wales.gov.uk/topics/olderpeople/publications/strategy2008-2013/;jsessionid=5176446FAB0976C594F2F9782F18439F?status=closed&lang=en.

41

THE UNITED STATES OF AMERICA

Sean Bulger, Emily Jones and Eloise Elliott

Physical activity and public health in the U.S.

Physical inactivity is identified as a primary risk factor for numerous chronic health conditions including coronary heart disease, Type 2 diabetes mellitus and insulin resistance, components of metabolic syndrome, colon and breast cancers, musculoskeletal problems, and psychological disorders like depression (Kraus et al., 2015). These chronic degenerative diseases and their related risk factors represent a significant economic burden in the U.S. and estimates of direct medical expenditures include: $313.8 billion in 2009 for cardiovascular disease, $89 billion for cancer in 2007, $116 billion for diabetes in 2007, and $61 billion for obesity in 2000 (U.S. Department of Health and Human Services [USDHHS] and Centers for Disease Control and Prevention [CDC], 2009). Despite the obvious importance of physical activity from a public health perspective and the corresponding potential impact on an individual's quality of life, available data describe that fewer than one-third (31%) of the global population, less than half (48%) of U.S. adults and only one quarter (25%) of U.S. adolescents meet the recommended amounts of physical activity (Hallal et al., 2012; CDC, 2014; USDHHS and CDC, 2009).

The problem of physical inactivity is a complex one with multiple contributing biological, psychological, social, and environmental factors that interact across levels of influence from an ecological perspective. Research on the determinants of physical activity demonstrates a positive relationship between physical activity, educational attainment, and socioeconomic status in Caucasian populations (Bauman, Sallis, Dzewaltowski, and Owen, 2002; Sherwood and Jeffery, 2000). However, an inverse relationship exists between obesity levels and demographic variables like socioeconomic status, educational attainment, gender, and race (Evans, Newton, Ruta, MacDonald, and Morris, 2007; Weintraub et al., 2011; White, O'Neil, Kolotkin, and Bryne, 2004). From a geographic perspective, lower-socioeconomic and high-minority regions document limited access to safe physical activity facilities, which in turn correlates with lower physical activity levels (Gordon-Larsen, Nelson, Page, and Popkin, 2006).

To attenuate these health disparities and reduce the inequalities that exist in disadvantaged populations, researchers in the U.S. have called for national and state-level policies targeting increased physical activity across multiple levels of influence (Story, Nanney, and Schwartz,

2009; Weintraub et al., 2011). The National Coalition for Promoting Physical Activity asserts that physical activity policies in various forms can positively impact community and infrastructure development, learning environments in schools, recreational opportunities, work productivity, competitiveness in a global economy, military recruitment, and national security. The purpose of this chapter is to provide insight into physical activity policy efforts in the U.S., alignment across national and state strategic planning efforts, and policy examples from a specific geographic region and state. Readers will be introduced to policy efforts at the national (Physical Activity Guidelines for Americans and U.S. National Physical Activity Plan) and state levels (West Virginia Physical Activity Plan). Specific policy examples include those targeting school physical education and physical activity, safety and active transportation, and promotion of shared-use of public facilities through limited liability.

The Physical Activity Guidelines for Americans and National Physical Activity Plan

In 2008, the Physical Guidelines for Americans were issued by the U.S. Department of Health and Human Services representing the federal government's first attempt to help Americans understand and achieve the recommended amounts of physical activity necessary for improved health and quality of life (USDHHS, 2008). The Physical Activity Guidelines for Americans provide lifestyle recommendations that emphasize the importance of physical activity for people of all ages and ability levels (e.g., yard work and gardening, active household chores, taking the stairs rather than the elevator, walking the dogs, active play with children). These guidelines are organized along a developmental continuum reflecting the unique requirements of individuals across the lifespan including active children and adolescents, adults, older adults, and people with special needs (e.g., chronic disease, disability, and pregnancy).

In the initial report, for example, children ages 6–17 were recommended to accumulate at least 60 minutes of moderate-to-vigorous physical activity each day in a variety of enjoyable and developmentally appropriate forms including aerobic, muscle-strengthening, and bone-strengthening activities (USDHHS, 2008). In its midcourse report targeting policymakers, health care, and public health professionals, the guidelines were extended to highlight evidence-based interventions and strategies that increase physical activity levels in five key settings: school, preschool and childcare, community, family and home, and primary health care (USDHHS, 2012).

Recognizing the numerous individual, social, and environmental barriers to increased physical activity participation at the population level and the resultant need for multi-disciplinary collaboration, the National Physical Activity Plan Alliance was formed "to facilitate this collective action, to help organizations from all sectors of society work together to increase physical activity in all segments of the American population" (Kraus et al., 2015, p. 1). Released in May 2010, the U.S. National Physical Activity Plan offers a comprehensive collection of policies, programs, and recommendations to facilitate this ambitious goal (Pate, 2009). The vision for the National Plan is that all Americans will be physically active, and they will live, work, and play in supportive environments that facilitate regular participation. Furthermore, the National Plan targets the development of a culture that supports personal achievement of the amounts of physical activity recommended in the previously described Physical Activity Guidelines for Americans as a mechanism for improved health, prevention and management of disease and disability, and enhanced quality of life.

The National Plan is not an official government plan, and it represents the result of a private and public sector collaborative planning process that invited multiple rounds of input and feedback from contributors across eight societal sectors: Business and Industry; Education; Health Care; Mass Media; Parks, Recreation, Fitness, and Sports; Public Health; Transportation, Land Use, and Community Design; and Volunteer and Non-profit (Bornstein, Pate, and Buchner, 2014). The National Plan is organized by these societal sectors and includes more than 250 recommendations for policy and evidence-based practice that users can adopt to promote physical activity based on the unique contextual constraints present within their communities, organizations, and/or programs. These recommendations are arranged in a collection of sector-specific strategies for physical activity promotion and related tactics that provide a basis for practical application of the National Plan in a flexible and non-prescriptive manner.

Given this ecological perspective, the importance of supportive policy at the national, state, local, and organizational level is reflected across all societal sectors. For example, the Education sector is recommended to "[d]evelop and implement state and school district policies requiring school accountability for the quality and quantity of physical education and physical activity programs [Strategy 2]." In Business and Industry, community and organizational leaders are called upon to "[d]evelop legislation and policy agendas that promote employer-sponsored physical activity programs while protecting individual employees' and dependents' rights [Strategy 4]." Public Health professionals are encouraged to "[e]ngage in advocacy and policy development to elevate the priority of physical activity in public health practice, policy, and research [Strategy 3]" and "[e]xpand monitoring of policy and environmental determinants of physical activity and the levels of physical activity in communities (surveillance), and monitor the implementation of public health approaches to promoting active lifestyles (evaluation) [Strategy 5]."

In addition to the strategies and tactics that align with each societal sector, plan developers recognized the importance of overarching strategies that intersect across all of the sectors. These overarching strategies include the following:

1 Initiate a national physical activity education program and promotion campaign that informs all Americans about the importance of physical activity and integrates well with other national health and disease prevention efforts.
2 Develop a national resource centre to distribute evidence-based physical activity promotion tools for use by professionals and organizational/community leaders.
3 Disseminate best practice models, programs, and policies for physical activity promotion that enable the broadest audience possible to achieve the federal guidelines.
4 Establish a centre for physical activity policy development and research that incorporates all societal sectors designated by the National Plan.
5 Launch "grassroots" advocacy and planning efforts at the state and local levels to facilitate support for and actual application of the numerous strategies and tactics included in the National Plan.

The final overarching strategy listed above is perhaps the most immediately actionable given its grassroots orientation and focus on state and local efforts rather than at a national level (Elliott, Jones, and Bulger, 2014; Elliott, Jones, Nichols, Murray, and Kohl, 2014). Due to the importance of state and local government in the U.S. and its diversity across geographic regions, comparable strategic planning efforts and policy modifications at the state and local level are likely to represent a more attainable next step than broader national initiatives given the related challenges associated with consensus-building on that scale, numerous competing national priorities, and limited amounts of federal and non-federal funding in the area of physical activity promotion.

Grassroots efforts and state-level plan development in West Virginia

The Appalachian Region is a 205,000-square-mile, 13-state region that spans the length of the Appalachian Mountains, extending from southern New York to northern Mississippi. More than 40 per cent of the Region's population is rural as compared to 20 per cent of the US population. West Virginia is the only state entirely classified as Appalachian, whereas only certain counties in the remaining 12 states classify. As a whole, the Region battles economic distress with 17 per cent of people in Appalachia living below the federal poverty line and 8.2 per cent being unemployed. The percentage of people living in poverty within WV exceeds both national and Regional rates, at 17.9 per cent (Pollard and Jacobsen, 2015). Related health disparities in rural Appalachia have been attributed to a combination of factors including poor living standards, lack of access to medical care and resources, and general lack of knowledge and awareness of health risks.

In 2004, mortality rates for persons over 35 years living in Appalachia exceeded that of the rest of the U.S. population about heart disease (651 deaths per 100,000 compared to 585 deaths per 100,000), cancers, stroke, lung cancer, diabetes, and motor vehicle accidents (Halverson, 2004). The prevalence of chronic diseases such as cardiovascular disease and cancers has been highly associated with risk behaviours such as smoking, poor nutrition, and physical inactivity. While these risk behaviours appear to be modifiable by individual behaviour change, social and behavioural risk factors including low socioeconomic status, lack of access to healthy foods, inadequate facilites for leisure-time physical activity, and poor public health infrastructure inhibits personal decision making. With many of these social factors well documented to exist in rural Appalachia, the prevalence of adult obesity, smoking, and physical inactivity in Appalachian counties is much greater than non-Appalachian counties (Halverson, 2004).

Adverse risk behaviours and related health outcomes are also evident in Appalachian children and adolescents. Societal conditions in rural WV communities limit access to structured physical activity opportunities for youth beyond what is offered before, during, or after school hours. Barriers to physical activity for children in Appalachia include lack of access to safe and usable play spaces, poor travel and road conditions, lack of availability of qualified persons to plan and deliver physical activity programming, multigenerational families raising children, poverty, and drug use and abuse (Jones et al., 2014; Kristjansson et al., 2015).

Based on recommendations from the U.S. National Physical Activity Plan highlighting the importance of state and local leadership and the facilitators and barriers to physical activity that present themselves in the Appalachian region, a state-wide strategic process was initiated to develop a physical activity plan unique to WV (Elliott, Jones et al. 2014; Elliott, Jones, Nichols et al. 2014). Modelled after the National Plan regarding process and product, the primary aim of the WV Physical Activity Plan (WVPAP) is to provide strategic and unified direction for physical activity promotion efforts across the state (Bulger et al., 2012). It is also expected that implementation of the WVPAP will increase the physical activity levels of children and adults to meet or exceed the national physical activity recommendations and to improve the health and quality of life of West Virginians. Borrowing from the National Plan, the WVPAP is organized around eight societal sectors identified as key contributors to promoting physical activity from a public health perspective. The target audience for the WVAP includes (a) policy leaders at the state, local, and organizational levels, (b) key stakeholders representing each societal sector, and (c) regular citizens who can promote active lifestyles in their communities and advocate for social, environmental, and policy change.

During plan development, participatory decision making was used to solicit input from key stakeholders (Elliott, Jones et al. 2014; Elliott, Jones, Nichols et al. 2014). Throughout 2011, West Virginians representing all societal sectors and geographic regions contributed to the generation of sector-specific strategies and tactics for implementation. These strategies and tactics were (a) initially developed during a state-wide symposium and multi-phase concept mapping process that included brainstorming of ideas, structuring of ideas through sorting and rating, and interpretation of results by experts, (b) further refined by key leaders and stakeholder teams from each societal sector, and (c) prepared for dissemination through the lens of the scientific evidence and recommendations summarized in the National Plan.

In addition to the determination of sector-specific strategies and tactics that are differentiated to meet the unique needs of West Virginians, this participatory planning process resulted in the identification of five overarching priority areas that provide a conceptual framework for the WVPAP: Priority Area 1 School-based Programs and Initiatives; Priority Area 2 Public Awareness and Social Marketing; Priority Area 3 Community Engagement and Environment; Priority Area 4 Institutional and Organizational Support; and Priority Area 5 Policy (Bulger et al. 2012).

The designation of policy at the state, local, and organizational level as a priority area is of particular interest to the current case study in that it has considerable potential to influence accessibility to physical activity opportunities for all citizens in WV. On this important priority area, plan developers recognized a clear need for better-networked leadership and advocacy efforts regarding programming, research, and policy. The value of evidence-informed policy decision making was also highlighted as a contributing factor to best practice in program planning, implementation, evaluation, and dissemination in a variety of physical activity settings. The information contained in Table 41.1 provides an overview of the key messages related to policy as a priority area, its influence on sectors, and brief summary of the related strategies.

The focus on policy within the WVPAP encompasses the collaboration of key stakeholders to recommend and advocate for policy change related to physical activity promotion. Strategies and tactics outlined within this priority area call for cross-sector policy development and implementation at both the state and local levels. In Public Health, for example, the sector team members highlighted the important role that their profession plays in advocating for more opportunities, educating for greater personal responsibility, informing policy, facilitating the use of evidence-based practices, and conducting surveillance and research on physical activity programs. The Public Health sector team generated the following strategy and tactics related to Policy:

Priority Area 5 Strategy: Engage in advocacy and policy development to elevate the priority of physical activity in evidence-based public health practice, policy, and evaluation. **Priority Tactics:** (1) Develop a series of white papers/technical reports to identify high-impact and evidence-driven policy guidelines; (2) Develop a policy framework that is used to allocate resources related to physical activity; (3) Look at current national standards (e.g., Healthy People 2020) and develop relevant policies at the state level; (4) Review successful effective health plans around the nation to inform physical activity policy in WV; and (5) Conduct timely and meaningful surveillance of physical activity and inactivity, and use the data to inform future policy and funding decisions.

As a second example, members of the Education sector team recognized that professionals in their field have an incredible opportunity and responsibility to impact the health and wellbeing of future generations. They also found it imperative that education professionals embrace the issue of accountability in designing and delivering opportunities within the

Table 41.1 Key messages, societal sectors, and summary of strategies for Priority Area 5 (Policy)

Key Messages	Societal Sectors	Summary of Strategies
Greater alignment and coordination of physical activity programming and policy efforts	Education Health Care Mass Media	• Form statewide leadership and advocacy network for physical activity research/policy • Promote unified public health messaging through a network of engaged individual partners, affiliate organizations, and advocates • Deliver comprehensive marketing campaign that influences policy maker priorities
Emphasis on evidence-informed policy decision making concerning physical activity	Public Health Parks, Recreation, Fitness, and Sports Non-profit and Volunteer	• Advocacy efforts to elevate the priority of physical activity in evidence-based public health practice, policy, and evaluation • Use best practices in physical activity program planning, implementation, and evaluation to leverage increased support • Sharing data about the benefits of physical activity to inform policymaker priorities
Specialized policy issues related to physical activity	Business & Industry Transportation, Land Use, and Community Design	• Use policy to advocate the importance of a physically active workforce and incentivize employers to develop healthy business climates and communities • Advocate for land-use plans that effectively address physical activity and health

school that facilitate youth participation in engaging, geographically and culturally relevant, accessible physical activity opportunities. Toward that important end, the following policy-related strategy and tactics were identified:

Priority Area 5 Strategy: Work within education and across societal sectors to establish a leadership/advocacy network for school physical activity and physical education research and policy development. **Priority Tactics:** (1) Educate key decision makers (e.g., school administrators, local wellness policy committees) of the need for physical activity and physical education for all; (2) Urge local and state policy makers to provide funding for physical activity and physical education resources (i.e., trails, physical activity/physical education equipment, playgrounds); (3) Encourage public policies that require cities and counties to establish well thought-out zoning policies that positively influence and encourage/allow physical activity; (4) Advocate for state/federal funding for population-based physical activity and school-based physical education programs; and (5) Provide grant funding to non-profit organizations that work with children to purchase physical activity and physical education resources and equipment.

As a final example from the WVPAP, the sector team in Transportation, Land Use, and Community Design recognized that the physical activity levels of West Virginians are impacted by transportation systems, strategic land use, and the built environment of their communities. Increased physical activity can be accomplished through the design and development of infrastructure within and across communities that accommodate all modes of transportation, including pedestrians, bicycles, and mass transportation. Accordingly, transportation, land use, and community design professionals must take an active role in informing and encouraging key decision makers to consider physical activity usage in all long-term land use and transportation plans:

Priority Area 5 Strategy: Advocate for land-use plans that effectively address physical activity and health. **Priority Tactics:** (1) Remind key decision makers in the state of their role in taking responsibility for creating opportunities for physical activity for all citizens; (2) Urge local and state policy makers to provide funding for local physical activity resources (e.g., parks, trails, community centres); (3) Establish zoning and subdivision rules requiring well-connected infrastructure to promote physical activity (i.e., sidewalks, walking trails, bike paths); (4) Adopt "complete streets" policies and provide related training to ensure transportation planners and engineers design and operate the entire roadway with all users in mind (i.e., bicyclists, public transportation vehicles, pedestrians of all ages and abilities); and (5) Support state staff and policy makers with the development, improvement or use of measurable criteria for assessing the health impacts of transportation and land-use decisions (i.e., air quality improvements, reduced or redirected vehicular traffic counts, pedestrian-vehicle and bicycle-vehicle accident data).

State-level physical activity policies in West Virginia

Although the WV Physical Activity Plan has served as a guide for state-wide physical activity programs, policies, and initiatives since 2012, a review of state legislation demonstrates that physical activity and healthy lifestyles related policy began to surface in 2005. Boehmer and colleagues (2007) indicate that approximately 25 per cent of legislation introduced between 2003 and 2005 in the United States involved physical activity or physical education policy changes in schools, and 28 per cent addressed safe routes to schools. The thrust of state-level policies (particularly in schools), however, was not accompanied by substantial funding or mandated evaluation requirements (Eyler et al., 2010). Since the launch of the WVPAP, three additional pieces of legislation have passed within West Virginia, two focusing on schools and one on active transit.

House Bill 2816 Healthy Lifestyles Act (2005)

In response to the well-documented poor health conditions of school-aged children, West Virginia state legislators passed House Bill 2816, the Healthy Lifestyles Act (HLA) in 2005 which outlined regulations for school nutrition and physical education guidelines. The HLA mandated a minimum physical education instruction time for elementary students (90 minutes per week) and middle school students (2,700 minutes per year) and required physical education credit for high school graduation. The HLA required schools to measure physical fitness scores and body mass index (BMI) for students in grades 4–12 on an annual basis and incorporate concepts of healthy eating and exercise to maintain a healthy weight into school health education and physical education curricula. With support from the State Department of Education implementation of the HLA began in 2006. A university-based research team funded by the Robert Wood Johnson Foundation conducted an evaluation of the HLA and indicated that 73 per cent of school-aged children were not accumulating the recommended amount of physical activity (West Virginia University, 2009). Furthermore, the report indicated 41 per cent of WV schools lacked the resources to implement one or more of the HLA requirements.

Senate Bill 158 Complete Streets Act (2013)

In 2013, the WV Senate passed Senate Bill 158 Complete Streets Act that takes account of the safety, mobility, and accessibility of public transportation areas such as streets, roads, and highways for all users. The focus of the bill is to make these areas accessible to pedestrians, bicyclists, and public transportation riders of all ages and abilities. The bill was developed based on research and data collected from the National Highway Traffic Safety Administration that reports close to 300 pedestrians and cyclists have been killed on WV roadways in the past decade as a result of motor vehicle-related traffic accidents. The Complete Streets Act encompasses all aspects of transportation planning, design construction, reconstruction, rehabilitation, maintenance, and operations of state, county, or local transportation facilities.

The Complete Streets Act strongly encourages the Division of Highways to use the latest design standards and federal, state, or local guidance documents published by the American Association of State Highway and Transportation Officials, the U.S. Access Board, and the Institute of Transportation Engineers, as they apply to bicycle, pedestrian, transit, and highway facilities. Unique to WV, the Act outlines the establishment of a governor-appointed Complete Streets Advisory Board that would make recommendations to the Division of Highways for restructuring procedures, updating guidance, providing education, and creating new measures for multimodal planning and design. The Board would also submit annual reports on the status of Complete Streets implementation, recommended changes to protocols, guidance, or standards, the status of performance indicator development, and available crash statistics.

West Virginia Board of Education Policy 2510 (2014)

The West Virginia Board of Education passed Policy 2510 in 2014 which is based on national recommendations for daily minutes of physical activity for children and evidence-based instructional practices through the use of whole-of-school approaches (Kohl and Cook, 2013; Story et al., 2009; Ward, 2011). Key features of the policy align with comprehensive or whole-of-school approaches to physical activity promotion recommended by several national and government organizations (e.g., Institute of Medicine, National Physical Activity Plan, the American Heart Association, National Association for Sport and Physical Education, Let's Move!). Policy 2510 extends the 2005 HLA by broadening school-time physical activity beyond physical education and establishing a criterion of time spent on physical education as health-enhancing. The policy requires elementary and middle schools to provide 30 minutes of daily physical activity beyond physical education that may include before or after-school programming, recess, and/or classroom activity breaks. Across all developmental levels, the new criterion for physical education is that at least 50 per cent of class time is to be spent in moderate-to-vigorous physical activity. No new funding was allocated for WVBE Policy 2510 implementation. However, programming efforts by the WV Office of Secondary Learning resulted in the training of approximately 200 classroom teachers and school administrators on classroom physical activity.

Senate Bill 238 Shared Use Limited Liability Protection for Schools (2015)

In 2015, West Virginia Senate Bill 238 Shared Use Limited Liability Protection for Schools passed to restrict the liability of county boards of education for loss or injury from the use of school property made available for unorganized recreation. The bill eliminates a major barrier for schools who want to open their doors to community groups, organizations, or associations to hold a discussion, study, recreation, and other activities. With this protection, county boards of education are not liable for any loss or injury arising from the use of school property that is made available for shared-use. County boards are, however, still liable for acts of gross negligence and wilful and wanton conduct which is the cause of injury or personal damage. Bill 238 provides local control and discretion for boards of education to establish shared use agreements with community members and groups and, in turn, increase access and availability to physical activity and sports facilities built and maintained by the school. This initiative is expected to be cost-effective and can promote stronger social connections revolving around the use of community schools.

Implications for future physical activity policy and practice

Physical activity policy initiatives, like those described above, have significant potential for equalizing access to safe and structured physical activity opportunities. Challenges remain, however, in prioritizing physical activity policy implementation amidst the varied contextual and cultural influences that exist within different localities in WV, and the tenuous status of state funding and financial support for education, training, implementation, and evaluation of policies. Practical implications exist for developing and passing activity-focused legislation and policies, and translating those policies into professional practice. Four key observations and lessons learned from state-level policy efforts in WV include: (1) stakeholder support is crucial to all phases of development, (2) intentional alignment is needed across levels of policy, and (3) policy implementation must be linked to training and education, and (4) on-going dissemination efforts are needed.

Stakeholder support at all phases

Grassroots efforts are often driven by like-minded individuals who share a common vision and can effectively bring together groups and organizations to collaborate and advocate for the cause. Key stakeholders were involved early and often in the planning, development, and dissemination of the state-wide physical activity plan. Having sector teams comprised of decisions makers, leaders, and legislators who were also proponents of physical activity allowed the WVPAP to reflect the unique cultural and contextual needs of the state. As policy emerged as a priority across all societal sectors, it became evident that sector team members and leaders would play a significant role in educating and advocating for local and state-level physical activity policy. The WVPAP did not hire lobbyists. However, sector team members became involved in drafting, proposing, and advocating for physical activity policies (including bills and resolutions) later introduced within the state. From the perspective of policy implementation and evaluation, the role of stakeholders is written into the WV Complete Streets Act with the Advisory Board designated to inform and educate the populace, make recommendations for best practice, and develop criteria for documenting implementation and impact. Garnering and maintaining support from stakeholders across the various phases of WVPAP development, implementation, and dissemination required clear communication of vision, process, and intended outcomes. As a function of these capacity building efforts, key stakeholders have been engaged in strategic decision making efforts that informed the WVPAP and continued to influence local and state-level policy decisions.

Alignment across levels of policy

For national recommendations to be effective, they must not only be evidence-based but offer concrete and realistic plans for implementation and evaluation (Phillips, Goodell, Philyaw-Perez, and Raczynski, 2014). These national recommendations can then better inform state planning initiatives such as the WVPAP that can, in turn, provide the science to inform and influence policy decision making concerning physical activity. From the WV examples previously shared, the Complete Streets Act originated from the National Complete Streets Coalition, who provides information on active transport and advocates at state, regional, and local levels. Complete Streets policies are enacted throughout the nation but are tailored to meet the needs of the particular context and environment. Although the WV policy has yet to be enacted at the state level, local policies and practices exist and are assessed by groups such as metropolitan planning organizations.

Training and implementation

A key challenge for any policy initiative is how to translate the mandates and priorities into meaningful, manageable, and coherent practices. Lack of public awareness, education, or training can be major impediments to policy implementation. Professional development and outreach training with leaders at regional and local levels are necessary at the onset of policy. Training for those who are responsible for the policy's implementation is critical to its success. Training is often needed related to communication and networking, linkages to current practices and resources, and examples of successful implementation strategies (Evenson, Brownson, Satinsky, Eyler, and Kohl et al., 2013). Additionally, guidance for overcoming barriers to policy implementation, including financial constraints, is imperative. Therefore, a comprehensive training plan needs to be in place at the initial stages of policy implementation (Chiang, Maegher, and Wan, 2014). In one of the examples provided, a commitment from state educational agencies helped to facilitate the translation of WVBE Policy 2510 into professional practice by offering whole-day training for school administrators and classroom teachers. The training educated school personnel on the policy requirements and reporting structure, and provided evidence-based practices and resources for classroom physical activity. Partnerships with regional universities shared expertise, resources, facilities, and evaluation of the policy training for teachers and administrators.

On-going dissemination efforts

Positive changes from policy implementation are often not realized immediately, so it is important to have a continued investment in awareness and dissemination. Without it, awareness of the physical activity plan or policy will slowly dissipate and eventually be forgotten. It is important to continue to recognize small victories, positive grassroots implementation efforts, and key movers and shakers. On-going promotional efforts, such as dissemination of promotional materials to local audiences, are critical, as is the use of print media (e.g., email, online newsletters, informational websites, and social media outlets). Local, state and national presentations are also important in plan and policy information dissemination because they promote further change moving forward. Again, stakeholders invested in the development and implementation of the plan and/or policy play a critical role in these promotional efforts. Opportunities for stakeholders to share their goals and successes can also facilitate additional cross-sector collaboration (Evenson and Satinsky, 2014). The WVPAP, for example, has been well-publicized and disseminated using these described strategies.

References

Bauman, A.E., Sallis, J.F., Dzewaltowski, D., and Owen, N. (2002) 'Toward a better understanding of the influences on physical activity: The role of determinants, correlates, causal variables, mediators, moderators, and confounders', *American Journal of Preventive Medicine, 23*(2): 5–14.

Boehmer, T.K., Brownson, R.C., Haire-Jshu, D., and Dreisinger, M.L. (2007) 'Patterns of childhood obesity legislation in the United States', *Prevention of Chronic Disease, 4*(3): A56.

Bornstein, D.B., Pate, R.R., and Buchner, D.M. (2014) 'Development of a national physical activity plan for the United States', *Journal of Physical Activity and Health, 11*(3): 463–469.

Bulger, S.M., Elliott, E., Jones, E., Fitzpatrick, S., Jones, D., Tompkins, N., and Olfert, M. (2012) *ActiveWV 2015: West Virginia physical activity plan*. Retrieved on January 6, 2016 from www.wvphysicalactivity.org.

Centers for Disease Control and Prevention (2014) 'Facts about Physical Activity', Retrieved on June 22, 2015 from www.cdc.gov/physicalactivity/data/facts.html.

Chiang, R., Maegher, W., and Wan, K. (2014) *State Physical Activity Policies, Implementing Physical Activity Strategies*, R.R. Pate and D. Buchner editors. Champaign, IL: Human Kinetics.

Elliott, E., Jones, E., and Bulger, S. (2014) 'ActiveWV: A systematic approach to developing a physical activity plan for West Virginia.' *Journal of Physical Activity and Health, 11*: 478–486.

Elliott, E., Jones, E.M., Nichols, D.C., Murray, T.K., and Kohl, H.W. (2014) *Chapter 29 State-Based Efforts for Physical Activity Planning: Experience from Texas and West Virginia, The National Physical Activity Plan: Implementing Physical Activity Strategies*, R.R. Pate and D.M. Buchner editors. Champaign, IL: Human Kinetics.

Evans, J.M.M., Newton, R.W., Ruta, D.A., MacDonald, T.M., and Morris, A.D. (2007) 'Socio-economic status, obesity and prevalence of Type 1 and Type 2 diabetes mellitus', *Diabetic Medicine, 17*(6): 478–480.

Evenson, K., Brownson, R., Satinsky, S., Eyler, A., and Kohl, H., III (2013) 'Initial dissemination and use of the United States National Physical Activity Plan by public health practitioners', *American Journal of Preventive Medicine, 44*(5): 431–438.

Evenson, K., and Satinsky, S. (2014) 'Sector activities and lessons learned around initial implementation of the United States National Physical Activity Plan', *Journal of Physical Activity and Health, 11*(6): 1120–1128.

Eyler, A.A., Brownson, R.C., Aytur, S.A., Cradock, A.L., Doescher, M., Evenson, K.R., Kerr, J., Maddock, J., Pluto, D.L., Steinman, L., and O'Hara Tompkins, N. (2010) 'Examination of trends and evidence-based elements in state physical education legislation: A content analysis', *Journal of School Health, 80*(7): 326–332.

Gordon-Larsen, P., Nelson, M.C., Page, P., and Popkin, B.M. (2006) 'Inequality in the build environment underlies key health disparities in physical activity and obesity', *Pediatrics, 117*(1): 417–424.

Hallal, P.C., Andersen, L.B., Bull, F.C., Guthold, R., Haskell, W., Ekelund, U., and Lancet Physical Activity Series Working Group (2012) 'Global physical activity levels: Surveillance progress, pitfalls, and prospects', *The Lancet, 380*(9838): 247–257.

Halverson, J.A. (November 2004) 'An analysis of disparities in health status and access to health care in the Appalachian Region', Appalachian Regional Commission: Office of Social Environment and Health Research. Retrieved on April 15, 2015 from www.arc.gov/research/researchreportdetails.asp?REPORT_ID=82.

Jones, E.M., Taliaferro, A.R., Elliott, E.M., Bulger, S.M., Kristjansson, A.L., Neal, W., and Allar, I. (2014) 'Feasibility study of comprehensive school physical activity programs in Appalachian communities: The McDowell CHOICES Project', *The Journal of Teaching in Physical Education, 33*: 467–491.

Kohl, H.W. and Cook, H.D. (Eds.) (2013) *Educating the Student Body: Taking Physical Activity and Physical Education to School*. Washington, DC: The National Academies Press.

Kraus, W.E., Bittner, V., Appel, L., Blair, S.N., Church, T., Després, J.P., Franklin, B.A., Miller, T.D., Pate, R.R., Taylor-Piliae, R.E., and Vafiadis, D.K. (2015). 'The national physical activity plan: A call to action from the American Heart Association a science advisory from the American Heart Association', *Circulation, 131*(21): 1932–1940.

Kristjansson, A.L., Elliott, E., Bulger, S., Jones, E., Taliaferro, A.R., and Neal, W. (2015) 'Needs assessment of school and community physical activity opportunities in rural West Virginia: The McDowell CHOICES planning effort', *BMC Public Health, 15*(327): 1–10.

Pate, R.R., (2009) 'A national physical activity plan for the United States', *Journal of Physical Activity and Health*, 6(Supplement 2): S157.

Phillips, M., Goodell, M., Philyaw-Perez, A., and Raczynski, J. (2014) Public school physical activity legislative policy initiatives: What we have learned. In R. Pate and D. Buchner (Eds.) *Implementing Physical Activity Strategies*. Champaign, Ill.: Human Kinetics.

Pollard, K. and Jacobsen, L.A. (April 2015) 'The Appalachian Region: A data overview from the 2009–2013 American Community Survey', Appalachian Regional Commission: Population Reference Bureau. Retrieved on April 15, 2015 from www.arc.gov/research/researchreportdetails.asp?REPORT_ID=114.

Sherwood, N.E., and Jeffery, R.W. (2000) 'The behavioral determinants of exercise: Implications for physical activity interventions', *Annual Review of Nutrition*, 20(1): 21–44.

Story, M., Nanney, M.S., and Schwartz, M.B. (2009) 'Schools and obesity prevention: Creating school environments and policies to promote healthy eating and physical activity', *The Milbank Quarterly*, 87(1): 71–100

United States Department of Health and Human Services (2008) '2008 physical activity guidelines for Americans', Retrieved on January 15, 2016 from http://health.gov/paguidelines/pdf/paguide.pdf.

United States Department of Health and Human Services (2012) 'Physical activity guidelines for Americans midcourse report: Strategies to increase physical activity among youth', Retrieved on January 15, 2016 from http://health.gov/paguidelines/midcourse/pag-mid-course-report-final.pdf.

United States Department of Health and Human Services and the Centers for Disease Control and Prevention (2009) 'The power of prevention: Chronic disease . . . the public health challenge of the 21st century', National Center for Chronic Disease Prevention and Health Promotion. Retrieved on June 22, 2015 from www.cdc.gov/chronicdisease/pdf/2009-Power-of-Prevention.pdf.

Ward, D. (October 2011) 'School Policies on Physical Education and Physical Activity. A Research Synthesis', Princeton, NJ: Active Living Research, A National Program of the Robert Wood Johnson Foundation. Retrieved on May 1, 2015 from www.activelivingresearch.org.

Weintraub, W.S., Daniels, S.R., Burke, L.E., Franklin, B.A., Goff, D.C., Hayman, L.L., Lloyd-Jones, D., Pandey, D.K., Sanchez, E.J., Schram, A.P., and Whitsel, L.P. (2011) 'Value of primordial and primary prevention for cardiovascular disease a policy statement from the American Heart Association', *Circulation*, 124(8): 967–990.

West Virginia University, Robert C. Byrd Health Sciences Center, Health Research Center (2009) 'West Virginia Healthy Lifestyles Act of 2005, Executive Summary', Retrieved on May 14, 2015 from www.rwjf.org/content/dam/web-assets/2009/02/west-virginia-healthy-lifestyles-act-of-2005.

White, A.M., O'Neil, P.M., Kolotkin, R.L., and Bryne, T.K. (2004) 'Gender, race, and obesity related quality of life at extreme levels of obesity', *Obesity Research*, 12(6): 949–955.

Index

Page numbers in bold refer to tables. Page numbers in italics refer to figures. Page numbers with 'n' refer to notes.